Teen Health
Course 3

Mary H. Bronson, Ph.D.

Michael J. Cleary, Ed.D.

Betty M. Hubbard, Ed.D., C.H.E.S.

Contributing Author
Dinah Zike, M.Ed.

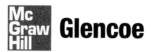

Glencoe

New York, New York   Columbus, Ohio   Chicago, Illinois   Peoria, Illinois   Woodland Hills, California

Meet the Authors

Mary H. Bronson, Ph.D., has taught health education in grades K–12, as well as health education methods classes at the undergraduate and graduate levels. As health education specialist for the Dallas School District, Dr. Bronson developed and implemented a district-wide health education program. She has been honored as Texas Health Educator of the Year by the Texas Association of Health, Physical Education, Recreation and Dance and selected Teacher of the Year twice, by her colleagues. Dr. Bronson has assisted school districts throughout the country in developing local health education programs. She is also the co-author of the *Glencoe Health* textbook.

Betty M. Hubbard, Ed.D., C.H.E.S., has taught health education in grades K–12 as well as health education methods classes at the undergraduate and graduate levels. She is a professor at the University of Central Arkansas, teaching classes in curriculum development, mental health, and human sexuality. Dr. Hubbard supervises student teachers and conducts in-service training for health education teachers in school districts throughout Arkansas. Her publications, grants, and presentations focus on research-based, comprehensive health instruction.

Michael J. Cleary, Ed.D., is Professor and School Health Education Coordinator at Slippery Rock University. Dr. Cleary taught at Evanston Township High School in Evanston, Illinois, and later became the Lead Teacher Specialist at the McMillen Center for Health Education in Fort Wayne, Indiana. Dr. Cleary has published and presented widely on curriculum development and portfolio assessment in K–12 health education. Dr. Cleary is the co-author of *Managing Your Health: Assessment for Action.* He is a Certified Health Education Specialist.

Dinah Zike, M.Ed., is an international curriculum consultant and inventor who has designed and developed educational products and three-dimensional, interactive graphic organizers for over thirty years. As president and founder of Dinah-Might Adventures, L.P., Dinah is the author of over 100 award-winning educational publications. Dinah has a B.S. and an M.S. in educational curriculum and instruction from Texas A&M University. Dinah Zike's *Foldables* are an exclusive feature of McGraw-Hill textbooks.

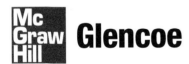

Glencoe

The McGraw-Hill Companies

Copyright © 2005 by Glencoe/McGraw-Hill, a division of the McGraw-Hill Companies. All rights reserved. Except as permitted under the United States Copyright Act, no part of this publication may be reproduced or distributed in any form or by any means, or stored in a database or retrieval system, without prior written permission from the publisher, Glencoe/McGraw-Hill.

Send all inquiries to:
Glencoe/McGraw-Hill
21600 Oxnard Street, Suite 500
Woodland Hills, California 91367

ISBN 0-07-861099-0 (Course 3 Student Text)
ISBN 0-07-861100-8 (Course 3 Teacher Wraparound Edition)

Printed in the United States of America.

5 6 7 8 9   071/043   08 07 06 05

Health Consultants

Christine A. Hayashi, M.A. Ed., J.D.
Attorney at Law, Special Education Law
Adjunct Faculty, Educational Leadership and Policy Studies Development
California State University, Northridge
Northridge, California

Patricia Sullivan, M.S., Special Education
Chair, Department of Language Arts
Meade Middle School
Fort Meade, Maryland

UNIT 1
Taking Charge of Your Health

Jill English, Ph.D., C.H.E.S.
Assistant Professor
California State University, Fullerton
Fullerton, California

Deborah A. Miller, Ph.D., C.H.E.S.
Professor and Health Coordinator
College of Charleston
Charleston, South Carolina

Alice Pappas, Ph.D., R.N.
Associate Professor/Associate Dean
Baylor University, Louise Herrington School of Nursing
Dallas, Texas

UNIT 2
Building Safe and Healthy Relationships

Kristin Danielson Fink
Executive Director
Community of Caring
Washington, DC

Jan King
Teacher
Neshaminy School District
Langhorne, Pennsylvania

J. Leslie Oganowski, Ph.D.
Professor of Health Education and Health Promotion
University of Wisconsin, La Crosse
La Crosse, Wisconsin

Howard S. Shapiro, M.D.
Associate Professor
University of Southern California School of Medicine
Los Angeles, California

UNIT 3
Physical Health and Fitness

Roberta Larson Duyff, R.D.
Food and Nutrition Consultant/President
Duyff Associates
St. Louis, Missouri

Mark L. Giese, Ed.D.
Chair, Health Science and Kinesiology Department
Northeastern State University
Tahlequah, Oklahoma

Tinker D. Murray, Ph.D.
Professor and Coordinator of the Exercise and Sports Science Program
Southwest Texas State University
San Marcos, Texas

Don Rainey
Instructor, Coordinator of the Physical Fitness and Wellness Program
Southwest Texas State University
San Marcos, Texas

UNIT 4
Making Safe and Drug-Free Decisions

Sally Champlin, C.H.E.S.
Faculty, Health Science
California State University, Long Beach
Long Beach, California

Taniesha Richardson, C.H.E.S.
Arkansas Department of Health
Office of Tobacco Prevention and Education
Little Rock, Arkansas

Peggy Woosley
Director of Curriculum
Stuttgart Public Schools
Stuttgart, Arkansas

UNIT 5
Understanding Your Body

Stephanie S. Allen
Senior Lecturer
Baylor University, Louise Herrington School of Nursing
Dallas, Texas

Victoria Bisorca, C.H.E.S.
Lecturer
California State University, Long Beach
Long Beach, California

Linda Stevenson, Ph.D., R.N.
Assistant Professor
Baylor University, Louise Herrington School of Nursing
Dallas, Texas

Health Consultants *(cont.)*

UNIT 6
Diseases and Disorders

Jennifer Weglowski, M.D.
Pediatrician/Senior Pediatric Resident
Children's Hospital of Pittsburgh
Pittsburgh, Pennsylvania

UNIT 7
Safety and Environmental Health

Jerry G. Hill
Agency Leadership Team
Arkansas Department of Health
Little Rock, Arkansas

David A. Sleet, Ph.D.
Associate Director for Science
Division of Unintentional Injury Prevention
Centers for Disease Control and Prevention (CDC)
Atlanta, Georgia

Reviewers

Beverly J. Berkin, C.H.E.S.
Health Education Consultant
Bedford Corners, New York

Donna Breitenstein, Ed.D.
Professor & Coordinator of Health Education
Director of North Carolina School Health
   Training Center
Appalachian State University
Boone, North Carolina

Julie Campbell-Fouch
Health Teacher, Department Chair
Stanford Middle School
Long Beach, California

Pamela R. Connolly
Subject Area Coordinator for Health and Physical
   Education, Diocese of Pittsburgh
Curriculum Coordinator for Health and Physical
   Education, North Catholic High School
Pittsburgh, Pennsylvania

Pat Freedman
Instructional Coordinator for Student Wellness
Humble Independent School District
Humble, Texas

Ginger Lawless, C.H.E.S.
Dyslexia and School Health Education Specialist
Fort Bend Independent School District
Sugar Land, Texas

Renee Rainey
Physical Education Teacher
Cowan Elementray School
Austin, Texas

James Robinson III, Ed.D.
Professor, Assistant Dean for Student Affairs
The Texas A&M University System
Health Science Center
School of Rural Public Health
College Station, Texas

Michael Rulon
Health/Physical Education Teacher
Johnson Junior High School
Adjunct Faculty, Laramie County Community
   College
Cheyenne, Wyoming

Jeanne Title
Coordinator, Prevention Education
Napa County Office of Education and Napa Valley
   Unified School District
Napa, California

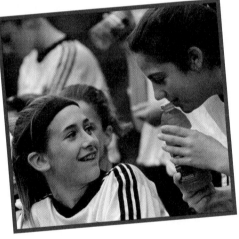
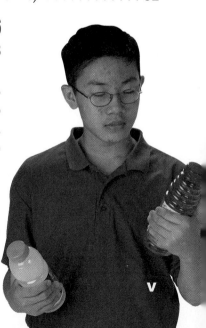

v

Building Safe and Healthy Relationships 82

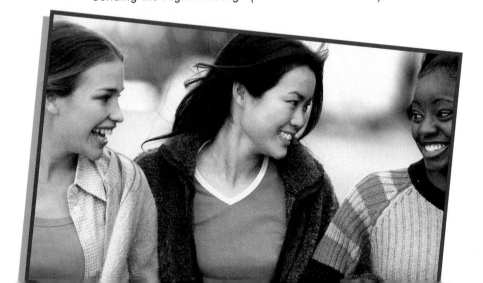

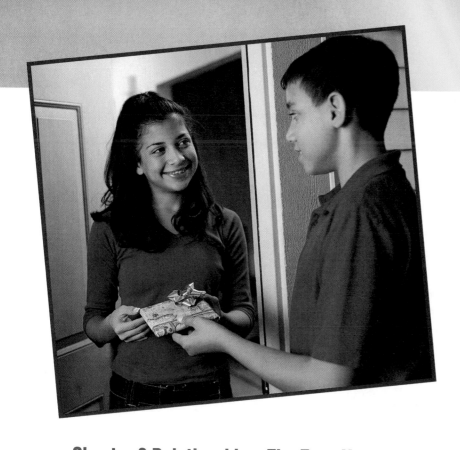

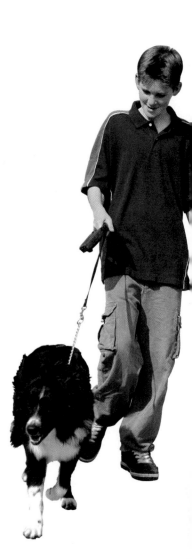

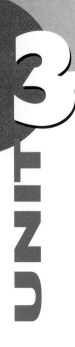

Physical Health and Fitness   188

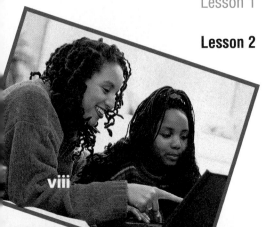

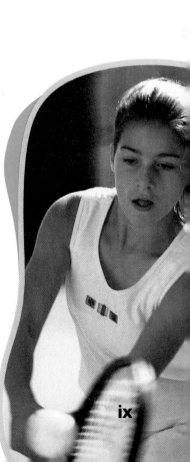

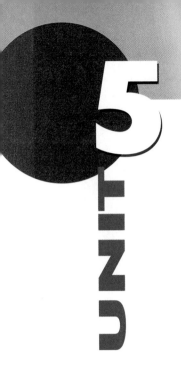

UNIT 5

Understanding Your Body   340

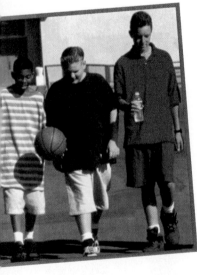

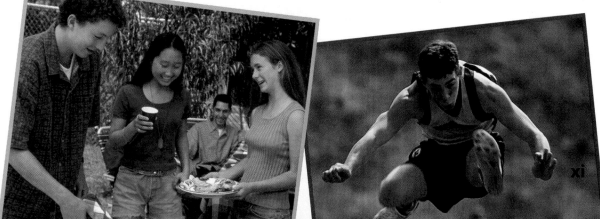

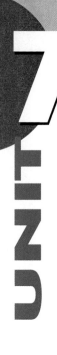

UNIT 7

Safety and Environmental Health 504

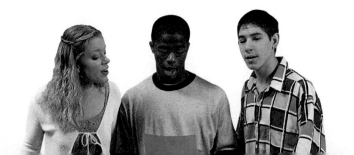

Hands-On Health

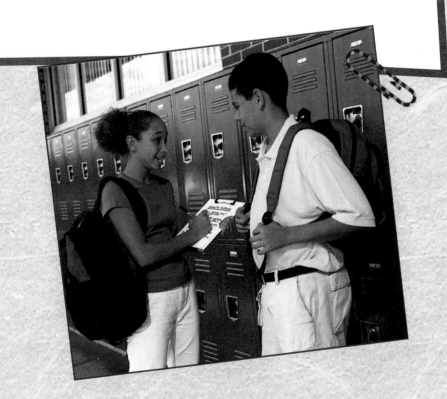

Getting the most out of *Teen Health*

Making healthy and responsible decisions is easy with *Teen Health*. Follow the guidelines below to make the most out of each lesson.

Do the Quick Write

This feature will help you start thinking about the information in a lesson.

Preview the Lesson

Get a preview of what's coming by reading the lesson objectives in the **Learn About....** You can also use this feature to prepare for quizzes and tests.

Review Key Terms

Find each vocabulary term in the text and read its definition. The terms appear in blue so you can locate them easily!

Lesson 2

Resolving Conflicts

Quick Write

Describe a personal situation in which you were able to resolve a conflict effectively.

LEARN ABOUT...

- skills for resolving conflicts.
- the importance of compromise in conflict resolution.
- peer mediation in schools.

VOCABULARY

- conflict resolution
- compromise
- win-win solution
- mediation

Conflict Resolution Skills

Conflict resolution involves *solving a disagreement in a way that satisfies both sides.* Some conflicts are easily resolved. For example, Saul and Jenna want to watch different television programs at the same time. They decide that Saul will record his program and watch it later.

Many conflicts are not so easily settled. People who have very different ideas or values may find it hard to reach agreement. Most conflicts can be resolved, however. The key to conflict resolution is having respect for the other person's rights.

Principles of Conflict Resolution

To reach agreement, people in conflict need to practice communication skills and self-control. They must also be willing to cooperate with one another and to compromise, or *give up something in order to reach a solution that satisfies everyone.* Most of all they must focus on the problem and not on the other person. **Figure 7.2** summarizes one approach to conflict resolution.

Reaching an agreement when both parties in a conflict strongly disagree is something to celebrate. *How did you resolve a recent conflict?*

168 CHAPTER 7: CONFLICT RESOLUTION

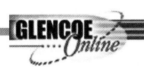

Use Glencoe's Health Web Site to Boost Your Health Smarts!

▶ Rate your health by taking the Health Inventory for each chapter. Jump-start your goals by filling out a Personal Wellness Contract.

▶ Check out Web Link Exercises for fun and interactive games and activities.

▶ Do some detective work on a particular health topic—Health Quests show you how.

▶ Get ready for tests by using the different Online Study Tools to review vocabulary terms and chapter content. E-flashcards, online quizzes, and interactive drag-and-drop games make studying fun!

▶ Building Health Skills features give you another chance to master important skills for wellness.

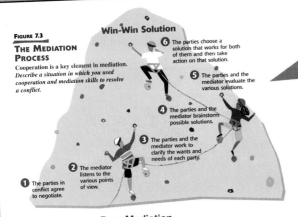

FIGURE 7.3
THE MEDIATION PROCESS
Cooperation is a key element in mediation. *Describe a situation in which you used cooperation and mediation skills to resolve a conflict.*

Win-Win Solution

❶ The parties in conflict agree to negotiate.

❷ The mediator listens to the various points of view.

❸ The parties and the mediator work to clarify the wants and needs of each party.

❹ The parties and the mediator brainstorm possible solutions.

❺ The parties and the mediator evaluate the various solutions.

❻ The parties choose a solution that works for both of them and then take action on that solution.

Peer Mediation

Many schools have peer mediation programs. In peer mediation, a student serves as the mediator for students who are involved in a conflict. Teens can be effective mediators because they understand their peers' attitudes and viewpoints. They can put the problem in language that students can relate to.

Students receive special training to become peer mediators. Training may be provided by teachers or by people from community mediation organizations. Training programs cover a number of topics that focus on the qualities, skills, and behaviors required of mediators. Here are some of the requirements of a peer mediator.

- Be trustworthy and keep the discussions confidential.
- Understand and analyze conflict.
- Listen carefully and express ideas clearly.
- Identify feelings.
- Remain completely neutral throughout the process.
- Handle anger in a positive way.
- Identify points of agreement.
- Brainstorm multiple solutions for a problem.
- Evaluate the consequences of various options.
- Take accurate notes.
- Once it has been agreed upon, describe a clear win-win agreement in writing.

170 CHAPTER 7: CONFLICT RESOLUTION

Study the Infographics

First, think about the overall message that the infographic is presenting. Then, read each callout carefully and determine what part of the image it is highlighting.

Try the Health Skills and Hands-On Health Activities

Develop valuable health skills by doing the Health Skills Activities that appear in each chapter. Conduct experiments, create ads, and try the other fun activities in the Hands-On Health features.

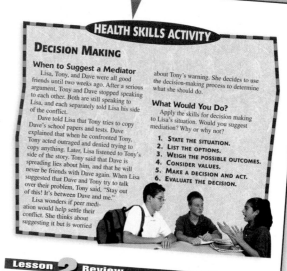

HEALTH SKILLS ACTIVITY

DECISION MAKING

When to Suggest a Mediator

Lisa, Tony, and Dave were all good friends until two weeks ago. After a serious argument, Tony and Dave stopped speaking to each other. Both are still speaking to Lisa, and each separately told Lisa his side of the conflict.

Dave told Lisa that Tony tries to copy Dave's school papers and tests. Dave explained that when he confronted Tony, Tony acted outraged and denied trying to copy anything. Later, Lisa listened to Tony's side of the story. Tony said that Dave is spreading lies about him, and that he will never be friends with Dave again. When Lisa suggested that Dave and Tony try to talk over their problem, Tony said, "Stay out of this! It's between Dave and me."

Lisa wonders if peer mediation would help settle their conflict. She thinks about suggesting it but is worried

about Tony's warning. She decides to use the decision-making process to determine what she should do.

What Would You Do?

Apply the skills for decision making to Lisa's situation. Would you suggest mediation? Why or why not?

1. STATE THE SITUATION.
2. LIST THE OPTIONS.
3. WEIGH THE POSSIBLE OUTCOMES.
4. CONSIDER VALUES.
5. MAKE A DECISION AND ACT.
6. EVALUATE THE DECISION.

Complete the Lesson Reviews

Completing the lesson reviews can help you see how well you know the material you have just studied. It also gives you a chance to apply what you've learned to different situations, as well as practice a health skill.

Lesson 2 Review

Using complete sentences, answer the following questions on a sheet of paper.

Reviewing Terms and Facts

1. **Vocabulary** Define *win-win solution.*
2. **Summarize** In your own words, summarize conflict resolution/mediation skills.
3. **Explain** What makes students effective mediators for their peers?

Thinking Critically

4. **Apply** Relate conflict resolution/mediation skills to personal situations: How have you used these skills in your life?
5. **Explain** How can a peer mediation program help make your school safer?

Applying Health Skills

6. **Conflict Resolution** With a partner, write a skit in which a conflict is resolved peacefully. Perform your skit for the class to demonstrate strategies for coping with problems related to conflict.

LESSON 2: RESOLVING CONFLICTS **171**

XV

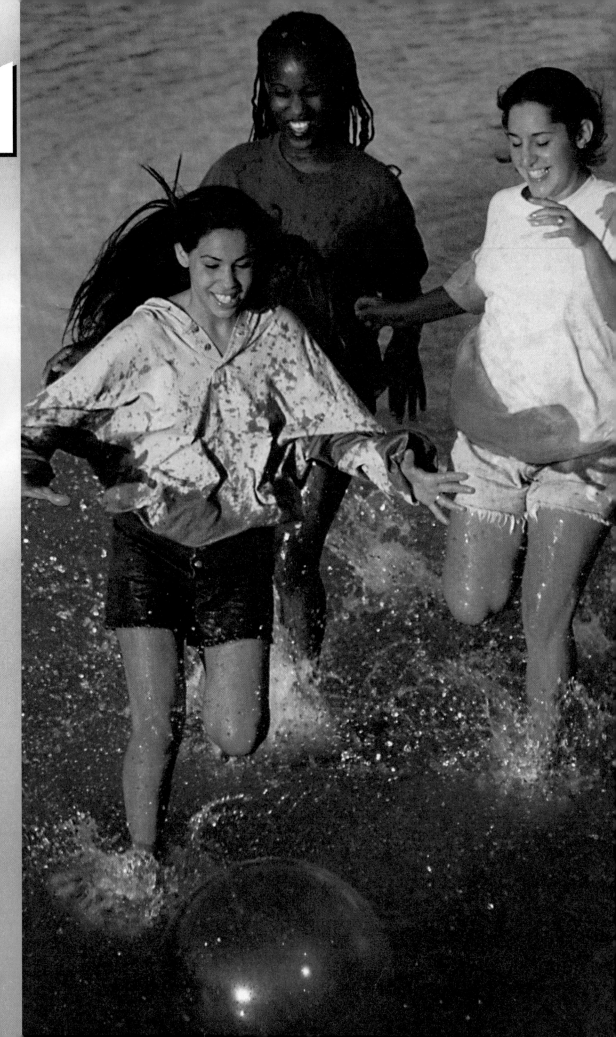

Taking Charge of Your Health

HEALTH in Action

The challenges you face in your teen years may seem bigger than an ocean, but you can develop the skills to meet them. You can learn to set goals, to make responsible decisions. You will be seeing many changes in the world around you— and in yourself—in the coming years. With the right skills and good habits on your side, however, you'll be prepared to make quite a splash!

How can taking care of yourself be like a day at the beach?

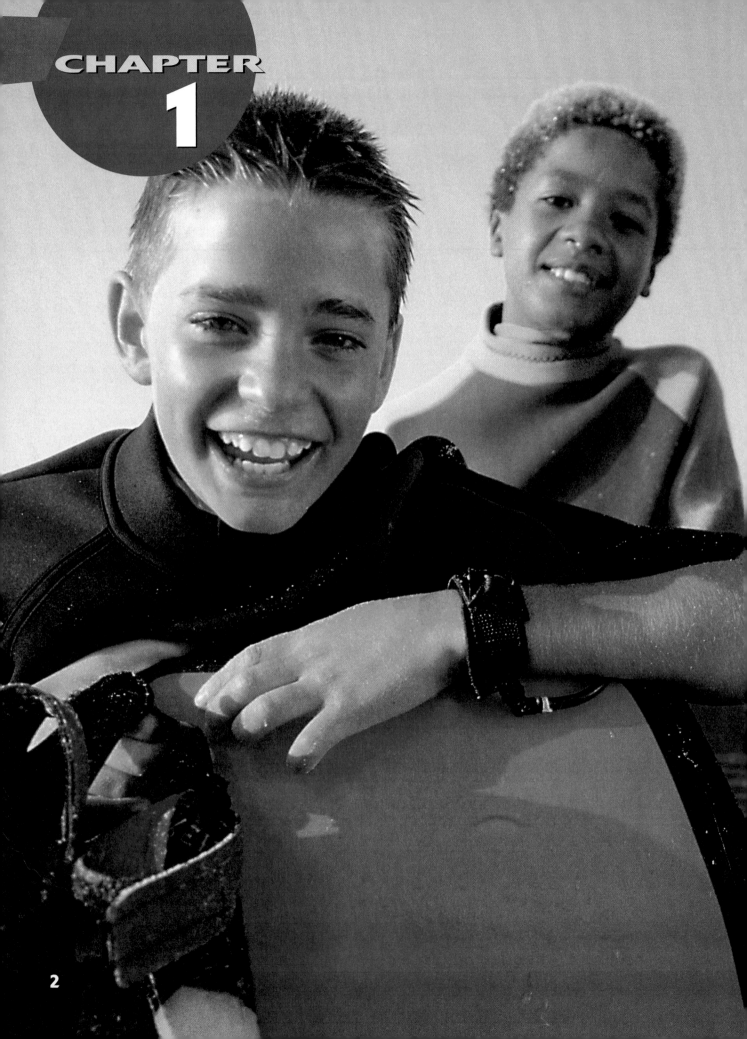

Understanding Your Health

HEALTH *Online*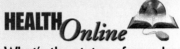

What's the status of your health—fair, good, or very good? Find out how you rate by taking the Chapter 1 Health Inventory at health.glencoe.com.

FOLDABLES™
Study Organizer

Before You Read

Make this Foldable to record what you learn about health and wellness in Lesson 1. Begin with a plain sheet of 11″ × 17″ paper.

Step 1

Fold the short sides of the sheet of paper inward so that they meet in the middle.

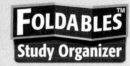

Step 2

Draw two circles—one that covers both sides of the Foldable, and one that covers only one side of the Foldable. Label as shown.

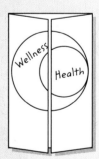

As You Read

On the back of each panel of your Foldable, take notes, define terms, and record examples of health and wellness. In the middle section, draw your personal health triangle.

What Is Health and Wellness?

Your Total Health

What do you think of when you hear the word *health*? Maybe you picture an athlete competing in a race. Perhaps you think of someone you know who never seems to get sick. Although being physically fit and being free from illness are important, there's much more to good health.

If you had a friend who was always putting herself down, would you think she was healthy? What about a classmate who was always picking fights with other students? Being healthy also involves feeling good about yourself and getting along with other people. **Health** is *a combination of physical, mental/emotional, and social well-being.*

You make choices every day that affect your health. You decide what to eat, how to spend your time, and who you will spend your time with. How can you tell which choices are best for your health? This book will help you recognize your health habits and decide whether you need to make any changes.

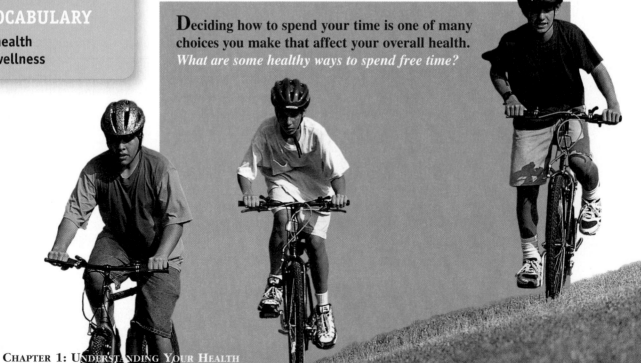

Deciding how to spend your time is one of many choices you make that affect your overall health. *What are some healthy ways to spend free time?*

The Health Triangle

Like a triangle, your health has three sides: physical, mental/emotional, and social. All three sides are interrelated. For example, a teen who skips meals and doesn't get enough sleep may feel irritable and have trouble concentrating. A teen who doesn't express emotions in healthy ways may have difficulty getting along with family and friends.

The key to good health is keeping a balanced health triangle. To have a balanced triangle, you need to keep each side of your triangle healthy. **Figure 1.1** provides more information about the three sides of the health triangle.

FIGURE 1.1

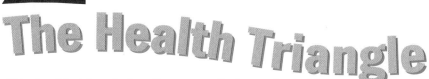

The health triangle has three equally important sides.
Which side deals with managing stress?

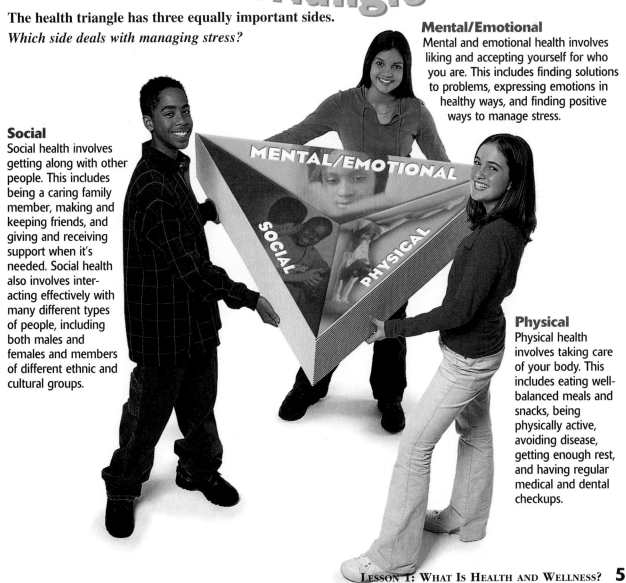

Social
Social health involves getting along with other people. This includes being a caring family member, making and keeping friends, and giving and receiving support when it's needed. Social health also involves interacting effectively with many different types of people, including both males and females and members of different ethnic and cultural groups.

Mental/Emotional
Mental and emotional health involves liking and accepting yourself for who you are. This includes finding solutions to problems, expressing emotions in healthy ways, and finding positive ways to manage stress.

Physical
Physical health involves taking care of your body. This includes eating well-balanced meals and snacks, being physically active, avoiding disease, getting enough rest, and having regular medical and dental checkups.

Reading Check

Understand purpose and focus. Which paragraph on this page makes a statement and gives an example? Which defines a term? Which poses a question to think about?

Maintaining a Balance

Each side of your triangle is equally important to good health. By working to keep the sides balanced, you will be on your way toward being a healthy person. **Figure 1.2** shows the health triangles of four teens. Three of these teens have unbalanced health triangles. What could they do to balance all the sides?

What Is Wellness?

Wellness is much more than just being healthy. **Wellness** is *an overall state of well-being, or total health.* To achieve wellness you need to make good health a part of your daily routine.

Every decision you make can affect your wellness. For example, healthy snack choices, such as fruit or yogurt instead of potato chips or candy, will satisfy your hunger and contribute to your wellness. Doing your homework and riding your bike are healthier ways to spend your time after school than playing video games. Keep in mind that developing good daily habits now will have positive long-term effects on your health and wellness.

FIGURE 1.2

Four Health Triangles

Each triangle reflects choices each person has made. *What does your triangle look like?*

Matthew

Matthew is an excellent student. He spends most of his free time on his computer, so he doesn't have much time for his family or friends. Matthew keeps physically fit by jogging alone several times each week.

Raj

Raj loves sports and plays on the soccer and basketball teams. He doesn't do very well with his schoolwork, though. Raj tries to avoid his problems by playing video games with his friends.

Karla

Karla spends a lot of time with her friends. They watch movies, listen to CDs, and go shopping. Karla gets good grades except in her physical education class. She doesn't get much physical activity and can't keep up with the rest of the class.

Chantelle

Chantelle has a few close friends and sees them mostly on weekends. Most weeknights she is busy with homework and spending time with her family. She bikes to school every day, and twice a week she has gymnastics class.

WELLNESS SURVEY

You may wonder why you should be concerned about staying healthy or becoming healthier. The reason is that the choices you make now could affect your health for years to come.

WHAT YOU WILL NEED
- pencil or pen
- sheet of paper

WHAT YOU WILL DO

1. With one or more classmates, develop a health survey. On a sheet of paper, list questions to find out how much students know about their physical, mental/emotional, and social health and the choices they make that affect their health triangles.
2. A few sample questions are: Is choosing nutritious foods important for good health? Are there healthy and unhealthy ways to express anger? Is physical activity necessary for good health? Do you need to know how to communicate with others to be healthy?
3. With the help of your teacher, make copies of the survey and distribute them to a sample of students in your school. Ask the students to return the survey to your teacher.

IN CONCLUSION

Tally the survey responses. How much did students know about good health? Write an article about the results of the survey for the school newspaper.

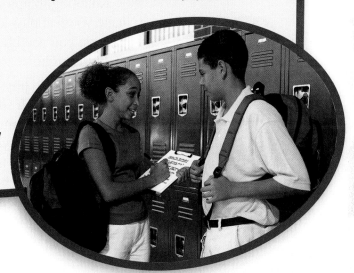

Lesson 1 Review

Using complete sentences, answer the following questions on a sheet of paper.

Reviewing Terms and Facts

1. **Vocabulary** Define the term *health.* Use it in an original sentence.
2. **Identify** Which side of the health triangle is concerned with taking care of your body?
3. **List** Name three characteristics of mental/emotional health.
4. **Explain** What does social health involve?

Thinking Critically

5. **Analyze** In your own words, analyze the interrelationships of physical, mental/emotional, and social health.

Applying Health Skills

6. **Practicing Healthful Behaviors** Draw your own health triangle. If your triangle is balanced, describe how you keep the three sides equal. If the triangle is unbalanced, list specific ways you can help balance it.

Changes During the Teen Years

Changing Times

The teen years involve changes that affect all sides of your health triangle. You might grow two inches, experience mood swings, and make new friends—all within a matter of months. Such changes can be challenging and even a bit scary, but they can also be exciting. These changing times signal that you're on your way to becoming an adult.

Adapting to and coping with changes during the teen years can make you feel physically tired and emotionally stressed. For these reasons, you need to pay careful attention to all sides of your health triangle:

- **Physical.** Be physically active, eat nutritious meals and snacks, and get enough sleep. Avoid tobacco, alcohol, and other drugs.
- **Mental/Emotional.** Use critical thinking skills. Find positive ways to express your feelings and manage stress. Ask for help and advice from trusted adults.
- **Social.** Do your best to get along well with others. Keep others' needs in mind and offer your support.

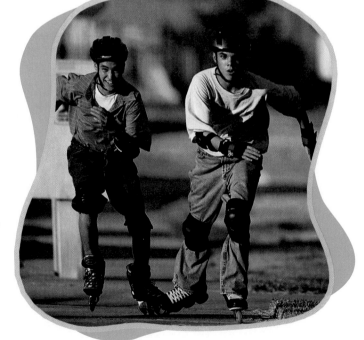

Your teen years are a time of growth and change. Remember to take care of your health and also take some time out to relax. *What do you like to do when you need to unwind?*

Adolescence

At the beginning of the school year, did you notice that some of your classmates had grown much taller over the summer while others remained the same height? Next to infancy, the fastest period of physical growth is adolescence. **Adolescence** is *the time of life between childhood and adulthood.* It usually starts any time between the ages of 11 and 15.

In addition to growing taller, you also experience other physical changes associated with adolescence. For example, you may have noticed new hair beginning to appear on parts of your body. You may have started perspiring more than before. These changes are all part of a growth spurt that occurs during adolescence. They are related to the release of **hormones**, which are *chemical substances, produced in glands, that help to regulate many body functions.* These hormones and the changes they cause are preparing you for adulthood. During adolescence, growth isn't just physical. You grow mentally, emotionally, and socially as well. Develop and use effective communication skills to discuss with parents or other trusted adults any questions you have about the changes that occur during adolescence.

Physical Development

How do you know when you have reached adolescence? You will know when you begin to develop the physical traits of adults of your gender. For example, boys may notice that their voices get deeper, and girls may find their figures are developing. These physical changes begin at different ages in different people. There are also differences in growth patterns among adolescents. Many girls begin their growth spurt between the ages of 11 and 14 and add about 3 inches to their height. For boys, the growth spurt usually begins between the ages of 13 and 16. Boys may grow 6 or 7 inches during those years.

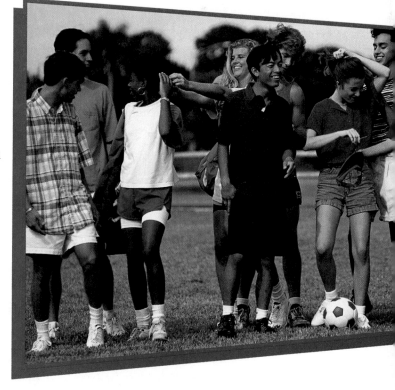

During the early teen years, you may grow at a faster or slower rate than your friends. *When do boys usually experience their first growth spurt?*

Social Studies

RITE OF PASSAGE
Many cultures and religions mark the beginning of adolescence with a special ceremony. In the Jewish faith, for example, boys and girls participate in a ceremony following their thirteenth birthday. For boys, it is called a bar mitzvah. For girls, it is called a bat mitzvah.

Reading Check

Think about these words from the chapter and what they have to do with stress and the changes of adolescence: *adapt, manage, coping.* Find two other words that fit with these to make a group.

Not only is physical development rapid during adolescence, but it is also uneven. Your hands and feet usually grow first, which may make them feel too big for the rest of your body. This makes some teens feel awkward or self-conscious. Keep in mind that every teen experiences these changes and they're completely normal.

Mental and Emotional Development

During adolescence, you also experience changes in the way you think and feel. As a child, you were able to solve only very basic kinds of problems. Now, you are able to solve increasingly complex problems.

Your new ability to reason and to think logically will enable you to think ahead and imagine possible outcomes of a situation. That way, you can weigh the consequences of a particular action. You will also be able to understand different points of view and see many possible solutions to a problem. **Figure 1.3** shows how new ways of thinking can help you with everyday situations.

FIGURE 1.3

New Ways of Thinking

Imagine possible outcomes.

Situation:
Tyler wants me to go with him to check out a construction site, even though there's a "No Trespassing" sign.

Possible consequences:
- I could get hurt.
- I could get in trouble with the law.
- I could get in trouble with my parents.

See many possible solutions.

Problem:
I need to study for a history test tomorrow, but I have band practice this afternoon and I have to baby-sit my little sister tonight.

Possible solutions:
- Ask the bandleader if I could skip practice this one time.
- Find out if someone else could baby-sit.
- Start studying after my sister goes to sleep.

Adolescence is also a time of great emotional changes. These changes include:

- **Mood swings.** Have you ever felt very happy one minute and suddenly sad the next? Many teens find these mood swings confusing and even disturbing. However, they're a common part of adolescence, related to the release of hormones.
- **New feelings toward others.** Have you recently started to see your family and friends in a new way? During adolescence, you recognize that the people around you have needs, just as you do. You may take a more active interest in helping to meet the needs of others, such as a friend who has a problem.
- **Increased romantic interest.** Do you find that you want to spend more time with someone you find attractive? Romantic interest develops at different times for different teens. Some teens find the new feelings they have confusing at times. Having them, however, is a normal part of growing up.
- **Increased interest in what is important to you.** You may begin to realize how important your family, friends, physical activity, and education are to you. You may also be aware of your growing sense of responsibility to yourself and to others.

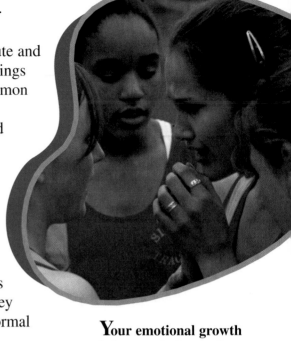

Your emotional growth helps you better understand what others are going through and to provide support. *How would you help a friend who is feeling sad?*

HEALTH SKILLS ACTIVITY

COMMUNICATION SKILLS

A Friend in Need

Recently, Heather has noticed that her friend Kyle seems unhappy. When Kyle's family moved into the apartment next door, Kyle and his brother Justin had to start sharing a bedroom. The two boys have not been getting along. Heather can see that Kyle is upset and frustrated with the situation. Heather wants to show Kyle that she supports him. What could she say to help him try to find a solution to his problem?

What Would You Do?

With a classmate, role-play a conversation between Heather and Kyle.

The teen taking the part of Heather should demonstrate good communication skills to help the teen playing Kyle.

Speaking skills:
- "I" messages
- Clear, simple statements
- Honest thoughts and feelings
- Appropriate body language

Listening skills:
- Appropriate body language
- Conversation encouragers
- Mirror thoughts and feelings
- Ask questions

Social Development

Social growth during the teen years affects the way you interact with your family, your friends, and your community. You may find, like many teens, that your friends become increasingly important to you during adolescence. As you begin to spend more time with friends, your relationship with your family could change. At the same time, you may begin to take a more active role in your community. Social growth involves relating to the people in your life in different ways:

- **Your Family.** During your childhood you were completely dependent on your parents or other family members. Now you are learning to act independently and to make decisions for yourself. It is only natural that this process may lead to differences between you and your family.
- **Your Friends and Peers.** During adolescence, you may prefer to share your thoughts and feelings with your friends rather than with family members. You may also find that your friends' opinions become more important to you. Your friendships may also change quite often, however, as you discover your own interests. If, for example, you become involved in soccer, you may make new friends on the team. That could leave less time for other friends who don't share your interest in soccer.

As a teen you will spend a great deal of time with your peers, or people your own age. Your peers will have a major effect on your social development. In fact, an important part of social growth is learning to benefit from the positive influence of peers while resisting any negative influence.

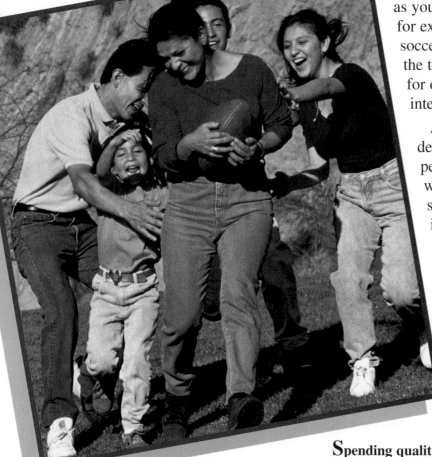

Spending quality time with your family is one way to develop mutual respect and maintain positive relationships. *What activities do you enjoy doing with your family?*

- **Your Community.** During the teen years, you will begin to recognize your role in the larger community that includes your school and your neighborhood. Social growth involves contributing to your community in a meaningful way. At school, for example, you might clean up litter or help other students with schoolwork. In your neighborhood, you might donate used clothing to the needy or support a local environmental group.

Developing positive relationships with family, peers, and role models and avoiding negative relationships is an important part of social growth. Analyze the positive and negative relationships in your life to determine how they might influence both individual and community health.

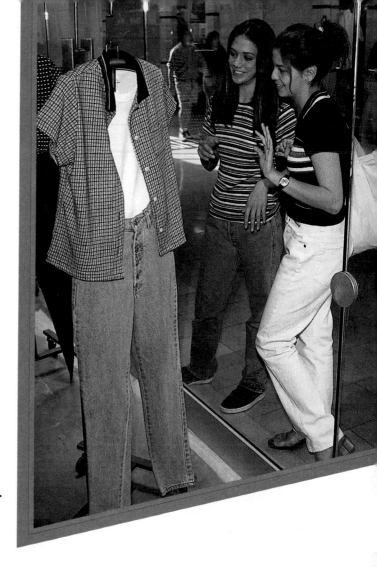

Your friends may influence many of your decisions during your teen years. *How have your friends had a positive influence on your behavior or actions?*

Lesson 2 Review

Using complete sentences, answer the following questions on a sheet of paper.

Reviewing Terms and Facts

1. **Vocabulary** Define *adolescence.*
2. **List** Examine some signs of physical and emotional development that occur during adolescence.
3. **Explain** What new mental skills do you develop during adolescence?
4. **Recall** How do relationships with family and friends change during the teen years?

Thinking Critically

5. **Analyze** How can positive and negative relationships influence individual health?

6. **Describe** Explain how differences in growth patterns among adolescents may affect personal health.

Applying Health Skills

7. **Communication Skills** Develop a dialogue in which a teen uses effective communication skills to discuss with parents or other trusted adults a concern about the changes that occur during adolescence.

Taking Responsibility for Your Health

Quick Write

What does the word *responsibility* mean to you? Write a brief definition, then list the ways you show that you are responsible.

LEARN ABOUT...

- how you can develop positive health habits.
- ways to recognize and avoid risk behaviors.
- why abstinence is the most responsible choice for teens.

VOCABULARY

- lifestyle factors
- risk behaviors
- sedentary lifestyle
- cumulative risks
- precaution
- abstinence
- attitude
- self-control

Choosing a Healthy Lifestyle

Do you eat nutritious foods even when you're not at home? Do you get at least eight hours of sleep each night? Do you wear a safety helmet every time you ride your bike or skateboard? You might be surprised to learn how such lifestyle factors affect your health. **Lifestyle factors** are *behaviors and habits that help determine a person's level of health.* **Figure 1.4** illustrates certain positive lifestyle factors. How many of them do you practice regularly?

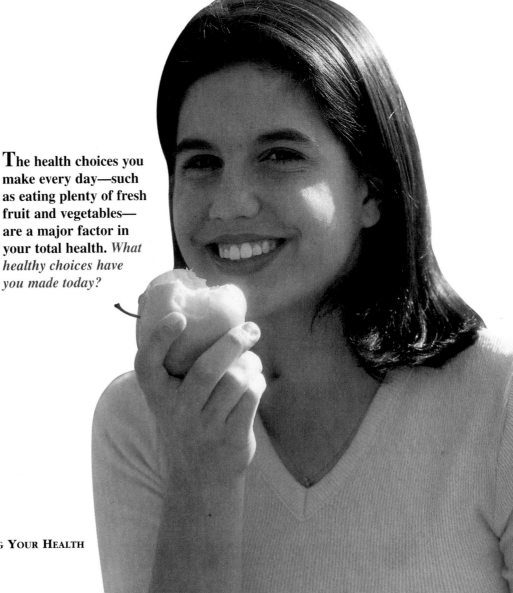

The health choices you make every day—such as eating plenty of fresh fruit and vegetables— are a major factor in your total health. *What healthy choices have you made today?*

FIGURE 1.4

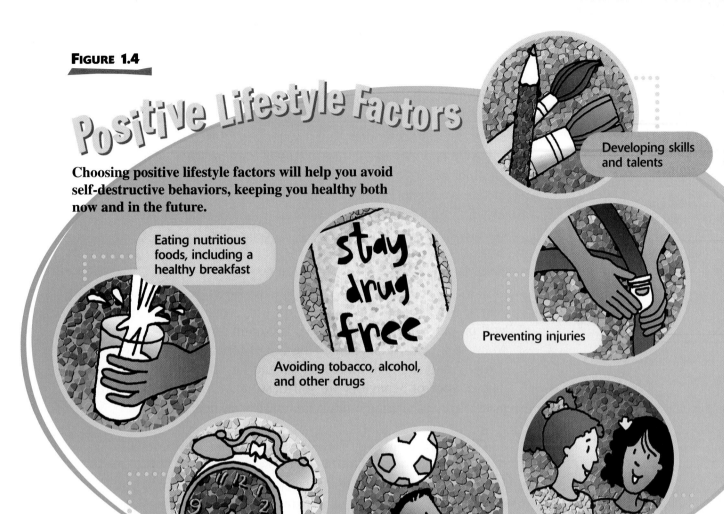

Positive Lifestyle Factors

Choosing positive lifestyle factors will help you avoid
self-destructive behaviors, keeping you healthy both
now and in the future.

Developing skills
and talents

Eating nutritious
foods, including a
healthy breakfast

stay
drug
free

Preventing injuries

Avoiding tobacco, alcohol,
and other drugs

Getting at least
eight hours of sleep
every night

Getting at least 60 minutes
of physical activity every day

Spending time with friends

Recognizing Risk Behaviors

Risks are an unavoidable part of life. For example, you may
need to cross a busy street on the way to school, or to use a
sharp knife when preparing food. Such risks are not likely to
injure you or someone else if you take reasonable care. Some
actions, however, involve a high level of unnecessary risk. A
risk behavior is *an action or behavior that might cause injury
or harm to you or others.*

Some risk behaviors are obvious. Diving into a river when
you don't know its depth is obviously risky. The chance of injury
is great and immediate. Other risk factors, however, are not so
obvious. For example, regularly eating foods high in fat and sugar
is a risk behavior. Even though you may not notice any immediate
effect, this unhealthy lifestyle factor may have a lasting negative
impact on your health.

Reading Check

Understand word parts. Investigate the words *consequence* and *unhealthy*. What are their prefixes? What are their roots? What does each mean?

Risk Behaviors and Teens

Certain risk behaviors are strongly associated with teens, according to the Centers for Disease Control and Prevention (CDC). These include the use of tobacco, alcohol, and other drugs; an unhealthy diet; and a sedentary lifestyle. A **sedentary lifestyle** is *a way of life that involves little physical activity.* Another negative risk factor for teens is sexual activity. Other unsafe behaviors include riding a bike without a helmet. Developing a healthy lifestyle is an effective strategy for counteracting these risk factors.

Risk Behaviors and Consequences

All risk behaviors carry consequences—some minor and some major. Not getting enough sleep for only one night, for example, will probably just make you feel tired and grouchy the next day. Many risk behaviors, such as the use of tobacco, alcohol, or other drugs, result in much more serious and far-reaching consequences. These types of behaviors are self-destructive—that is, harmful to your physical, mental/emotional, and social health.

Consider Jason's story. He was running late for baseball practice, so he hopped on his bike without putting on his helmet. He took a shortcut on a busy street and crossed the road without looking first. A car hit him, causing a deep gash on his head and a concussion. Now he is angry with himself for taking an unnecessary risk, for ruining his bike, and for upsetting his parents. He won't be able to play baseball for the rest of the season.

This teen knows that a sedentary lifestyle is a risk behavior. By staying physically active, she protects her health. *What are some ways that you stay physically active?*

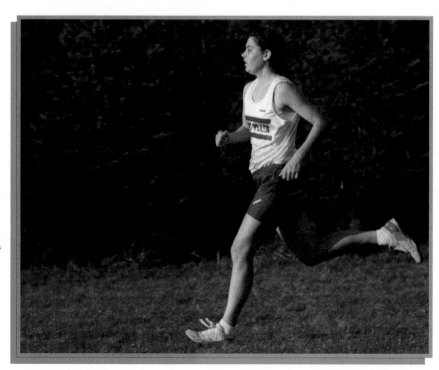

Jason's story is also an example of **cumulative risks**. These are *related risks that increase in effect with each added risk*. Jason's first risk behavior was not wearing a helmet. His second was riding his bike on a busy street. His third was crossing the street without looking. With each additional risk behavior, Jason's chances for serious consequences increased.

Abstaining from Risk Behaviors

How can you avoid serious consequences like Jason's? One effective strategy is taking precautions. A **precaution** is a *planned action taken before an event to increase the chances of a safe outcome.*

In addition to taking precautions, you can stay safe and avoid negative consequences by practicing healthful behaviors and abstinence. **Abstinence** is *not participating in high-risk behaviors.* You may be familiar with the word *abstinence* used to discuss avoiding sexual activity. Abstinence, however, means avoiding all high-risk behavior, including the use of tobacco, alcohol, and other drugs.

Abstinence from risk behavior is the wise choice for teens. It shows that you are responsible and that you respect yourself and others. By practicing abstinence, you protect all three sides of your health triangle. You protect your physical health by avoiding injury. You protect your mental/emotional health by avoiding the stress and worry involved with taking risks. In addition, you protect your social health by not disappointing family members and friends and by maintaining their trust.

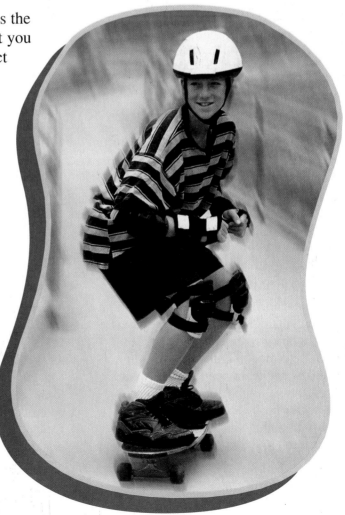

This teen is protecting himself from injury by wearing protective gear. *How else can teens abstain from risk behaviors?*

Developing Good Character

Self-discipline

Developing a healthy lifestyle takes commitment, but the rewards are worth the effort. For example, you may have to decide to watch less TV and instead select entertainment that promotes physical health. *How have you shown self-discipline in the past week?*

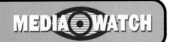
HEALTH IN THE NEWS

You've probably seen a headline like this: "Amazing pill lets you shed 10 pounds in 10 days!" *To protect your health, how would you determine if this information is true?*

Taking More Responsibility

Taking responsibility for your health involves more than just recognizing healthy choices and risk factors. Your personal **attitude**—your *feelings and beliefs*—also plays a role. You need to believe that making wise choices and developing good health habits can have a positive effect on your health.

Your attitude also includes the way you feel about yourself. If you like and respect yourself and believe that other people like and respect you, you will want to take care of yourself. To look, feel, and do your best, you will make choices that protect and promote your health. Taking responsibility for your health also requires **self-control**, or *control of your own emotions and desires*. For example, instead of slamming a door when you are angry, you could take a walk to cool off.

Having a positive attitude and using self-control will help show that you are ready to take on greater responsibility. Your family members can offer advice and support, but only your actions show that you're ready for more freedom. Being responsible for your own health is an important step toward becoming an adult.

HEALTH SKILLS ACTIVITY

PRACTICING HEALTHFUL BEHAVIORS

Making Health a Habit

A first step toward improving yourself and your total health is to take an honest look at your behavior. Do you feel that you're a responsible person? Do you show that you're ready for more responsibility? You can demonstrate your readiness in several ways. For example:

● Do your schoolwork and turn it in on time.
● Do your share of the household chores without being reminded.
● If you see something that needs to be done, do it without waiting to be asked.
● Be on time.
● Keep your promises.
● Finish tasks that you start, and clean up after yourself.

You can also improve yourself by following the positive lifestyle factors shown in **Figure 1.4** on page 15. Are all of those habits part of your current daily routine? If not, try the following:

● Identify a good health habit that you would like to develop. Write down the habit and the benefits that you could gain from making it part of your daily routine.
● Practice the habit several times during the next week. Each time, put a check mark next to the habit and the benefits you gained from practicing the habit.

ON YOUR OWN
Think about the ways that you demonstrated responsibility in the past week. Record the number of times you perform these actions during the week.

Staying Informed

How much do you really know about health? Where can you find more information? Because good health is part of a happy, satisfying life, learning how to get and stay healthy should be an important part of your life.

That's why health education is essential. Health education is more than just learning health facts. It can help you gain the tools you need to maintain and improve your total health and wellness. You can use health facts you learn in all areas of your life.

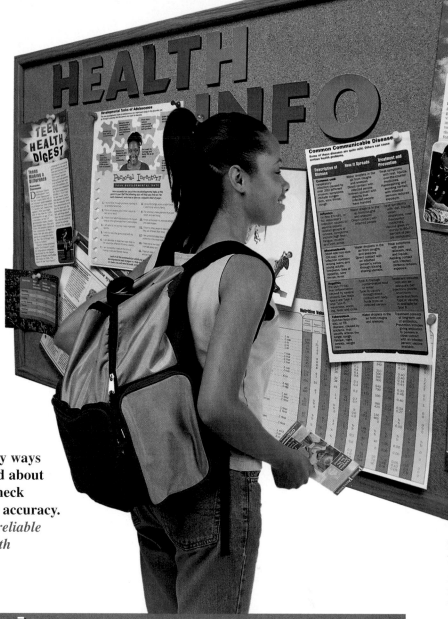

There are many ways to stay informed about health and to check information for accuracy. *What are some reliable sources for health information?*

Lesson 3 Review

Using complete sentences, answer the following questions on a sheet of paper.

Reviewing Terms and Facts

1. **Vocabulary** In the context of health, what are *lifestyle factors?*
2. **Vocabulary** Define *risk behaviors.*
3. **Give examples** What health risks are particularly associated with teens?
4. **Explain** How can you avoid the consequences associated with cumulative risks?
5. **Identify** Name two personal qualities that demonstrate that you are ready for more responsibility.

Thinking Critically

6. **Analyze** Look at the list of positive lifestyle factors in **Figure 1.4** on page 15. Choose one and think of ways you could develop it as a personal habit.
7. **Explain** Why is it important to be well informed about health?

Applying Health Skills

8. **Advocacy** Write a public service announcement that emphasizes the importance for teens of practicing abstinence.

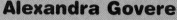

Teens with a Mission

Alexandra Govere
14, from Fullerton, California. Founder of Assisting AIDS Orphans

THE CHARITY: "I created the organization last year to provide clothing, toys, and school supplies to AIDS orphans in villages across Africa. With my younger sister, Saunsuray, I've brought together young people across the world to gather donations and send packages to kids in need."

WHY IT'S PERSONAL: "Zimbabwe is a peaceful place, but very poor. Living there until I was nine, I was extremely sad to see people in our village—even close friends and relatives—die of AIDS and leave their children behind. Many end up with no choice but to live in the streets and beg for money."

THE PAYOFF: "I was invited to speak at the first International Students Conference on HIV/AIDS and the Youth, but it was in Uganda and I couldn't afford to go. I was honored when one of the organizers wound up reading my speech for me. I felt that my effort to be an AIDS activist was finally being recognized."

HOW SHE'LL MAKE THE WORLD A BETTER PLACE: "The Assisting AIDS Orphans project is something I'd like to do for the rest of my life. I want to get more members and start helping worldwide. AIDS orphans aren't just in Africa, they're everywhere."

These three teens are out to make the world a better place.

Roxanne Tingir
17, from Port Washington, New York. Student cancer researcher

WHAT SHE DID: "I developed a diagnostic tool, called an ELISA, for a certain colon cancer treatment developed by the lab where I had an internship during high school. Basically my research will help doctors make sure that these colon cancer treatments are working."

WHY CANCER: "On Long Island, where I grew up, we have one of the highest breast cancer rates in the nation. Everyone knows of someone who's had it. My dad is a physician, and medical research has always interested me because you get such visible results."

ON HER ACCOMPLISHMENTS: "I really haven't done anything that extraordinary. When I read about what other teenagers have done, I'm absolutely amazed."

HOW SHE'LL MAKE THE WORLD A BETTER PLACE: "I really am not sure. I plan on attending Georgetown University. I'm leaning toward a major in government. I think our generation's biggest problem right now is globalization and how we're going to deal with September 11 and what's happened since. Everyone else's issues have really become our issues. The entire world is connected and we can't ignore that anymore."

Hans Lee
17, from Carmel, California. Inventor of a car safety system

THE INVENTION: "I built a safety system for a car that greatly improves its handling. [When a car goes out of control] the system will correct its trajectory and bring it back under control. I'm working at M.I.T. to implement the system in a full-size race car."

KEEPING AT IT: "I've always liked to build things. In sixth grade I decided to build a hybrid car from scratch. I worked on it in my garage for four years. Eventually it progressed into this project."

BEST MOMENT: "As I was walking up to receive my first award at the Intel International Science & Engineering Fair, I suddenly saw my face on two 40-foot screens on either side of the stage."

HOW HE'LL MAKE THE WORLD A BETTER PLACE: "I want all of my projects to improve people's lives, to make them easier and safer, and to advance society." ■

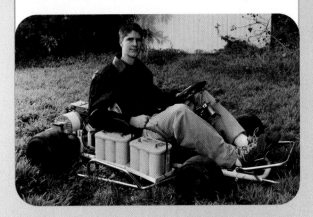

TIME TO THINK...

About Teens Making a Difference

Pair off with a classmate and interview each other about your goals for the future. Using the style and format of the above article, write a brief description of your interview subject's goals. Read your article aloud.

LOOKING AT HEALTH INFLUENCES

Model

Your friends and family are two of the many influences that affect the physical side of your health triangle. Other influences include your environment, your culture, the media, and your role models. Personal influences—such as what you know, your interests, and your hopes and fears—affect your physical health too. As you read about Cassidy, notice the influences that affect her physical health.

Cassidy has enjoyed being physically active since she was very young. She used to play soccer every weekend. Now she is more involved in track and bicycling.

Her best friend, Jacy, is a bicycling fanatic. Cassidy and Jacy often talk about becoming famous athletes. Cassidy knows that even if she never becomes famous, she wants to do something that involves sports.

Cassidy has learned a lot about sports from her family. Her sister is a high school athlete, and her dad played several sports in college. Around the dinner table, a common topic of conversation is healthful foods and training for competition.

Practice

Read about Lyle, who is learning Spanish. Then complete the three items about the influences on his mental/emotional health.

Lyle's favorite class is Spanish. He hopes to travel when he gets older. The idea of visiting Spanish-speaking countries is very exciting to Lyle. He has written "Visit Spain" on his list of "Things to Do Before I'm 30." One reason Lyle is so interested in Spanish is that his mom's family emigrated from Spain. When he visits his grandmother, Lyle looks through her scrapbook and listens to her stories about growing up in Barcelona.

1. Make a list of the influences that affect Lyle's goal to learn Spanish.
2. How do these influences affect Lyle's mental/emotional health?
3. In your opinion, which influences have the most effect on Lyle? Explain.

Apply/Assess

Think about your social health. Who are your friends and why did you choose them? How well do you get along with members of your family? Which family activities do you enjoy? Do you participate in clubs, extra-curricular activities, or community groups? When you answer these questions, you discover some influences that affect your social health. Identifying these influences will help you understand many of the health choices you make.

Write a newspaper article on your social health. In your article, describe your social life and analyze positive and negative relationships that influence your health, such as families, peers, and role models. Describe the factors that affect you most and tell how they influence your health.

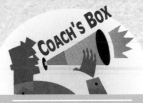

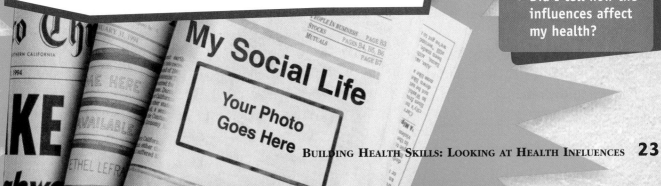

My Social Life

Your Photo Goes Here

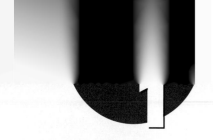

After You Read

Use your completed Foldable to review the information on health and wellness.

FOLDABLES™
Study Organizer

Reviewing Vocabulary and Concepts

On a sheet of paper, write the numbers 1–10. After each number, write the term from the list that best completes each statement.

- physical
- adolescence
- balanced
- growth spurt
- health triangle
- hormones
- mental/emotional
- social
- mood swings
- peers

Lesson 1

1. The three sides of health are physical, mental/emotional, and _____.
2. Each side of the _____ is as important as the others.
3. The key to good health is a _____ health triangle.
4. Your _____ health involves liking and accepting yourself for who are.
5. Your _____ health involves taking care of your body.

Lesson 2

6. _____ is the time of life between childhood and adulthood.
7. Chemical substances, produced in glands, that help to regulate many body functions are called _____.
8. During adolescence, boys and girls experience a _____ and add several inches to their height.

9. Having _____, or feeling happy one minute and sad the next, is a common emotional change that occurs during adolescence.
10. Your _____, or people your own age, have an important effect on your social growth.

Lesson 3

On a sheet of paper, write the numbers 11–15. After each number, write the letter of the answer that best completes each statement.

11. A way of life that includes little physical activity is called a
    a. cumulative risk.
    b. sedentary lifestyle.
    c. consequence.
    d. benefit.
12. Which of the following will increase the chances of a safe outcome if taken before an activity?
    a. a deep breath
    b. your blood pressure
    c. a nap
    d. precautions
13. You avoid all high-risk behavior if you practice
    a. abstinence.
    b. social growth.
    c. communication skills.
    d. adolescent behavior.
14. What are formed from your feelings and beliefs?
    a. mood swings
    b. hormones
    c. attitudes
    d. growth spurts
15. Going for a jog when you would rather just watch television is an example of
    a. a risk behavior.
    b. dependence.
    c. advocacy.
    d. self-control.

Thinking Critically

Using complete sentences, answer the following questions on a sheet of paper.

16. **Analyze** How will the mental abilities that you develop during adolescence help you throughout life?
17. **Apply** How might your personal attitudes influence your lifestyle?
18. **Suggest** What are some precautions you can take in your life to reduce risks?
19. **Apply** What factors might cause a teen to engage in a risk behavior such as sexual activity or illegal substance use? List three effective strategies that a teen could develop to counteract these risk factors.

Career Corner

Registered Nurse Registered nurses are health care professionals who want to help people. To become a nurse, you need at least a two-year nursing degree from a junior or community college. Many nurses complete a four- to five-year degree in nursing. To see whether you would enjoy this type of work, volunteer at a local hospital. Learn more about nursing and other health careers by clicking on Career Corner at health.glencoe.com.

Standardized Test Practice

Reading & Writing

Read the paragraphs below and then answer the questions.

Taking a bicycle tour is a fun way to see the country and improve your fitness level. Planning in advance will help ensure a safe and enjoyable trip.

Make sure your bike is in good condition and is equipped with a light, a repair kit, and a water carrier. Begin an exercise program to build your endurance. Prepare for weather changes by packing clothing that will protect you from strong winds, rain, and the cold. Plan your route before you leave by consulting experienced cyclists and by reading books and magazine articles about bike touring. When biking, always wear your helmet.

1. What is the passage mostly about?
   A bicycle safety
   B keeping your bike safe
   C planning for a bike tour
   D traveling fast on a bike

2. Why did the author probably write the passage?
   A to explain the rules of bike touring
   B to express feelings about bike touring
   C to explain how to begin bike touring
   D to persuade readers to bike safely

3. Write a paragraph describing some steps you might take to ensure your health and safety before you begin a new activity.

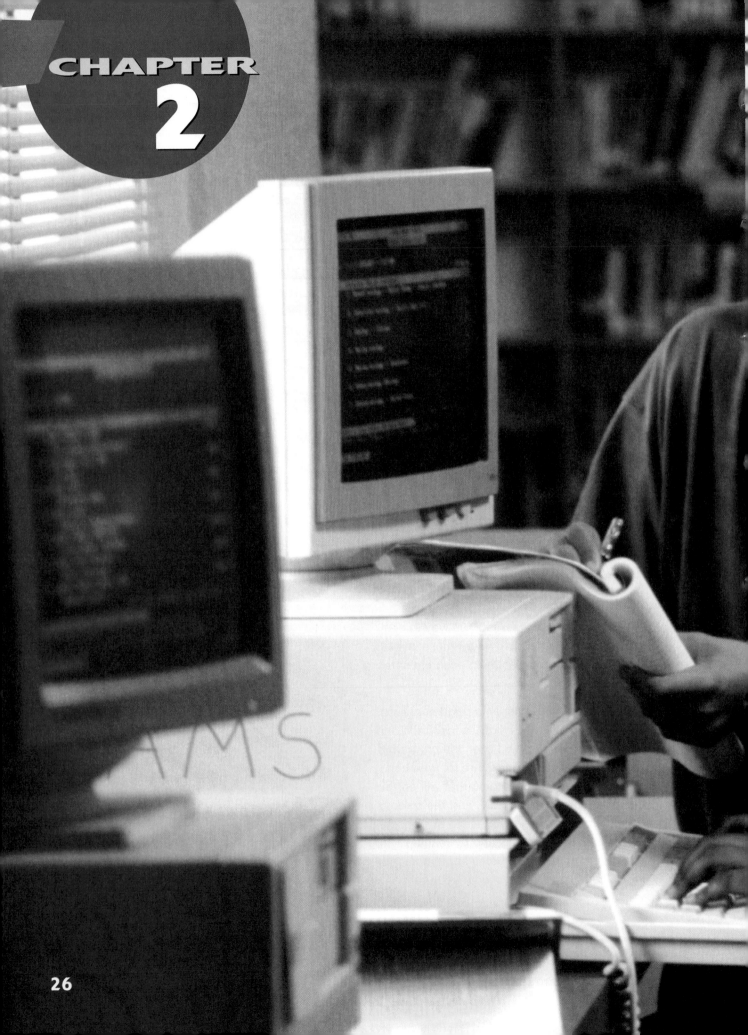

Health Skills: The Foundation

HEALTH *Online*

Do you have a strong foundation of health skills? Find out by taking the Health Inventory for Chapter 2 at health.glencoe.com.

FOLDABLES ™
Study Organizer

Before You Read

Make this Foldable to help you progress through the six steps of the decision-making process. Begin with a plain sheet of notebook paper.

Step 1

Fold the sheet of paper from side to side, leaving a ½″ tab along the side.

Step 2

Turn the paper, and fold it into thirds.

Step 3

Unfold and cut the top layer along both folds. Then cut each tab in half to make six tabs.

Step 4

Label the tabs as shown.

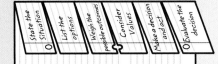

State the Situation · List the options · Weigh the possible outcomes · Consider Values · Make a decision and act · Evaluate the decision

As You Read

Under the appropriate tab of your Foldable, define terms and record information about each step in the decision-making process.

1

Making Decisions and Setting Goals

LEARN ABOUT...

- how decisions affect your health and the health of others.
- ways to make healthy, responsible decisions.
- the benefits of setting health goals.

VOCABULARY

- decision making
- values
- evaluate
- goal setting

Decisions and Goals

Decision making and goal setting are two important health-related skills. Decision-making skills will help you make the best choices and find healthy solutions to problems. Goal-setting skills will help you take control over your life and give it purpose and direction. Making decisions and setting goals also help you to develop a focus on the future.

When it comes to health, even a decision that may seem small can have great significance. Daniel, for example, persuaded his older brother to drive him to the video store. Because they were driving only around the corner, Daniel did not bother to fasten his safety belt. The car skidded on ice and Daniel hit his head against the windshield. What Daniel thought was a minor decision has left him with scars for life.

It's also important to develop strategies for setting long-term personal and health-related goals. Achieving goals that help you stay physically active and prevent injury will provide health benefits throughout your life. Moreover, people who set and achieve goals feel better about themselves and about their lives.

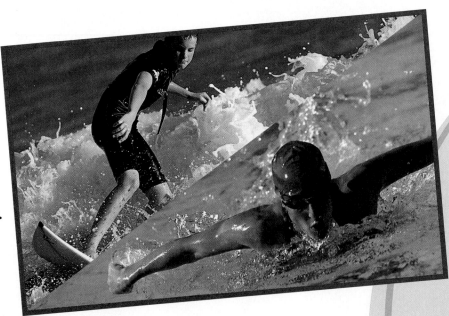

Deciding to stay physically active is one decision that will have positive lifelong benefits. *Appraise the risks and the benefits of decision making about personal health.*

The Decision-Making Process

Decision making is *the process of making a choice or finding a solution.* It involves a series of six steps. **Figure 2.1** relates the practices and steps that are necessary for making decisions, including health decisions.

Step 1 is to identify the situation. What choice do you need to make? Steps 2 and 3 are to think through your options and consider the possible outcomes of each option. When evaluating your choices, follow the H.E.L.P. criteria to keep you focused on critical issues:

- **H (Healthful)** Will it contribute to your health?
- **E (Ethical)** Does it show respect for yourself and others?
- **L (Legal)** Is someone your age allowed by law to do this?
- **P (Parent Approval)** Would your parents approve?

FIGURE 2.1

The Decision-Making Process

What should Kendra do? Go through the six-step decision-making process to help her decide.

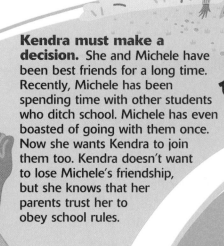

Kendra must make a decision. She and Michele have been best friends for a long time. Recently, Michele has been spending time with other students who ditch school. Michele has even boasted of going with them once. Now she wants Kendra to join them too. Kendra doesn't want to lose Michele's friendship, but she knows that her parents trust her to obey school rules.

1 State the situation.

2 List the options.

3 Weigh the possible outcomes.

4 Consider values.

5 Make a decision and act.

6 Evaluate the decision.

Reading Check

Understand cause and effect. Complete this analogy: Showing respect is to earning trust as showing disrespect is to _____.

In Step 4 you consider your values and the values of society. **Values** are *the beliefs and ideals that guide the way a person lives.* For example, keeping a positive relationship with your family is probably one of your personal values. You know that if you decide to stay out past your curfew, family members may lose trust in you. By considering your values, and getting home on time, you show respect and earn your family's trust. Respect and trust are also core ethical values, which means they are shared by people around the world.

Evaluating Your Decision

After Step 5—making your decision and taking action—Step 6 will have you evaluate the results. **Evaluate** means *to determine the value of something.* To evaluate your decision, ask yourself the following questions:

- What was the outcome of my decision? Was it what I expected?
- How did my decision make me feel about myself?
- How did my decision affect others?
- How did my decision affect each side of my health triangle?
- What did I learn? Would I make the same decision again?

As with any skill, decision making gets easier with practice. For example, you might think about some problems that you or your family may face. Think through all six steps of the decision-making process to find a healthy solution for each problem. This practice will help you with future decisions.

HEALTH SKILLS ACTIVITY

DECISION MAKING

What to Do? What to Do?

Andy has been swimming since he was five years old. He loves to swim because it's fun, it makes him feel healthy, and it helps him keep physically fit. Now he has a place on the local swim team, and that requires regular practice.

However, Andy has been so busy with his sport that his grades have begun to fall. If they slip too far, he could lose his place on the team, but cheating on homework and tests could also get him kicked off. What should Andy do?

WHAT WOULD YOU DO?

Apply the six steps of the decision-making process to Andy's situation. Compare your outcome to the solutions of your classmates.

1. **STATE THE SITUATION.**
2. **LIST THE OPTIONS.**
3. **WEIGH THE POSSIBLE OUTCOMES.**
4. **CONSIDER VALUES.**
5. **MAKE A DECISION AND ACT.**
6. **EVALUATE THE DECISION.**

Why Set Goals?

Do you feel that you do all you can do to protect your health, or are you aware that there is room for improvement? Perhaps you need to work on family relationships, or ways to better protect yourself from injury or infection. Setting goals will help you focus on the behaviors you want to change. **Goal setting** is *the process of working toward something you want to accomplish.* Achieving a goal requires planning and effort, and it can give you a great sense of accomplishment and pride.

Goals that you set for one area of your life often lead to the achievement of goals in other areas. For example, if you work toward the goal of becoming a black belt in karate, you will achieve fitness goals, too. Along the way, you may also reach other goals such as making new friends, gaining more self-confidence, and learning more ways to manage stress.

The Benefits of Setting Goals

Goals help you identify what you want out of life. They also help you use your time, energy, and other resources wisely. Setting goals and working to reach them is an acceptable method of gaining attention. Your peers may admire your success and be inspired to set and achieve their own goals. Receiving positive attention and recognition from others can also encourage you to set new goals.

You will most likely have both long-term goals and short-term goals. Short-term goals often help you reach your long-term goals.

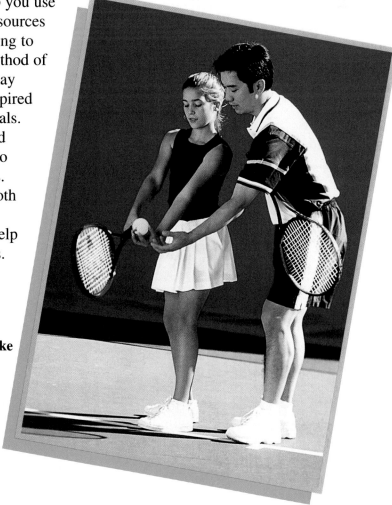

This teen wants to make the tennis team. *How will short-term goals help her achieve this long-term goal?*

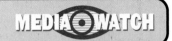

It took many short-term goals along the way for this teen to reach her long-term goal of playing in front of an audience. *What are some of your long-term goals?*

Short-Term Goals

Some short-term goals are just that: goals that you want to achieve in the next few days or weeks. Your short-term goals may, for example, include finishing a homework assignment and writing an e-mail to your grandfather.

Other short-term goals are stepping-stones to long-term goals. Suppose, for example, that your long-term goal is to take part in a local charity 5-K run. Your short-term goals might be to run several times a week, to gradually increase the distances that you run, and to eat more nutritious foods.

Long-Term Goals

Some goals take several weeks, months, or even years to achieve. For example, you might want to go on a rafting trip next summer, or to reach a vocational (career) goal such as becoming a professional baseball player. These are long-term goals. They will take time, planning, and dedication. Short-term goals will help you meet these long-term goals.

Building Goal-Setting Skills

Goal setting is a skill that will benefit you in many areas of life. A good way to ensure that you reach the goals you set for yourself is to make a plan. **Figure 2.2** shows the steps one teen used to reach his goal of making the school basketball team. Follow these steps to develop strategies for setting your own long-term personal and vocational goals.

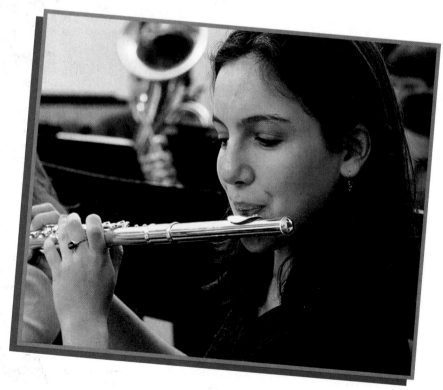

FIGURE 2.2

The Goal-Setting Process

Here is one teen's plan to meet his goals.

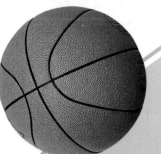

1 Identify a specific goal and write it down.
Making the school basketball team.

2 List the steps you will take to reach your goal.
Run at least 2 miles four times each week.
Practice basketball every day.

3 Get help and support from others.
Ask my friends and my brother (who plays on the high school team) to play basketball with me whenever they can.
Get advice from the basketball coach about my training routine.

4 Set up checkpoints to evaluate your progress.
After 2 weeks of training, play a game of one-on-one against my brother.

5 Give yourself a reward once you have achieved your goal.
If I make the team, I will buy myself a new pair of basketball shoes.

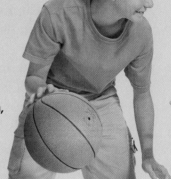
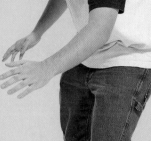

Lesson 1 Review

Using complete sentences, answer the following questions on a sheet of paper.

Reviewing Terms and Facts

1. **Vocabulary** Define *decision making*.
2. **Relate** What are the necessary steps and practices of the decision-making process?
3. **Recall** What are three questions you can ask yourself when you evaluate a decision?
4. **Summarize** What are the benefits of setting goals?

Thinking Critically

5. **Analyze** Think of a personal health decision you made in the past month. Appraise the risks and benefits of making that decision.
6. **Suggest** What are some goals that you could set to improve your level of health?

Applying Health Skills

7. **Goal Setting** Develop strategies for setting long-term personal and vocational goals: Think of one personal health goal and one career goal that you would like to achieve over the long term. Use the goal-setting steps to develop strategies for achieving each goal.

Practicing Communication Skills

Quick Write

Write down five questions that you could use to start a conversation with someone you just met.

LEARN ABOUT...

- how body language can help you communicate.
- why "I" messages are more effective than "you" messages.
- how to improve your speaking and listening skills.
- how to use refusal skills.

VOCABULARY

- interpersonal communication
- body language
- mixed message
- eye contact
- active listening
- feedback
- refusal skills

How Well Do You Communicate?

Some people are much better communicators than others. They have the ability to get their message across, listen to what others have to say, and keep the lines of communication open. In short, they have good interpersonal communication skills. **Interpersonal communication** involves *the exchange of thoughts, feelings, and beliefs between two or more people.*

Like other skills, interpersonal communication must be learned and practiced. It is an important skill because you use it in all of your relationships. Think about how often you talk with family members, friends, teachers, and classmates. Effective interpersonal communication involves body language and careful word choice as well as speaking and listening skills.

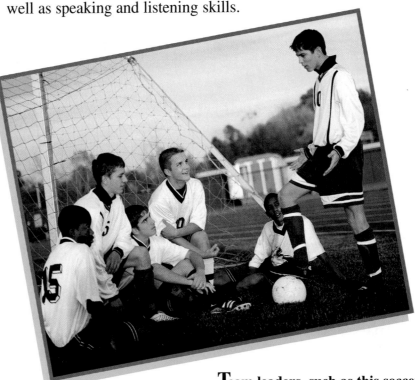

Team leaders, such as this soccer captain, use communication skills to get the best performance from their players. *Why are communication skills important for leadership?*

Body Language

Interpersonal communication involves more than words. Your body helps to communicate your thoughts and feelings too. **Body language** is *a form of nonverbal communication.* For example, raised eyebrows might reflect curiosity, surprise, or interest. Drooping shoulders might indicate sadness, insecurity, or fear.

It is important for speakers and listeners to be aware of body language. Some forms of body language such as smiling and nodding encourage communication. Other forms such as frowning and crossing arms tightly across the chest discourage communication.

Sometimes your words and your body language don't communicate the same message. A **mixed message** occurs *when your words say one thing but your body language says another.* For example, you might say, "I'm not angry," but your frown and clenched jaw convey a different message. Your body language gives your true feelings away.

Using "I" Messages

Imagine your reaction if a friend said to you, "You're never on time!" or "You're so bossy!" These types of "you" messages place blame on the other person and often cause hurt or angry feelings. Using "I" messages instead is a much more effective way to communicate. An "I" message is a statement in which a person uses the pronoun I to express an opinion or comment.

A well-crafted "I" message is a powerful communication tool. It states the situation and how you feel about the situation. It also offers an explanation for your feelings. Finally, it states what you need. For example, you might say, "When you were late for the movie I felt disappointed. I'd heard that the opening sequence was funny and I didn't want to miss it. Next time we go to the movies let's make sure we're early so we don't miss anything."

Your body language and your words tell someone if you are interested in what he or she has to say. *What body language tells you that the teen on the right is interested in what the other teen is saying?*

CULTURAL CONTEXTS
The use of eye contact varies among different cultures. In some cultures, eye contact means that the listener is interested in the speaker and that the message is getting across. In other cultures, however, eye contact is considered rude.

Speaking Skills

Interpersonal communication involves both giving and receiving messages. Speaking is the giving part. Good communication involves speaking clearly and carefully. Here are some tips for improving your speaking skills.

1. **Use "I" messages.** Consider how your words will affect the other person, and express your concerns in terms of your own feelings. You'll be less likely to make others feel defensive.
2. **Make clear, simple statements.** Stick to the point and be specific. Make sure the other person understands what you're saying.
3. **Be honest with thoughts and feelings.** Say what you want to say. Be truthful and direct about your values while showing respect for your listener's values.
4. **Use appropriate body language.** Make sure your facial expressions, gestures, and posture match your message. Use **eye contact**, or *direct visual contact with another person's eyes,* to show that you are sincere.

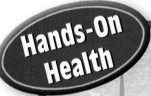

SENDING "I" MESSAGES

This activity will give you the opportunity to practice sending "I" messages. The more you practice this skill, the better communicator you will become.

WHAT YOU WILL NEED
- pencil or pen
- index cards

WHAT YOU WILL DO
1. Working in pairs, imagine everyday situations in which "you" messages might occur. Write the situation across the top of the card. Then write the "you" message below on the left. Change that same message into an "I" message, and write the "I" version on the right. A sample card is shown here.
2. Here are a few sample situations:
   - Your older brother was an hour late in picking you up at the mall.
   - Your friend told a lie about you.

3. Read each "you" message to the class. Then read the corresponding "I" message.

IN CONCLUSION
1. Which types of messages did you think were the most effective? Why?
2. Think of a recent disagreement that you had with a family member or friend. How could using "I" messages have helped resolve the conflict?

Situation:
Your friend always chooses what you'll do together

You
"You always get your own way."

"I'll go along with your choice this time if I can pick what we do the next time."

Listening Skills

Good listening skills are just as important to interpersonal communication as speaking skills. A speaker's message has meaning only if the listener receives it. Good communication involves active listening. **Active listening** means *hearing, thinking about, and responding to the other person's message.* Here are some effective listening skills.

1. **Use appropriate body language.** Pay attention to what the speaker has to say. Make eye contact, and use facial expressions and gestures that show that you are listening.

2. **Use conversation encouragers.** Show that you're listening by nodding or asking questions. Say things like "Really?" or "What happened next?" to show that you are paying attention.

3. **Mirror thoughts and feelings.** Repeat what the person said as a way of confirming what you heard. Offer feedback when appropriate. **Feedback** is *a response by the listener to what the speaker has said.*

4. **Ask questions.** After the person has finished speaking, ask questions or add your own comments or opinions.

Refusal Skills

During your teen years, there may be times when friends or acquaintances want you to do something that you do not want to do. Maybe you're just not interested. Maybe you don't have the time or the money. Maybe it's something that is unhealthy or that goes against your values. In these situations, refusal skills are useful. **Refusal skills** are *communication strategies that help you say no effectively.*

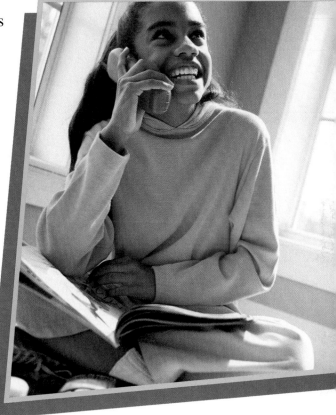

Good communication skills help you form healthy relationships. *How do the speaking and listening skills apply when you talk on the telephone?*

Using refusal skills will help you be true to yourself. You can resist without feeling guilty or uncomfortable. Other people will respect you for being honest about your needs and wants. An easy way to remember refusal skills is to keep in mind the letters in the word *stop.*

- **S**ay no in a firm voice.
- **T**ell why not.
- **O**ffer other ideas.
- **P**romptly leave.

When you need to refuse someone, it is important to show that you mean what you say. Your body language, including eye contact, helps you to do this. **Figure 2.3** illustrates how body language can show refusal.

FIGURE 2.3

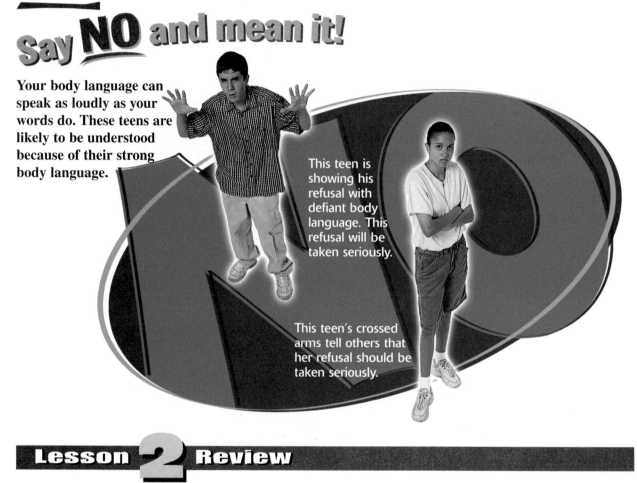

Say **NO** and mean it!

Your body language can speak as loudly as your words do. These teens are likely to be understood because of their strong body language.

This teen is showing his refusal with defiant body language. This refusal will be taken seriously.

This teen's crossed arms tell others that her refusal should be taken seriously.

Lesson 2 Review

Using complete sentences, answer the following questions on a sheet of paper.

Reviewing Terms and Facts

1. **Vocabulary** Define *interpersonal communication.*
2. **Recall** Give three examples of ways people use body language.
3. **Identify** List four tips for improving speaking skills.
4. **Explain** What is meant by *active listening?*

Thinking Critically

5. **Analyze** Choose someone you consider a particularly good communicator. Identify the skills that person uses to communicate so well.
6. **Compare** Distinguish between effective and ineffective listening, such as paying attention to the speaker versus not making eye contact.

Applying Health Skills

7. **Communication Skills** Make a videotape that demonstrates the power of nonverbal communication. Tape the body language of some volunteers and narrate the tape, explaining how body language sends messages. Ask the audience to interpret each person's message from his or her body language.

Managing Stress

What Is Stress?

The teen years are a time of many changes. Your body is changing, you are gaining new responsibilities, and you are forming new kinds of relationships. Because of such changes, teens may experience stress. **Stress** is *your body's response to change* and is a normal part of life.

Stress is not necessarily bad. *Positive stress,* called **eustress**, can make your life more pleasurable. It can help you reach your goals and motivate you to do your best. Eustress is an exciting feeling. It might help you find the energy to score the winning goal in a soccer match or do exceptionally well on a school project.

Some stress can have a negative effect on personal health, however. This type of *negative stress* is called **distress**. You might react to distress by having an upset stomach before giving a report, or by losing sleep after you argue with your parents. You can't always avoid negative stress, but you *can* learn to manage it.

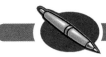

Quick Write
Jot down the types of situations that are most likely to cause you to feel stress.

LEARN ABOUT...
- the causes of stress.
- how your body responds to stress.
- positive ways to manage the stress in your life.

VOCABULARY
- stress
- eustress
- distress
- stressor
- fight-or-flight response
- adrenaline
- fatigue
- stress management skills
- time management

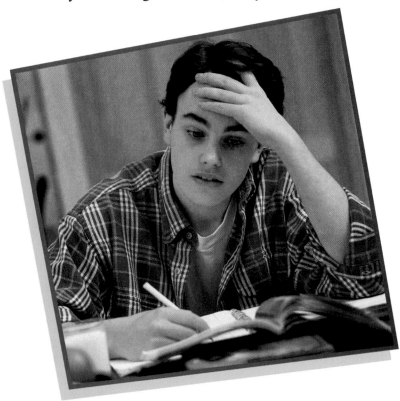

Learning to manage your time and planning ahead are coping strategies that can help you avoid stressful situations. *What steps do you take to manage stress in your life?*

What Causes Stress?

To handle stress, you need to know what causes it. *Anything that causes stress* is called a **stressor**. Stressors range from everyday annoyances to serious personal problems. They also affect different people in different ways. Whereas you might feel nervous about auditioning for the choir, your friend might find the same situation exciting. **Figure 2.4** shows some of the things that cause stress for teens.

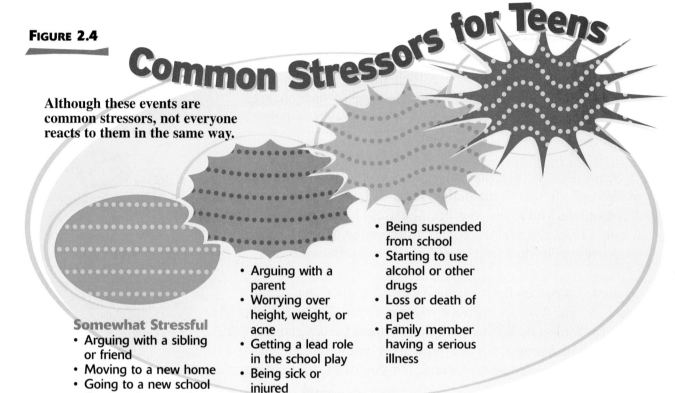

FIGURE 2.4

Common Stressors for Teens

Although these events are common stressors, not everyone reacts to them in the same way.

Somewhat Stressful
- Arguing with a sibling or friend
- Moving to a new home
- Going to a new school
- Getting glasses or braces

- Arguing with a parent
- Worrying over height, weight, or acne
- Getting a lead role in the school play
- Being sick or injured

- Being suspended from school
- Starting to use alcohol or other drugs
- Loss or death of a pet
- Family member having a serious illness

How Your Body Responds to Stress

When a person experiences a great deal of stress, the body reacts as though it is in danger. The natural way to deal with a danger is either to fight it or to flee from it. *The process by which the body prepares to deal with a stressor* is, therefore, known as the **fight-or-flight response**. One part of this response is the release of adrenaline. **Adrenaline** is *a hormone that gives the body extra energy.*

There's a limit to how much stress your body can handle. Too much stress can result in headaches, digestive problems, and high blood pressure. It can make you feel anxious, depressed, angry, or irritable. Over time, you might experience **fatigue**, or *exhaustion,* and a lower resistance to infection. This is your body's way of telling you that you need to rest and reduce your stress.

Ways to Manage Stress

To handle stress you need a variety of **stress management skills**, or *ways to deal with and overcome problems*. One of the basic ways to manage stress is to follow a healthy lifestyle. Problems are always easier to deal with if you feel well. More specific skills for dealing with stress include knowing how and when to relax, keeping a positive outlook, being physically active, and managing your time.

Relaxation

Relaxation reduces stress by slowing your heart rate and making you feel less tense. Try some of these strategies for coping with stress:

- **Relax your muscles.** Tighten and then relax one group of muscles at a time. Start at your toes and work your way up to your head.
- **Slow your breathing.** Take deep, even breaths for five minutes. Inhale through your nose and exhale through your mouth.
- **Get enough sleep.** Feeling tired can make a stressful situation seem worse. Everything looks better after a good night's sleep!

Keep a Positive Outlook

When you are under stress, it is easy to feel hopeless. In fact, stress can affect your emotions, causing you to feel depressed, anxious, or afraid. A minor problem can seem major. Remind yourself to look at the big picture and keep things in perspective. Is it *really* the end of the world if you don't get to stay out as late as some of your friends? Is your homework assignment *really* as difficult as you think? Following are some tips for keeping a positive outlook at times of stress.

Reading Check

Eustress and *distress* are antonyms. Think of words or phrases that are opposites, or close opposites, for *stressor, fatigue, benefit,* and *worry.*

Laughter is a great stress reliever. *Describe the relationship between emotions and stress.*

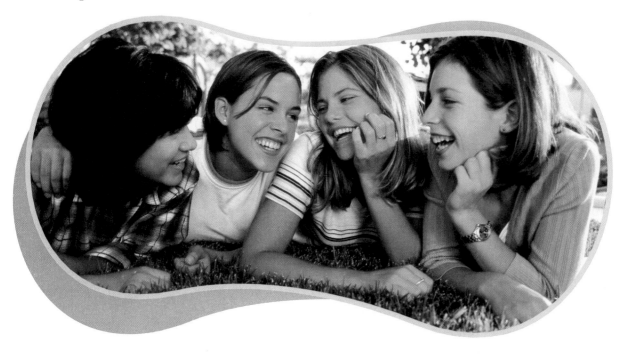

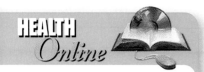
- **Think positively.** If you tell yourself that you will fail at something, you will increase your stress. Instead, tell yourself that you will do a great job.
- **Keep your sense of humor.** Don't let stress prevent you from seeing the funny side of things. A good laugh is a great stress reliever.
- **Have some fun.** Take a little time out to do something enjoyable and relaxing. Listen to your favorite CD, read a book, or watch a funny video.

Remember that some stress can be helpful. It can motivate you to take action. Say, for example that you're nervous about doing well in team tryouts. The stress that you feel might motivate you to put in plenty of practice.

Physical Activity

Being physically active is one of the healthiest ways to manage stress. Physical activity can bring about physical and emotional changes that can offset the effects of stress and give you a more positive outlook. **Figure 2.5** shows some of these changes.

FIGURE 2.5

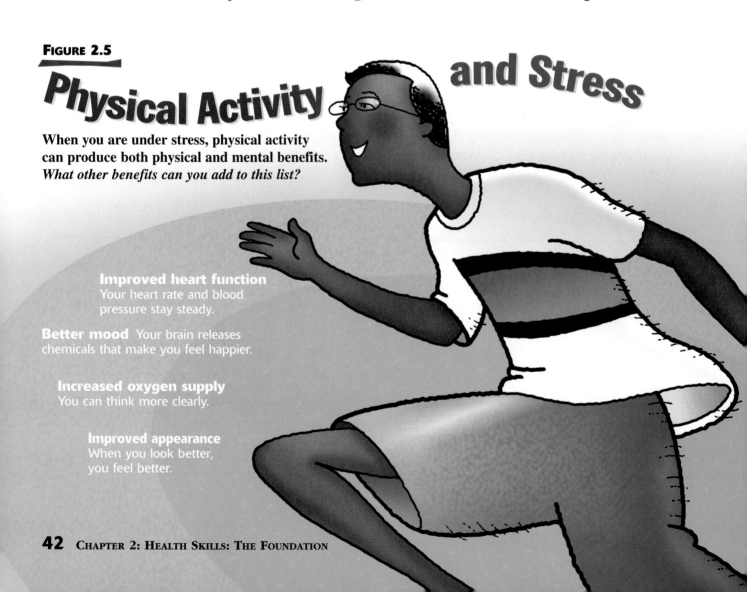

Physical Activity and Stress

When you are under stress, physical activity can produce both physical and mental benefits. *What other benefits can you add to this list?*

Improved heart function Your heart rate and blood pressure stay steady.

Better mood Your brain releases chemicals that make you feel happier.

Increased oxygen supply You can think more clearly.

Improved appearance When you look better, you feel better.

Managing Your Time

Learning time-management skills can help you reduce stress and get more done. **Time management** means *using your time wisely*. It combines planning and self-discipline.

Managing your time involves figuring out which activities are most important to you. When you have a task to finish, stay focused. Avoid distractions such as phone calls and visitors until you are ready to take a break.

HEALTH SKILLS ACTIVITY

STRESS MANAGEMENT

Balance Your Schedule

One strategy for coping with stress is to use your time wisely and balance your schedule. Try these tips for managing a busy schedule.

- **SET PRIORITIES.** Figure out which tasks are required and which are optional.
- **PUT IT IN WRITING.** Include both required and optional tasks, but make sure you list (and do) the required tasks first.
- **PLAN YOUR TIME.** Allow enough time for each task, but also set aside some time for something you enjoy.

- **THINK AHEAD.** Think through all the details before you start a task.
- **USE REFUSAL SKILLS.** You won't always have time to do everything you want to do. Learn to say no to things you don't have time for.

WITH A GROUP
In small groups, devise your own list of time-management skills for busy teens. Demonstrate these time-management skills for the rest of the class.

Lesson 3 Review

Using complete sentences, answer the following questions on a sheet of paper.

Reviewing Terms and Facts

1. **Vocabulary** What is the difference between *eustress* and *distress?*
2. **Explain** What is the process known as the *fight-or-flight response*?
3. **Identify** Name four skills that can help you deal with stress.
4. **Summarize** What does time management involve?

Thinking Critically

5. **Interpret** Describe some possible effects of stress on personal and family health.
6. **Explain** Why are planning and self-discipline important to time management?

Applying Health Skills

7. **Stress Management** Choose one of the strategies for coping with stress described on pages 41–43. Create a skit about a teen who uses that strategy. Perform your skit for the class to demonstrate this strategy for coping with stress.

Developing Other Health Skills

Quick Write

What influences your decisions about health? List the people, media, and other factors that you think have the strongest influence on the decisions you make about your health.

LEARN ABOUT...

- ways to get the health information you need.
- behaviors that enhance the way you look and feel.
- internal and external influences on your health.

VOCABULARY

- support system
- environment

Health Skills: An Overview

Health skills are practices that help you maintain, protect, and improve your health. At the same time, they help you understand how and why your decisions, choices, and attitudes influence your health.

Health skills are also called life skills. That's because they will benefit you not only during the teen years but also throughout your life. The skills already discussed in this chapter—decision making, goal setting, communication skills, refusal skills, and stress management—are examples of health skills. **Figure 2.6** shows a complete list of health skills.

FIGURE 2.6

THE HEALTH SKILLS

Practicing these health skills will provide a lifetime of benefits.

* **Accessing Information**
* **Self-Management**
  —Practicing Healthful Behaviors
  —Stress Management
* **Analyzing Influences**
* **Interpersonal Communication**
  —Communication Skills
  —Refusal Skills
  —Conflict-Resolution Skills
* **Decision Making/Goal Setting**
* **Advocacy**

Accessing Information

This skill involves finding reliable health information and using health resources. "Reliable" means that the information comes from sources you can trust. Where can you find reliable information? Sources include parents, teachers, counselors, school nurses, and other trusted adults. You can also access printed and published information from a wide variety of sources available to the public. **Figure 2.7** shows some of these sources.

Analyzing and Using Health Information

Although you can obtain health information from a variety of sources, not all of it is accurate and reliable. Some information is misleading or even completely false. Sources that you should treat with caution include supermarket tabloids, advertisements, rumors, e-mail, and the Internet. Use critical-thinking skills to interpret media messages about health information.

FIGURE 2.7

Where to find Health Information

Which of these sources have you used recently? Explain the role of media and technology in influencing individual and community health.

Library
encyclopedias, nonfiction books, magazines, and health-related CD-ROMs

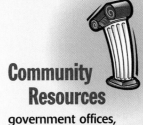

Print and Broadcast Media
newspaper articles, magazine articles, special interest magazines, health newsletters, television shows, and radio reports

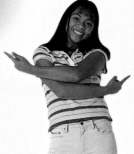

Internet
Web sites for government agencies, health organizations, and educational institutions

Community Resources
government offices, such as the county health department, and health organizations, such as the American Heart Association

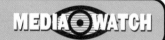

How can you tell the reliable information from the unreliable? You need to consider the source and make sure that it is trustworthy. Say, for example, that you read about a weight modification program on the Web. Check it out first. For accurate, up-to-date health information, you can count on agencies run by the government. Their Web addresses usually end in *.org* or *.gov.* Examples include the National Institutes of Health, the Food and Drug Administration, and the Centers for Disease Control and Prevention.

Practicing Healthful Behaviors

This skill applies to all sides of your health triangle—physical, mental/emotional, and social health. Practicing healthful behaviors involves taking care of yourself and avoiding risky situations. It means developing lifelong habits that increase your level of health and protect you from illness and injury.

Make Health a Habit

What health habits do you practice every day? Habits are things you do regularly and almost without even thinking about

HEALTH SKILLS ACTIVITY

PRACTICING HEALTHFUL BEHAVIORS

Personal Health Inventory

Take your personal health inventory by considering these lists of good habits for each area of your health triangle.

PHYSICAL HEALTH

● I eat well-balanced meals, including breakfast, and choose healthful snacks.
● I get regular physical activity and at least 8 hours of sleep each night.
● I avoid using tobacco, alcohol, and drugs.
● I stay within 5 pounds of my healthy weight.
● I practice good personal hygiene habits.
● I get regular physical checkups.

MENTAL/EMOTIONAL HEALTH

● I can name several things I do well.
● I generally keep a positive attitude.
● I express my emotions in healthy ways.

● I ask for help when I need it.
● I take responsibility for my actions.
● I take on new challenges to improve myself.

SOCIAL HEALTH

● I relate well to family, friends, and peers.
● I have several close friends.
● I can disagree with others without becoming rude.
● I treat others with respect.
● I use refusal skills to avoid risk behaviors.
● I get along with all kinds of people.

ON YOUR OWN

Give yourself 2 points for each habit that you always practice and 1 point for each one that you usually practice. If you scored 5 or less in any area, make a list of ways to improve your health habits.

them. Making health a priority and establishing good habits are key elements for good health.

Do you understand the health benefits of brushing and flossing your teeth every morning after breakfast and every night before bedtime? Do you understand the benefit of putting on your safety belt every time you enter a car? Brushing your teeth and wearing a safety belt are habits that promote your physical health. You can also practice habits that promote the other areas of your health triangle. For example, managing stress in healthy ways and planning your time wisely are habits that promote mental/emotional health. Greeting people in a friendly manner and spending time with friends are good social health habits to develop.

Build a Support System

Having a solid support system is essential for good health. A **support system** is *a network of people available to help when needed.* If you have health questions or problems, the people in your support system can provide reliable information, advice, and encouragement. They care about you and your health. Your support system might include the following people.

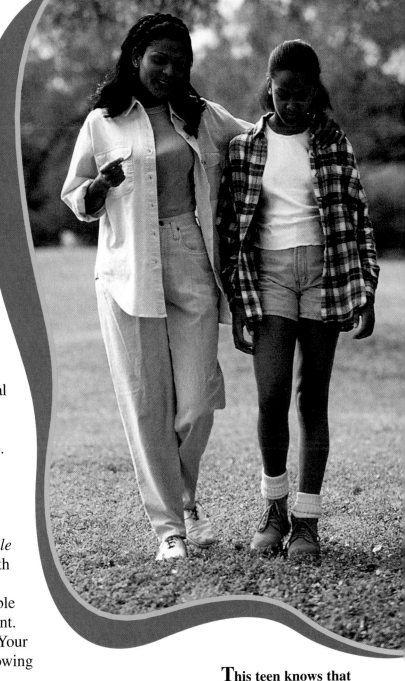

This teen knows that she can always turn to her aunt when she needs advice and support. *Analyze other positive relationships that influence individual health, such as peers and role models.*

- **Parents and other relatives,** such as grandparents and older brothers or sisters, are a built-in support system. Your family members can provide guidance and encouragement.
- **Teachers, coaches, and school counselors** whom you respect and trust can offer support and advice. School nurses can also help. These people are trained to understand situations faced by teens.
- **Health care providers,** such as doctors and nurses, are trained to deal with health-related issues and concerns. They can give you professional advice.
- **Religious leaders,** such as ministers, priests, mullahs, and rabbis, often are trained in counseling. They can listen to your questions and problems and offer answers and guidance.

Analyzing Influences

This skill is based on an awareness of all the factors that affect your health. Understanding these internal or external factors enables you to choose behaviors that will contribute to improved health.

Internal Influences

Internal influences on your health come from within you. You have a great deal of control over these factors, which include:

- **Your knowledge.** How much do you know about health? The more knowledge you have, the better able you will be to make wise decisions and evaluate health information.
- **Your likes and dislikes.** What foods do you like and dislike? What types of activities do you enjoy in your free time? If you like fruits and vegetables and if you stay physically active, for example, you are well on your way to a healthy lifestyle.
- **Your values.** What beliefs and ideals are important to you? Placing value on good health can influence your decisions, such as avoiding drugs and practicing abstinence.
- **Your desires.** What are your plans and goals? If you hope to enjoy good health and to lead an active life, you will make decisions that lead you in that direction.
- **Your curiosity.** It's natural to be curious about things you haven't tried before. Be sure to focus your curiosity on healthful concerns, such as new sporting activities or foods that are unfamiliar to you, and to steer clear of harmful substances.
- **Your fears.** What health-related fears do you have? Concerns about the health of a relative who smokes cigarettes, for example, can influence your decision never to smoke.

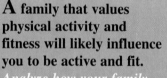

A family that values physical activity and fitness will likely influence you to be active and fit. *Analyze how your family has a positive influence on your health.*

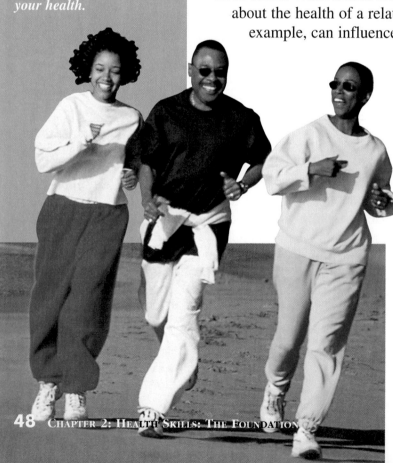

External Influences

External influences on your health come from outside sources. Being aware of these influences can help you make the right choices for you. External influences include:

- **Your family.** Your family influences what you do and how you behave. If family members help out in the community, for example, you will probably want to help others too. However, your health behaviors and knowledge may differ from those of your parents.

- **Your friends and peers.** Your friends and classmates can have either a positive influence or a negative influence on your health. For example, a friend who encourages you to go bike riding instead of watching television has a positive influence.
- **Your environment.** Do you live in a house or an apartment? In a small town or a big city? In a warm or cold climate? Your **environment** is *the sum total of your surroundings.* It includes both physical and social factors. It includes your home and the school you attend. Your environment also includes such factors as the air quality, available recreational facilities, crime rate, and available health care.
- **Your culture.** What are your family's cultural background and traditions? Your culture can influence the way you live, the foods you eat, your values, and your goals.
- **Federal, state, and local laws.** What are the health-related federal, state, and local laws? For example, federal laws make buying cigarettes and drinking alcohol illegal for teens. Respecting these laws influences your decision not to use these substances.
- **The media and technology.** What TV shows do you watch? Which magazines and newspapers do you read? What Web sites do you visit? Media and technology can have a major influence on individual and community health. Just remember, though, to evaluate the source before making any decisions.
- **Your role models.** Who do you admire? Perhaps you look up to a favorite teacher or coach. Your role models show you how people with good character behave in situations that you might encounter.

Reading Check

Analyze the internal and external influences listed here and write an *If . . ., then. . .* statement for each. For example: *If you know a lot about health, then you will be better able to make decisions.*

Lesson 4 Review

Using complete sentences, answer the following questions on a sheet of paper.

Reviewing Terms and Facts

1. **List** Give four sources where you might find printed and published health information.
2. **Explain** What is a *support system?* How can a support system contribute to your health?
3. **Identify** What are six types of internal influences on your health?
4. **Vocabulary** Define the term *environment.*

Thinking Critically

5. **Describe** How are your personal health behaviors and knowledge different from those of your parents and grandparents? How might your behaviors and knowledge differ from a teen who lives in another part of the world?
6. **Relate** How does your physical environment influence your health?

Applying Health Skills

7. **Accessing Information** Prepare a survey of the available sources of health information in your community. Report your findings in the form of a pamphlet.

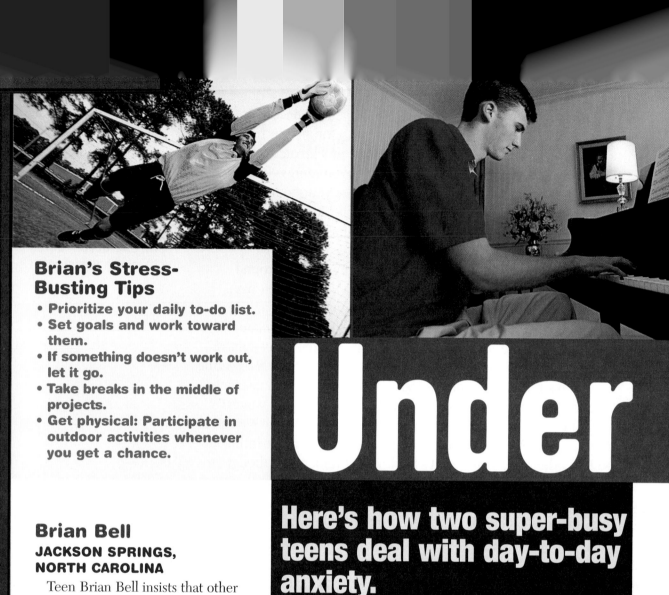

Brian's Stress-Busting Tips

- **Prioritize your daily to-do list.**
- **Set goals and work toward them.**
- **If something doesn't work out, let it go.**
- **Take breaks in the middle of projects.**
- **Get physical: Participate in outdoor activities whenever you get a chance.**

Under

Here's how two super-busy teens deal with day-to-day anxiety.

Brian Bell
JACKSON SPRINGS, NORTH CAROLINA

Teen Brian Bell insists that other people have schedules that are just as hectic as his is. However, one look at his jam-packed plans makes that pretty hard to believe. Over the past three years, Brian has participated in 10 projects to help the elderly in his community and to raise funds for starving kids in third-world countries. "Knowing that what I'm doing will actually make a difference to someone is what keeps me motivated," he says.

Brian's motivation knows no limits. He played varsity soccer and also took part in his church's basketball league. All the activity proves to be a healthy distraction for him. "Getting out in the fresh air takes my mind off whatever I'm worried about," he says.

Physical activity isn't the only remedy for a stressed-out student: Playing the piano also helps. Brian says, "Playing it in a room where the lights are dim really relaxes me."

Brian designs Web sites and spends three or four nights a week working part-time at a computer store. On his evenings off, after he's finished his homework, Brian usually tinkers with his own Web site. "I certainly don't get to watch much television," he says, laughing.

These days, Brian does his best to hit the sack early. "There was a time when I was staying up until 3:00 A.M. every night, and I was so tired and worn out," he says. "My mom made a list of things for me to get done by a certain time. She showed me how to work toward a goal, which really helped. These days, I'm trying to focus on the long-term and not sweat the little stuff."

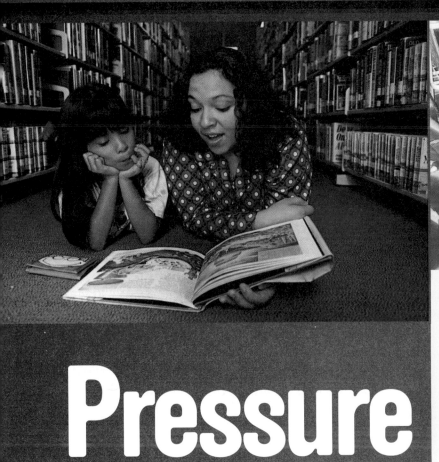

Pressure

Adriana Cantu

MISSION, TEXAS

Ask Adriana Cantu to name her top priority in life and she'll answer, "I have to get an academic scholarship if I want to go to college." Adriana is faced with having to finance her own education. "My dad just retired, and that money isn't going to stretch for too long," she says. She adds that her parents' love and support is worth more to her than any amount of money.

"I get really frustrated when my grades start to sink," she says. "I just want to quit, but my mom sits with me while I do my homework."

To escape the tension, Adriana performs with a local theater company. "It takes you away from real life because you have to concentrate hard in order to become another person," says Adriana.

What happens when Adriana heads home after rehearsal? "I do my homework, then go to sleep by 10:30," she says. Adriana knows that lack of sleep can pose a problem, especially during football season. She plays flute in the school marching band, which means she gets up at 5:00 A.M. to make 6:45 practice.

Fortunately, Adriana has learned ways to maintain her energy. "Sometimes I read for a while, then take a nap," says Adriana, who enjoys books so much that she reads to children at her town's public library. She adds, "Other days I'll go for a run in the park, listen to Celtic music on my Walkman, or go shopping at the mall with friends." Adriana keeps it all together with one simple quote: "Believe and you can succeed." ◢

TIME TO THINK...

About Managing Stress

How do you relieve stress in your life? Choose one or two of your own stress-busting tips and create an antianxiety ad campaign around them. Think of a catchy slogan that can help teens remember to stay calm when things get hectic. Create a visual aid, such as a poster, that features your slogan, and present your ad campaign to the class.

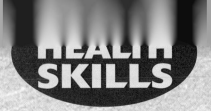
SAY NO TO PEER PRESSURE

Model

Laurel knows that she must honor her own sense of right and wrong instead of just going along with her peers. She realizes that refusing to do things that don't feel right can protect her health. Read how Laurel used refusal skills to stand up for her own beliefs.

Sara and Bethany think it's fun to tease other students at school. They want Laurel to distract James so they can play a practical joke on him. Laurel knows that James would be upset by the joke.

SARA: Here's the plan. Laurel, you get James's attention and we'll take his math homework out of his backpack.

LAUREL: No, Sara. James would be upset when he gets to class and can't find his assignment. *(Say no in a firm voice; tell why not.)*

BETHANY: That's the point. Come on, it'll be funny, and James will get over it.

LAUREL: I'd rather do something else that won't get us in trouble. Why don't we go watch the guys try out for the basketball team? *(Offer another idea.)*

BETHANY: No, that's not the same.

LAUREL: I agree, it's not the same. It's better! Are you guys coming with me?

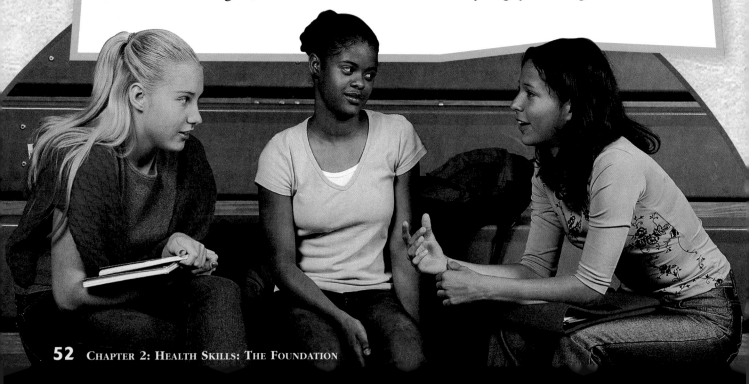

Practice

Divide into groups of three or four students and read the situation below. Write statements based on the S.T.O.P. strategies that show how you would use the refusal skills.

Alejandra is with friends at the mall. One of the girls dares her to take some makeup without paying for it. Show how Alejandra can refuse by using the S.T.O.P. criteria.

Apply/Assess

Read the following situations. Choose the situation that seems most realistic for you. Work with a partner to write a script that shows how you would refuse. Use as many of the refusal skills as you can. Act out your script for other students in your class.

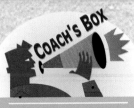

COACH'S BOX

Refusal Skills

You can use just one skill or combine several. You could:

S Say no in a firm voice.

T Tell why not.

O Offer another idea.

P Promptly leave.

Self-√Check

- Did my refusal reflect how I usually talk and interact with others?
- Did my refusal show a firm stand?
- Was my refusal realistic for the situation I chose?

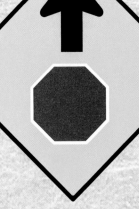

No Adults in Sight.

You have permission from your parents to attend a party at your friend's house on Saturday. At school, you learn that your friend's parents will be away for the weekend and no adults will be present.

It's a Bargain.

Someone you know offers to sell you a CD at a bargain price. You suspect that the bargain CD has been stolen.

STOP

STOP AHEAD

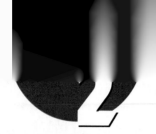

After You Read

Use your completed Foldable to review the information on the decision-making steps.

FOLDABLES™
Study Organizer

Reviewing Vocabulary and Concepts

On a sheet of paper, write the numbers 1–11. After each number, write the term from the list that best completes each statement.

> long-term goal
> active listening
> eye contact
> value
> feedback
> decision making
> "I" messages
> interpersonal communication
> mixed message
> goal setting
> refusal skills

Lesson 1

1. The first step in _____ is to state the situation.

2. To evaluate means to determine the _____ of something.

3. The process of working toward something you want to accomplish is _____.

4. Achieving a _____ might take several weeks, months, or even years.

Lesson 2

5. Using _____ instead of "you" messages shows respect for other people.

6. Nodding and smiling are examples of _____, which shows a speaker that you are listening.

7. If a friend wants you to do something that you don't want to do, use _____ to say no.

8. _____ involves hearing, thinking about, and responding to a speaker's message.

9. If you say one thing with your words but something else with your body language, you are sending a(n) _____.

10. _____, or direct visual contact, shows a listener that you mean what you say.

11. The exchange of thoughts, feelings, and beliefs is called _____.

On a sheet of paper, write the numbers 12–22. Write *True* or *False* for each statement below. If the statement is false, change the underlined word or phrase to make it true.

Lesson 3

12. The hormone that gives the body extra energy is <u>adrenaline</u>.

13. <u>Speaking skills</u> are ways to deal with and overcome problems.

14. Another word for exhaustion is <u>feedback</u>.

15. The process by which the body prepares to deal with a stressor is <u>fight-or-flight</u>.

16. The body's response to change is <u>stress</u>.

17. A cause of stress is a <u>mixed message</u>.

18. When you practice <u>time management</u>, you use your time wisely.

Lesson 4

19. <u>Reliable</u> information comes from sources you can trust.

20. Parents, teachers, and health care providers are part of your <u>support system</u> and can offer help when needed.

21. Your knowledge is an example of an <u>external</u> influence on your health.

22. Your <u>environment</u> includes your school.

Thinking Critically

Using complete sentences, answer the following questions on a sheet of paper.

23. **Apply** Identify a health decision that a teen might have to make. Relate the practices and steps of the decision-making process to that situation to make a healthy choice.

24. **Explain** How do the goal-setting steps help you to accomplish your goals?
25. **Hypothesize** When might a teen need to use refusal skills with someone other than a peer?
26. **Analyze** Name three events that act as stressors for you. Why do you find them stressful? How can you manage your response to them?
27. **Describe** Choose one of the health skills discussed in this chapter. Write a short paragraph describing how developing that skill can help a person gain a high level of physical, mental/emotional, or social health.

Career Corner

Physician's Assistant Do you think you'd like to be a doctor, but you're not sure you want to spend the required years in medical school? Consider a career as a physician's assistant. These professionals work under a doctor's supervision examining and treating patients. You'll need to complete a four-year physician's assistant program. You'll also need experience in the field to be licensed. Any health care experience will help you prepare for this career. Learn more about this and other health careers by clicking on Career Corner at health.glencoe.com.

Standardized Test Practice

Reading & Writing

Read the paragraphs below and then answer the questions.

It's time to rethink the traditional five-day school week, which we have been familiar with for years. By adding extra hours to four school days, the school could be closed on the fifth day. This would give teachers and students the time they need for other activities and would save energy.

Having one day off a week would leave teachers an entire day for rest or to prepare lessons. Students would also have an extra day for rest, to practice extracurricular activities, and to work on research projects. Less energy would be used for heating and lighting the building. School buses traveling four days instead of five would cut down on gas consumption. This would save money and reduce pollution.

1. Which phrase in the first paragraph helps you understand the meaning of the word *traditional*?
   - **A** adding extra hours to four school days
   - **B** school could be closed on the fifth day
   - **C** it's time to rethink
   - **D** which we have been familiar with for years

2. The second paragraph is important to the editorial because it
   - **A** supports the arguments made in the first paragraph.
   - **B** compares and contrasts the two sides of the argument.
   - **C** explains why the idea won't work.
   - **D** makes a prediction about the future.

3. Write a paragraph making your own argument about a four-day school week or another issue.

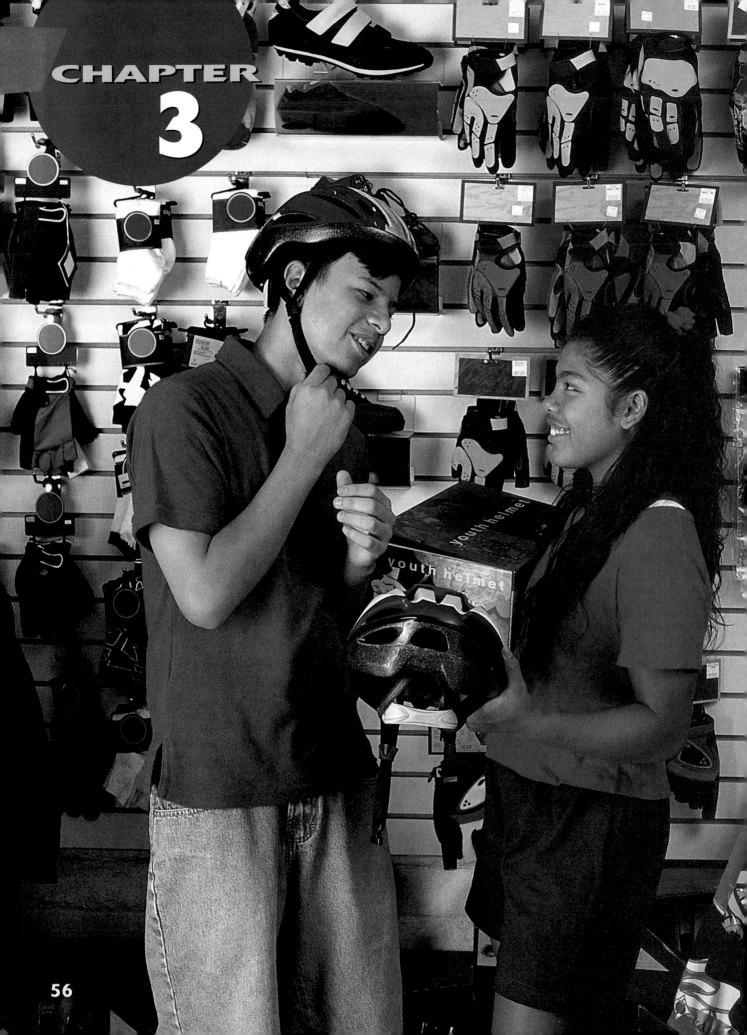

Being a Health Consumer

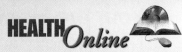

HEALTH *Online*

Are you a wise consumer? Find out by taking the Chapter 3 Health Inventory at health.glencoe.com.

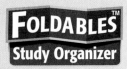

FOLDABLES™ Study Organizer

Before You Read

Make this Foldable to record what you learn in Lesson 1 about being a wise health consumer. Begin with two sheets of notebook paper.

Step 1

Fold one sheet in half from top to bottom. Cut about 1″ along the fold at both ends, stopping at the margin lines. ✂

Step 2

Fold the second sheet in half from top to bottom. Cut or shave off the fold *between* the margin lines. ✂

Step 3

Insert the first sheet through the second sheet and align folds.

Step 4

Fold the bound pages in half to make a booklet, and label the cover as shown. Then label each page as instructed by your teacher.

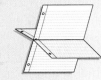

Chapter 3,
Lesson 1:
Healthy Consumer
Habits

As You Read

Define terms and take notes on being a health consumer on the appropriate page of your Foldable.

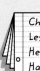

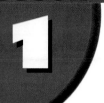
Healthy Consumer Habits

Quick Write

Identify three health products you use. Explain what or who influenced you in choosing these products.

Learn About...

- being an informed health consumer.
- effective health advocacy.
- new buying options for health consumers.

Vocabulary

- consumer
- media
- advertising
- comparison shopping
- warranty
- health advocacy
- online shopping

You, the Health Consumer

Teen consumers in the United States spend millions of dollars every year. A **consumer** is *anyone who purchases products or services.* Many of the products and services that teens purchase can affect their health. Toothpaste, sunscreen, eyeglasses, sporting goods, food, and sports drinks are examples of health-related products. You purchase health-related services when you get your teeth cleaned or have a health screening.

Becoming an Informed Consumer

Informed consumers base their choices on reliable information. When shopping for health products they compare quality, effectiveness, and safety as well as cost. Informed consumers also know how to resolve problems with products or services that they buy.

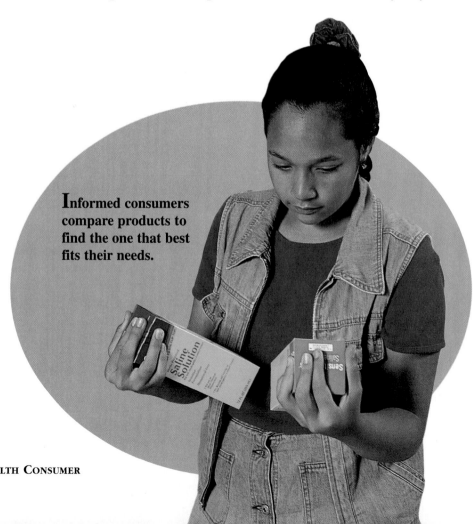

Informed consumers compare products to find the one that best fits their needs.

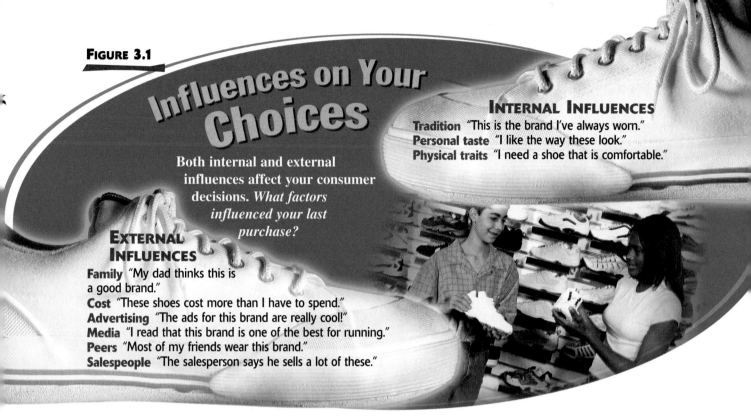

FIGURE 3.1

Influences on Your Choices

Both internal and external influences affect your consumer decisions. *What factors influenced your last purchase?*

INTERNAL INFLUENCES

Tradition "This is the brand I've always worn."
Personal taste "I like the way these look."
Physical traits "I need a shoe that is comfortable."

EXTERNAL INFLUENCES

Family "My dad thinks this is a good brand."
Cost "These shoes cost more than I have to spend."
Advertising "The ads for this brand are really cool!"
Media "I read that this brand is one of the best for running."
Peers "Most of my friends wear this brand."
Salespeople "The salesperson says he sells a lot of these."

What Influences Your Buying Decisions?

Many factors influence your buying decisions. Some are internal—they originate with you. Your personal taste is an example of an internal factor that influences your buying. External factors (those from outside sources) can also influence you. You may be influenced by what you see on TV, in newspapers and magazines, or on the Internet or billboards. Together, these *various methods for communicating information* are known as the **media**. Identifying the factors that influence you can help you understand why you buy a particular product or service. **Figure 3.1** illustrates the influences on one teen's purchasing decision.

Understanding Advertising Appeals

Many companies use advertising to promote health products and services. **Advertising** involves *sending out messages designed to interest consumers in buying a product or service.* Media advertising includes magazine and other print ads, TV and radio broadcast commercials, infomercials, and Internet advertising. Be aware that advertisers work closely with TV programmers and movie marketers to influence your buying decisions.

Ads let you know what products or services are available. Many ads provide good basic information. However, remember that the first goal of advertising is to get your attention and the second is to get you to buy. To reach these goals, advertisers use a variety of techniques to appeal to potential buyers. **Figure 3.2** on the next page explains some advertising techniques.

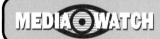

MEDIA WATCH

UNBIASED INFORMATION

Many people turn to Consumers Union for reliable information when planning a purchase. Consumers Union tests products and researches services. It reports its findings in various ways, such as in *Consumer Reports* magazine and Consumer Reports Online.

FIGURE 3.2

DECODING HIDDEN MESSAGES IN ADVERTISING

Advertisements often include a hidden message designed to appeal to consumers' emotions. *How might these media messages influence a consumer's decision to purchase a health product?*

Technique	Example	Hidden Message
Bandwagon	Group of people using product or service.	Everyone is using it--don't be left behind.
Rich and famous	Expensive car driven by attractive person.	It will make you feel rich and famous.
Free rewards	Redeemable coupons for merchandise.	It offers great value because you get something for free.
Great outdoors	Scenes of nature.	It is associated with nature so it must be healthy.
Good times	People smiling and laughing.	It will add more fun to your life.
Testimonial	Celebrity	It will make you be like this person.

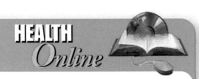

HEALTH Online

Topic: Consumer education

For a link to more information on consumer education, go to health.glencoe.com.

Activity: Using the information provided at this link, create a fact sheet on consumer awareness.

Identifying Hidden Advertising

Advertising is sometimes disguised as informative articles. A prominently displayed product logo worn by a sports figure during a media interview also sends consumers an advertising message. Increasingly, advertisers are getting their products into movies and TV programs in a process called product placement. Aware consumers ask: What is the message here? Who is creating it? What might advertisers want consumers to believe or do?

Comparing Choices

Comparison shopping is *a method of judging the benefits of different products or services by comparing several factors, such as quality, features, and cost.* The factors that are most important to you in a particular product will determine your choice.

When buying health-related products and services, safety should always be a priority. If you were buying sunglasses, for example, you might begin by comparing safety features. Find out if the lenses are unbreakable and protect from UV rays. Then you might compare other features, such as weight, durability, appearance, and cost. For some types of products you can compare warranties. A **warranty** is *a written promise to handle repairs if the product fails to work properly.*

Health Advocacy

Health advocacy involves *taking action to influence others to address a health-related concern or to support a health-related belief.* A major goal of health advocacy is to help friends, family, and members of the community to be healthy. Health advocates also help others become informed and aware consumers.

When you practice the skill of advocacy, you make a difference by taking action. Follow these guidelines to be an effective health advocate:

- **Identify your values.** Why are you proposing this action?
- **Understand the purpose of your message.** What result do you want to achieve?
- **Make your message appropriate to your audience.** What is important to the audience? What will appeal to them? What will make a difference to them?
- **Give convincing reasons why your message will benefit health.** How will your advice improve or protect the health of others?
- **Provide reliable supporting data to back up your proposal.** What facts and figures support your position?

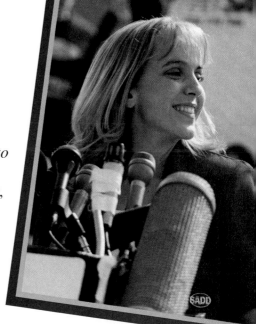

Speaking for Students Against Destructive Decisions, this teen advocates for the health of others. *How can you help others make healthy decisions?*

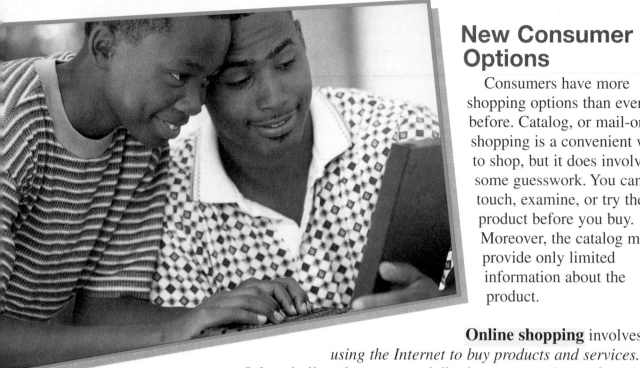

New Consumer Options

Consumers have more shopping options than ever before. Catalog, or mail-order, shopping is a convenient way to shop, but it does involve some guesswork. You cannot touch, examine, or try the product before you buy. Moreover, the catalog may provide only limited information about the product.

Online shopping involves *using the Internet to buy products and services.* It has similar advantages and disadvantages to those of catalog shopping. Both mail-order and online shoppers often pay a lower price than they would pay in a store. However, that gain may be lost if shipping charges are added to the price. Additional shipping charges may be incurred if a product needs to be returned.

Teens who shop online usually need their parents' permission since many online stores allow only credit card purchases.

Lesson 1 Review

Using complete sentences, answer the following questions on a sheet of paper.

Reviewing Terms and Facts

1. **Vocabulary** Define the word *consumer.*
2. **List** Give two examples of internal influences on consumer choices and two examples of external influences.
3. **Recall** What is the purpose of comparison shopping?
4. **Explain** What is health advocacy?

Thinking Critically

5. **Apply** What criteria would you develop to select or reject a health product or service such as sunscreen or a dental exam?

6. **Analyze** Think about the last health care product you bought. Identify a variety of influences on that purchase. Analyze how each affected your decision.

Applying Health Skills

7. **Advocacy** Encourage others to become involved in health-promotion efforts at many different levels. Think of a health-related issue. Create a flyer that lists ways to advocate for that issue. For example, if you select tobacco-use prevention, your flyer might say that choosing not to smoke, supporting the school as a tobacco-free environment, and supporting local efforts to reduce smoking in the community are some ways to advocate for that issue.

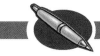
Choosing Health Services

The Role of Health Care

David is having a physical examination as required by his school. After checking David's immunization record, Dr. Lee gives him a booster shot for tetanus. When David tells her that he is having pain in his right knee, Dr. Lee carefully examines the knee. Then she writes out an order for tests on David's knee at the hospital X-ray department.

Dr. Lee, the hospital, and the X-ray technician are all part of the health care system. A **health care system** includes *all the medical care available to a nation's people, the way they receive the care, and the way the care is paid for.* The original role of the health care system in the United States was to treat people who were sick or injured. Today the role has expanded to include **preventive care**, which involves *keeping disease or injury from happening or getting worse.*

Quick Write

Make a list of the people who provide you and your family with health care. Beside each name, write what that person does.

LEARN ABOUT...

- different kinds of health care providers.
- why teens need regular health screenings.
- how people pay for health care.
- trends in health care.

VOCABULARY

- health care system
- preventive care
- primary care physician
- specialist
- health insurance
- health maintenance organization (HMO)
- preferred provider organization (PPO)
- point of service plan (POS)

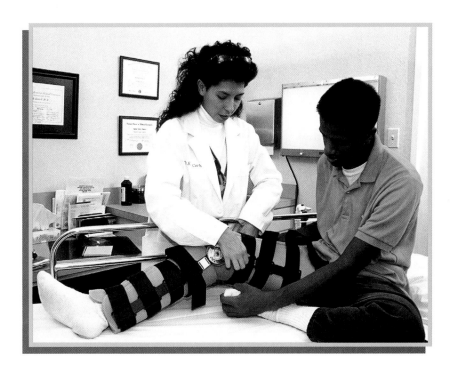

A health care professional's responsibilites include treating many different types of injuries.

The Health Care System

To be an informed consumer of health care services, you need to understand how the health care system works. Physicians, nurses, dentists, dental hygienists, optometrists, pharmacists, and laboratory technicians are just a few of the professionals who work in the health care system. Health care providers work in a variety of settings.

Who Provides Health Care?

Health care can be divided into general care and specialized care. **Primary care physicians** are *the medical doctors who provide physical checkups and general care.* School nurses, nurse practitioners, and physician's assistants are also part of primary care.

Patients who need a specific type of care are referred to specialists. **Specialists** are *doctors trained to handle particular kinds of patients or medical conditions.* Pediatricians (peed·ee·uh·TRISH·uhnz), for example, deal with infants and children, and dermatologists deal with problems and diseases of the skin. Have you had experience with a health specialist?

You and Your Health Care

It is recommended that teens get annual health screenings for preventive care. Sometimes called wellness exams, these screenings are designed to promote wellness and detect any health problems early. The recommended ages for these physicals are between 11 and 14 years, between 15 and 17 years, and between 18 and 21 years.

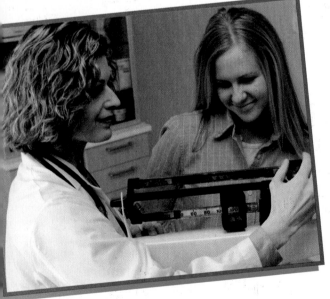

Nurse practitioners perform many routine medical examinations. *Explain the role of wellness exams in disease prevention.*

A wellness exam for teens might include:

- testing hearing and vision.
- checking for sports injuries, especially in the knee.
- checking for scoliosis, which is a disorder of the spine.
- screening for high blood pressure.
- screening for eating disorders and obesity.

In addition to the annual wellness exam, teens need to get other regular health screenings and to cooperate with the health care provider's recommendations for treatment. Types of health care teens might receive are listed in **Figure 3.3**.

FIGURE 3.3

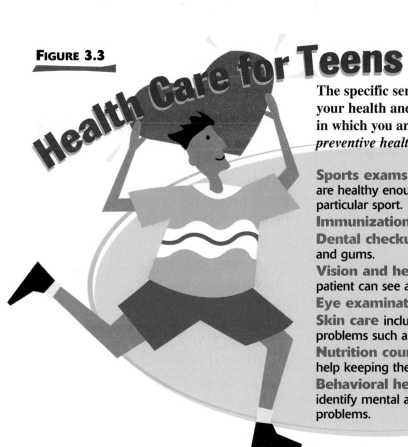

Health Care for Teens

The specific services that you receive will depend on your health and, possibly, on the health care plan in which you are enrolled. *Explain the role of these preventive health measures in disease prevention.*

Sports exams ensure that teens are healthy enough to participate in a particular sport.

Immunizations protect against specific diseases.

Dental checkups determine the health of the teeth and gums.

Vision and hearing testing determine how well the patient can see and hear.

Eye examinations check for eye diseases and disorders.

Skin care includes screening and treatment for problems such as acne and skin cancer.

Nutrition counseling assists those who need help keeping their weight within a healthy range.

Behavioral health assessment helps identify mental and emotional problems.

Where Do You Go for Health Care?

Health care facilities provide inpatient care and outpatient care. Inpatient care is for patients who have serious illnesses or injuries and who need to stay at the facility. A person recovering from major surgery, or one who needs constant monitoring, would receive inpatient care. Outpatient care is for less serious conditions or procedures. Examples are treating sprains, stitching up wounds, and extracting teeth. Patients get the care they need and then return home. Many routine tests are also provided on an outpatient basis.

Health services are available in most communities in a variety of forms. Facilities in your community may include the following:

- **Clinics.** Primary care physicians and specialists may provide outpatient care in a community clinic. Local clinics often receive government funding.
- **Private practice.** Primary care physicians and specialists who work in private practice work for themselves.
- **Group practice.** Often two or more physicians join together to offer health care in a group practice. Doctors in group practice share office space, equipment, and support staff.
- **Hospitals.** Most hospitals offer both inpatient and outpatient care. Some doctors work only in a hospital. Others have offices elsewhere and use the hospital facilities when their patients need them.

Science

MAGNETIC RESONANCE IMAGING
Modern technology plays an important role in medicine. Thanks to magnetic resonance imaging (MRI), doctors can now examine images of a patient's soft tissue. The images make it possible for doctors to detect tumors and other abnormalities. Finding such abnormalities early often makes it possible to treat them before they develop into serious problems.

How People Pay for Health Care

Many people have some form of **health insurance**, which is *a plan in which private companies or government programs pay for part of a person's medical costs.*

With private insurance, a person pays a monthly fee to the insurance company. In return, the company pays part or most of that person's medical costs. Many people have private insurance through their employers. Common types of private insurance plans include:

- **Health Maintenance Organizations (HMOs).** An **HMO** is *an organization that provides health care for a fixed price.* People who belong to an HMO pay a monthly fee regardless of how much health care they need. Usually they must see only doctors who have signed a contract with the HMO.
- **Preferred Provider Organizations (PPOs).** A **PPO** is *a type of insurance in which medical providers agree to charge less for members of the plan.* Members who choose doctors outside the plan pay more.
- **Point of Service (POS) plans.** A **POS** is *a health plan that allows members to choose providers inside or outside the plan.* Choosing an outside provider often results in greater out-of-pocket costs to members.

Reading Check

Brainstorm. Think about what *health care* means to you. List as many details as you can.

HEALTH SKILLS ACTIVITY

ACCESSING INFORMATION

Health Care in the Community

Most communities have a variety of health care services. Examples include:

- home nursing care for patients who need medical help in their own home.
- relief support for people who are caring for an ill or injured family member.
- Alateen and Al-Anon groups for family members who live with alcoholics.
- community health screenings.
- flu shots for the elderly and other at-risk individuals.
- recreational sports and activity programs, providing supervised physical activity sessions.

WITH A GROUP

Make a list of health care resources offered at your school and in your community. You can obtain the information from parents and from local media. Then create a brochure that includes the name and number of each resource you found.

Trends in Health Care

The health care community is constantly looking for ways to improve the quality of health care or to reduce its cost. Here are some trends that reflect those goals.

- **Birthing centers** are homelike settings that involve the entire family in the delivery of the baby. Birthing centers are usually less expensive than hospitals.
- **Drug treatment centers** specialize in treating people with drug and alcohol problems.
- **Continuing care and assisted living facilities** provide care for people who need help with daily tasks but who do not require skilled medical care. Many older people need this kind of care.
- **Hospices** provide care for people who are terminally ill. Hospice workers are experts at managing pain and providing emotional support for the entire family.
- **Telemedicine** is the practice of medicine over distance through the use of telecommunications equipment. A specialist located hundreds of miles away can be brought electronically into an examination room via a live interactive system.

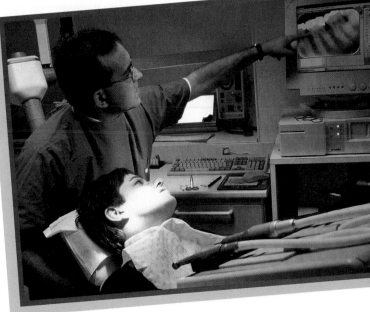

Computerized technology makes it possible for this teen to see images of the inside of his mouth as the dentist explains what he finds. *Explain the role of technology in influencing individual and community health.*

Lesson 2 Review

Using complete sentences, answer the following questions on a sheet of paper.

Reviewing Terms and Facts

1. **Vocabulary** Define the term *preventive care* and use it in an original sentence.
2. **Compare** What is the difference between a *primary care physician* and a *specialist*?
3. **Contrast** What are the differences in the ways HMOs, PPOs, and POS plans pay for health care?

Thinking Critically

4. **Hypothesize** Why do you think there is more emphasis on preventive care now than there was in the past?

5. **Summarize** Name four things a typical teen could expect his or her doctor to check for during a preventive medical checkup.

Applying Health Skills

6. **Advocacy** You've learned about the importance of preventive health measures. Prepare an announcement in which you explain why teens need to get regular health screenings. Be sure to mention wellness exams, dental checkups, immunizations, and treatment. If possible, arrange for your announcement to be delivered at school.

Managing Consumer Problems

Let the Buyer Beware

You may have heard the saying "Let the buyer beware." It is used to warn people to watch out for products and services that don't do what sellers claim they will do. Most products *do* work, and most sellers *are* honest. Some individuals and businesses, however, sell faulty or useless products and services.

Health Fraud

Fraud is *deliberate deceit or trickery.* One of the worst types of fraud is **health fraud**, involving *the sale of worthless products or services claimed to prevent diseases or cure other health problems.* **Figure 3.4** illustrates some examples of health fraud.

To protect yourself from health fraud, watch for these signs:

- Cure-all products. There is no such thing as a product that cures everything.
- Instant results. The human body does not change appearance or shape overnight.
- Suggestions that the usual treatment offered by doctors is wrong and that this product or procedure is better.
- Testimonials from "satisfied customers" as proof of the effectiveness of the product or procedure.
- Phony medical claims such as "detoxify your body" and "boost nerve energy," which are impossible to measure.
- Claims that the health care system is trying to keep this product or service off the market.

Problems with Products

It is always a good idea to find out the seller's return policy before you buy. Follow these steps if you find you have bought a defective item.

1. Reread the instructions to make sure you followed them correctly and to ensure that the item is defective.

2. Decide whether you want a replacement or your money back.

3. Read the warranty that came with the product and follow the instructions in the warranty.

Figure 3.4

EXAMPLES OF FRAUD

Type of Product	Typical Advertisement	Facts
Weight Management Products Pills Fad diets Exercise equipment	LOSE WEIGHT FAST! Get the slim body you want without changing what you eat. Just a few minutes a day with our Body Shaper will change fat into firm tissue. Why wait? Order now.	A good weight-management plan includes a sensible eating plan and regular physical activity. Losing weight takes time. False weight-loss programs and fad diets can damage your health.
Beauty Products Acne creams Hair enhancers Teeth whiteners	ERASE PIMPLES AND BLACKHEADS FOREVER. Don't hide behind makeup. With this breakthrough formula made from all-natural ingredients, you can have permanently clear skin in a few days. Send for a Free Sample. Enclose $10.00 shipping and handling.	Many products can help your skin temporarily. No product, however, can make your skin blemish-free permanently. Products that have not been approved by the FDA may actually harm your skin.
Miracle Cures Arthritis Cancer Depression	CONFUSED? DEPRESSED? IN PAIN? I can help! Benefit from the ancient healing techniques learned during 12 years of travel and study in remote areas of the Andes Mountains. Call today for a phone therapy session. Credit card required. Dr. Westfall, Healer.	Worthless products and phony cures often give seriously ill patients false hope. Using useless therapies may keep people from seeking the medical treatment they need.

"Let the Buyer Beware"

4. If you are to return the item to the store, take the item and your sales receipt back to the store. Ask a clerk to direct you to the returns department.
5. If you are to send the item to the manufacturer, repack the item in its original packaging and write a letter explaining the problem. Keep a copy of your letter.
6. If you are shipping the item to the manufacturer, get a shipping receipt to prove you sent it.

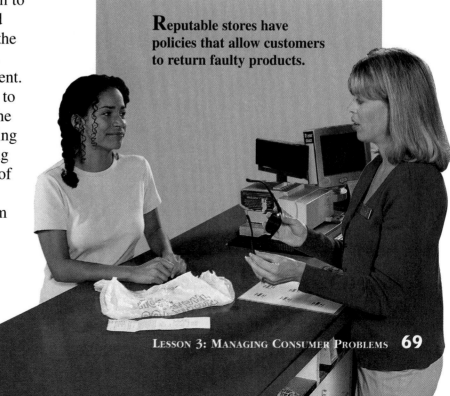

Reputable stores have policies that allow customers to return faulty products.

FACT VS. OPINION

Some ads contain statements of fact and statements of exaggerated opinion, also called hype. In this activity, you will use critical-thinking skills to analyze marketing and advertising techniques and their influences on the selection of health-related services and products by separating fact from hype.

WHAT YOU WILL NEED
- two print ads for different health-related services or products
- paper and pencil

WHAT YOU WILL DO
1. Divide a sheet of paper vertically into two columns. In column 1, list the words used to describe the product (*great, smooth, breakthrough,* and so forth).
2. Still in column 1, skip two lines, then list the words that tell what the product claims to do (*stop dandruff, whiten, give shine,* and so forth).
3. Decide if each of the words listed in column 1 is fact or opinion. Is it something that can be verified, or proven to be a fact? Is it something that cannot be verified and that is,

therefore, an opinion? In column 2, write *fact* or *opinion* beside each word listed in column 1.
4. Write a brief summary of your findings. Compare your finished sheet with those of your classmates.

IN CONCLUSION
1. Remember that the goal of advertising is to get you to buy. With your classmates, prepare a master list of some typical hype words to watch out for.
2. Write a newspaper article warning against advertising hype aimed at teens.

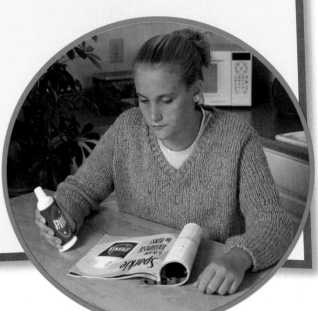

Consumer Groups

Problems with defective products are usually not difficult to solve. Most businesses want their customers to be satisfied. Satisfied customers keep coming back. Sometimes, though, to get satisfaction, a consumer needs to take additional action. Several consumer groups can help.

- **Consumer advocates** are people or groups who help consumers with problems. The Consumers Union and local consumer groups are examples of such groups.
- **Business groups**, such as the Better Business Bureau, can help with disputes.

- **Government offices**, such as consumer affairs offices, make sure that consumers' rights are upheld in disputes.
- **Small claims courts** are state courts in which people can present their own cases without an attorney. A judge hears both sides and decides who wins.

Problems with Health Services

Some people experience problems with health services. If a person feels that a doctor does not spend enough time answering questions, he or she may simply decide to change doctors. Some concerns about the quality of health care are more complicated, however. One patient may feel that a doctor took too long to identify an illness. Another may think that the treatment the doctor recommends is not the best choice.

When patients have doubts about their doctor's diagnosis or about the treatment plan their doctor suggests, they should seek a second opinion. A second doctor will examine the patient, look over the patient's test results, and give an opinion about the patient and about the proposed treatment. Many insurance companies pay for a second opinion before major surgery.

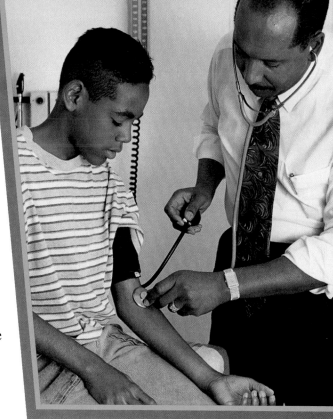

A patient who is unhappy about recommended treatment should request a second opinion.

Lesson 3 Review

Using complete sentences, answer the following questions on a sheet of paper.

Reviewing Terms and Facts

1. **Vocabulary** Define the term *fraud* and use it in an original sentence.
2. **Summarize** Briefly outline the steps to take when you buy a defective product.
3. **Describe** What happens in a small claims court?

Thinking Critically

4. **Apply** Imagine that you had a serious complaint about a local store that had sold you defective products. What organization could you take your complaint to?
5. **Interpret** Suppose a doctor misdiagnosed a patient's illness. How might the patient solve this problem? What critical issues might arise?

Applying Health Skills

6. **Communication Skills** Write a dialogue in which a teen uses effective communication skills to return a faulty health product to a store.

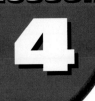
Public Health

Government Health Services

Certain aspects of health need to be managed as part of a larger effort. This larger effort, managed by federal, state, and local governments, is referred to as public health. **Public health** involves *the protection and promotion of health at the community level.* In this context, the community may be a small town, a large city, a state, or even the nation. Many organizations are involved in administering public health at these different levels.

Federal Health Agencies

The main health organization of the federal government is the Department of Health and Human Services (HHS). HHS is responsible for more than 300 programs that protect the health of all Americans. These programs include two federal health insurance programs—Medicare and Medicaid. **Figure 3.5** lists some of the HHS public health divisions.

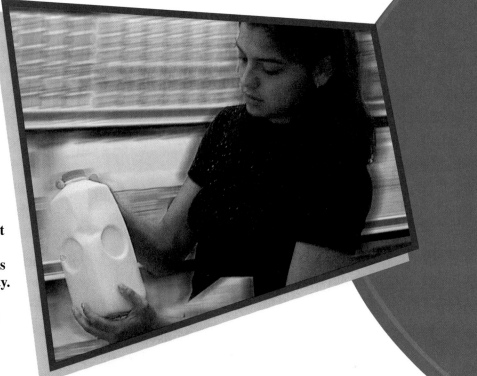

Making sure that milk is kept refrigerated in warehouses, during transport, and in stores is a public health responsibility. *What action can you take to ensure that the milk you buy is safe to drink?*

Other federal agencies work to protect and enforce consumer rights. These include:

- **Consumer Product Safety Commission (CPSC).** The CPSC works to reduce the risk of injury or death from unsafe products. It can ban products it finds dangerous and can order manufacturers to notify people who have bought an unsafe product.
- **Food Safety and Inspection Service (FSIS).** The FSIS oversees the safety of meat and poultry.
- **Federal Trade Commission (FTC).** The FTC protects consumers from unfair trade practices. It also regulates advertising in order to prevent advertisers from presenting misleading information.

Reading Check

Which agency listed here would provide service for a teen with drug addiction? A doctor looking for information about a patient's unusual illness?

FIGURE 3.5

Federal Public Health Services

THE DEPARTMENT OF HEALTH AND HUMAN SERVICES (HHS)

HEALTH RESOURCES AND SERVICES ADMINISTRATION (HRSA)
Provides access to essential health services for people who are uninsured, who have lower income, or who live in rural and urban neighborhoods where health care is scarce.

NATIONAL INSTITUTES OF HEALTH (NIH)
Supports about 35,000 research projects nationwide in cancer, diabetes, arthritis, heart disease, AIDS, and other diseases.

CENTERS FOR DISEASE CONTROL AND PREVENTION (CDC)
Monitors disease trends, investigates outbreaks of disease, promotes safe and healthful environments, and takes actions to prevent and control illness and injury.

SUBSTANCE ABUSE AND MENTAL HEALTH SERVICES ADMINISTRATION (SAMHSA)
Works to improve the quality and availability of substance abuse prevention, addiction treatment, and mental health services.

INDIAN HEALTH SERVICES (IHS)
Provides medical and dental services through hospitals and health centers to nearly 1.5 million American Indians and Alaska Natives.

FOOD AND DRUG ADMINISTRATION (FDA)
Makes sure that foods and cosmetics are safe and that product labels are truthful. Makes certain that medicines and medical devices are safe and effective.

Social Studies

HEALTH-RELATED LAWS, POLICIES, AND PRACTICES
Public health laws, policies, and practices have had a positive impact on many health-related issues. For example, laws on the proper disposal of solid waste help keep drinking water safe. Policies such as requiring restaurant workers to wash their hands after using the restroom help prevent the spread of communicable diseases; so do practices such as regular inspections of restaurant kitchens. *Analyze local law, policy, or practice on a health-related issue.*

State and Local Health Agencies

State and community health organizations also offer services independently. All states and most cities have health departments. The work of these departments varies from place to place, but all help to control and prevent disease. Some of the tasks performed by local health departments include the following:

- Provide basic health care services to people with low incomes.
- Monitor the safety of water and sewage systems.
- Make sure that garbage is removed and properly handled and disposed of.
- Set standards of cleanliness and sanitation for restaurants.
- Offer health education and promotion programs.

HEALTH SKILLS ACTIVITY

ADVOCACY

Public Health

Use your advocacy skills to influence others to support a public health-related law, ordinance, goal, or project. Here are some of the many ways that teens can practice public health advocacy:

- Set an example by following health and safety laws and ordinances.
- Never take an action that could endanger the health or safety of others.
- Volunteer to help charitable organizations that sponsor public-health events.
- Learn which groups in your community deal with public-health issues. Identify their current goals and support them.
- If you notice a condition or activity that threatens public health, notify the proper authorities.

WITH A GROUP

Brainstorm a list of public health issues in your community. From your list, choose one issue to work on. Make an advocacy plan to bring about change. Interpret any critical issues related to solving this public health problem.

Nongovernmental Health Organizations

Governmental public health organizations are funded by the taxes people pay. Nongovernmental health organizations rely mostly on contributions and volunteers to provide important public health services. Some of these organizations focus on one type of disease. Examples are the American Heart Association, the Asthma and Allergy Foundation of America, and the American Cancer Society. They pay for research for ways to prevent and cure the disease. They also help people who have the disease, and they provide programs that teach ways to prevent it.

The American Red Cross is one of the first organizations on the scene after a natural disaster. Its workers are trained to respond quickly to a large-scale emergency. The Red Cross collects blood from volunteers and distributes it to hospitals for people who need transfusions. It also offers courses on first aid, safety, and health.

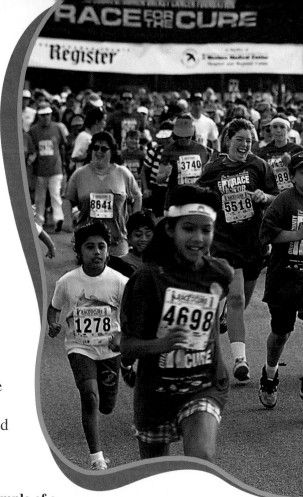

Race for the Cure is an example of a community-based event that raises money for cancer research. *What events like this take place in your community?*

Lesson 4 Review

Using complete sentences, answer the following questions on a sheet of paper.

Reviewing Terms and Facts

1. **Vocabulary** Define the term *public health* and use it in an original sentence.
2. **Recall** What is the name of the main health organization of the federal government?
3. **Identify** Which federal agency is authorized to ban the sale of unsafe products?

Thinking Critically

4. **Apply** Name the HHS division you would contact for information on safe ways to store and prepare food.

5. **Investigate** Which nongovernmental health organizations would you contact for information on the latest cancer research? On where to find a safe place to stay after a serious storm?

Applying Health Skills

6. **Accessing Information** Interview the manager of your school cafeteria or the manager of a local public swimming pool. Find out what state and local health laws the manager must obey. Share your information with your classmates.

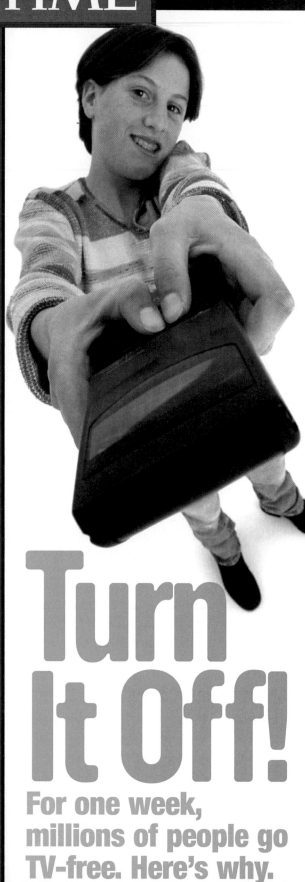

Turn It Off!

For one week, millions of people go TV-free. Here's why.

In April, millions of television sets around the world will go blank. Instead of fiddling with the remote or calling the cable company, those thwarted TV watchers will take drastic action. Entire families will go outside to ride bikes; groups of friends will play games. Will other television addicts turn off their sets and join in—or will they just watch?

TV-Turnoff Network, a nonprofit organization, has promoted the annual TV-Turnoff Week since 1995. In the beginning, only a few thousand people took part. Now there are participants in every state and in more than 12 countries.

TV and Violence

Each year, kids in the United States spend more time glued to the tube than doing anything else—except for sleeping! People have worried about the effects of TV ever since the 1940s, when television first became popular. Over the years, health-care groups like the American Academy of Pediatrics and the American Medical Association have voiced their concern. They point to studies that link excessive TV viewing to such problems as poor eating habits, a sedentary lifestyle, obesity, and violent behavior.

A study published in the journal *Science* claims that there is evidence of a connection between TV viewing and violence. Psychologist Jeffrey G. Johnson and his research team followed children in 707 families for 17 years. The researchers found that kids who watched more than one hour of television a day were more likely than other kids to show aggressive and violent behavior as they grew older.

Other TV Turnoffs

Others worry about the impact of commercials on kids. One study found that during four hours of Saturday-morning cartoons, television networks ran 202 ads for empty-calorie foods. The nonstop reminders to buy sugary sodas, cereals, and candy may be one reason that more than one in eight American kids is overweight. Long hours sitting in front of the tube is probably another reason. "Almost anything uses more

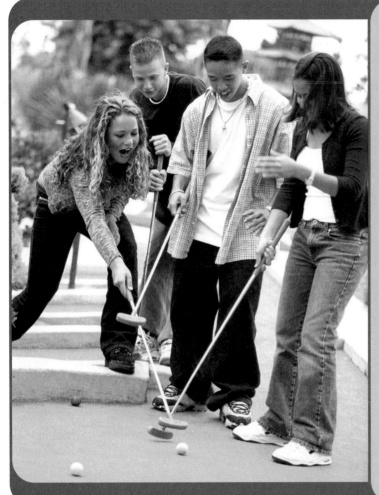

TV By The Numbers

1,023 Hours per year the average American child watches television

900 Hours per year spent in school

1,180 Minutes per week the average kid watches TV

38.5 Minutes per week parents say they spend in meaningful conversation with their kids

41 Percent of U.S. households with three or more TV sets

49 Percent of Americans who say they watch too much TV

6 million Number of videos rented daily in the United States

3 million Public library items checked out daily

200,000 Average number of violent acts Americans see on TV by age 18

91 Percent of kids polled who said they felt upset by TV violence

Source: TV-Turnoff Network

energy than watching TV," says Dr. William H. Dietz of the Centers for Disease Control and Prevention in Atlanta, Georgia.

Enjoying Life, Unplugged

TV-Turnoff Network wants to encourage life outside the box. "We're not anti-TV," says the group's director, Frank Vespe. The goal is to help kids tune in to real life so that "they won't have time for TV."

Is it really possible to live without your favorite TV shows? Sarah Foote, a middle-school student in Burke, Virginia, says she made it through TV-Turnoff Week last year—and actually enjoyed herself! Sarah says that after a few days without TV, "I thought, 'Why did I ever need TV?'" Her brother, Nathaniel, agrees: "There are about 8,000 other things you can do."

Still, some kids can't picture life without television. Christian Cardenas of New York City

doesn't plan on tuning out. "It entertains you on rainy days," he says.

Could you go without TV for a whole week? Says TV-Turnoff veteran Carly Cara of Niles, Illinois: "You're doing so many fun things that before you know it, it's over!"

TIME TO THINK...

About Turning Off the TV

Figure out the number of hours that you watch television during an average week. Then, using a map and the map's scale, start at your hometown and see how far you could travel in that amount of time if you were moving 50 miles per hour. Report to your class what cities you could visit.

FINDING RELIABLE SOURCES

The extension ".gov" identifies a site run by a government agency. Glenn considers most information from these sites to be valid.

Model

Glenn is working on a report for health class about different kinds of pain relievers. He has decided to search the Internet for up-to-date information. Glenn knows, however, that not all information on the Internet is reliable. As he looks at different Web pages, he pays attention to their addresses, or URLs. Most URLs contain an extension that identifies the nature of the site. Glenn knows that some types of sites are more likely to be reliable than others.

U.S. DEPARTMENT OF HEALTH AND HUMAN SERVICES
FOOD AND DRUG ADMINISTRATION
FDA

Hot Topics

Buying Medicines Online

Antibiotic Resistance

BSE ("mad cow disease")

LASIK Surgery

Liver Toxicity

Search | A-Z Index | Site Map | About FDA

FDA NEWS

New Test Detects HIV, Hep C Virus Sooner in Plasma Donors.
FDA has licensed the first nucleic acid test systems, expected to further ensure the safety of plasma-derived products by permitting... action of HIV and the hepatitis C virus in ...make products such as clotting donors, ...factors...

Citizens for Accurate Labeling

Who We Are

Our Programs

Links

Site map

The purpose of most sites that end in ".com" is to sell a product or service. Glenn is always cautious when viewing these sites because he knows that companies may make false or exaggerated claims about their products. He does not use information from these sites unless he can find another source to support it.

The ".org" extension is often used by nonprofit organizations. Some organizations, such as the American Cancer Society, are valid sources of health information. However, information from nonprofit organizations may be biased, or slanted toward a particular point of view. When Glenn views these pages, he looks for information about the organization and its purpose. He also checks to see whether a Web site is endorsed by public health and medical organizations. If it is, he considers it reliable.

Sayers Pharmaceuticals
"Healing the World through Science"

Our Products

Research

Investments

Job Opportunities

Buying Prescription Medicines Online: A Consumer Safety Guide

The Internet is rapidly changing the way we live, including how we work and shop. The growth of the Internet in recent years has enabled many consumers to purchase medicines online. There are online pharmacies that provide legitimate prescription services. Unfortunately, there are also questionable sites that make purchasing medicines online risky.

Practice

Read the following scenario and answer the questions at the end. Share your answers with the class.

While watching television, Dawn sees an infomercial about a new weight-loss program. The creator of the program is a doctor who has written a book about his "medical breakthrough." He explains the basis for his program in technical-sounding language, but Dawn cannot tell whether his information is accurate.

1. Is this infomercial a valid source of health information? Why or why not?
2. What steps could Dawn take to verify the claims in the infomercial?

Apply

In a small group, look through several magazines for health-related claims in articles and advertisements. For example, an ad might claim that a particular food supplement will help prevent colds. Choose one of these claims to research, interpret, and analyze. As a group, discuss the sources you could use to verify the claim. You might start by checking the sources listed in the original article. You can also use reference works in the library, articles from other magazines and journals, and Internet sources.

Work as a group to develop evaluation criteria, then research your health claim. Try to find at least three reliable sources of information. Is the claim accurate? Why or why not? When you are done, present your findings to the class. List the sources you used and explain why you think they are reliable.

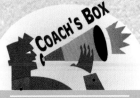

COACH'S BOX

Accessing Information

When evaluating health information, ask yourself these questions:

- Is it based on scientific research?
- Does it give only one point of view?
- Is it trying to sell something?
- Does it agree with other reliable sources?

Self-√ Check

- Did we find at least three sources to support or contradict our health claim?
- Did we identify the sources we used and explain why they are reliable and valid?

After You Read

Use your completed Foldable to review the information on being an informed consumer.

FOLDABLES™
Study Organizer

Reviewing Vocabulary and Concepts

On a sheet of paper, write the numbers 1–10. After each number, write the term from the list that best completes each statement.

- comparison shopping
- advertising
- health maintenance organization (HMO)
- media
- online shopping
- health care system
- health insurance
- warranty
- primary care physicians
- preventive care

Lesson 1

1. Messages designed to interest consumers in buying a product or service are known as _____.

2. A written promise from a company to handle repairs if the product fails to work properly is a(n) _____.

3. _____ is a method of judging the benefits of different products or services by comparing several factors.

4. Together, various methods for communicating information are known as the _____.

5. If you buy products on the Internet, you are participating in _____.

Lesson 2

6. The U.S. _____ includes all the medical care available to Americans, the way they receive the care, and the way the care is paid for.

7. _____ involves keeping disease or injury from happening or getting worse.

8. An organization that provides health care for a fixed price is a(n) _____.

9. Medical doctors who provide physical checkups and general care are called _____.

10. _____ is a plan in which private companies or government programs pay for part of a person's medical costs.

On a sheet of paper, write the numbers 11–16. Write *True* or *False* for each statement below. If the statement is false, change the underlined word or phrase to make it true.

Lesson 3

11. <u>Fraud</u> is deliberate deceit or trickery.

12. <u>Second opinions</u> involve the sale of worthless products or treatments claimed to prevent diseases or cure other health problems.

13. People or groups who help consumers with problems are known as <u>consumer advocates</u>.

Lesson 4

14. The main federal health agency is the <u>Department of Health and Human Services</u>.

15. The Food Safety and Inspection Service oversees the safety of <u>milk and eggs</u>.

16. <u>The Centers for Disease Control and Prevention</u> monitor disease trends and investigate outbreaks of disease.

Thinking Critically

Using complete sentences, answer the following questions on a sheet of paper.

17. **Hypothesize** Explain how programmers develop media to influence purchasing decisions.

18. **Analyze** Select an ad for a health-related product or service. Use critical-thinking skills to analyze the marketing and advertising techniques used in the ad and their influence on the selection of the health-related service or product.

19. **Apply** Develop and apply criteria for the selection or rejection of health products, services, and information. Create a list of guidelines for consumers to follow.

20. **Judge** Should people who practice health fraud by selling worthless products or treatments be allowed to advertise in magazines and on television? Give reasons for your answer.

Career Corner

Health Services Administrator Nursing homes, hospitals and outpatient care facilities provide important community health services. It is the job of each facility's health services administrator to understand the needs of the consumer (the patient), while also maintaining and supervising health employees. Find out more about this challenging health career on Career Corner at health.glencoe.com.

Standardized Test Practice

Reading & Writing

Read the paragraphs below and then answer the questions.

Most fast-food choices tend to be high in fat, salt, or sugar, but low in vitamins and fiber. However, you don't have to give up fast food completely if you want to be healthy. You just need to be willing to make a few changes in the way you usually order.

First, look carefully at the menu before ordering. Burgers and fries are not the only items you will find there anymore. Fast-food restaurants are starting to offer healthier foods, such as salads and baked potatoes. Next, consider if you really need that jumbo portion. Big portions may seem like a great deal, but they can provide too many calories and contribute to unhealthful weight gain.

1. The author probably wrote this passage to
   A explain how fast-food restaurants trick customers into ordering expensive food.
   B persuade readers to change their eating habits at fast-food restaurants.
   C describe the different types of food to be found in fast-food restaurants.
   D persuade readers to give up eating at fast-food restaurants.

2. From the information in the second paragraph readers can conclude that
   A people will always eat what they want.
   B there are few choices at fast-food restaurants.
   C it is up to you to decide what to eat.
   D fast foods are always healthy.

3. Write a paragraph in which you try to persuade a friend or family member to take a specific action to improve his or her health.

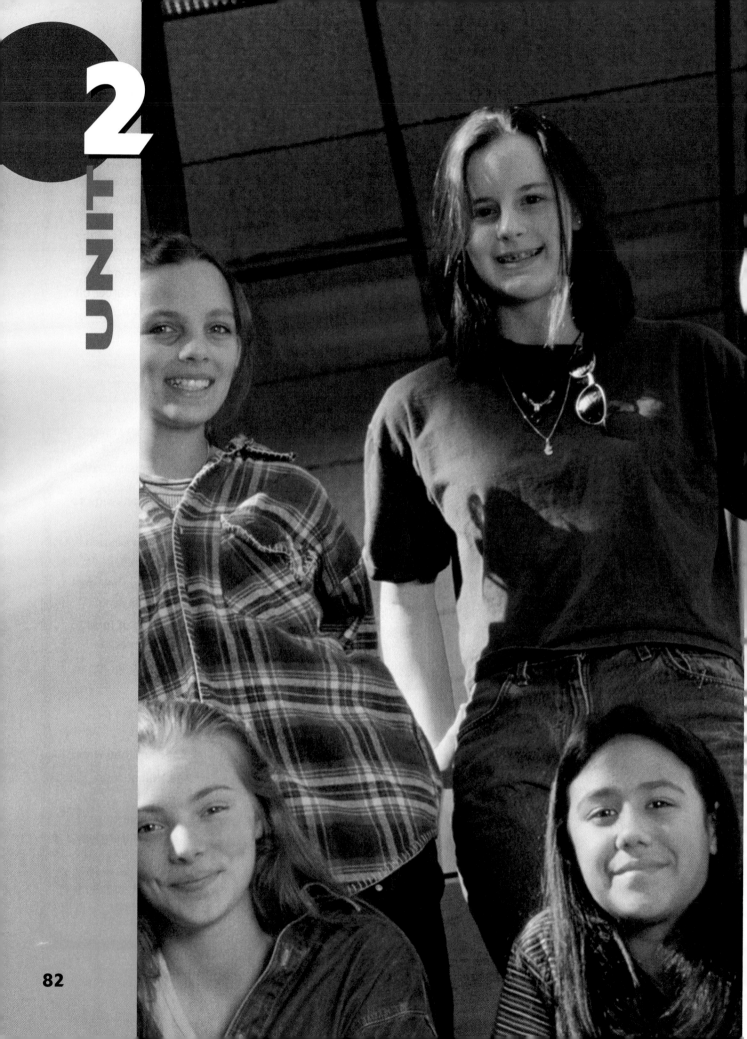

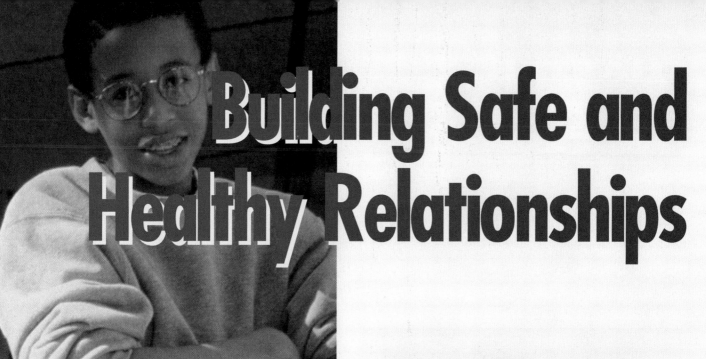

Building Safe and Healthy Relationships

HEALTH *in Action*

When is hanging out helping out?

When you spend time with friends and family, you're not just having fun. You're learning to express your own needs and feelings, and you're listening to others who want to share theirs. This helps you build new relationships. It also helps you handle conflicts and problems when they arise. That means you can be there to help your friends and your family when they need a hand!

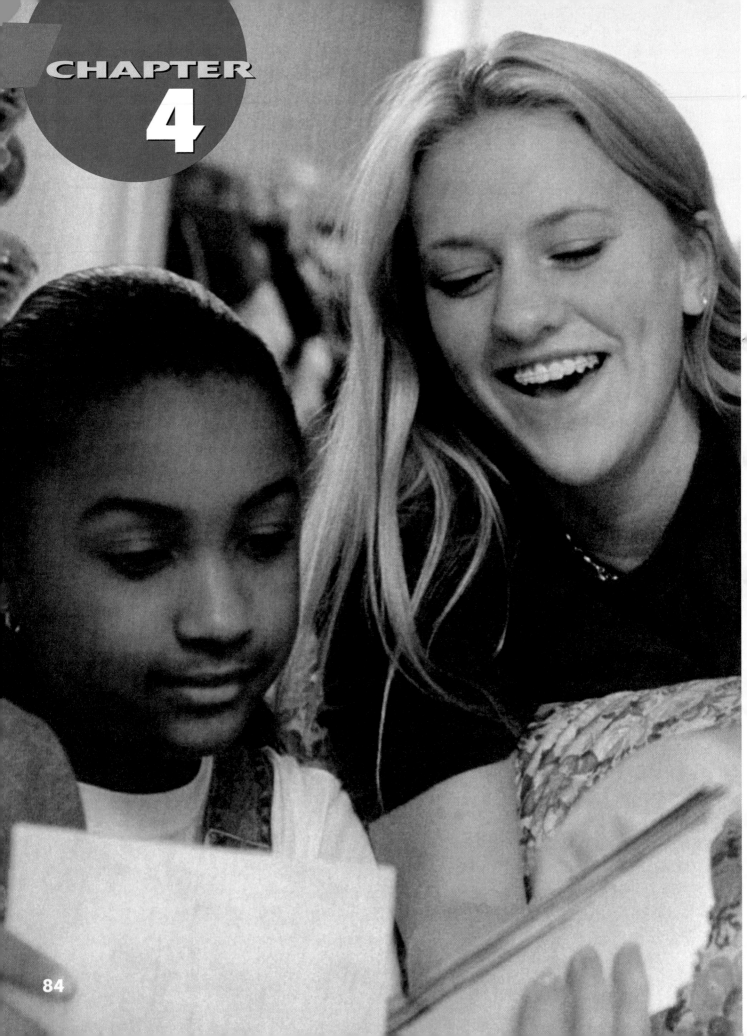

Mental and Emotional Health

HEALTH Online

Go to health.glencoe.com and take the Health Inventory for Chapter 4 to assess your mental and emotional health.

FOLDABLES™ Study Organizer

Before You Read

Make this Foldable to help you organize the main ideas on mental and emotional health in Lesson 1. Begin with a plain sheet of 8½" × 11" paper.

Step 1

Line up one of the short edges of a sheet of paper with one of the long edges to form a triangle. Fold and cut off the leftover rectangle.

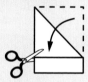

Step 2

Fold the triangle in half, then unfold. The folds will form an X dividing four equal sections.

Step 3

Cut up one fold line, and stop at the middle. This forms two triangular flaps. Draw an X on one tab, and label the other three as shown.

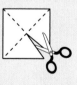

Step 4

Fold the X flap under the other flap, and glue together to make a three-sided pyramid.

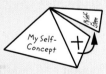

As You Read

Write the main ideas on mental and emotional health on the back of the appropriate side of the pyramid.

Your Mental and Emotional Health

Quick Write

What do you think it means to be mentally and emotionally healthy? List at least three traits that suggest good mental and emotional health.

LEARN ABOUT...

● **the signs of good mental and emotional health.**
● **ways to improve your self-esteem.**
● **how your thoughts, behaviors, and attitudes affect the way you feel about yourself.**

VOCABULARY

● **mental and emotional health**
● **personality**
● **self-concept**
● **self-esteem**

Mental and Emotional Health

Think about some of the people whose company you most enjoy. It's likely that you enjoy being around them because you have fun with them, they make you laugh, and they listen to your concerns. They may also have a positive outlook on life. A positive outlook is just one of the signs of mental and emotional health. **Mental and emotional health** is *the ability to accept yourself and others, adapt to and cope with emotions, and deal with the problems and challenges you meet in life.*

There are several signs you can look for in yourself and in others that indicate good mental and emotional health.

● You see yourself, and life in general, in positive ways.
● You face life's challenges with confidence.
● You accept the fact that situations and events will not always go your way.
● You can motivate yourself to achieve goals.
● You understand and cope with your feelings.
● You can focus on your strengths.
● You accept constructive criticism and learn from your mistakes.
● You have a healthy sense of humor.
● You bounce back from disappointments.

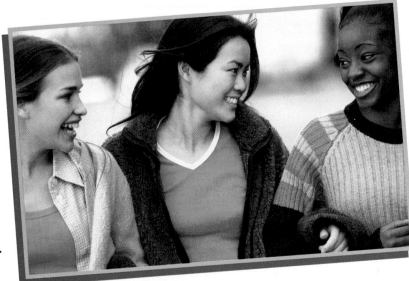

Your mental and emotional health affects every aspect of your life—your happiness, your success in school, and your relationships with other people.

What Makes You Who You Are?

The early teen years are a time to learn more about who you are. You find out about your physical and mental abilities. You discover the kinds of people you like to be with and the kinds of activities you enjoy and do well. You begin to determine what is really important to you.

Your Personality

Your personality has a big impact on your mental health. Your **personality** is *the unique combination of feelings, thoughts, and behavior that makes you different from everyone else.* Your personality helps determine how you react to problems, new situations, and other events. How would you feel about moving to a new school, for example? Would you feel excited and confident, or nervous and a little afraid? Different people react in different ways to the same situation.

Your Self-Concept

If you were asked to choose three words that best describe you, would you focus on your strengths? People who recognize their strengths and strong qualities generally have a positive self-concept. Your **self-concept** is *the view you have of yourself.* It is basically how you see yourself as the unique person you are.

Some teens and adults tend to focus on their limitations rather than on their strengths. People who focus on their limitations can begin to feel inadequate and can develop a negative self-concept. When teens who have a positive self-concept make a mistake, they are likely to say, "Okay, so I'm human." Those who have a negative self-concept might say, "I never do anything right." A positive self-concept is an important part of good mental and emotional health.

Your Self-Esteem and Self-Confidence

Your **self-esteem**, *the way you feel about yourself, and how you value yourself,* is closely related to your self-concept. Often a negative self-concept leads to low self-esteem. For example, if you aren't chosen for the track team after practicing for months, you might look upon yourself as a failure, even though you excel in other activities. This unrealistic picture of yourself could negatively affect your self-esteem.

Self-confidence, the belief you have in your abilities, is closely tied to self-esteem. People with good self-esteem usually have self-confidence. Characteristics that contribute to self-esteem and self-confidence include honesty, integrity (standing up for your values), responsibility, and respecting the dignity (worth) of other people.

FIGURE 4.1

How High Self-Esteem Leads to Success

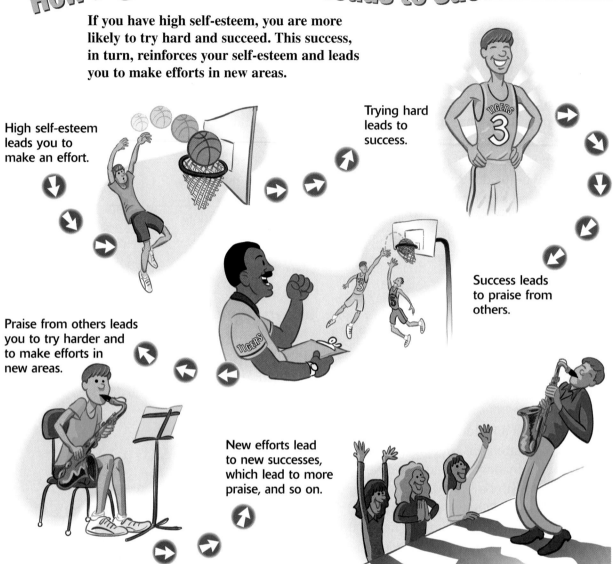

If you have high self-esteem, you are more likely to try hard and succeed. This success, in turn, reinforces your self-esteem and leads you to make efforts in new areas.

High self-esteem leads you to make an effort.

Trying hard leads to success.

Success leads to praise from others.

Praise from others leads you to try harder and to make efforts in new areas.

New efforts lead to new successes, which lead to more praise, and so on.

How do you feel when you think about the kind of person you are? Do you like and respect yourself? Do you accept yourself for who you are? Do you have confidence to try new things even though you might fail? If you do, you have high self-esteem. **Figure 4.1** shows how high self-esteem leads to success.

Improving Your Mental/Emotional Health with Coping Skills

Mental/emotional health will go through ups and downs throughout life. Fortunately, you can apply the effective coping skills that follow to improve your self-esteem and your overall level of mental/emotional health.

Motivate Yourself

Being able to motivate yourself is a key to success. It means setting healthful, realistic goals and working to achieve them. Motivation helps you focus on your goals. You will be willing to set aside short-term pleasures to achieve important long-term goals. Imagine, for example, that your long-term goal is to play in your city's youth orchestra. Because you are motivated, you make time for lessons and for practice even though it means that you miss out on other activities with your friends. Motivating yourself to engage in healthful, rewarding activities is one of the best ways to combat boredom. Managing boredom effectively will contribute to your mental/emotional health.

Focus on Your Strengths

Seeing yourself in a more positive way can help improve your self-esteem. Start by listing all your strengths and your successes. Work to improve your talents and abilities. Recognize your limitations and develop realistic expectations—no one is perfect. All these actions are effective strategies for coping with feelings of inadequacy.

Understand and Manage Your Feelings

Managing your feelings is another important part of your mental and emotional health. For example, suppose that you find

Reading Check

Consider these words: *motivated, lazy, determined, doubting, confident, positive.* **What do they have to do with mental and emotional health? Categorize these words under high and low self-esteem.**

HEALTH SKILLS ACTIVITY

PRACTICING HEALTHFUL BEHAVIORS

Improving Your Self-Esteem

There are many ways to take action to improve your self-esteem.

- Make a list of your good qualities. Include adjectives such as *honest, kind, fair, hardworking,* and so on.
- Make a list of everything you do well. You may include sports, problem-solving skills, artistic abilities, academic skills, ability to get along with people, and so on.
- Find something you enjoy doing that gives you a feeling of success.
- Spend time with people who accept you as you are and who support you.
- Offer to help someone who needs help.
- Set realistic goals.

ON YOUR OWN

Choose one of the tips listed here. Demonstrate ways to use this health information to help yourself by putting this tip into action.

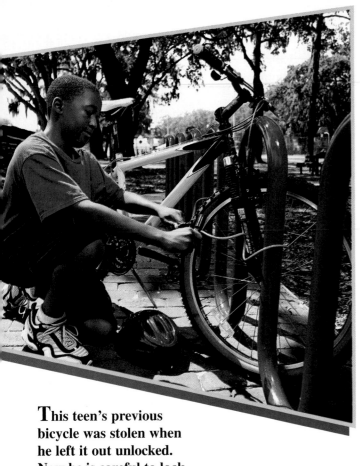

This teen's previous bicycle was stolen when he left it out unlocked. Now he is careful to lock his new bike whenever he has to leave it. *Which coping skill has he applied to his situation?*

yourself losing your temper with friends for no apparent reason. You may realize that you are nervous because you have a track meet coming up. Recognizing the cause of your anxiety will help you manage your interactions with friends.

Develop a Positive Attitude

Your thoughts and behavior have a strong influence on your mental and emotional health. If you believe that you cannot handle new situations, your mental and emotional health will suffer. If, on the other hand, you see challenges as obstacles that you can overcome, your mental health will be affected in a positive way.

Learn from Your Mistakes

You can also improve your self-esteem by learning from your mistakes. This means that you take responsibility for your actions and behavior and recognize when you are wrong. It also means that you see mistakes as opportunities to grow and improve.

Lesson 1 Review

Using complete sentences, answer the following questions on a sheet of paper.

Reviewing Terms and Facts

1. **Vocabulary** Define *self-concept* and *self-esteem.* Use both in a sentence that shows their relationship.
2. **Summarize** List four things you can do to improve your mental and emotional health.
3. **Describe** How does a positive attitude help you?

Thinking Critically

4. **Apply** Rebecca was so embarrassed when the teacher criticized her report that she

hardly listened to the criticism. Although she wasn't sure what the teacher meant, she said nothing. Describe some techniques Rebecca could have used to respond to the criticism.

Applying Health Skills

5. **Communication Skills** With a partner create a skit showing how a teen might demonstrate one of the characteristics that contribute to self-confidence and self-esteem: honesty, integrity, responsibility, and respecting others' dignity. Perform your skit for the class.

Understanding Your Emotions

What Are Emotions?

Your **emotions** are your *feelings created in response to thoughts, remarks, and events.* The basic emotions are happiness, love, jealousy, sadness, anger, fear, anticipation, and joy. Emotions can influence most aspects of your life, including how you behave. For example, do sad movies make you cry? How do you react to being teased? How do you express extreme happiness?

Understanding Emotions

Emotions are neither good nor bad, right nor wrong. How you express your emotions is another matter. You can't always choose when an emotion will well up inside you, but you can choose how to handle it. People with good mental and emotional health seek healthy, responsible ways to express their emotions.

Important steps in learning how to express your emotions are described in **Figure 4.2** on page 92.

Quick Write

Briefly describe in writing two situations in which you experienced one of the following: fear, anger, love, guilt, mixed emotions.

LEARN ABOUT...

- expressing emotions in healthy ways.
- meeting emotional needs in healthy ways.

VOCABULARY

- emotions
- empathy
- anxiety
- panic
- resilience
- emotional needs

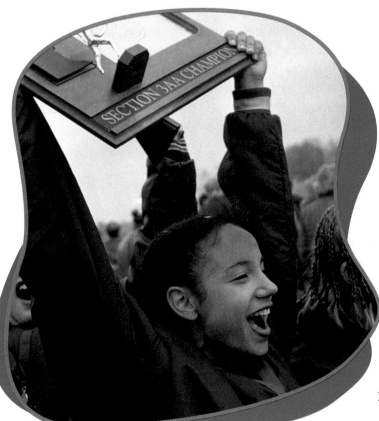

Expressing your happiness about an achievement is appropriate. *How do you celebrate your accomplishments?*

FIGURE 4.2

Expressing Your Emotions

Expressing your emotions in healthy ways helps improve your overall mental health.

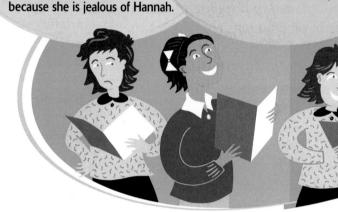

① Identify the Emotion
Amy and Hannah used to be best friends. Now Amy feels angry with Hannah and avoids her. She realizes that it is because she is jealous of Hannah.

② Understand the Cause
Amy had expected to get the lead role in the school play. Instead Hannah got the lead, and Amy has just a small part.

③ Respond in a Healthy Way
Amy recognizes that her jealousy is ruining a good friendship. She congratulates Hannah and offers to help her learn her lines.

Identifying Your Emotions

Recognizing the emotions that you experience will help you deal with them. Which emotions listed below are familiar to you?

- **Happiness** is a sense of well-being. When you are happy, you feel good about life in general.
- **Sadness** is a normal, healthy reaction to an unhappy event, such as a good friend moving away or a loved one dying. When you are sad, you may feel easily discouraged and have less energy.
- **Fear** is an emotion that can help keep you safe from danger. However, some fears, such as the fear of failure, may keep you from doing things you want or need to do.
- **Anger** is a common reaction to being emotionally hurt or physically harmed.
- **Love** is a combination of caring and affection that binds one person to another.
- **Empathy** affects your social health. **Empathy** is *the ability to understand and share another person's feelings.*
- **Sympathy** means understanding and sharing another's problems or sorrow.
- **Anxiety** can keep you from doing your best. **Anxiety** is *an overwhelming feeling of dread, much like fear.*
- **Jealousy** is a feeling of resentment or unhappiness at another's good fortune.

Reading Check

Complete a cause-and-effect chart listing emotions in the first column and possible effects of each emotion in the second column. In the third column, determine whether the effect was positive or negative.

Expressing Emotions

People express emotions in different ways. We often learn how to express them from watching others who are close to us, such as family members. Learning to understand emotions and to express them in healthy ways is an important part of good mental and emotional health.

Expressing Anxiety and Fear

Have you ever felt anxious before giving a report or taking a test? When you are anxious or fearful, you take shorter breaths, your heart beats faster, and your muscles tense. Anxiety can help you accomplish more by releasing energy. However, too much anxiety and fear can cause you to lose sleep or even to panic. **Panic**, *a feeling of sudden, intense fear,* may be accompanied by physical symptoms such as dizziness and a pounding heart.

Hands-On Health

COMMUNICATING EMOTIONS

This activity will give you practice in communicating positive feelings.

WHAT YOU WILL NEED
- paper
- pen or pencil

WHAT YOU WILL DO
1. In a small group, develop a list of situations that could produce positive feelings for teens. An example might be receiving recognition from a coach after winning a track event.
2. Choose one of the situations on your list and write a skit in which someone expresses positive feelings to a friend.
3. Perform your skit for your classmates.
4. Have classmates evaluate your skit and, if necessary, describe a more effective method of communicating the positive emotions.

IN CONCLUSION
1. Draw conclusions from the skits. Were students comfortable expressing positive emotions? Did the audience have useful suggestions?
2. Overall, what did you learn from this activity? How will it affect your behavior in the future?

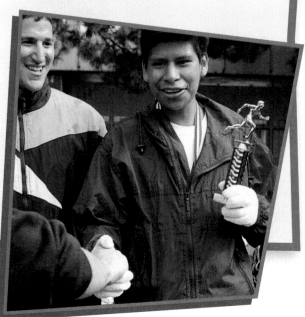

Be responsible, and
take these steps to
become more resilient:

- **Join your peers in
  healthful activities
  at school.**
- **Develop positive
  bonds with your
  family members
  and others in the
  community.**
- **Set worthwhile
  goals for the
  future.**

Protective factors
such as these can
help you "bounce
back" from
difficulties.

Sometimes just admitting to a family member or friend that you feel anxious helps. Other people may give you the reassurance and encouragement that you need. Overcoming your anxiety will help build your resilience. **Resilience** is *the ability to adapt to and recover from disappointment, difficulty, or crisis.* Resilience is also known as the "bounce-back" factor. People who develop resilience can bounce back from setbacks and disappointments.

Expressing Anger

It is normal to feel angry at times, but some people express their anger in unhealthy ways. Yelling, hitting, and threatening are not healthy ways to express anger. It is also not healthy to hold anger inside or to deny how you feel. Try these steps when you feel angry.

- Exercise self-control—take a deep breath and stay calm.
- Focus on exactly what made you angry.
- Think of words to communicate your true feelings.
- Calmly tell the other person how you feel and what action has caused you to feel this way.
- Tell the person what you expect from him or her in the future.

Understanding Your Emotional Needs

Everyone has physical needs, such as water, food, and sleep. You also have **emotional needs**. These are *needs that affect your feelings and sense of well-being.* Your basic emotional needs include the following:

- **The need to feel worthwhile.** You need to feel that you make a difference in the world—that you are making a contribution. Working toward short-term and long-term goals will give you a sense of accomplishment.
- **The need to love and be loved.** You need to feel that you are cared for and that you are special to people—family, friends, and classmates.
- **The need to belong.** You need to know that others accept and respect you as you are. Find friends who are accepting, reliable, and trustworthy.

Teens who participate in team sports often form strong bonds with coaches and teammates. The sense of belonging adds to their enjoyment of the sport.

Meeting Emotional Needs in Healthy Ways

Recognizing your emotional needs will help you meet them in healthy ways. You might, for example, offer to help someone without being asked. You could ask a friend how his or her day went and really listen to the answer. You can show affection for family members or volunteer for a good cause.

Meeting your emotional needs in healthy ways means making the choice to engage in healthful behavior. It also means abstaining from unhealthful behavior. Some teens may try to meet their emotional needs for love and affection by engaging in sexual activity. This behavior carries many risks, including the risks of an unplanned pregnancy or sexually transmitted diseases. By choosing sexual abstinence teens show respect for themselves and for the health of others. Caring and affection can be shown in other positive ways, such as getting to know the other person better and sharing everyday experiences.

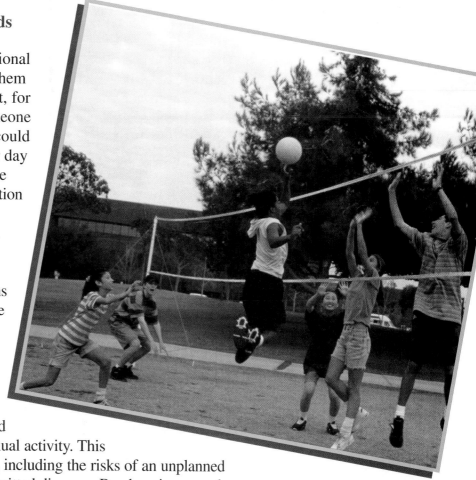

Choose friends who share your values and abstain from risky behaviors. *How do your friends help you practice healthful behaviors?*

![Lesson 2 Review banner]

Using complete sentences, answer the following questions on a sheet of paper.

Reviewing Terms and Facts

1. **Vocabulary** Define *emotions*. List five basic emotions.
2. **Compare** What is the difference between *empathy* and *sympathy?*
3. **Explain** Why is *resilience* sometimes called the "bounce-back" factor?

Thinking Critically

4. **Explain** What do you need to do before you express your anger?
5. **Summarize** What are the basic emotional needs that everyone has?

Applying Health Skills

6. **Advocacy** Write a public service announcement that informs students of volunteer opportunities in your community.

Mental and Emotional Problems

LEARN ABOUT...

- types of mental and emotional problems.
- recognizing when a person is seriously depressed.
- the warning signs of suicide.

VOCABULARY

- anxiety disorder
- phobia
- personality disorder
- schizophrenia
- mood disorder
- clinical depression
- suicide

Kinds of Mental Health Problems

Everyone has problems from time to time. Most people overcome their problems and are able to function well at home, school, and work. About one person in five cannot cope, however. Such people need treatment in order to regain their mental health. As with most illnesses, the earlier treatment begins, the more effective it can be. Early identification and treatment can prevent long-term disability.

The three most common types of mental health problems are anxiety disorders, personality disorders, and mood disorders. People with these disorders are troubled by worries, fears, or other emotions that interfere with their daily lives.

Anxiety Disorders

Most people experience anxiety from time to time. It's a normal reaction to challenging and worrying situations. Some people, however, have unreasonable or excessive anxiety. These people have an **anxiety disorder**, *a condition in which intense anxiety or fear keeps a person from functioning normally.* **Figure 4.3** describes common anxiety disorders and their symptoms.

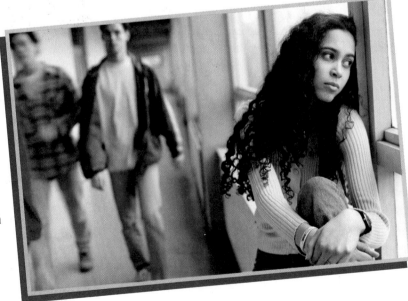

Anxiety disorders, such as post-traumatic stress disorder, can make a person feel isolated.

FIGURE 4.3

TYPES OF ANXIETY DISORDERS

Anxiety disorders are grouped into the five categories shown here.

Disorder	Symptoms
Generalized Anxiety Disorder	Restlessness, tiredness, difficulty concentrating, irritability, muscle tension, sleep disturbance
Panic Disorder	Pounding heart, sweating, trembling, shortness of breath, nausea, fear of losing control
Phobia	*Intense and exaggerated fear of a specific situation or object.* Examples: fear of spiders, fear of flying
Obsessive-Compulsive Disorder	Obsessions such as a need to perform behaviors over and over; compulsions such as handwashing, counting, hoarding, and arranging possessions
Post-Traumatic Stress Disorder	Withdrawal or depression after a distressing experience such as sexual abuse, natural disaster, accident, or witnessing violence

Personality Disorders

Personality disorders include *a variety of psychological conditions that affect a person's ability to get along with others.* People with personality disorders behave in unexpected ways. These disorders affect their thinking, moods, personal relationships, and control of sudden urges.

One of the most serious personality disorders is schizophrenia. **Schizophrenia** (skit·zoh·FREE·nee·uh) is *a severe mental disorder in which people lose contact with reality.* They may experience hallucinations in which they see or hear things that are not actually there. They may have delusions involving false personal beliefs that are unreasonable. People who have schizophrenia may not be able to sort out what is important from what is not. They may also be unable to separate what is really happening from what they imagine. For example, they may believe that they are other people, such as celebrities or historical figures.

Mood Disorders

People who feel sad when life is good, or happy for no apparent reason, may suffer from a mood disorder. A **mood disorder** is *a disorder in which a person undergoes changes in mood that seem inappropriate or extreme.* Mood disorders include bipolar disorder (formerly called manic-depressive disorder) and clinical depression. People with bipolar disorder go from feeling upbeat and energetic to feeling desolate and tired for no apparent reason.

CONNECT TO
Science

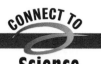

MOOD AND THE BRAIN
No one knows for sure why certain people get depressed. It is known, though, that depression starts in the brain. Brain chemicals called neurotransmitters regulate mood in the brain. Reduced activity of certain kinds of neurotransmitters results in depression. Check reliable mental health sources to learn about current research on and treatment of depression.

Teen Depression

Everyone feels "down" or "blue" from time to time. Many teens, for example, become depressed because they feel lonely or isolated from their peers. This kind of depression usually passes. At such times it's a good idea to examine the situation that led to the feelings of depression and to talk about it with a trusted adult.

Clinical depression, also known as major depression, is much more serious. **Clinical depression** is *a mood disorder in which people lose interest in life and can no longer find enjoyment in anything.* The National Institute of Mental Health estimates that every year about 5 percent of teens experience clinical depression. Some depressed teens abuse alcohol, other drugs, or both. Some try to harm themselves. Symptoms of clinical depression are described in **Figure 4.4.**

If depression persists, seek appropriate assistance right away—you might be clinically depressed. Discuss your feelings with a parent, coach, religious leader, or other trusted adult. These adults can help you obtain appropriate health care to treat the condition.

Suicide

Suicide, or *intentionally killing oneself,* is a serious problem in the United States, especially among teens. Suicide is one of the

FIGURE 4.4

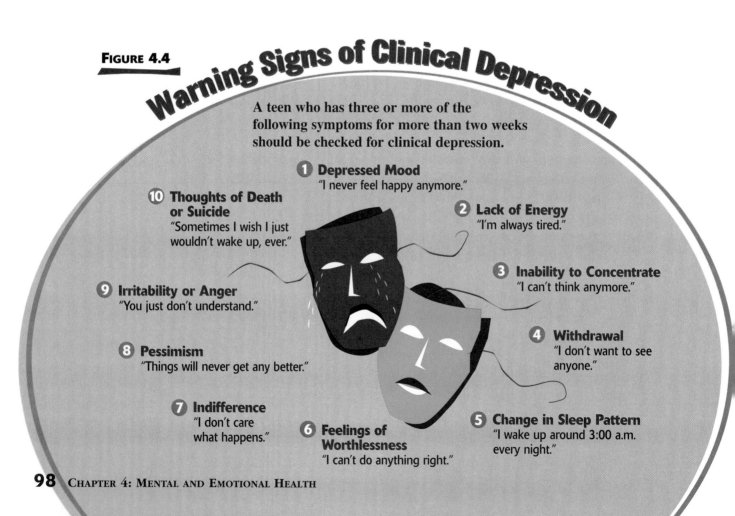

Warning Signs of Clinical Depression

A teen who has three or more of the following symptoms for more than two weeks should be checked for clinical depression.

1 Depressed Mood
"I never feel happy anymore."

2 Lack of Energy
"I'm always tired."

3 Inability to Concentrate
"I can't think anymore."

4 Withdrawal
"I don't want to see anyone."

5 Change in Sleep Pattern
"I wake up around 3:00 a.m. every night."

6 Feelings of Worthlessness
"I can't do anything right."

7 Indifference
"I don't care what happens."

8 Pessimism
"Things will never get any better."

9 Irritability or Anger
"You just don't understand."

10 Thoughts of Death or Suicide
"Sometimes I wish I just wouldn't wake up, ever."

DECISION MAKING

If a Friend Seems Depressed

Leon has noticed that Keith just doesn't seem like Keith anymore. They have been friends since fifth grade. A month ago Keith's parents told him that the family will be moving to another state in the summer. At first Keith was excited about the move, but now he seems depressed about it. Nothing interests him, and he seldom smiles.

Leon is worried that Keith is showing the warning signs of suicide. However, he is afraid that if he says something, Keith might actually attempt it.

WHAT WOULD YOU DO?

Apply the decision-making skills to Leon's situation. Demonstrate the strategy that you would use to help Keith.

1. **STATE THE SITUATION.**
2. **LIST THE OPTIONS.**
3. **WEIGH THE POSSIBLE OUTCOMES.**
4. **CONSIDER VALUES.**
5. **MAKE A DECISION AND ACT.**
6. **EVALUATE THE DECISION.**

leading causes of death among young people. Every day, 14 young people between the ages of 15 and 24 years take their own lives.

Warning Signs of Suicide

You may know someone who has said things like: "The world would be better off without me," or "I'd be better off dead." Most people who commit suicide talk about it beforehand. Anyone who talks about suicide should be taken seriously. Tell a trusted adult immediately.

People who are thinking about suicide may show signs of depression at first. Once they decide to end their lives, they may feel better because they think that they have solved their problems. They may give away valued possessions. People who reach this point are in great danger. Other warning signs of suicide include:

- Lack of energy
- Withdrawal from friends and family
- No longer taking interest in favorite activities
- No longer taking interest in personal appearance
- Taking unnecessary risks
- Expressing suicidal thoughts or talking a lot about death

Family and friends can be a source of help and support for teens who are having difficulty handling their problems.

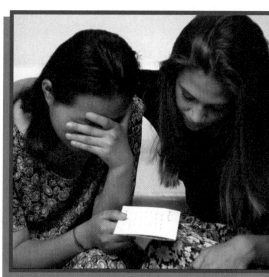

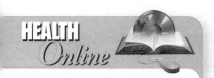
What You Can Do

With most people, a suicide attempt is a cry for help. They don't really want to die, but they feel so much emotional pain that they can't see any other course of action. They need to be convinced that even though the pain seems unbearable, it will not last forever. If anyone you know talks of suicide:

- Try to react calmly and let the person talk out his or her feelings. Listen without interrupting.
- Don't make comments that challenge the person's intent, such as "You'd never have the nerve," or "You just want attention."
- Offer comfort and support. Tell the person how important she or he is to you and to other people.
- Urge the person to get help right away.
- Don't promise to keep a friend's talk of suicide secret. Tell an adult who will help. Telling could save a life.

Things to Remember When You're Down

Everyone has tough times and feels depressed now and then. Here are some points to remember next time you feel down.

- You are not alone. There are people who understand how you feel.
- Take care of your physical needs—get enough sleep, eat regular and healthful meals, and take time to relax.
- Participate in regular physical activity. Aerobic exercise is particularly effective in boosting mood.
- Avoid alcohol and other drugs, even caffeine. They will only add to your problems.
- Don't wait. Talk to someone about how you feel.

Lesson 3 Review

Using complete sentences, answer the following questions on a sheet of paper.

Reviewing Terms and Facts

1. **Vocabulary** Define *anxiety disorder*.
2. **Identify** What kind of mood disorder is characterized by extreme mood swings?
3. **Compare** What is the difference between clinical depression and the normal depression that most people feel from time to time?

Thinking Critically

4. **Restate** Explain why clinical depression is a serious mental disorder.
5. **Identify** Describe two lifetime strategies for the prevention of disorders such as depression and anxiety that may lead to long-term disability.

Applying Health Skills

6. **Communication Skills** With a classmate, role-play a situation in which one person is depressed and the other reaches out to help. The person offering help should use effective communication skills.

Getting Help

Knowing When to Get Help

Talking about your thoughts and feelings may be difficult at first. You may feel frightened or embarrassed. You may feel that the adult will be shocked or annoyed by what you have to say. Realize that most adults understand and want to help. Sometimes all you need to do is let someone know that you need help. Needing help is nothing to be ashamed of. It is a mistake *not* to ask for help.

Quick Write

List at least five adults to whom teens can go for help at your school or in your community.

LEARN ABOUT...

- how to know if you need professional help for a mental or emotional problem.
- the kinds of treatments that are available.
- kinds of professionals who help people with mental health problems.

VOCABULARY

- therapy
- family therapy
- psychologist
- psychiatrist

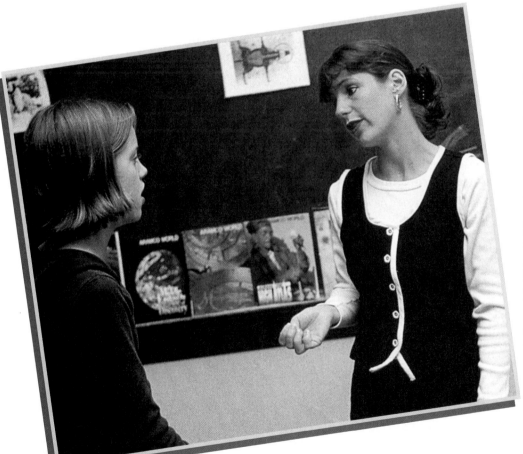

The first step toward solving a problem is to let someone know that you want help. *When was the last time you shared a problem with your parents, guardians, or a trusted adult?*

Seeking Professional Help

How can you tell if a problem is serious enough to discuss with a mental health professional? Learning the warning signs of mental health problems will help. **Figure 4.5** shows some signs that may indicate a mental health problem for which a professional's help is needed.

Therapy Methods

There are various methods of **therapy**, or *treatment,* for mental health problems. These fall into two broad types: talk therapy and biological therapy. Talk therapy includes a variety of counseling methods. Biological therapy involves using medication to treat mental health problems.

The goal of all mental health treatment is to help patients change so that they can handle their problems better. Some professionals use only counseling, others rely mostly on medication, and still others use both types of therapy. A teen who is clinically depressed after the death of a close friend may be given medication to help improve his or her mood. The teen may also receive counseling to help her or him deal with the loss.

FIGURE 4.5

SIGNS THAT YOU MAY NEED PROFESSIONAL HELP

If you experience several of these signs, and if they last a long time, you may need to talk to a professional. Getting help is an important lifetime strategy for early identification of mental health problems such as depression and anxiety.

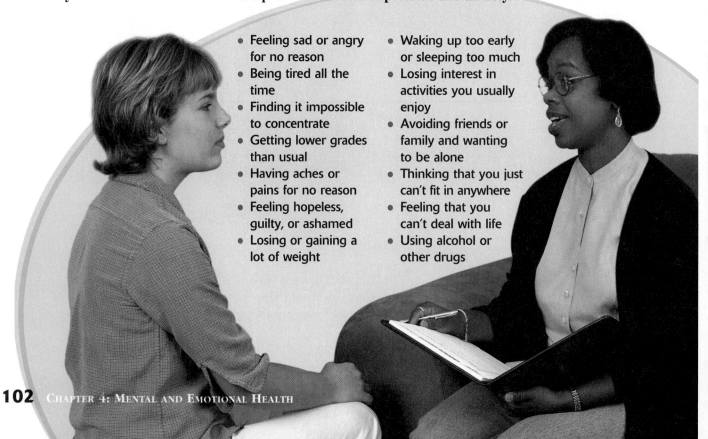

- Feeling sad or angry for no reason
- Being tired all the time
- Finding it impossible to concentrate
- Getting lower grades than usual
- Having aches or pains for no reason
- Feeling hopeless, guilty, or ashamed
- Losing or gaining a lot of weight

- Waking up too early or sleeping too much
- Losing interest in activities you usually enjoy
- Avoiding friends or family and wanting to be alone
- Thinking that you just can't fit in anywhere
- Feeling that you can't deal with life
- Using alcohol or other drugs

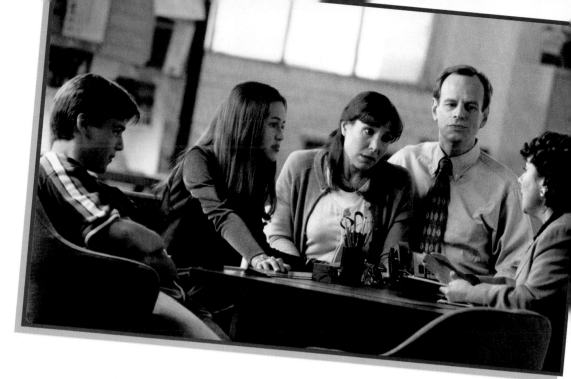

Counseling

In counseling, an individual talks with a mental health professional to learn new ways of thinking or behaving. Changing thoughts or behavior leads, in turn, to changes in feelings. By learning to think and behave in healthy ways, the person improves his or her mental and emotional health. Some people feel much better after just a few sessions with a mental health professional. Others may need months of counseling.

Some people choose to talk alone with a counselor. Others prefer to take part in group counseling. In group therapy, the counselor meets with several people at once who have the same or similar problems. Some people find that they benefit from the empathy and support that comes from other members of the group.

A variation on group therapy is family therapy. **Family therapy** is *counseling that seeks to improve troubled family relationships.* Family therapists are trained to help relieve family problems, strengthen family relationships, and solve small problems before they get bigger. The therapy sessions may involve all or some family members.

Family therapy is helping this family learn better ways to communicate with one another. *Describe how effective communication contributes to family health.*

Counseling Methods

One form of counseling focuses on helping people think more positively about themselves. This kind of therapy can be especially helpful for people who experience depression. The professional helps the depressed person identify negative thoughts that are contributing to the depression. From that point, the person can be guided to more positive ways of thinking. Teens who are depressed because they focus on their weaknesses or mistakes, for example, can learn to focus on their strengths and achievements instead.

Another form of counseling focuses on changing behavior. This type of therapy is especially helpful to people with anxiety disorders such as phobias. The individual learns to stay calm while facing the situation he or she fears. Imagine, for example, a girl who has a severe fear of giving speeches. She might begin by learning to stay calm while giving a brief talk to a few friends. Her therapist might then encourage her to speak for a little longer and to more people. Eventually, she might be able to speak in front of a large group without feeling any fear.

Drug Treatments

Some mental health disorders can be treated with drugs. Different types of drugs are used to treat different kinds of illnesses. People with anxiety disorders may take antianxiety drugs, which affect the central nervous system. Those who have clinical depression may take antidepressant drugs, which affect brain activity. Drug treatment is highly individual. A drug or dose that may help one person could seriously harm another. The medications used to treat mental disorders can be prescribed only by a medical doctor.

Sources of Help

People in a variety of roles and professions can help with mental health problems. Teens often seek help from the following people:

● **Parent or other adult family member.** You might be able to get all the help you need by talking with a parent or guardian, older brother or sister, or other adult family member. Family members have a special bond and care very deeply for one another.

School psychologists are trained to listen to students and help them find a way of dealing with their problems. *How could teens and their families seek a cure for a mental or emotional problem from a school-linked service such as a school psychologist or a school nurse?*

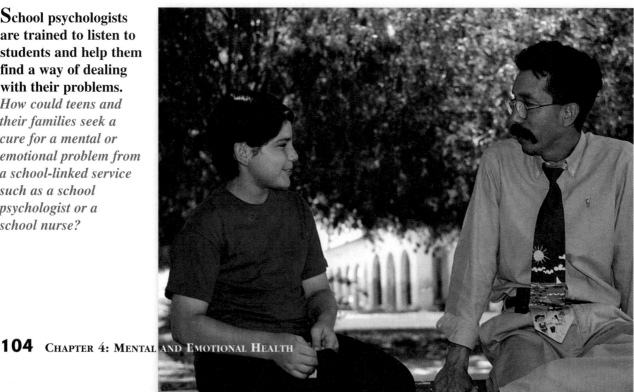

- **Clergy member.** A religious leader may have formal training in counseling. Even those who do not have such training usually have a lot of experience in counseling people of all ages.
- **Teacher or school counselor.** Many teachers and all school counselors are trained to help students with mental and emotional problems.
- **Family counselor.** Family counselors see family members together. Most family counseling sessions focus on improving communication among family members.
- **School nurse.** If you are not sure what kind of help you need, seek care from the school nurse with your family. School nurses are trained to deal with all types of health problems. A nurse can guide you to the help you need.
- **Social worker.** Many schools have social workers who help students and their families with social and personal problems that interfere with learning. Students experiencing these types of problems should seek care from school-linked services with their families when appropriate.
- **Psychologist.** A **psychologist** (sy·KAH·luh·jist) is *a mental health professional who is trained and licensed by the state to counsel.* Psychologists treat mental health problems by using one or several types of counseling.
- **Psychiatrist.** A **psychiatrist** (sy·KY·uh·trist) is *a medical doctor who treats mental health problems.* A psychiatrist is the only mental health professional who can prescribe drugs.

Reading Check

Increase comprehension. Complete a T-chart that shows what you know about getting help.

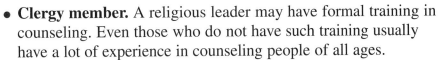

Lesson 4 Review

Using complete sentences, answer the following questions on a sheet of paper.

Reviewing Terms and Facts

1. **Identify** Name the two broad types of therapy for mental health problems.
2. **Recall** What are some of the benefits of group therapy?
3. **Vocabulary** Define the term *family therapy* and use it in a sentence.

Thinking Critically

4. **Compare** Compare and contrast thought and behavior therapy.

5. **Apply** What factors might determine which person an individual should talk to about a mental health problem?

Applying Health Skills

6. **Accessing Information** Research mental health disorders that are common in teens. In a report, identify and describe lifetime strategies for early identification and treatment of these disorders.

Lesson 5

Coping with Loss

Quick Write

Write about what you might do to help a close friend or relative deal with the loss of a loved one.

LEARN ABOUT...

- the stages people go through when they are dying.
- the stages of grieving.
- strategies for dealing with loss.

VOCABULARY

- grief
- hospice care
- grief counselor

Different Kinds of Loss

Have you ever lost something that was really important to you? Maybe a close friend moved away or a beloved family pet died. Whenever you experience loss, you feel sorrow.

The greatest sorrow usually occurs when a loved one dies. Although dying and death are part of the life cycle of human beings, at such times everyone experiences some kind of grief. **Grief** is *the sorrow caused by loss of a loved one.* The length of time a person grieves after a death depends on the individual.

Elisabeth Kübler-Ross, a noted Swiss-American doctor, studied the experiences of dying people and their families. Dr. Kübler-Ross identified five stages that people go through when they face death. Some people experience these stages in different sequences. The stages provide guidelines that help us understand how people experience dying.

- **Stage 1: Denial.** Refusing to accept that one is dying. Telling oneself that "it is all a mistake" and hoping to wake up from this "nightmare."

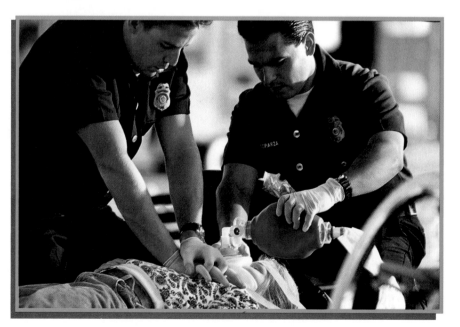

Rescue workers are among the first on the scene during emergencies. Their efforts can mean the difference between life and death.

- **Stage 2: Anger.** Angrily asking, "Why me?" Often directing the anger toward friends, family members, doctors, and nurses.
- **Stage 3: Bargaining.** Looking for ways to prolong life. Hoping for a medical miracle or praying to be spared in exchange for living a better life.
- **Stage 4: Depression.** Feeling deep sadness for loss of life and other losses. Realizing that one will not live to keep promises or realize goals.
- **Stage 5: Acceptance.** Accepting the reality of death and making peace with the world.

Hospice Care

Many dying people and their families choose to have hospice care during the last few weeks or months of the dying process. **Hospice care** is *care provided to the terminally ill that focuses on comfort, not cure.* The goal of hospice care is to provide support, relief from pain, and comfort for dying people and their families. Some people receive hospice care in a hospital, nursing home, or an inpatient hospice center. Most often, though, hospice care is provided in the patient's home to maintain peace, comfort, and dignity.

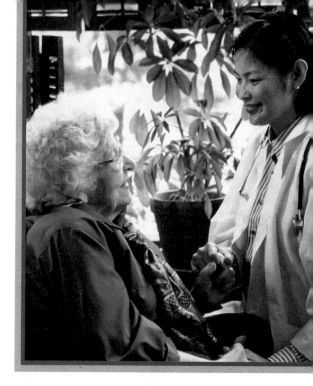

Hospice workers are specially trained to help people who are dying. *Where is hospice care provided?*

HEALTH SKILLS ACTIVITY

COMMUNICATION SKILLS

Writing a Sympathy Note

If a close friend or relative loses a loved one, you may wish to write a sympathy note. Your words will be a loving gift to your grieving friend and will also help you deal with the sorrow yourself.

Consider the following guidelines.

- Mention the special qualities of the person who died.
- Share a favorite memory about the person who died.
- Avoid comments such as: "Just be happy that he is out of pain," or "Think of all that you still have to be thankful for." Such comments can be hurtful and can make the grief process more difficult.

- Understand that your friend's grief is unique. Different people respond to death in different ways.
- Don't try to take away the hurt. You can't, but your sincere acknowledgment of your friend's sorrow can help.

ON YOUR OWN
Write a sympathy note to an imaginary friend who has suffered the loss of a loved one. Your note should be kind and comforting.

When a friend is grieving, you can help simply by listening. Your friend may want to go over the death or events that led up to the death. Let your friend tell the story as often as necessary. Remember that tears are a natural way to express grief. *What else can you do to comfort a grieving friend?*

The Grief Process

Understanding that death is part of the life cycle of human beings does not mean that the death of someone you care about won't be painful. Knowing how to grieve, however, can help you handle the hurt.

Grief often has stages similar to the stages of death. Like the stages of death, the stages of grief may be experienced in various orders. Not all people experience all of the following stages:

- **Shock.** Shortly after the death of a loved one, people tend to feel separated from their emotions. They may feel numb or empty or seem to have no feelings at all.
- **Anger.** Sometimes the survivors feel angry. The anger may even be directed at the dead person for leaving them.
- **Yearning.** The survivors ache. The loss of the loved one has left a great empty place in their lives. They wish that the loved one could come back.
- **Depression.** The survivors begin to accept the reality of their loss. The person has died and will not be coming back.
- **Moving on.** The survivors are able to go forward with their lives. They have not forgotten the one who died, but the deep pain over the loss has lessened.

In a national or local crisis in which people die, the community shares in the grieving process. *How does the bonding of communities provide support for individuals and families?*

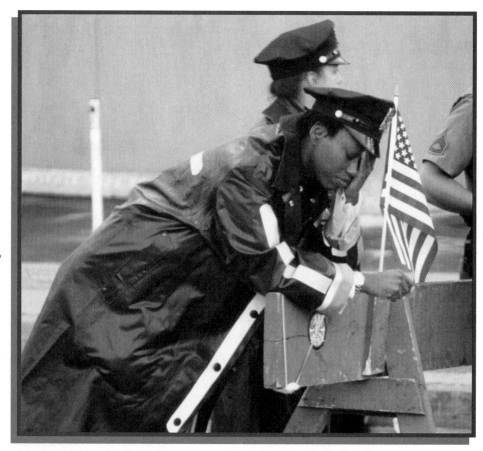

Coping with the Death of a Loved One

Grieving people often need to share their feelings with others. Sometimes trained counselors help people cope with their loss. **Grief counselors** are *counselors who teach people coping strategies to deal with grief.* They often help whole communities cope with a disastrous event such as an airplane crash.

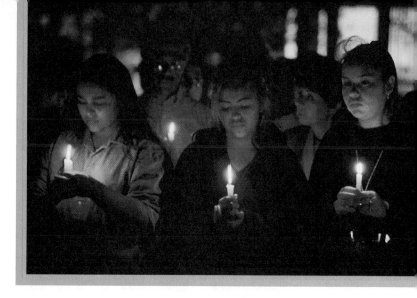

Memorial services provide an opportunity to deal with loss and to start the healing process. *Have you attended a memorial service? How did it seem to comfort people?*

Coping strategies suggested by grief counselors include the following.

- **Remember what was good about the person.** Focus on happy times and on ways in which the person was special.
- **Don't run away from your feelings.** The hurt from the loss cannot be denied. It is best to let the feelings out.
- **Share your feelings with others.** Telling someone about the hurt you are feeling will remind you that you are not alone.
- **Join a support group.** Most communities offer support groups in which people who have suffered a loss can share their pain with others. These groups are usually sponsored by churches, synagogues, and other organizations.

 Lesson 5 Review

Using complete sentences, answer the following questions on a sheet of paper.

Reviewing Terms and Facts

1. **Vocabulary** Define the term *grief.*
2. **Explain** List and describe the five stages of dying.
3. **Recall** Describe three effective coping strategies for dealing with the loss of a loved one.

Thinking Critically

4. **Compare** How are the stages of dying and stages of grief similar? How are they different?

5. **Synthesize** How might you comfort a child whose pet had died?

Applying Health Skills

6. **Communication Skills** Active listening is important when you talk with a grieving person. With a classmate, write and perform a skit that demonstrates the use of listening skills to help a person who has lost a close friend. Demonstrate correct use of body language, conversation encouragers, mirroring thoughts and feelings, and asking questions.

Dealing with Anxiety

There's more than one kind of therapy when it comes to relieving anxiety.

Behavioral Therapy

When the brain sets off anxiety alarms, our first instinct is to find the off switch. Behavioral scientists (therapists who focus on changing a person's behavior) take the opposite approach. They want you to get used to the noise so that you don't hear it anymore. In this type of therapy, the standard treatment for anxiety conditions such as phobias is to expose patients to a tiny bit of the very thing that causes them anxiety. The exposure is increased over a number of sessions until the brain gets used to the fear.

A patient suffering from a blood phobia, or fear of blood, for example, might first be shown a picture of a scalpel or syringe, then a real syringe, then a vial of blood, and so on. The patient is taken up the anxiety ladder until there are no more rungs to climb. There is a risk that if

treatment is cut short (before the patient has become used to the anxiety triggers), the anxious feelings could be made worse. Done right, however, behavioral therapy can bring relief from specific phobias in as little as two or three sessions. Social anxiety takes somewhat longer to treat, and other conditions may take a good deal longer still.

Cognitive Therapy

Cognitive therapists don't expect patients to surround themselves with anxiety. They ask patients to use the power of the mind to think their way through it. Cognitive therapy teaches people who are anxious or depressed to rethink their view of the world. This helps patients develop a more realistic idea of the risks or obstacles they face.

Patients suffering from social-anxiety disorder, for example, might see a group of people whispering at a party and assume the gossip is about them. A cognitive therapist would teach them to rethink that assumption.

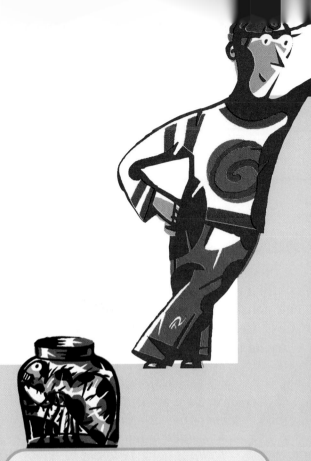

Physical Activity

Before turning to therapy, many people try to bring their anxiety under control on their own. Unlike most emotional or physical conditions, anxiety disorders can respond well to such self-medication. One of the most effective techniques is physical activity. It's no secret that a good workout or a brisk walk can take the edge off even the most severe anxiety. Scientists once believed that this positive effect was due to the release of natural chemicals known as endorphins. New research, however, has called this idea into question. Regardless, being physically active on a regular basis may well help ease the anxious brain.

Breathing Exercises

One way to quiet the mind is by focusing attention on breathing. Breathing exercises can help calm anxiety by slowing a racing heart and lengthening the short, shallow breaths of a panic attack.

Lifestyle Changes

If all else fails, go back to basics and try cleaning up your lifestyle. For starters, you can cut back on sugar and caffeine. Ask yourself: Am I eating right and getting enough physical activity, sleep, and time to relax? ■

Generalized Anxiety Disorder

What it is: Excessive anxiety or worry, occurring regularly for at least six months.
What it isn't: Occasional serious worry that doesn't noticeably decrease quality of life.

Specific Phobia

What it is: Intense and exaggerated fear of a specific situation or object, often accompanied by extreme anxiety symptoms.
What it isn't: Strong dislike of certain places or things.

Panic Disorder

What it is: Recurrent, unexpected attacks of acute anxiety, peaking within 10 minutes. Such panic may occur in a familiar situation, such as a crowded elevator.
What it isn't: Occasional episodes of extreme anxiety in response to a real threat.

TIME TO THINK...

About Coping with Anxiety

People suffer from many different types of anxiety. This article mentions one specific example: blood phobia. Think of another kind of anxiety that a person might have. Now imagine that you are a behavioral therapist. Write down a step-by-step treatment plan for your patient's anxiety, using the method described in this article. Share your plan with the rest of the class.

PUT STRESS IN ITS PLACE

Model

Teens experience many different and often conflicting emotions. These sudden emotional changes can become a source of stress. Read about a teen named A.J., who is trying to deal with many emotions at once.

A.J. has been friends with Paige for many years. Recently, he began to think of her as more than a friend. He wanted to tell her about his feelings but was afraid he might lose her friendship if he did. Then he found out that she was interested in another boy, Malcolm. Now he feels even more conflicting emotions. He still likes Paige and is happy when he's with her, but he feels angry about her feelings for Malcolm. He also feels jealous of Malcolm.

A.J. knows that he can't change his emotions, but he can deal with the stress they are causing in his life. He tries to think positively and keep matters in perspective. Paige is still his friend, and he is lucky to have her in his life. He also knows that Paige may not always like Malcolm as much as she does now. In the meantime he tries to ease the stress by spending time on activities he enjoys, such as listening to music. He also talks to other friends about his problems. This helps him feel better.

Practice

The physical changes of adolescence can be a source of stress for teens. Rapid physical changes can lead to problems with body image, causing anxiety and low self-esteem. Read the scenario below, and answer the questions that follow. Compare answers with your classmates. How many stress-management skills can you suggest?

Kelsey spends a lot of time looking in the mirror and worrying about her appearance. She feels that her feet are too big, her legs are too long, and her mouth is too small. Kelsey's mom keeps telling her, "You're beautiful the way you are." Kelsey knows that she has some attractive features, but she just can't seem to feel comfortable with her changing appearance.

1. What is the cause of Kelsey's stress?
2. Suggest three ways Kelsey can manage her stress.

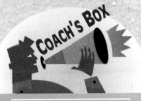

Stress Management

Ways to manage stress include:
- Relaxing
- Connecting with others
- Keeping a positive outlook
- Staying physically active
- Managing your time

Apply/Assess

Use what you've learned about emotional stress to develop a TV or radio announcement. Your announcement should tell teens what they need to know about managing emotional stress. Work with a small group to write an announcement between 30 and 60 seconds long. Describe some common emotions that teens experience, and explain how they can cause stress. Then suggest some strategies for coping with stress. If you have access to video or recording equipment, tape your announcement to demonstrate these strategies for other students.

Self-√ Check

- Does our announcement describe emotions that teens experience?
- Do we explain how emotions can lead to stress?
- Do we suggest ways to manage stress?

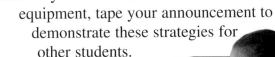

After You Read

Use your completed Foldable to review the information on self-concept, self-esteem, and personality.

FOLDABLES™
Study Organizer

Reviewing Vocabulary and Concepts

On a sheet of paper, write the numbers 1–7. After each number, write the term from the list that best completes each sentence.

- self-concept
- empathy
- resilience
- anxiety
- personality
- panic
- mental and emotional health

Lesson 1

1. Your _____ is the unique combination of feelings, thoughts, and behavior that makes you different from everyone else.

2. Your self-esteem is closely related to your _____.

3. A positive outlook is a sign of _____.

Lesson 2

4. Your ability to bounce back from disappointments and difficulties is called _____.

5. Dizziness and a pounding heart can accompany _____.

6. If you understand and share another person's feelings, you have _____.

7. _____ is an overwhelming feeling of dread, much like fear.

On a sheet of paper, write the numbers 8–15. Write *True* or *False* for each statement below. If the statement is false, change the underlined word or phrase to make it true.

Lesson 3

8. <u>Mood disorders</u> are a variety of psychological conditions that affect a person's ability to get along with others.

9. A person with <u>anxiety</u> loses contact with reality.

10. One of the warning signs of suicide is giving away <u>valued possessions</u>.

11. <u>Phobia</u> is an intense and exaggerated fear of a specific object or situation.

12. Bipolar disorder and depression are examples of <u>therapy</u>.

Lesson 4

13. There are two broad types of <u>therapy</u>, or treatment, for mental health problems.

14. A mental health professional who is trained and licensed by the state to counsel is a <u>hospice caregiver</u>.

15. The only kind of mental health professional who can prescribe drugs is a <u>psychiatrist</u>.

Lesson 5

On a sheet of paper, write the numbers 16 and 17. After each number, write the letter of the answer that best completes each statement.

16. Which of the following cares for the terminally ill?
    a. resilience
    b. hospice
    c. mood disorders
    d. heredity

17. What is the term for a person who teaches people coping strategies to deal with grief?
    a. therapist
    b. psychiatrist
    c. psychologist
    d. grief counselor

Thinking Critically

Using complete sentences, answer the following questions on a sheet of paper.

18. **Relate** How is self-esteem related to self-motivation?
19. **Hypothesize** What are some ways you can show resilience that set an example for younger students to follow?
20. **Compare** How are anxiety disorders and mood disorders similar and different?

Career Corner

Mental Health Counselor Do you enjoy helping others solve personal problems? Then you might consider a career as a mental health counselor. These professionals have four years of college and a two-year advanced degree in counseling. They must also have supervised counseling experience to become licensed. Learn more by clicking on Career Corner at health.glencoe.com.

Standardized Test Practice

Math

Read the paragraph below and then answer the questions.

Teens who are severely depressed might consider suicide as a way out. What can you do to help someone before he or she reaches this point? Be aware of signs such as changes in sleeping and eating patterns and withdrawal from family and friends and activities that were once enjoyed. Tell the person that you care and listen to him or her. Encourage the person to get professional help.

1. Suicide is the third leading cause of death in the United States among people ages 15 to 24. In 1990, about 13 out of every 100,000 people in this age group committed suicide. According to this ratio, how many young people in a group of 525,000 young people would commit suicide? Use a proportion to solve.

   (A) 9 young people
   (B) 24 young people
   (C) 53 young people
   (D) 68 young people

2. Out of a group of 498 troubled young people, suppose 67 percent of them got counseling and medical help. How many of these young people received needed help?

   (A) 33 young people
   (B) 164 young people
   (C) 334 young people
   (D) 378 young people

3. What is meant by the statement that four times as many young males commit suicide as females, but young females attempt suicide four times more frequently than males?

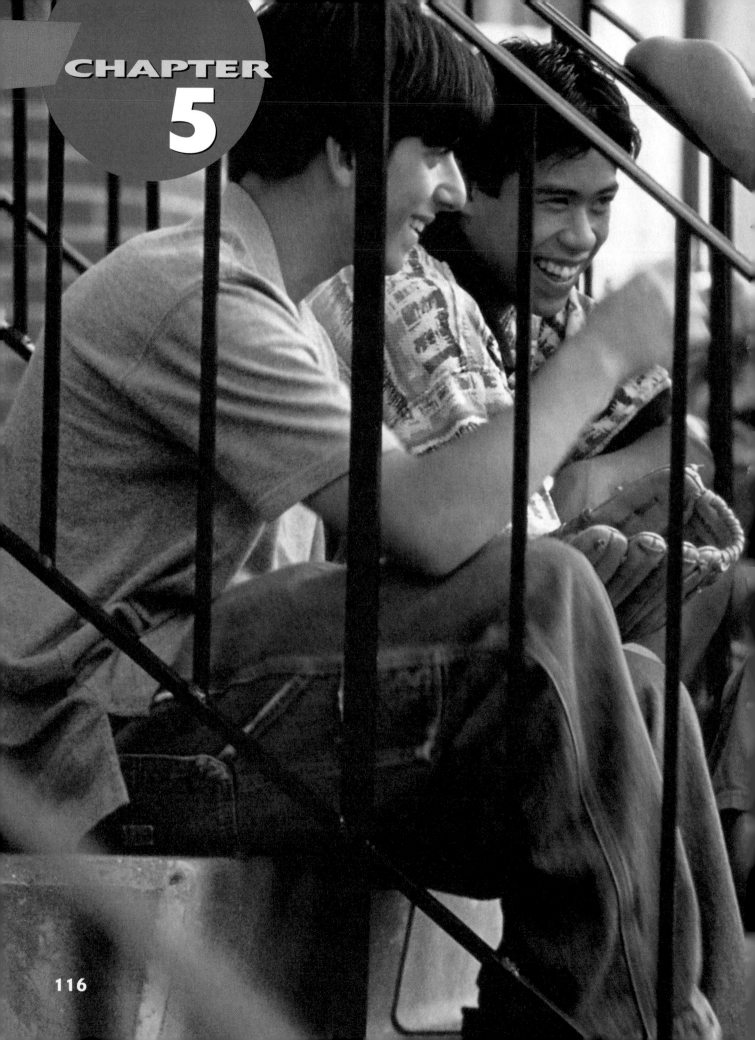

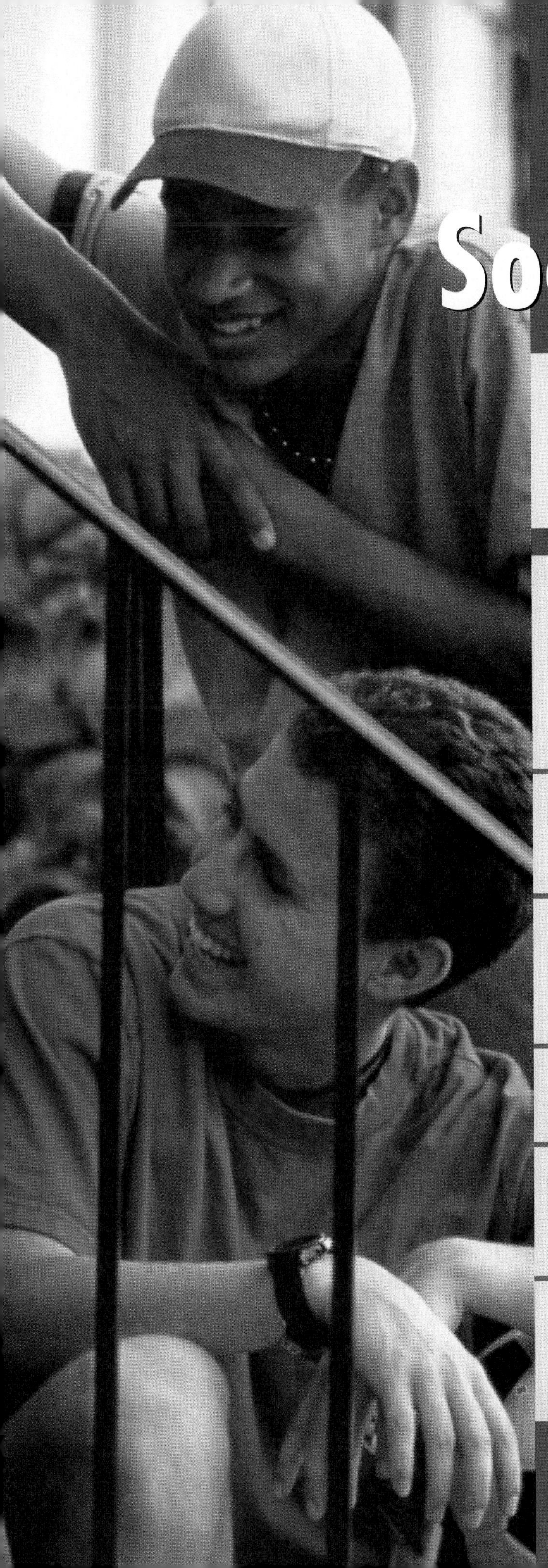

Promoting Social Health

HEALTH *Online*

Do you have a strong character? Find out by taking the Health Inventory for Chapter 5 at health.glencoe.com.

FOLDABLES™
Study Organizer

Before You Read

Make this Foldable to record what you learn in Lesson 1 about the six traits of good character. Begin with a plain sheet of 11″ × 17″ paper.

Step 1

Fold a sheet of paper into thirds along the short axis. This forms three columns.

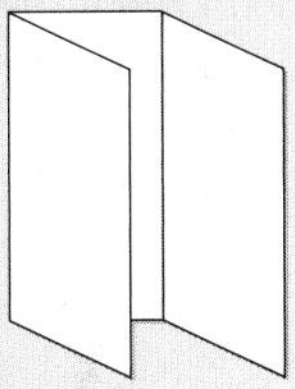

Step 2

Open the paper and fold it in half along the long axis. Fold in half lengthwise two more times to form eight rows.

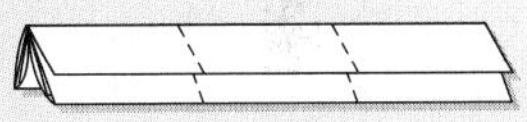

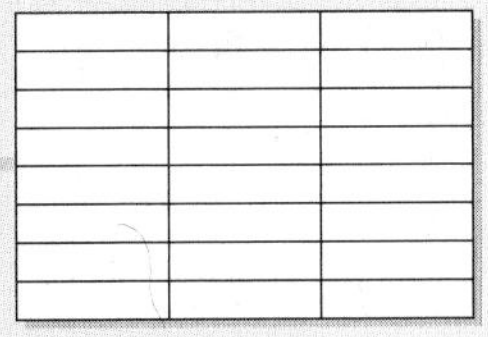

Step 3

Unfold and draw lines along the folds.

Step 4

Label the chart as shown.

Character Trait	My Traits	Others' Traits
Trustworthiness		
Respect		
Responsibility		
Fairness		
Caring		
Citizenship		
Additional Notes		

As You Read

Analyze and write about your own character traits and those of people you admire in the appropriate column of the chart.

Your Character and Your Relationships

Quick Write

Make a list of the qualities that you look for in a friend. How do you demonstrate those qualities to your friends?

LEARN ABOUT...

- different types of relationships.
- why character is important to relationships.
- the traits of good character.
- ways to demonstrate good character.
- ways to strengthen relationships.

VOCABULARY

- social health
- relationships
- character
- values
- character trait
- citizenship

Different Kinds of Relationships

One side of your health triangle is social health. **Social health** is *your ability to get along with the people around you.* Your social health is tied directly to your relationships. **Relationships** are *the connections you have with other people and groups in your life.*

People have many different kinds of relationships. As a teen, your relationships are mainly with family, friends, and peers. As you get older, you will develop other relationships, such as those you form at work.

A relationship with one person is distinct from those with others. For instance, you might have a closer bond with one cousin than with another cousin whom you don't see as often. No matter what kinds of relationships you have, they should be healthy and based on strong character traits.

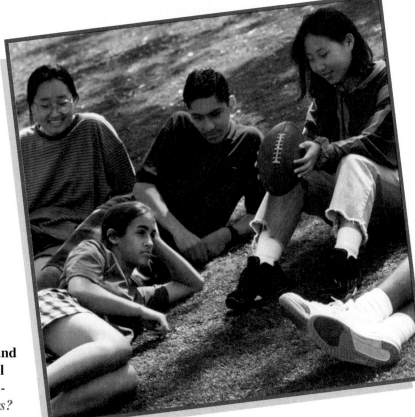

Your relationships with family and friends contribute to your overall social health. *How can you demonstrate positive actions toward others?*

Character—The Foundation of Relationships

How would you describe your character? **Character** is *the way in which a person thinks, feels, and acts.* Character is essential to all of your relationships and to your overall social health. It is the foundation of relationships. The greatest influence on the kinds of relationships you have with other people is your own character.

Whom do you enjoy spending time with? Whom do you trust in your everyday life? Perhaps you trust your parents or other family members, your friends, your teacher, and even your school bus driver. Why do you trust these people? Most likely, you trust them because, through their behavior and actions, they show that they understand, care about, and act upon what they believe is important.

Character, then, is concerned with understanding, caring about, and acting upon certain values. **Values** are *the beliefs and ideals that guide the way a person lives.* Certain core ethical values, such as trust, respect, responsibility, and fairness, are shared by people around the world.

What Is Good Character?

Many different character traits contribute to good character. A **character trait** is *a quality that demonstrates how a person thinks, feels, and acts.* **Figure 5.1** on the next page shows six primary traits of good character.

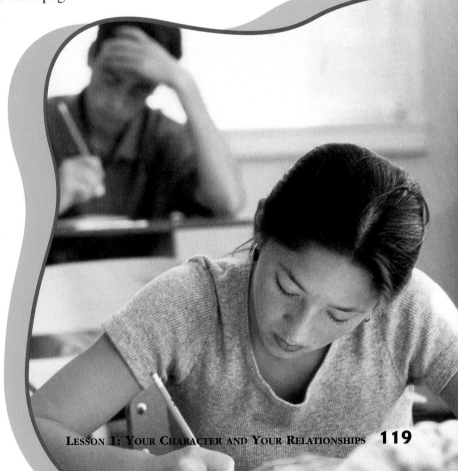

Your values guide your behavior and actions. By not cheating on tests or lying to your parents, you show that you are honest. *What are some other ways you show that you can be trusted?*

FIGURE 5.1

Traits of GOOD Character

A person with these traits has good character. *How do you demonstrate these character traits?*

Trustworthiness

A trustworthy person is honest, loyal, and reliable. He or she has the courage to do the right thing and doesn't deceive, cheat, or steal.

What you might hear: "I know that you can talk to the P.E. coach. She never lets me down."

Respect

Showing respect means being considerate of others and tolerant of differences. It also means using good manners and dealing peacefully with anger or disagreements. You make decisions that show you respect your health and the health of others. You treat people and property with care.

What you might hear: "I'm getting along better with my parents since I stopped talking back to them."

Responsibility

Showing responsibility means using self-control, thinking before you act, and being accountable for your choices. It also involves doing what is expected of you and always doing your best.

What you might hear: "I'm calling to let you know I'll be late."

Fairness

Being fair means playing by the rules and practicing good sportsmanship. Fairness also involves taking turns, sharing, and being open-minded.

What you might hear: "We've been using this basketball court for a while now. Why don't we let those other kids have a turn?"

Caring

A caring person is kind and compassionate. If you care about others, you are sensitive to their needs.

What you might hear: "She's my friend, so I'm going to be there to listen when she needs me."

Citizenship

The way you conduct yourself as a member of a community is called **citizenship**. Showing good citizenship means doing your part to advocate for a safe and healthy school and community. It also involves obeying the rules and laws and respecting authority.

What you might hear: "We recycle in our house—I know my efforts can make a difference."

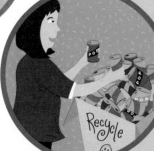

Character and Your Health

Your character affects all three sides of your health triangle—your physical, mental/emotional, and social health. Respecting yourself, for example, helps your physical health because you take care of your body by eating nutritious foods and keeping physically active. When you act responsibly and consider consequences, you protect your physical health by staying safe. Being kind and generous and helping people in need enhances your mental/emotional health because you feel good about yourself. When you treat people with respect and compassion, you get along well with others and improve your social health.

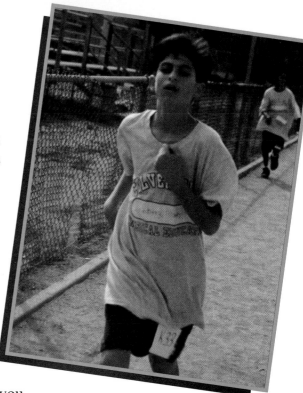

Character in Action

When you demonstrate good character traits, you promote not only your own health but also the health of other people. In addition, demonstrating good character through your actions is an acceptable method of gaining attention. You can make a difference in all areas of your life—at home, at school, and in your community.

When you practice healthful behaviors such as jogging, you show that you care about your health. *How can you show that you care about the health of others?*

HEALTH SKILLS ACTIVITY

DECISION MAKING

A Matter of Character

Jay met Brian a few months ago when Brian first moved into town, and the two teens hit it off right away. Today, Brian came over to Jay's house to work on a social studies report. When Jay suggested that they start with an outline, Brian said, "Hey, there's a much easier way to do this." Then he described how they could go on the Internet and find anything they might need on a subject without having to write the report themselves.

Jay likes Brian, but he knows that this is cheating and it's wrong. Besides, he could get in trouble if he goes along and his teacher finds out.

WHAT WOULD YOU DO?

Apply the six steps of decision making to Jay's situation. What are the possible outcomes? How might Jay's decision affect other people? How could he use this situation to demonstrate good character?

1. STATE THE SITUATION.
2. LIST THE OPTIONS.
3. WEIGH THE POSSIBLE OUTCOMES.
4. CONSIDER VALUES.
5. MAKE A DECISION AND ACT.
6. EVALUATE THE DECISION.

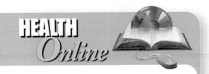
When people care about their community, everyone benefits. *How do you show that you care for others in your community?*

Making a Difference at Home

How do you demonstrate good character at home? You can show that you are responsible by getting up on time in the morning and telling your parents where you will be when you go out. You can also settle disagreements with your brother or sister without arguing. Doing your household tasks without being told and keeping your room neat are good ways to demonstrate responsibility at home. When you remember a family member's birthday or help make dinner, you show that you care about others.

Making a Difference at School

At school, you demonstrate good citizenship by understanding and following school rules and respecting teachers and other adults. You show caring by not bullying or harassing others. If you play a school sport, you can demonstrate fairness by being a responsible team player and a good sport. Refusing to use tobacco, alcohol, and other drugs shows that you are trustworthy.

Making a Difference in Your Community

There are many ways to demonstrate good character in your community. Some teens make a difference by participating in walkathons and supporting food drives. Many teens find ways to volunteer their time for such programs as the Special Olympics. By greeting your neighbors in a friendly manner or helping an older neighbor with her groceries, you show that you're a caring person. By reporting suspicious behavior and keeping a watchful eye on your neighborhood, you can help prevent crime and be ready to assist others.

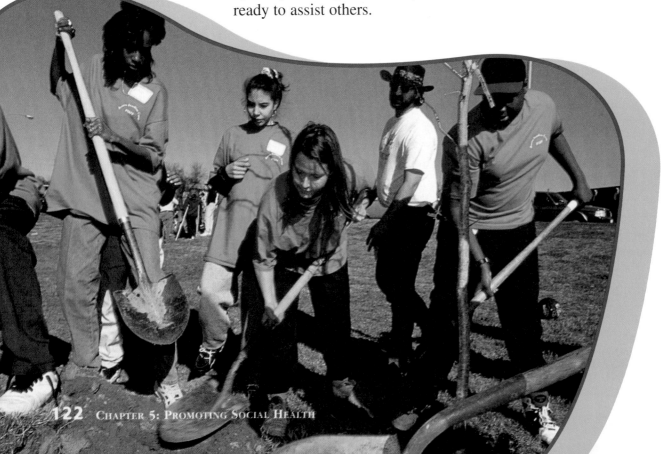

Strengthening Relationships

The best way to build the foundation of healthy relationships is to demonstrate good character traits. Here are some ways to work on improving your relationships:

- **Show respect.** Use good manners and treat others kindly. Avoid directing demeaning statements (those that are meant to insult a person) toward others.
- **Use open and honest communication skills.** By communicating, you get to really know another person's ideas and beliefs. Communication also enables you to share your thoughts and feelings and to have a good time with someone else.
- **Spend quality time and share common interests.** Plan fun outings based on common interests, such as bike riding, hiking, or seeing a movie.
- **Demonstrate affection and admiration in healthful ways.** Let friends and family members know that you care about them and appreciate them. Give compliments and encouragement.
- **Understand and accept individual differences.** No two people are exactly alike. Good social health involves accepting people of different ages, religions, and ethnic and cultural groups. It also involves respecting people who have physical impairments, behavior disorders, or learning disabilities. Understanding and accepting individual differences will help you interact effectively with many different people. This, in turn, can help you form rewarding relationships.

Lesson 1 Review

Using complete sentences, answer the following questions on a sheet of paper.

Reviewing Terms and Facts

1. **Vocabulary** Define the term *relationship*. Use it in an original sentence.
2. **List** Name the six basic traits of good character.
3. **Give Examples** What are three ways to show good character at school?
4. **Summarize** Give four examples of ways to strengthen relationships.

Thinking Critically

5. **Evaluate** How can understanding and accepting individual differences help you interact effectively with many different people? Give two examples.
6. **Apply** Think of three school rules related to health. Why is it important to understand and follow these rules? How does this show good character?

Applying Health Skills

7. **Advocacy** Demonstrate how showing good character is an acceptable method of gaining attention. With a classmate, write a skit involving one or more of the traits of good character illustrated in Figure 5.1 on page 120. Perform your skit for the class.

Getting Along with Your Family

Quick Write

Jot down all the words that come to mind when you think of your family. What have you learned from your family members?

LEARN ABOUT...

- how families meet each other's physical, mental/emotional, and social needs.
- changes that affect families.
- ways to strengthen family bonds.

VOCABULARY

- family
- extended family
- stepparent
- blended family

The Importance of Families

What activities do you enjoy doing with your family? Perhaps you enjoy camping, biking, or playing board games. As humans, we need to feel that we belong to a group. Although you will belong to many groups in your lifetime, the first group to which you belong is your family. The **family** is *the basic unit of society.*

Families come in all shapes and sizes. Your immediate family consists of you, your parents or guardians, and any brothers and sisters. Your **extended family** is *your immediate family plus other relatives such as grandparents, aunts, uncles, and cousins.*

Members of a family have special emotional bonds with one another. The family provides for the health and safety of its members. It is also responsible for teaching them values, or right from wrong. The family provides emotional support for its members.

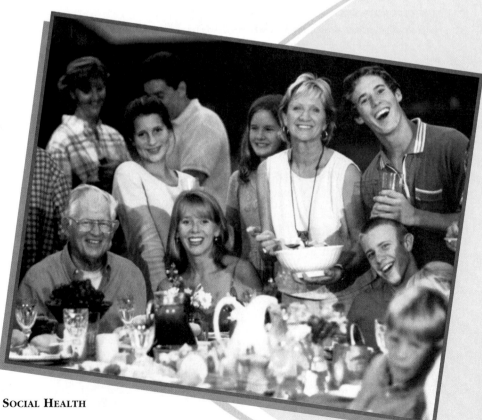

This extended family gets together for a reunion every summer. *What other family traditions can you describe?*

Functions of the Family

One of the most important roles of the family is to meet the physical, mental/emotional, and social needs of its members. **Figure 5.2** shows how families accomplish these essential tasks.

Practicing health-promoting behaviors with the family, such as preparing nutritious meals together or going for a walk after dinner, improves the health of each family member. This in turn strengthens the health of the family unit. Another role of the family is to support and encourage other family members to practice positive health behaviors. For example, parents or older siblings may help younger children brush their teeth and choose nutritious snacks. Families also keep and build traditions. Sharing celebrations and traditions strengthens family bonds.

FIGURE 5.2

Families and the Health Triangle

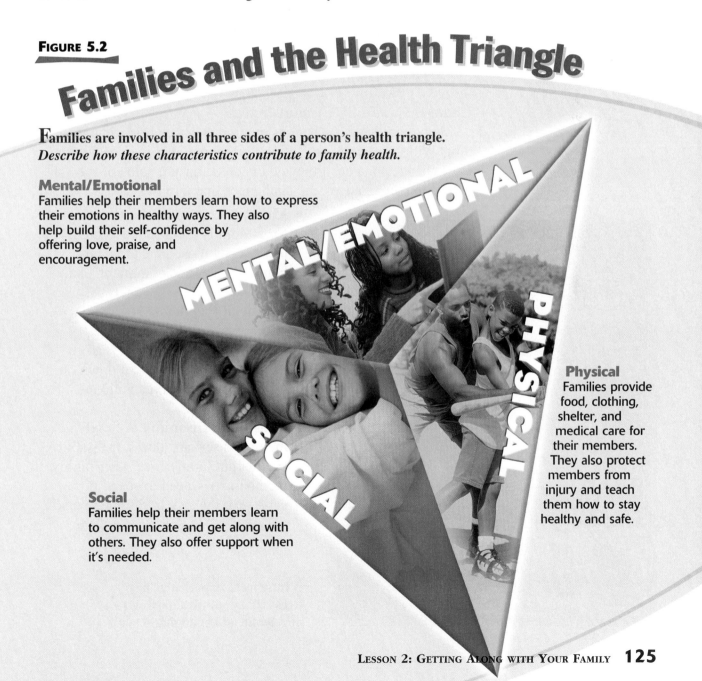

Families are involved in all three sides of a person's health triangle. *Describe how these characteristics contribute to family health.*

Mental/Emotional
Families help their members learn how to express their emotions in healthy ways. They also help build their self-confidence by offering love, praise, and encouragement.

MENTAL/EMOTIONAL

PHYSICAL

SOCIAL

Physical
Families provide food, clothing, shelter, and medical care for their members. They also protect members from injury and teach them how to stay healthy and safe.

Social
Families help their members learn to communicate and get along with others. They also offer support when it's needed.

✔

Reading Check

Contrast types of families. Look over the family structures described on this page. What are some of the ways families differ?

Changes in the Family

Change is a normal part of life, and it affects all families. A family may experience changes in structure and in circumstances. Some of these changes can be stressful.

Changes in Family Structure

In recent years, the structure of American families has been changing. Here are some of the trends affecting families:

- **More single-parent families.** More than one-fourth of all children live with only one parent.
- **More divorces.** Compared to the past, divorces occur more frequently today. This change in family structure can pose many challenges for family members.
- **More blended families.** The increase in the number of divorces and remarriages has created more blended families. A **stepparent** is *someone who marries a child's mother or father.* A **blended family** is *a family that consists of a parent, a stepparent, and the children of one or both parents.*

Changes in Family Circumstances

Many families face changes in circumstances from time to time. With good communication, family members can deal with most changes in a healthy way. Listed below are some of the most common changes and challenges that families face:

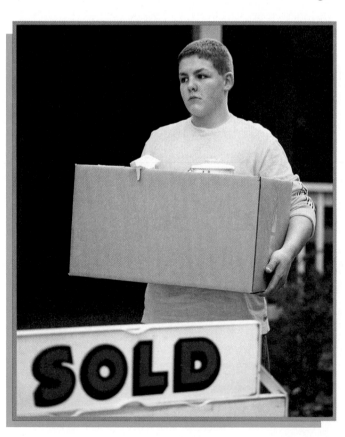

- **Moving.** A move can be stressful for all family members, especially teens. They must adjust to a new home, school, and community, and make new friends.
- **Financial Problems.** For a variety of reasons, a family may have trouble making ends meet. Family members may need to cut down on expenses and take on additional responsibilities.
- **Illness and Disability.** A family member's serious illness or disability can disrupt family life. Other family members may need to spend time caring for the sick or disabled person.

Many teens experience the stress that goes with moving to a new home and changing schools.

- **Unemployment.** Sometimes a parent loses his or her job. If that parent provided the family's main or sole income, family members may have to change their way of living.
- **Substance Abuse.** A family member may become dependent on, or addicted to, alcohol or other drugs. This person's addiction may cause tension and stress for other family members.
- **Physical Abuse.** More than three children die every day as a result of parental abuse. More than three-fourths of those who die are under five years old.

A teen may need to seek assistance to cope effectively with some of these changes. For example, someone who is being physically abused should tell a parent or other trusted adult who is part of his or her support system. The teen may require professional counseling to cope with this situation.

Hands-On Health

POSITIVE FAMILY INTERACTIONS

Children and teens can do their part to help support positive family interactions. Encouraging the family to spend time together and improving communication among family members are two good ways to do this.

WHAT YOU WILL NEED
- pencil or pen
- several sheets of paper

WHAT YOU WILL DO
1. In groups of three or four, brainstorm ideas for keeping family members informed about what is happening in one another's lives and for spending quality time together. Have one person record your group's ideas on a sheet of paper. A few examples are: eat at least one meal together every week, schedule regular family meetings, have a family movie or game night, plan family outings.

2. Write a skit that demonstrates ways in which children and teens can help support positive family interactions. Include the communication and activity ideas that your group came up with. Create a role for each member of your group. Then perform your skit for the class.

IN CONCLUSION
1. Think about the ways you and your family communicate. Do you think you set aside enough time to talk things over? Identify and write down the obstacles to good communication in your family. How could you improve communication within your family?
2. Make a plan to implement one of your communication or activity ideas with your family. Discuss it with your family members. Then make it happen.

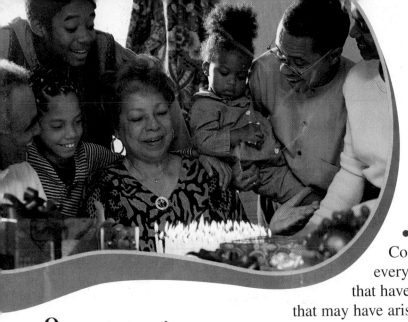

Coping with Family Changes

Use these effective strategies to strengthen the family unit and cope with family changes:

- **Show respect.** Show consideration for family members. Be honest and follow through on your promises.
- **Share your thoughts and feelings.** Communicate with your family members every day. Tell them about the good things that have happened, as well as any problems that may have arisen. Ask for help if you need it and be a good listener if someone else has a problem.
- **Show that you support and value all family members.** Compliment family members on a job well done. Tell them that you appreciate them. Offer to help when needed.
- **Accept responsibility.** Do your household tasks without being reminded. Complete self-initiated activities beyond assigned chores to help support your family. For example, do the dishes without being asked.
- **Safely demonstrate care and concern toward an ill family member.** Make an effort to spend time with the person. Help out caregivers by taking over some of their household tasks.

One way to strengthen the family is to share special events with family members. *For each of the bulleted suggestions on the right, give an example.*

Lesson 2 Review

Using complete sentences, answer the following questions on a sheet of paper.

Reviewing Terms and Facts

1. **Recall** What are three changes in family structure that affect families?
2. **Explain** What is the difference between an extended family and a blended family?
3. **List** Give three examples of common changes and challenges that families may face.

Thinking Critically

4. **Apply** Give two examples of health-promoting behaviors that you could practice with your family.

5. **Hypothesize** What strategies might a teen use to effectively cope with a serious change within the family, such as an older sibling's substance abuse?
6. **Analyze** Describe characteristics and actions that contribute to family health.

Applying Health Skills

7. **Analyzing Influences** With a group of classmates, compile a list of traditions and rituals that families might share. Discuss your list. Which of the traditions and rituals does your family take part in? How do each of the traditions enhance a family's sense of unity?

Marriage and Parenthood

Marriage

At some point in their lives, the majority of adult Americans will decide to marry. Marriage is a serious, long-term commitment. A **commitment** is *a pledge or a promise.*

Reasons for Marrying

Most people decide to marry because they are in love. Marriage involves more than just love, however. Getting married shows that two people have made a commitment to live together and care for each other for the rest of their lives.

In addition to love, people get married for other important reasons. Many people who want to have a family feel that marriage is a stable environment in which to raise children. Most people enjoy the companionship and comfort that marriage brings. Some make choices based on religious beliefs. Being married also brings certain financial benefits.

Quick Write

Make a list of the words that come to mind when you think of parents and children. Compare your list with those of your classmates.

LEARN ABOUT...

- why people marry and the factors that affect marriage.
- the responsibilities involved in being a parent.
- the consequences of being a teen parent.

VOCABULARY

- commitment
- adjustment
- divorce
- parenting
- unconditional love

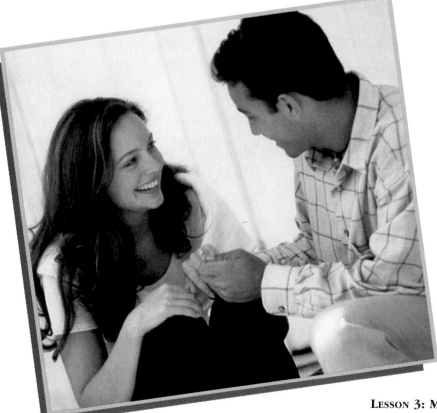

Couples who are ready to marry have a strong commitment to each other. *Why do you think that commitment is so important?*

Reading Check

Write three to five words or phrases from these pages that fit under the heading *What Helps Marriages Succeed?* Then write three to five words or phrases that fit under the heading *Causes of Problems in Marriages.*

Factors Affecting Marriage

What makes a marriage successful? One of the most important factors is emotional maturity. Emotionally mature people bring commitment and effort to a marriage. They try to understand their partner's needs and are willing to make any necessary adjustments. An **adjustment** is *an adaptation or change in behavior.* In addition to emotional maturity, several other factors help a marriage succeed:

- **Good communication.** As with any relationship, good communication is essential in a marriage. Couples need to be able to share their feelings, needs, and concerns.
- **Similar values.** Sharing values such as the importance of good health, religious beliefs, cultural pride, family, and friendships brings two people closer. A couple is more likely to stay together if they hold the same values.
- **Realistic expectations.** Issues involving such things as money, children, and where to live can cause disagreements in a marriage. Solving problems as a couple and learning to compromise gives the marriage a better chance of success.
- **Similar interests.** Sharing interests such as physical activity, nutrition, and travel can help a couple spend more time together. This, in turn, can strengthen the bond of marriage.

Problems in a Marriage

Even the strongest marriage occasionally has problems. Because no two people are exactly alike, no married couple will ever agree on every issue. There is a difference, however, between couples who sometimes disagree on minor issues and those who continually disagree on major issues. Examples of major issues that may cause problems include money, work, whether to have children, how to raise children, and how to spend free time. Some couples seek counseling to help them with their problems. If married people can't resolve their problems, however, they may decide that separation or divorce is the right choice. A **divorce** is *a legal end to a marriage contract.*

Teen Marriages

More than 60 percent of teen marriages end in divorce within five years. The main reason so many teen marriages fail is that the two people are usually too young to understand what is

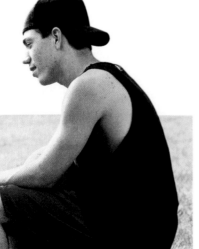

This couple thought they were ready for marriage, but they now realize they are too young to make the commitment. *What are some factors couples should talk about before they consider marriage?*

important to them. In addition, many teens marry because of an unplanned pregnancy. Caring for a baby is a serious responsibility. It puts a great deal of stress on a teen marriage that may have already been fragile.

Choosing Parenthood

After getting married, many couples decide to start a family. Parenthood can be a wonderful experience, and most parents find great joy in loving and caring for a child. They watch with pride as the child grows and develops.

A parent is the mother or father of a child. Being a parent is not the same as parenting, however. **Parenting** means *the process of meeting a child's physical, mental/emotional, and social needs.* Many people, including grandparents, aunts and uncles, and baby-sitters, use parenting skills.

Responsibilities of Parenthood

Parenthood can be rewarding, but it can also be very challenging. Parents are responsible for helping their children become happy, productive, and caring individuals. They need qualities such as patience, understanding, and a sense of humor. Parents have an obligation to give their children the necessary love and care.

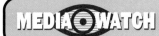

MARRIAGE ON TV

Think about the characters on some of your favorite television sitcoms. Consider how the married couples are portrayed. Identify the qualities that you think make a strong marriage and explain your choices.

HEALTH SKILLS ACTIVITY

ANALYZING INFLUENCES

Identifying Role Models

People learn parenting skills by watching how other people act with their own children. That is why it's so important to have role models who can demonstrate good parenting techniques. Here are some ways that role models might show the qualities of good parenting.

- Provide children with nutritious foods, clean clothes, and adequate shelter.
- Make sure that children get enough physical activity, plenty of rest, and good medical care.
- Stimulate children's thinking and learning abilities, and help them get a good education.
- Teach children how to make responsible decisions and solve problems.
- Give children unconditional love and make them feel accepted and valued.
- Teach children right from wrong, how to get along with others, and how to care for others.

ON YOUR OWN
Write a letter to your future child. Explain what you would do to meet the child's needs and be a good parent.

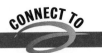

CONNECT TO

Science

HIGH-RISK BABIES
Babies born to teen mothers are more likely to be born prematurely, or too early. This means that many of the babies will be born at a low birth weight, which increases the risk of mental retardation, blindness, and deafness. *What are some ways to publicize this information so that more teens would be aware of the risks?*

One of the most important responsibilities of parenthood is to provide unconditional love for a child. **Unconditional love** is *love without limitation or qualification.* In other words, the child is loved regardless of whether he or she is good or bad, happy or cranky, healthy or sick. A child who receives unconditional love is more likely to grow into a caring, well-adjusted adult.

Teen Parenthood

Each year in the United States, more than half a million babies are born to teen mothers. About 79 percent of these teen mothers are not married. Some teens want a baby so that they'll have someone to love who loves them back. Most of these teens, however, don't realize how demanding a baby can be. Many overlook the fact that raising a child is a full-time and long-term commitment.

Risks of Teen Parenthood

Teen pregnancy and parenthood create health risks for both the young mother and the baby. A female teen's body is still developing and may not be completely ready to support and nourish an unborn child. Many pregnant teens do not get adequate nutrients, which can be unhealthy for both the teen and the baby.

Because teen mothers are themselves young, they may not know how to take care of themselves during pregnancy. For example, many pregnant teens receive inadequate prenatal care. As a result, children born to teen mothers are more likely to have low birth weights, which can lead to serious health problems as the baby grows and develops.

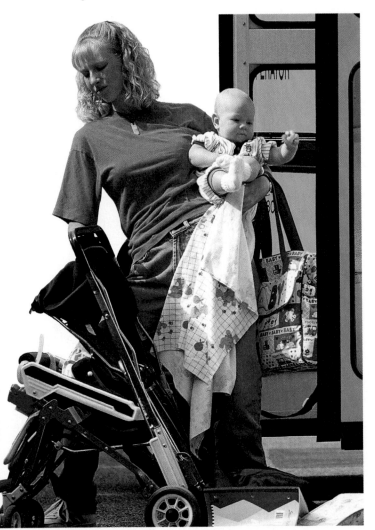

Raising a child is challenging for any parent but especially so for a teen who is not prepared to handle the financial and emotional responsibilities. *What challenges might this teen face?*

Consequences of Teen Parenthood

Parenthood is a challenging task for anyone. For teen parents, however, the task is especially difficult. Teen parents generally lack money, education, and emotional maturity. For them, parenthood creates consequences in nearly every aspect of their lives:

- **Financial problems.** Raising a child costs a great deal of money. In the first year alone, parents need to buy thousands of dollars worth of baby clothes, food, and supplies. Most teen parents have difficulty meeting even the minimal expenses.
- **Effects on education and career plans.** Teen parents often must put aside their plans for education and a fulfilling career. They may have to quit school to care for their child or to earn money to support the child. Teens without a high school diploma have limited career choices and little chance of getting a well-paying job.
- **Emotional stress.** During adolescence, teens struggle to discover who they are and where they fit in. Coping with the normal anxieties of adolescence is challenging enough for many teens. Adding the responsibility of caring for a baby creates even more stress.
- **Effects on personal and social life.** Parenting is a time-consuming job. Teen parents will have less time to spend with their friends, or they may be too tired for social activities. Many teen parents begin to resent having limited their personal freedom.

Lesson 3 Review

Using complete sentences, answer the following questions on a sheet of paper.

Reviewing Terms and Facts

1. **Vocabulary** Use the term *commitment* in a sentence to show that you understand its meaning.
2. **Explain** In your own words, explain what factors help a marriage succeed.
3. **Summarize** What does *parenting* involve?
4. **Identify** What health risks are associated with teen pregnancy?

Thinking Critically

5. **Evaluate** Why is providing unconditional love one of the important responsibilities of parenting?

6. **Hypothesize** In what ways might a teen's life change if she or he became a parent?

Applying Health Skills

7. **Analyzing Influences** Observe young children and their parents in a public place such as a park, playground, or shopping mall. Notice instances in which the parent uses effective parenting techniques. Keep a list of these techniques and share your findings with your classmates.

Friendly Persuasion

Teens are finding that peer counselors give great advice. Here are three examples.

Changing Lives

Liz Treganowan knows firsthand how much impact one person can have. In sixth grade, she watched a movie on television that changed her life. It was about Ryan White, a teen who contracted HIV, survived the cruel taunts of neighbors, and became an activist before dying of AIDS. "He really inspired me," says Liz, now a high-school student in Boston. "I started educating myself, keeping my eyes peeled for science articles or TV stories about AIDS."

Years later, Liz put her knowledge to work—reaching out to help others learn about the disease (and other STDs) through Boston HAPPENS, a peer-counseling organization based at Boston's Children's Hospital.

Boston HAPPENS trains local teens to speak honestly with their peers about the dangers of STDs and AIDS at health fairs, at schools, and even when they're just hanging out. Liz says

Liz Treganowan

teens often feel more comfortable asking a peer touchy questions. "I'm the same age, so I can relate to their problems much better than an adult or a doctor," she explains.

It's well worth the effort, she says, because she knows she's making a difference. "Boston HAPPENS has given me all these resources and education," she says, "so I feel like I should take a stand."

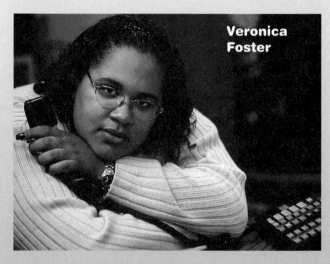

Veronica Foster

Help on the Line

By the time 15-year-old Veronica Foster started manning the phones at Teen Line, a California-based crisis hot line, she'd completed

13 weeks of training. Still, she wasn't entirely prepared for her first call—from a guy who said he was considering ending his life. "He was having problems at home," she recalls. "He felt [suicide] was the only way out."

Veronica was scared. "What if I say the wrong thing?" she wondered. She calmed the caller down, then transferred the call to a professional therapist on duty. A week later, the guy called back to thank Veronica for her help. "That was really gratifying," she says.

Veronica is among the more than 100 teens who answer some 14,000 calls from peers each year about such issues as gang activity and eating disorders. The situation is often intense: One girl called just after her boyfriend physically abused her. Veronica told her how to get help. "I know I made a difference in her life," says Veronica.

Veronica's age makes her an effective counselor, and she's moved up to Teen Line's suicide outreach team. It trains the Los Angeles Police Department in dealing with suicidal youth. Working with Teen Line, she says, has helped her as well as those she's counseled. "Listening to the callers helped me know I wasn't the only one going through problems," she says. "If it weren't for Teen Line, I don't know where I'd be."

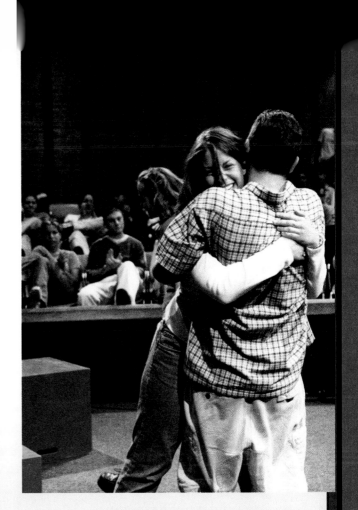

Not Just Playing Around

Coming To Alternative Recovery is a unique theater group that brings its antidrug message to schools around the country. The cast of each Coming To show is made up of teens. These young actors perform dramatic scenes that show other teens how alcohol and drugs can destroy their lives.

The idea is that teens will find their peers' stories more powerful than the same old speeches—and it's working. After each performance, the young cast is surrounded by teens who want to talk and ask more questions. In fact, a Stanford University study of Coming To audiences found that 21 percent of viewers sought more information after seeing the presentation.

That's not to say everyone is so enthusiastic: The performers are often hassled by audience members. However, they have an answer for everything—even the boy who once responded to a performance by yelling, "This is stupid!" Instead of asking "problem kids" to leave, the group members question them onstage about their own behavior. Some audience members have broken down and admitted to being uncomfortable with the performance because they found the antidrug issues confusing. That's when the group shows the person how to get answers. ▰

TIME TO THINK...

About Positive Peer Pressure

You probably hear a lot about negative peer pressure. However, you've also learned that peer pressure can be positive. With your class, brainstorm possible ways that a teen can have a positive influence on his or her peers. Your teacher will list these ideas on the board. Choose one of the ideas and write a short story about how a teen had a positive influence on his or her peers.

SENDING THE RIGHT MESSAGE

Model

Communication is an essential part of a healthy relationship. Read the conversation between Ellen and Chris, two teens who are working together on a health project. Identify the skills that help them communicate their ideas and feelings about what kind of project to do.

USE "I" MESSAGES.
"I think we should look up information on the Internet and write a report."

MAKE CLEAR, SIMPLE STATEMENTS; ASK QUESTIONS.
"Everyone's doing that. Can't we do something different, like a poster?"

BE HONEST WITH THOUGHTS AND FEELINGS; USE "I" MESSAGES.
"I don't draw very well, so I couldn't help much with a poster. Besides, I think it's important to get current information for our project."

MIRROR THOUGHTS AND FEELINGS; USE APPROPRIATE BODY LANGUAGE; USE CONVERSATION ENCOURAGERS.
"You're right, we need current information that's reliable, too. So what if you do the research and decide what to put on the poster?"

"Right! Then you could draw the poster."

"But let's work together to choose the colors and paint it, okay?"

Practice

Practicing your communication skills can make your relationships stronger. Working with a partner, choose one of the following situations. Write a script that shows how you would use communication skills in that situation. When you're finished, act out your script for other students in your class.

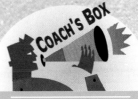

Coach's Box

Communication Skills

Speaking Skills:
- "I" messages
- Clear, simple statements
- Honest thoughts and feelings
- Appropriate body language

Listening Skills:
- Appropriate body language
- Conversation encouragers
- Mirror thoughts and feelings
- Ask questions

> Alec has asked Elizabeth to go to a movie with him. Elizabeth likes Alec, but not as a boyfriend.

> Rosemary asks to borrow Tyra's math homework so she can copy it during study hall. Tyra worked hard on the assignment and doesn't think it's fair for Rosemary to copy her work.

> Sharon tells Lynetta that she thinks their classmate Carlos is "stuck up." Lynetta really likes Carlos and thinks he is very nice. She believes in speaking up for her friends.

Apply/Assess

Demonstrate your communication skills by having a conversation with a classmate. Get together with two partners. Two of you will have a conversation while the third person observes. Before you start, the observer should write down the speaking and listening skills shown in the Coach's Box. Then the other two partners should select a topic from the list below and have a one-minute conversation about it. The observer will check off all the speaking and listening skills that are used in the conversation. When the conversation is over, the observer will report the skills that he or she observed. Hold two more conversations so each person gets to observe.

Self-√Check

- Did we use several communication skills in our conversation?
- Was our conversation an example of good communication?

Topics for conversation:

- My first friend
- Why friendships are important
- What I've learned from my family
- What I look for in a friend
- A funny family story
- What I learned from a friend

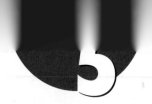

After You Read

Use your completed Foldable to review the information on character traits.

FOLDABLES™
Study Organizer

Reviewing Vocabulary and Concepts

On a sheet of paper, write the numbers 1–9. After each number, write the term from the list that best completes each statement.

- character trait
- character
- blended family
- values
- social health
- stepparent
- extended family
- citizenship
- family

Lesson 1

1. The beliefs and ideals that guide the way a person lives are called _____.
2. A(n) _____ is a quality that demonstrates how a person thinks, feels, and acts.
3. Your ability to get along with the people around you is called your _____.
4. The way you conduct yourself as a member of a community is _____.
5. A person's _____ describes the way in which she or he thinks, feels, and acts.

Lesson 2

6. A(n) _____ consists of a parent, a stepparent, and the children of one or both parents.
7. The basic unit of society is the _____.
8. A(n) _____ is someone who marries a child's mother or father.

9. Parents, two children, aunts, and grandparents is an example of a(n) _____.

Lesson 3

On a sheet of paper, write the numbers 10–15. After each number, write the letter of the answer that best completes each statement.

10. Meeting a child's physical, mental/emotional, and social needs is part of
    a. citizenship.
    b. parenting.
    c. making adjustments.
    d. teen relationships.

11. A legal end to a marriage contract is a(n)
    a. defense mechanism.
    b. arrangement.
    c. character trait.
    d. divorce.

12. A modification in behavior that is a sign of emotional maturity is called a(an)
    a. adjustment.
    b. divorce.
    c. relationship.
    d. character trait.

13. To be a parent, it is important to have
    a. a sense of humor.
    b. understanding.
    c. patience.
    d. all of the above.

14. Which of the following is a consequence of teen parenthood?
    a. more time to spend with friends
    b. financial security
    c. less time to spend with friends
    d. less responsibility

15. One of the most important responsibilities of parenting is to provide a child with
    a. early education opportunities.
    b. unconditional love.
    c. many companions of the same age.
    d. a large house.

Thinking Critically

Using complete sentences, answer the following questions on a sheet of paper.

16. Apply How could you demonstrate care and concern toward an ill family member?

17. Describe What are some strategies to show respect for individual differences, including age differences and differences in ethnic and cultural backgrounds?

18. Analyze How might positive and negative relationships influence community health? Give three examples of positive and negative influences on health in your community.

Career Corner

Social Worker Would you like to help children and families in need? Then a career as a social worker might be for you. Social workers help with problems related to poverty, sickness, and family crises. These professionals may also find foster homes for children or begin legal action in child abuse cases.

To become a social worker, you need a college education and a master's degree in social work. To find out more about this and other health careers, visit the Career Corner at health.glencoe.com.

Standardized Test Practice

Reading & Writing

Read the paragraphs below and then answer the questions.

Whenever my friends and I want to hang out and eat good food, we head to Angelo's, which is just around the corner from school. Angelo's looks like it's been there forever. On the outside is an ancient and dingy sign. Inside are booths with chipped tables and imitation leather seats. On each table are a vase of plastic flowers, a container of grated cheese, and another container of red pepper.

The first thing that greets us when we open the door to Angelo's is the smell of pizza coming from the big brick oven at the back of the restaurant. We usually crowd into one booth and place our order with a patient, but rushed waitress. While we're waiting for our pizza, we talk about school. Some of us like to watch the pizza maker at the back

of the restaurant as he tosses the dough, pours on the sauce, and slides our pizza into the oven.

1. From the description of Angelo's in the passage, the reader can tell that the writer

   Ⓐ never goes to the restaurant.

   Ⓑ is fond of the restaurant.

   Ⓒ goes to the restaurant every day.

   Ⓓ dislikes the restaurant.

2. In the passage, the author uses description to

   Ⓐ give details about the restaurant's location.

   Ⓑ compare the restaurant to others.

   Ⓒ create a picture of the restaurant.

   Ⓓ encourage readers to eat at the restaurant.

3. Write a paragraph describing a place where you or you and your friends feel comfortable.

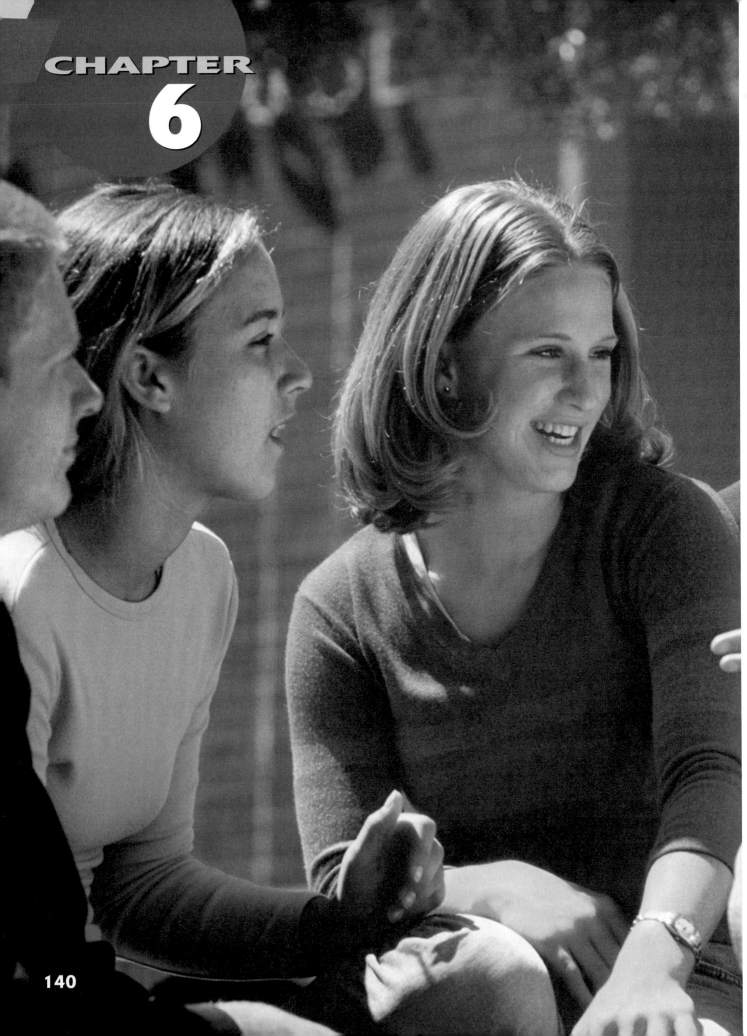

Relationships: The Teen Years

HEALTH *Online*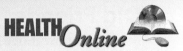

Before you begin Chapter 6, discover how well you rate as a friend. Take the Health Inventory at health.glencoe.com.

FOLDABLES™
Study Organizer

Before You Read

Make this Foldable to help you organize the information about friendships in Lesson 1. Begin with a plain sheet of 11″ × 17″ paper.

Step 1

Fold the short sides of a sheet of paper inward so that they meet in the middle.

Step 2

Fold the top to the bottom.

Step 3

Open and cut along the inside fold lines to form four tabs.

Step 4

Label the tabs as shown.

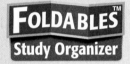

Who	When We Met
What I Admire	Why We're Friends

As You Read

Write down the qualities of a good friendship on the back of the Foldable. Then, describe the Who, What, When, and Why of a close friend under the appropriate tab.

Friendships: Growing and Changing

Quick Write

There's a saying: "To have a friend, you must be a friend." Write what you think this saying means. Give examples.

LEARN ABOUT...

- the qualities of a good friend.
- how to make new friends.
- what a clique is.
- the advantages of group dating.

VOCABULARY

- empathetic
- clique

Old Friends, New Friends

As you now move from childhood into your teen years, life starts to change. Friendships take on greater importance, and relationships with friends become deeper and more complex. You and your friends still talk about having fun, as you did when you were younger. However, you also begin to share thoughts and feelings about more serious matters.

You might also find that during the early teen years, friendships are often very changeable. Someone who was your best friend only a few months ago may not be your friend now. Teens grow and change at different rates, a fact that also affects their relationships. They often develop new interests and look for new friends to share these interests. They may see old friends less often in order to fit into a certain group. Changing relationships are a normal part of growing up.

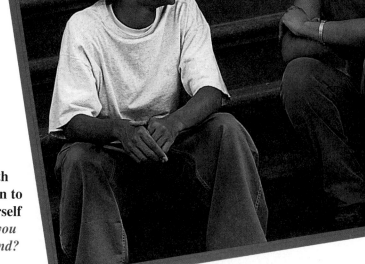

Through your relationships with friends, you learn to understand yourself better. *What do you look for in a friend?*

Qualities of a Good Friendship

All good friends share similar qualities:

- **Trust.** Good friends trust and believe in one another.
- **Reliability.** Good friends know that they can count on each other to keep their word.
- **Empathy.** Good friends are **empathetic** (em·puh·THE·tik), or *able to identify and share another person's feelings.*
- **Caring.** Good friends care for and about each other.
- **Respect.** Good friends respect each other's decisions and opinions.

The Changing Social Scene

Social groups can form and change throughout your life. For example, your school might have students who come from many different neighborhoods. That gives you the opportunity to meet new people and perhaps expand your circle of friends. By interacting with various social groups, you may learn new ideas, understand different perspectives, and gain important skills that will be helpful in adulthood.

Making New Friends

Making new friends is a skill that anyone can learn. Getting acquainted with new people is not easy for everyone, but it gets easier with practice. **Figure 6.1** shows four ways you could make new friends.

Reading Check

Cause and effect relationships. Look for the connection between cause and effect in the paragraphs on these pages.

FIGURE 6.1

Ways to Make New Friends

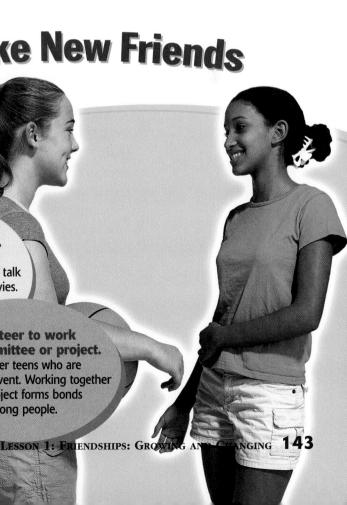

It's important to know and use appropriate ways to make new friends. *Appraise the importance of social groups.*

Join a school club or community group that interests you. Your school and community offer many activities for young people, such as sports teams, volunteer groups, and local plays.

Start a conversation. Ask a question or give a compliment. You can always talk about school, sports, or movies.

Offer to help someone. Show a classmate or neighbor how to solve a problem or fix something. Reaching out to others lets them know that you want to be friends.

Volunteer to work on a committee or project. Join other teens who are planning an event. Working together on a project forms bonds among people.

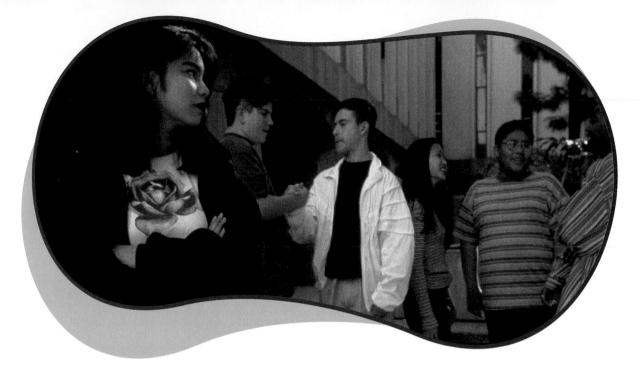

The desire for a sense of belonging is common to all teens. *How do cliques help fill this need? How can they be harmful?*

Cliques

A **clique** is *a group of friends who hang out together and act in similar ways.* Cliques are a common feature of the teen years. Members of a clique usually have certain things in common. For example, they might all play on the same team or belong to the same club or group, or they might all be good students. Membership in a clique is limited. Not everyone who wants to belong can join.

Cliques can have a positive or negative influence. Because most teens have a strong need to belong, they want to feel that they fit into a group. Cliques can help them meet this need. Sometimes teens feel unsure of themselves, and they use a clique to gain approval of what they wear or how they act.

Cliques can become harmful, however, if they pressure members to conform to the group in behavior that may damage their health. Cliques may discourage members from making their own decisions, presenting their own opinions, or having other friends who aren't accepted by the clique. Cliques may even pressure members to act in ways that go against their individual values and beliefs, such as lying to parents or teachers. Cliques can also hurt people outside the group. For example, members might make fun of a teen who isn't in the clique.

If you find yourself under this type of pressure from a clique, here are some actions you can take to improve your situation.

- **Suggest other activities.** Offer ideas that don't involve hurting others or putting anyone at risk.
- **Find new friends.** If staying in the clique is becoming a negative experience, you will be better off with new friends.

Peer Relationships

In your early teen years, your relationships with both boys and girls may be changing. Some teens become interested in spending more time with people they find attractive.

However, not all young teens share these feelings of attraction. They might be shy and uncomfortable when they are around others of the opposite gender without the support of a group of friends. Still other teens have interests—such as sports, clubs, and hobbies—they prefer for the time being. Family customs and values also may influence with whom a teen is permitted to spend time. Whatever your situation, remember that you have options about how you spend your social time and with whom.

Going Out in a Group

Many teens prefer to go out in a mixed group of boys and girls. Going out in a group can be a good way to feel more comfortable with teens of both genders. For example, it may be more comfortable to go to parties, movies, and dances in groups. In those situations, you don't have to worry about making conversation. If you can't think of something to say, someone else in the group almost certainly will keep the conversation going. In a group you get an opportunity to practice social skills, and just being together can be lively and fun, too. **Figure 6.2** shows some ways to have fun with a group.

FIGURE 6.2

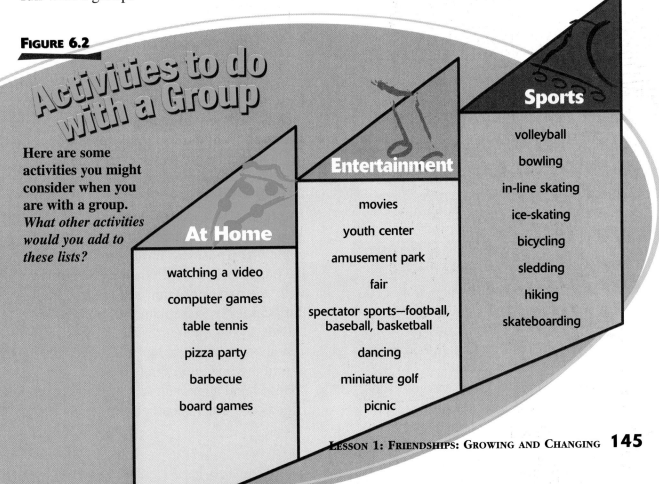

Activities to do with a Group

Here are some activities you might consider when you are with a group. *What other activities would you add to these lists?*

At Home
- watching a video
- computer games
- table tennis
- pizza party
- barbecue
- board games

Entertainment
- movies
- youth center
- amusement park
- fair
- spectator sports—football, baseball, basketball
- dancing
- miniature golf
- picnic

Sports
- volleyball
- bowling
- in-line skating
- ice-skating
- bicycling
- sledding
- hiking
- skateboarding

Individual Dating

Eventually you may begin to develop an interest in one person. Individual dating is a way to get to know that person better. Make sure that you go out on a date because you want to, and not because you feel pressured or because you want to win the approval of friends. This is part of responsible dating.

In a responsible dating relationship, you want to spend time with someone who demonstrates positive qualities. Here are some examples of traits to look for in a dating partner, with examples of actions and words that match those traits:

- **Respect.** "Your musical talents are really great! No wonder you made the choir."
- **Responsibility.** "We should call home and let our parents know that the game ran late, so they won't be worried."
- **Trustworthiness.** "I'll be there because I know how much this speech means to you."
- **Reliability.** "Don't worry—I'll make sure I'm on time so that you don't miss the bus."
- **Caring.** "I saved this seat for Janet because I knew she would be late getting out of practice."
- **Fairness.** "Before we decide to see this movie, let's make sure that the others agree on it."

Lesson 1 Review

Using complete sentences, answer the following questions on a sheet of paper.

Reviewing Terms and Facts

1. **Recall** List four ways to make new friends.
2. **Vocabulary** Define the term *clique*.
3. **Identify** What is the main advantage of going out in a group?

Thinking Critically

4. **Apply** Use the Qualities of a Good Friendship list on page 143 to develop three strategies for monitoring positive and negative peer relationships that influence health.
5. **Suggest** Choose a group activity from each column in Figure 6.2 on page 145.

Describe how you would adapt activities to include a variety of individuals.

6. **Analyze** Why do you think some teens begin dating before they feel they are ready?

Applying Health Skills

7. **Analyzing Influences** Draw four concentric circles (like a target) to represent your circle of friendships. Write your name in the innermost circle. In the second circle write the names of your best friends. In the third circle write the names of your good friends and in the fourth, the names of casual acquaintances. Write a paragraph describing how your circle of friends has changed and appraising the importance of friends and other social groups.

Peer Pressure and Refusal Skills

Recognizing Peer Pressure

Relationships with peers are very important during the teen years. They begin to take on a special role, and as a group, your peers can also have a strong influence on you. **Peer pressure**, *the influence to go along with the beliefs and actions of your peers,* may come from the group either directly or indirectly. It can have a positive or negative effect on decision making.

Positive Peer Pressure

Peer pressure may be positive when it inspires you to do something worthwhile. For example, you may have acting talent but feel afraid to try out for the school play. Pressure from your friends may encourage you to audition for the play. A contest to see which classroom can bring the most canned food for a local charity can also create positive peer pressure. Positive peer pressure uses encouraging words and expressions.

Teens may use positive peer pressure to encourage others to engage in health-promoting behaviors. For example, someone who enjoys jogging may persuade a sedentary friend to try it.

Quick Write

Write a paragraph describing a time when someone your age tried to persuade you to do something that you felt was wrong or risky. Tell how this experience made you feel.

LEARN ABOUT...

- the difference between positive and negative peer pressure.
- the risks of negative peer pressure.
- how to develop and use refusal skills and assertiveness.

VOCABULARY

- peer pressure
- refusal skills
- assertive

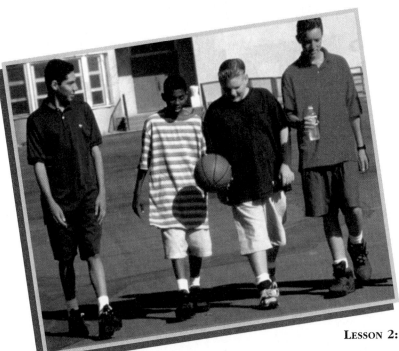

Positive peer pressure can encourage you to acquire new skills, such as learning a new sport. *How can a teen promote positive behaviors among peers? Give two examples.*

Developing Good Character

Responsibility

Working with your classmates, give examples of situations that involve negative peer pressure. Then brainstorm strategies for resisting the negative peer pressure. Practice these strategies in the form of role-plays or skits.

Negative Peer Pressure

Peer pressure becomes a negative social influence when people are trying to get you to do something that could hurt you or others. It could be something dangerous or illegal, something you're just not ready for, or something that goes against your values or your family's values. Teens who use tobacco, alcohol, or other drugs, for example, often do so because of negative peer pressure. Some peers may also pressure you to cheat, steal, lie, or show disrespect for others.

Negative peer pressure may involve threats, bribes, teasing, and name-calling. It may also take more subtle forms, such as facial expressions or gossip. When someone challenges your beliefs or encourages you to make an unhealthy or unsafe decision, it's important to know how to stand your ground and to resist negative peer pressure.

Learn to recognize and respond to negative peer pressure by avoiding this negative social influence. If you do find yourself in a situation in which you need to further resist negative peer pressure, you can use refusal skills. **Refusal skills** are *communication strategies that help you say no effectively.* **Figure 6.3** shows some refusal skills you can apply to effectively cope with negative peer pressure.

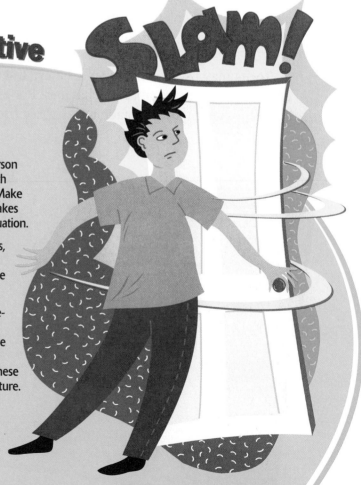

FIGURE 6.3

Closing the Door on Negative Peer Pressure

SLAM!

State reasons. You don't have to apologize or defend your position, but if you wish to, state your reasons clearly. You might practice saying no in front of a mirror so that you are ready to be firm and confident.

Don't agree to meet the other person halfway. You have the right to say no. Giving in a little is still giving in, and it leaves you open to continued pressure.

Use strong body language. Look the person in the eye when you're speaking to show that you're serious.

Suggest alternatives. Try to interest the other person in doing something else with which you're comfortable. Make sure that your suggestion takes you away from the risky situation.

Walk away. If all else fails, walk away. Your actions will match your words and make it clear that you mean no.

Plan ahead. Talk to someone you trust—a parent or counselor— about the people who pressure you. Trusted adults can help you avoid these pressure situations in the future.

Effective Refusal Skills

When you feel pressured to do something you don't want to do, you need to use effective refusal skills. Effective refusal skills let others know that you mean what you say. Like other skills, they take practice.

It's important to be assertive when you use refusal skills. **Assertive** means *behaving with confidence and clearly stating your intentions.* Show with words and actions that you mean what you say. Speak clearly, calmly, and in a firm tone of voice.

Be sure that your body language and gestures match your words. If you stare at the floor or shift your weight from one leg to another, you won't seem very assertive. If you have a smile on your face and a teasing look in your eyes, the person pressuring you won't believe that you're serious. Instead, use eye contact, put a serious or neutral look on your face, and stand or sit up straight.

Hands-On Health

RECOGNIZING PEER PRESSURE

Learning to recognize peer pressure will help you decide whether to go along with the group or to act as an individual.

WHAT YOU WILL NEED
- pencil or pen
- several sheets of paper

WHAT YOU WILL DO
1. During the next week, observe peer pressure around you. Try to identify one example of peer pressure in your life, one in the lives of others in your family, and one on television or in other media.
2. For each observation, divide a sheet of paper into two columns. Head the columns with the words *Observation* and *Analysis.*
3. In the Observation column, describe the situations you observed.

4. In the Analysis column, write your interpretation of the event. Describe how peer pressure was involved. Differentiate between positive and negative peer pressure. Note how the person handled the pressure. If the pressure was handled poorly, what could the person have done?

IN CONCLUSION
At the end of the week, share your observations and analyses with your classmates. Discuss the consequences of giving in to negative pressure and ways of resisting it.

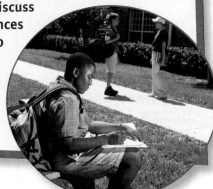

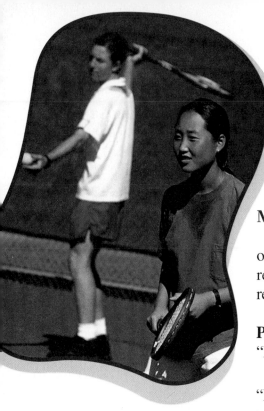

The next time you're in a pressure situation, think of the word *stop*. It will help you remember the four steps of effective refusal skills. Here's what the letters represent:

- **S**ay no in a firm voice.
- **T**ell why not.
- **O**ffer other ideas.
- **P**romptly leave.

More Ways to Refuse

Peers who try to persuade you to act against your judgment often use pressure lines such as "Everybody's doing it." To resist negative peer pressure, you should be ready with responses to these pressure lines. Here are some examples.

Pressure Lines	What You Can Say
"Everybody's going."	"Well, I'm not everybody. Besides, I don't believe that everybody's going."
"If you're my friend, you'll do it."	"I am your friend. If you were my friend, you wouldn't ask me to do it."
"Oh, come on—just this once."	"It only takes once to get into trouble."

Effective refusal skills can earn you the respect of others. You certainly will be able to respect yourself. Remember, you have the right to make safe and healthful choices for yourself and others.

Teens can have fun together in ways that do not involve risky situations. *What are some ways you and your friends have fun together safely?*

Lesson 2 Review

Using complete sentences, answer the following questions on a sheet of paper.

Reviewing Terms and Facts

1. **Vocabulary** Define the term *peer pressure.*
2. **Compare** Differentiate between positive and negative peer pressure.
3. **List** Give three examples of refusal skills.
4. **Describe** How can you be assertive in using refusal skills?

Thinking Critically

5. **Describe** Examine and describe the effects of peer pressure on decision making.

6. **Analyze** Predict the consequences of using refusal skills in various situations.

Applying Health Skills

7. **Advocacy** In a small group, decide on a worthwhile improvement for your school. For example, you might want trash-free school grounds, new sports equipment, or a recycling program. Plan a campaign to achieve your goal. Include ways to use positive peer pressure to persuade other students to join your campaign. If possible, put your plan into action.

Practicing Abstinence

Setting Limits

Limits are *invisible boundaries that protect you.* Setting limits protects you from risky or unhealthy behavior. There may be limits, for example, on the amount of television you are allowed to watch or on how late you can stay up on a school night. That's because if you watch too much television, you don't have time for anything else. If you stay up too late, you can't stay awake in school the next day.

Limits are important when it comes to dating. As a young teen, you need limits on the kinds of people you date, the places you go, your activities, and even the transportation you take. Such limits protect you from getting hurt. They also help you avoid sexual activity. Parents or guardians set limits because they love their children and want them to be safe.

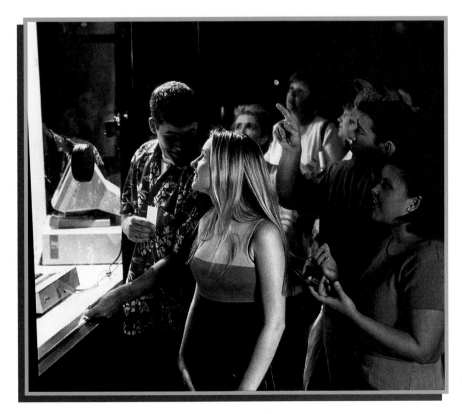

Quick Write

List examples of limits your parents or other adults place on you or limits you place on yourself. Explain at least one health-related benefit of these limits.

Learn About...

- the importance of setting limits in dating situations.
- ways to practice abstinence.
- the benefits and rewards of abstinence.

Vocabulary

- limits
- self-respect
- consequences

Trust your judgment and spend your time with people who share your values. *Who are the people you trust and like to go out with?*

MEDIA WATCH

AVOIDANCE TECHNIQUES

Avoidance techniques are actions or phrases you can use to avoid risky situations. With your classmates, recall successful avoidance techniques you have seen in movies or on television. ***How many of them involved humor? Role-play some avoidance techniques that use humor to deal with a difficult situation.***

Some guidelines for setting limits include:

- **Plan ahead.** Planning ahead can help make dating safe and fun. For example, if you're going to a party, find out who will be there and whether adults will be present to supervise. For any date, decide ahead of time what you will do and how long the date will last. This will make it easier to stay in control of a situation.
- **Avoid risky situations.** Teens need to be able to recognize and avoid situations that may place them at greater risk of participating in sexual activity. For example, a party where there will be alcohol or drugs is a risky situation. These substances impair judgment and reduce inhibitions. A teen who gives in to peer pressure to use alcohol or drugs might end up engaging in sexual activity. It is also wise to avoid being home alone or in an isolated spot with a date.

Practicing Abstinence

You've learned that *abstinence* means not participating in high-risk behaviors, including sexual activity. Responsible teens abstain from sexual activity before marriage.

Practicing sexual abstinence shows that you respect your health and the health of others. You may begin to experience strong physical attraction to another person. Sexual feelings are normal and healthy, and they can be managed. Use effective communication skills to discuss with parents or other trusted adults any questions you have about sexual feelings or other aspects of sexuality. Adults can offer useful suggestions for dealing with these issues. Exercise self-control by setting limits, planning ahead, and avoiding risky situations.

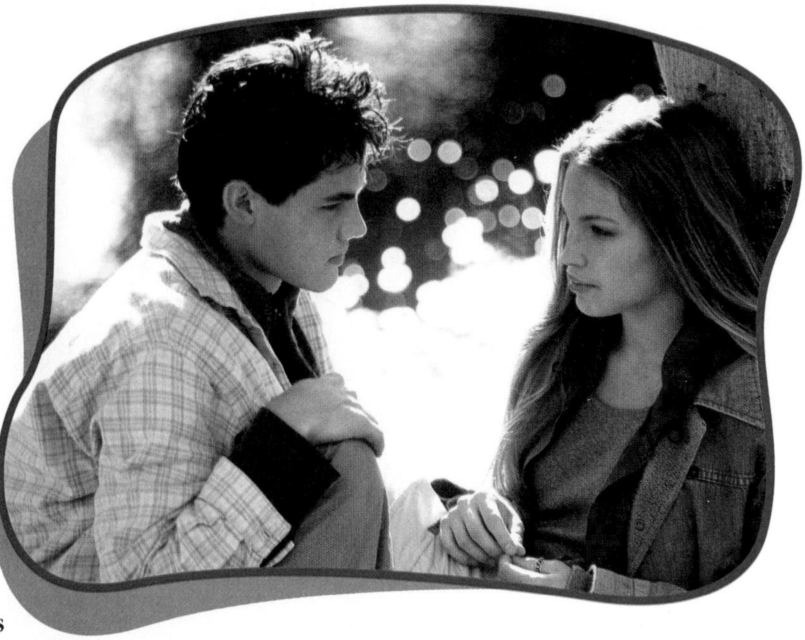

These teens have made a conscious decision to practice abstinence and to give themselves time for their friendship to develop. ***Discuss why abstinence from sexual activity is the only method that is 100 percent effective in preventing the emotional trauma associated with adolescent sexual activity.***

Showing Affection

Some teens may think that they must engage in sexual activity to show that they love or care for someone. This isn't true. Sexual activity isn't the same as love. It is one way to express love, but it isn't the only way. Here are a few ways to be close to someone and show affection without being sexually active.

- Listen to each other's problems.
- Give or get a hug.
- Study together at the kitchen table.
- Go for a long walk and hold hands.
- Do something nice for each other.
- Put affectionate notes in each other's locker or books.

You can show someone that you care in hundreds of different ways. *What are some ways in which you would show your affection for a special person?*

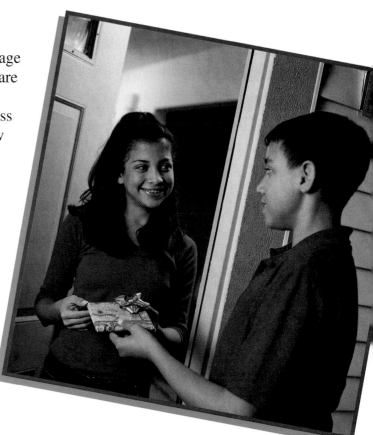

HEALTH SKILLS ACTIVITY

ADVOCACY

Supporting Abstinence

You can be an advocate for sexual abstinence by telling other teens why you've made a decision to protect your health in this way. Being an advocate for abstinence strengthens your own commitment. At the same time, you can be a role model to friends who are looking for ways to make abstinence easier. Here are a few ideas.

- Join a program or group that supports teen abstinence.
- Socialize with other teens who share your beliefs.
- Talk to parents and other trusted adults about your decision to be abstinent.
- Find out the facts about pregnancy and sexually transmitted diseases so that you are informed.
- Participate in group dates.

ON YOUR OWN

In a paragraph, analyze why abstinence from sexual activity is the preferred choice of behavior for unmarried persons of school age. Then list ways to practice abstinence.

Reading Check

List the contractions on these pages and explain what the apostrophe indicates. Then list possessive forms and explain what the apostrophe shows.

Reasons to Practice Abstinence

More and more teens are choosing to abstain from sexual activity. These teens also are willing to talk about their decision. They want others to know that abstinence makes it easier for them to remain physically and emotionally healthy.

Respect for Self and Others

Teens who practice sexual abstinence gain self-respect. **Self-respect** is *the positive feeling you have about yourself when you live up to your beliefs and values.* We learn our beliefs and values from our families, through religious instruction, and in school. Many teens have been taught that sexual intimacy should be postponed until a couple is married. They also strongly believe that a relationship should be based on trust, caring, and friendship, not on physical attraction alone. Teens who are abstinent for these reasons honor their ideals.

Teens also may decide on abstinence to show respect for the beliefs and values of their parents and other family members. They may feel that sexual activity would disappoint or hurt people who are important to them. In addition, there are legal implications regarding sexual activity as it relates to minor persons.

Avoiding Possible Consequences

Consequences are *outcomes or effects that may occur as a result of a decision or an action.* Sexual activity among teens is likely to have several consequences, any of which may have a serious and long-lasting impact on a teen's life:

- **Unplanned pregnancy.** Most teens who are sexually active don't use birth control, or they use it inconsistently. Pregnancy and childbearing can damage a teen mother's physical health. Teens generally aren't prepared emotionally or financially to raise a child. These situations can also prevent or hinder future goals, such as going to college.
- **Sexually transmitted diseases (STDs).** Teens who are sexually active often fail to protect themselves against STDs. STDs can lead to lifelong health problems, and in the case of HIV/AIDS, even death. They can cause sterility, increase the risk of some cancers, and pose serious health risks to future children.

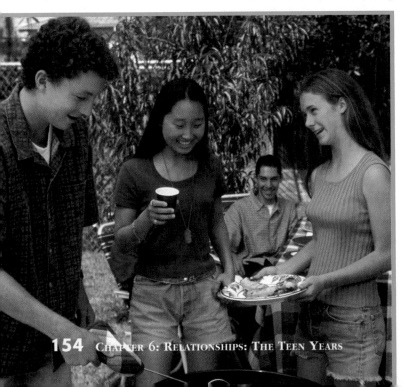

Practicing abstinence enables you to focus on your friends and the ways in which they are special. *How could a sexual relationship with a boyfriend or girlfriend interfere with other friendships?*

- **Emotional trauma.** Sexual activity affects emotional as well as physical health. The stress of lying and the guilt caused by behavior that must be hidden from parents is painful. Teens also might regret behavior that doesn't bring them love, respect, or acceptance.

Rewards of Abstinence

Abstinence from sexual activity provides teens with many rewards. Here are just a few of the many benefits of deciding to be sexually abstinent:

- **Peace of mind.** Abstinence is the only method that is 100 percent effective in preventing pregnancy; sexually transmitted diseases, including HIV infection; and the emotional trauma associated with adolescent sexual activity.
- **Self-respect.** Abstinence allows you to be in control of your own body. Others will know you as a confident, responsible person.
- **Time for personal growth.** A sexual relationship can complicate life and keep teens from achieving their goals. Abstinence gives you more time to pursue your interests and develop your talents and skills.
- **Healthy relationships.** Abstinence lets you avoid the pressure of a sexual relationship. Teens who are abstinent can develop meaningful relationships based on mutual respect and shared interests.

Lesson 3 Review

Using complete sentences, answer the following questions on a sheet of paper.

Reviewing Terms and Facts

1. **Explain** Why does setting limits in dating help teens to show responsibility?
2. **Recall** Give an example of a risky dating situation.
3. **Vocabulary** Define *self-respect*.
4. **List** Describe three possible consequences of failure to practice abstinence.

Thinking Critically

5. **Evaluate** List the advantages of abstinence. Then study your list and determine which items you consider most important. Explain your choices.

6. **Apply** Discuss the legal implications regarding sexual activity as it relates to minor persons.

Applying Health Skills

7. **Goal Setting** Having clear goals for your future can help you practice abstinence. Make a list of goals you want to accomplish. Then write a paragraph describing how early sexual activity might keep you from reaching your goals.

Cliques
—Good or Bad?
What do you think about cliques? Join the debate!

Pro

"Too many people hear about cliques and immediately think of a social circle that's as secure as Fort Knox, where only the most beautiful, rich, and popular kids can be included. I think this idea is totally false and extremely outdated. Teenagers are looking for somewhere to belong. The word 'clique' is simply a label that gets attached to a circle of friends as soon as they find a few people who they're comfortable around. In my opinion, finding that niche is a very positive thing and an important element of being a teenager. For me, being in a group is part of what makes school so great—through thick and thin, 'my girls' and I are always there for one another. I believe that today's teens are forming cliques not for the purpose of exclusivity, but to find other kids who they can connect with. As far as I'm concerned, there's absolutely nothing wrong with that."

—*Kerisha Harris, 15*
Paterson, New Jersey

Con

"While Hollywood tends to make cliques seem fashionable, the truth is, there's nothing glamorous about them. For kids who can't seem to fit in anywhere (and whose self-esteem gets shattered in the process), cliques are one of the most devastating parts of school. Granted, it's normal for teens to be drawn to people who are like them, and that may automatically make a group of friends seem like a clique. I'm not saying it's bad to have close friends, but that stops being OK when you're not accepting of others. If you're hurting your peers or putting them down just because they're not as 'cool' or they're different from you, that's when it's time to take a closer look at yourself. Most likely there's something wrong with you, not the other people."

—*Nick Casey, 15, Brentwood, California.*

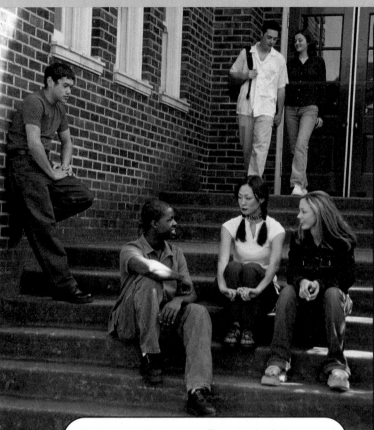

Making Things "Click"

School violence has raised people's awareness of the problems cliques can cause—and moved more teens to find ways to help turn things around. That's where SHINE365 (Seeking Harmony in Neighborhoods Everyday) comes in. The youth organization's Get Yourself Connected Speak Outs, held at malls nationwide, are getting teens talking about what causes clique intolerance and how to solve it. Inspired, young people have also formed school-based diversity organizations and channeled aggressive energy into art projects. "The mall forums get a whole cross section of teens," says SHINE365 coexecutive director Jennifer Kahn. "If we can expose [them] to different points of view, hopefully we can start making a difference in their lives."

Many teens think overcoming barriers starts with acceptance. "When you see someone [all alone], go up and ask about something that happened that day. It makes them feel more accepted," says SHINE365 member Melissa Mercier, 14, of Springfield, Massachusetts. Kahn suggests "embracing uniqueness," instead of passing judgment on people who are not like you. ▰

Other Teens Speak Up

"Some people believe that being dependent on a small group of people is harmful or can create peer pressure. I think trusting and knowing someone well is exactly what makes friends into best friends."
—*Maria Marchenkova, 16, Columbus, Ohio*

"[At my school] everyone watches out for each other, so we are in essence one big clique."
—*Katie Chamberlain, 16, Huntsville, Alabama*

"A clique, by definition, is a group of friends, so I don't think that they're necessarily bad. However, the 'group-think' mentality of cliques concerns me."
—*Tony Pham, 16, Bellevue, Washington*

"Cliques tend to discriminate against other cliques or individuals. I've seen situations where people join a clique simply to be part of the crowd and end up hurting themselves or their true friends in the end."
—*Amanda Hughes, 14, Goshen, Ohio*

TIME TO THINK...

About Cliques

Hold a class debate on whether cliques have a positive or negative influence on teens. Start by defining the term *clique* on the board. Your teacher will then divide the class in half, assigning one half to argue for cliques, the other against them. Before the debate, each group—through research and discussion—should develop at least five strong arguments to support its position.

KNOW YOUR LIMITS

Model

Claudia recently began dating. She knows that she does not want to become sexually active, and she wants to avoid situations where she might be pressured. Claudia decides to set some firm limits for herself. She uses the goal-setting steps to plan ahead.

1. **Identify a specific goal.** "I want to avoid being pressured to be sexually active."

2. **List the steps you will take.** "I will insist that my first date with anyone be a group situation. I will always let my parents know where I am and when I will be home. I will not go to parties or other places where alcohol is present."

3. **Get help and support from others.** "My older sister can help me decide how to tell my dates about my limits. I will ask my parents to come pick me up if I ever need to leave in the middle of a date."

4. **Set up checkpoints.** "Each time I begin dating someone, I will tell that person what my limits are. I will not go out with anyone who does not agree to respect them."

5. **Reward yourself.** "I will feel good about myself because I am sticking to my limits."

Practice

Read the paragraph below. Then show how Lawrence could use the goal-setting steps to structure the time he spends with Mimi. Write your plan on a separate piece of paper.

Lawrence has been dating Mimi for several months, and he likes her very much. He also finds her very attractive. He values their relationship and wants it to last for a long time. Lawrence feels that in order to practice abstinence with Mimi, he must set limits for himself. He decides to use the goal-setting steps to help him plan for the time he spends with Mimi.

Apply/Assess

Make a contract with yourself in which you set a goal to remain abstinent. Remember to include limits that you set for yourself. Use the goal-setting steps to write your contract. First, state your goal. Then list the limits you will set to help you reach your goal. Include the names of people who can help you stick to your limits, and describe checkpoints you can use to make sure that you are staying on target. Finally, describe the rewards you will gain by choosing these limits. Use the sample contract here as a model.

I, the undersigned, am setting a goal to practice abstinence. In order to reach this goal, I intend to _____.
I will also _____. I will ask _____ to help me by _____.
Every _____ I will remind myself of my goal and set new limits if I think they are needed. By being abstinent, I will receive the rewards of _____.

Lawrence Whitaker
11/04/05

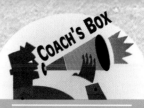

Goal Setting

1. **Identify a specific goal.**
2. **List the steps you will take.**
3. **Get help and support from others.**
4. **Set up checkpoints.**
5. **Reward yourself.**

Self-✓Check

- Does my contract include all the steps for goal setting?
- Did I list the personal rewards of setting limits?

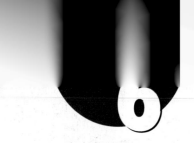

After You Read

Use your completed Foldable to review the information on the qualities of a good friendship.

Reviewing Vocabulary and Concepts

On a sheet of paper, write the numbers 1–10. After each number, write the term from the list that best completes each statement.

- individual date
- assertive
- clique
- volunteer
- negative peer pressure
- peer pressure
- positive peer pressure
- refusal skills
- group date
- empathetic

Lesson 1

1. Friends are said to be _____ when they are able to identify and share another person's feelings.
2. A group of friends who hang out together and act in similar ways are a(n) _____.
3. One way to feel more comfortable around teens of both genders is to go out on a(n) _____.
4. One way to make new friends is to _____ to work with others.
5. When you go on a(n) _____, you get to know one person better.

Lesson 2

6. _____ is the influence other teens have on you to act and think like them.
7. Classmates who encourage another student to stop smoking are using _____.

8. _____ occurs when other teens ask you to do something that will hurt you or others.
9. _____ can help you get out of uncomfortable situations.
10. When you behave with confidence, you are being _____.

Lesson 3

On a sheet of paper, write the numbers 11–15. After each number, write the letter of the answer that best completes the sentence or answers the question.

11. Which of the following is another word for invisible boundaries that protect you?
    a. distress
    b. limits
    c. crowd
    d. clique
12. Living up to your values and beliefs helps you have
    a. self-respect.
    b. sympathy.
    c. peer pressure.
    d. guilt.
13. Having an accident or getting a speeding ticket because of driving too fast would be a
    a. limit.
    b. group date.
    c. consequence.
    d. conversation.
14. Which of the following might be a consequence of early sexual activity?
    a. refusal skills
    b. group dating
    c. trust
    d. a sexually transmitted disease
15. The only method that is 100 percent effective in preventing pregnancy and STDs is
    a. abstinence from sexual activity.
    b. going on group dates.
    c. responding to peer pressure.
    d. being assertive.

Thinking Critically

Using complete sentences, answer the following questions on a sheet of paper.

16. **Hypothesize** When might a teen need to use refusal skills with someone other than a peer? Predict the consequences of refusing in this situation.

17. **Apply** How would one of your long-term goals be negatively affected by an unplanned pregnancy or an STD?

18. **Explain** How can you determine if relationships are a positive or negative influence on your health? Develop strategies for monitoring these relationships.

Career Corner

School Counselor Many teens will go to a school counselor for help in handling emotions or resolving conflicts. School counselors help students with school, family, or personal problems. They also work with students to help plan their futures.

This profession requires a four-year degree and two years of graduate training in counseling. If you think you might like to help young people solve problems, visit the Career Corner at health.glencoe.com to find out more about this career.

Standardized Test Practice

Math

Read the paragraph below and then answer the questions.

Surveys have shown that many teens don't wear safety belts when riding in a car. One of the main reasons that teens gave for not wearing safety belts was peer pressure.

1. In 2001, more than 5,000 teens were killed in traffic accidents. Two-thirds of these teens were not wearing safety belts. How many of the teens were not wearing safety belts?
   - **A** 1,667 teens
   - **B** 2,500 teens
   - **C** 3,333 teens
   - **D** 4,500 teens

2. Of the students surveyed, 32 percent of students who didn't wear safety belts said that they did not wear them because of peer pressure. Suppose there are 194 students in your school who say they don't wear safety belts. How many of these students do not wear safety belts because of peer pressure?
   - **A** 45 students
   - **B** 62 students
   - **C** 132 students
   - **D** 149 students

3. Suppose you surveyed teens who rode with adults and those who rode with teen drivers about safety belt use. For which group do you think the percentage of teens not wearing a safety belt is higher? Explain.

CHAPTER 7

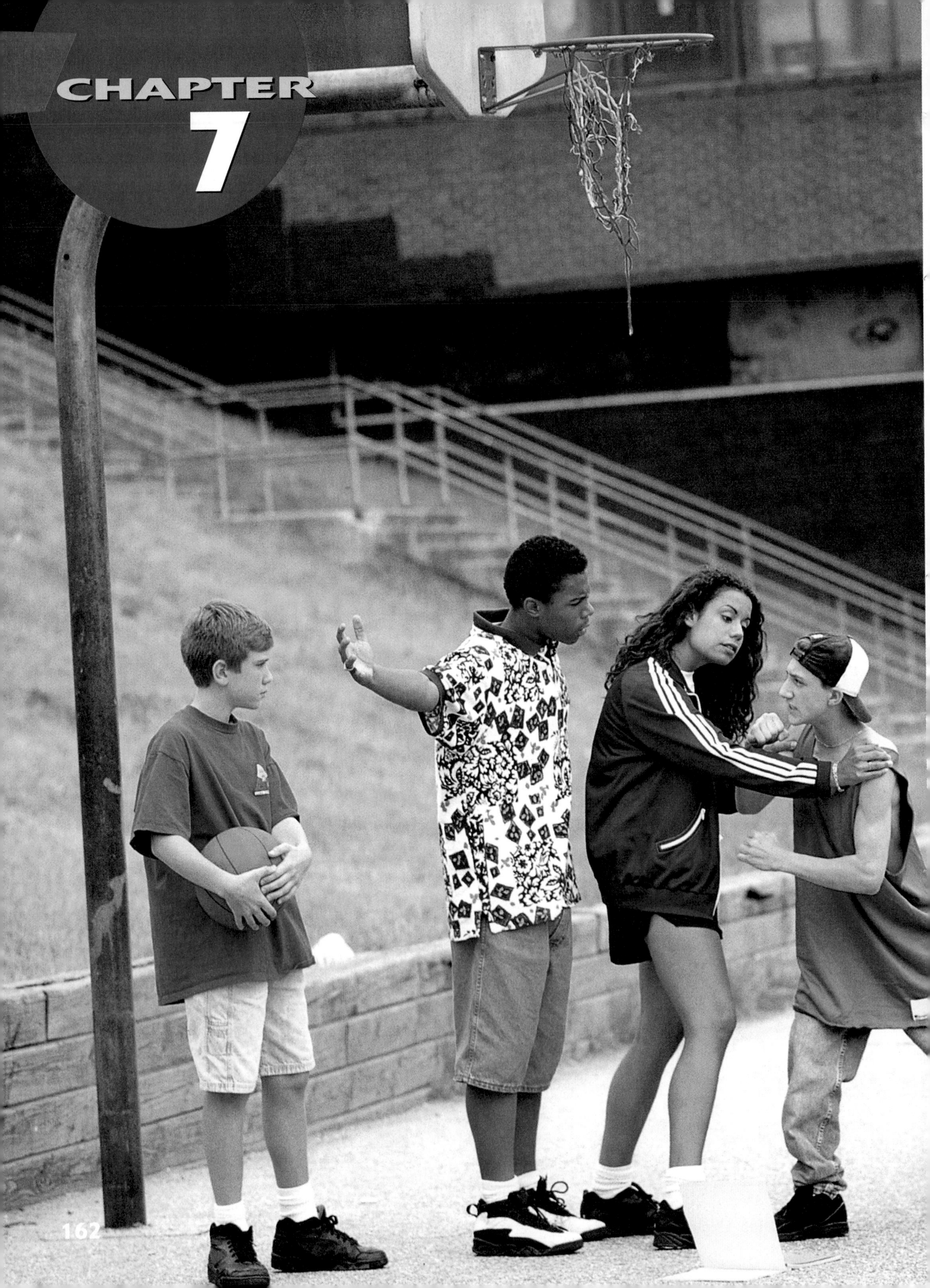

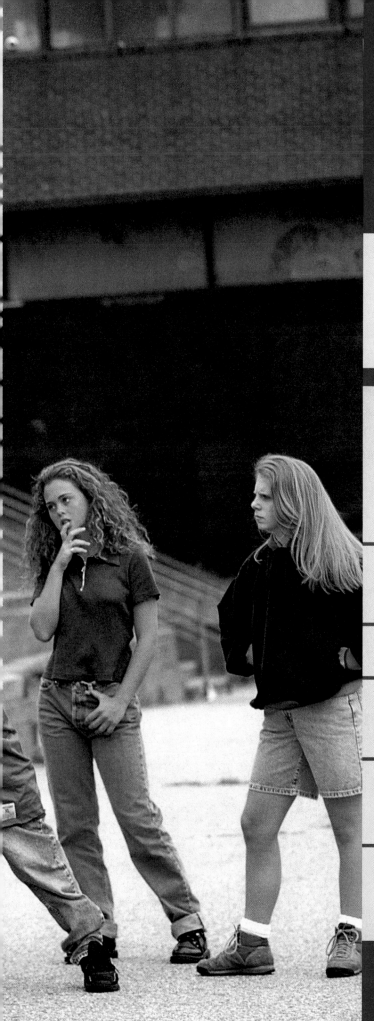

Conflict Resolution

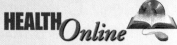

HEALTH *Online*

Discover what you know about the nature of conflicts and violence prevention. Go to health.glencoe.com and take the Chapter 7 Health Inventory.

FOLDABLES™
Study Organizer

Before You Read

Make this Foldable to help you organize what you learn in Lesson 1 about the nature of conflict. Begin with a plain sheet of 8½″ × 11″ paper or notebook paper.

Step 1

Fold the sheet of paper from top to bottom, leaving a 2″ tab at the bottom.

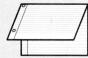

Step 2

Fold in half from side to side.

Step 3

Unfold the paper once. Cut along the center fold line of the top layer only. This makes two tabs.

Step 4

Label the tabs as shown.

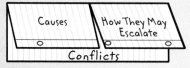

As You Read

Under the appropriate tab, record information on some common causes of conflict and the factors that may cause them to escalate.

The Nature of Conflict

Quick Write

Describe an incident that you witnessed in which someone's words or actions resolved a conflict peacefully.

LEARN ABOUT...

- how conflicts occur.
- why some conflicts get out of hand.
- positive ways to manage anger.
- factors that can cause conflicts to escalate.

VOCABULARY

- conflict
- escalate
- prejudice

How Conflicts Occur

Conflict is *a disagreement between people with opposing viewpoints, ideas, or goals.* It is a normal part of life. Conflict can arise among friends, family members, and groups in a community. Sometimes a conflict can be positive and can produce needed change. A conflict does not have to be a contest in which one side wins and the other loses. The best solution is a fair one, in which both sides win. There are many reasons for conflict, but the three major ones are competition for resources, clashes over values, and exchanges involving emotional needs.

- **Conflicts over Resources.** You can peacefully handle conflict over resources by sharing. To share resources without conflict, the people involved must respect one another's needs. For example, two sisters argued daily because they both borrowed each other's clothing without asking permission. Eventually each girl realized that the best way to gain respect was to show respect. The sisters agreed not to borrow again without asking.
- **Conflicts over Values.** Your values are the beliefs and ideals that guide your decisions and behavior. A conflict over values, for example, may involve you and your parents disagreeing about what you wear, how you spend your money, or who you spend your time with.

Conflicts often begin over competition for resources, differences in values, and emotional needs. *What caused a recent conflict you had with a friend?*

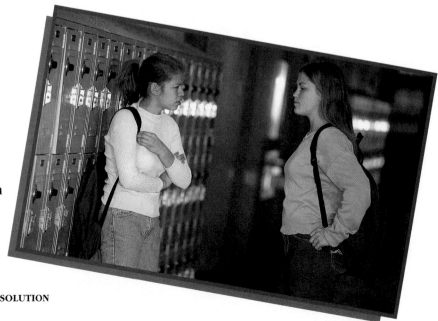

A Survey of Conflicts

Analyzing conflicts you have had in the past can give you insight into effective ways to manage future conflicts.

WHAT YOU WILL NEED
- notebook paper
- pen or pencil

WHAT YOU WILL DO
1. Use the paper to create a record sheet. Make four columns and label them *Location, Number of People Involved, Problem, What Happened.*

2. In the next two days, observe one conflict in school or among friends and write your observations on the record sheet.

IN CONCLUSION
In a small group, discuss what you observed with your classmates. Choose conflicts that were not resolved or that were poorly managed. Brainstorm ideas for ways in which they could have been managed better. Write a new plan for a healthier resolution.

- **Conflicts Involving Emotional Needs.** People's basic emotional needs include the need to belong and the need to feel respected and worthwhile. Conflicts may arise when people are excluded from groups they would like to join. Also, when someone shows disrespect to another person or group, disagreements are bound to occur. A frequent source of conflict for teens is spreading rumors about others.

Why Some Conflicts Get Out of Hand

The best time to resolve a conflict is in its early stages. If a disagreement isn't managed peacefully, the conflict can **escalate**, or *become more serious.* Certain factors, such as anger, bullying, and group pressure, can increase the chance that a minor argument will escalate into a major dispute.

Anger

People become angry when they are frustrated or believe that they are being mistreated. Everyone feels angry now and then. When you are angry, your heart beats faster than usual. Blood rushes to your face and your muscles tense as your body prepares for action. If you can channel your energy into something positive, you have a better chance of avoiding violence.

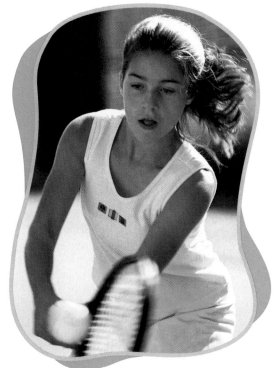

Vigorous physical activity is a positive way to release your anger.

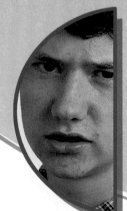

Reading Check

Understand suffixes. The suffix *-ing* can be used to turn a verb into the subject of a sentence. Find as many examples as you can on this page.

Anger that is not managed well can make a conflict worse. It's important to exercise self-control so that your anger does not get out of hand. One strategy is to stop focusing on how angry you are. Dwelling on whatever is making you angry can build anger into rage. Rage, in turn, can lead to violence. Fortunately, there are several effective ways to manage anger. **Figure 7.1** shows some positive strategies for dealing with anger.

Bullying and Teasing

Some people seek power and attention by bullying. Bullies can be males or females of any age. Groups sometimes bully individuals or even whole neighborhoods. Bullying may take the form of pushing, shoving, or other physical abuse. Teasing, taunting, using ethnic slurs, and making sexual comments or gestures are other forms of bullying.

One way to deal with bullies is to walk away with your head held high. Bullies want victims to react with fear or anger. Walking away sends the message that you don't care. Ignoring the bully or pretending the bully doesn't exist are other ways to stop aggressive behavior. Bullying is serious and no one needs to put up with it. If you become aware of bullying in your school or neighborhood, talk with a school counselor, parent, or other adult.

Group Pressure

When Tanya found out that Alison had started a rumor about her, she was furious. She confronted Alison, and as they argued, their voices became louder. A crowd gathered. Someone began to shout, "Fight! Fight!" Although Tanya and Alison had been ready to stop, both now felt pressured to keep the argument going.

FIGURE 7.1

Positive Ways to Manage Anger

You don't have to give in to anger. Coping skills can help you manage anger.
Describe some strategies you have applied to effectively manage anger.

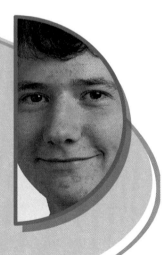

- Take time to cool down.
- Walk, run, swim, or do something active.
- Listen to music, or just sit quietly.
- Identify exactly what triggered your anger.
- Attack the problem, not the person.

- Brainstorm ways to handle the situation.
- Ask yourself if you have taken the situation too personally.
- Explain to the other person how you feel.
- Try to imagine the other person's point of view.
- Talk over the situation with a parent, friend, or trusted adult.

Pressure from a group can cause a small conflict to escalate into a big one. Once a crowd gets involved, the people in conflict may ignore their own thoughts and give in to the crowd. Group pressure can also encourage people to express prejudice. **Prejudice** is *a negative and unjustly formed opinion, usually against people of a different racial, religious, or cultural group.*

Alcohol and Other Drugs

Alcohol and other drugs play a major role in violent crimes. According to the U.S. Department of Justice, about 35 percent of victims of violent crimes report that their offender had been drinking.

People under the influence of alcohol and other drugs may not think clearly. They may make unreasonable judgments and lose the ability to control their anger. A person who has been drinking or taking other drugs is also much more susceptible to negative group pressure. Avoiding situations where drugs and alcohol are likely to be present is a good way to avoid violence.

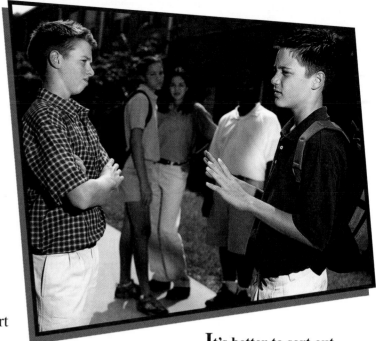

It's better to sort out differences on your own than to involve a whole group. *Why do some conflicts get bigger when a crowd is involved?*

Lesson 1 Review

Using complete sentences, answer the following questions on a sheet of paper.

Reviewing Terms and Facts

1. **Vocabulary** Define the term *conflict* and use it in a sentence that demonstrates its meaning.
2. **Identify** What are three main causes of conflicts?
3. **Explain** What factors can make a conflict escalate?
4. **List** Give three examples of positive ways to manage anger.

Thinking Critically

5. **Apply** Each day in school Ned purposely bumps Phil as he passes him in the hallway. Phil's books fall to the floor. Then Ned makes an exaggerated apology to Phil. Phil's face turns red. Ned loudly calls Phil a baby. How would you describe what Ned is doing? What can Phil do?
6. **Explain** Why are people who have been drinking alcohol or using drugs more likely to become violent?

Applying Health Skills

7. **Practicing Healthful Behaviors** Give examples of the kinds of events or remarks that make you angry. Make a list of activities that would help you release anger in healthful ways at such times. Demonstrate one of these strategies for the class.

Resolving Conflicts

Quick Write

Describe a personal situation in which you were able to resolve a conflict effectively.

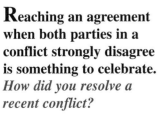

LEARN ABOUT...

- skills for resolving conflicts.
- the importance of compromise in conflict resolution.
- peer mediation in schools.

VOCABULARY

- conflict resolution
- compromise
- win-win solution
- mediation

Conflict Resolution Skills

Conflict resolution involves *solving a disagreement in a way that satisfies both sides.* Some conflicts are easily resolved. For example, Saul and Jenna want to watch different television programs at the same time. They decide that Saul will record his program and watch it later.

Many conflicts are not so easily settled. People who have very different ideas or values may find it hard to reach agreement. Most conflicts can be resolved, however. The key to conflict resolution is having respect for the other person's rights.

Principles of Conflict Resolution

To reach agreement, people in conflict need to practice communication skills and self-control. They must also be willing to cooperate with one another and to **compromise**, or *give up something in order to reach a solution that satisfies everyone.* Most of all they must focus on the problem and not on the other person. **Figure 7.2** summarizes one approach to conflict resolution.

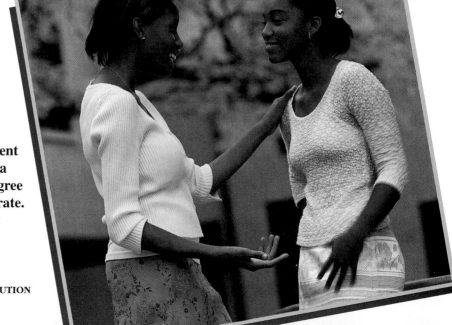

Reaching an agreement when both parties in a conflict strongly disagree is something to celebrate. *How did you resolve a recent conflict?*

FIGURE 7.2

Conflict Resolution Skills

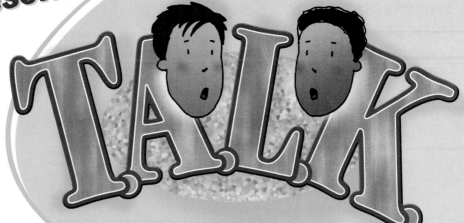

Try following the T.A.L.K. strategies the next time you are involved in a conflict. *Why do you think the first recommendation is to take a time out?*

Take a time out, at least 30 minutes.
Go for a walk, listen to some music, or read something that interests you.

Allow each person to tell his or her side uninterrupted.
Listen actively and make sure you understand what the other person has said.

Let each person ask questions.
Many conflicts are based on misunderstandings. Asking questions and listening to the answers may be all that is needed to clear up a conflict.

Keep brainstorming to find a good solution for both parties.
Be prepared to examine different ideas. Don't let your anger keep you from thinking clearly or from examining different options.

Mediation

The best kind of solution to a conflict is a win-win solution. A **win-win solution** is *an agreement that gives each party something they want.* When each party gets something they want, they are more likely to honor the agreement they have made.

In many cases, people can reach a win-win solution on their own. Sometimes, however, they cannot and they may resort to mediation. **Mediation** is *a process in which a third person, a mediator, helps those in conflict find a solution.*

In a typical mediation process, the two conflicting parties sit down in a private place with the mediator. The mediator listens to both sides, asks questions to clarify issues, and makes sure that both parties have a chance to tell their side and understand each other's viewpoint. Finally, the mediator may guide the parties to a win-win solution.

To be an effective mediator you need certain qualities and skills. The most important is that you must remain neutral, meaning that you do not favor one side over the other. You need to listen to and understand the issues. Then you need to restate and summarize them in clear statements. **Figure 7.3** on the next page shows the six stages in the mediation process. Each step depends on successful completion of the previous step.

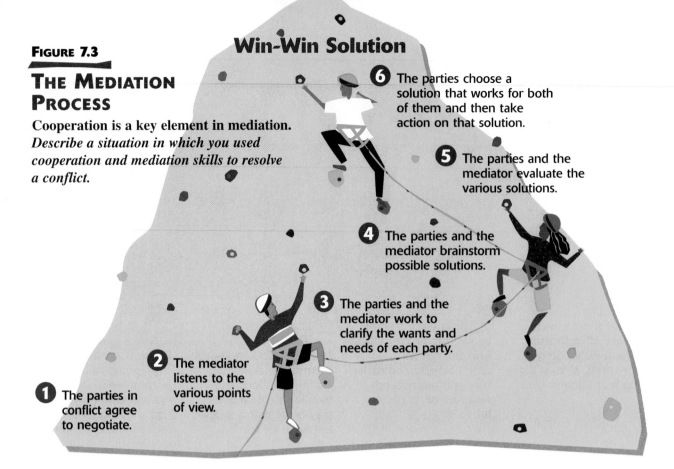

FIGURE 7.3

THE MEDIATION PROCESS

Cooperation is a key element in mediation. *Describe a situation in which you used cooperation and mediation skills to resolve a conflict.*

Win-Win Solution

6 The parties choose a solution that works for both of them and then take action on that solution.

5 The parties and the mediator evaluate the various solutions.

4 The parties and the mediator brainstorm possible solutions.

3 The parties and the mediator work to clarify the wants and needs of each party.

2 The mediator listens to the various points of view.

1 The parties in conflict agree to negotiate.

Peer Mediation

Many schools have peer mediation programs. In peer mediation, a student serves as the mediator for students who are involved in a conflict. Teens can be effective mediators because they understand their peers' attitudes and viewpoints. They can put the problem in language that students can relate to.

Students receive special training to become peer mediators. Training may be provided by teachers or by people from community mediation organizations. Training programs cover a number of topics that focus on the qualities, skills, and behaviors required of mediators. Here are some of the requirements of a peer mediator.

- Be trustworthy and keep the discussions confidential.
- Understand and analyze conflict.
- Listen carefully and express ideas clearly.
- Identify feelings.
- Remain completely neutral throughout the process.
- Handle anger in a positive way.
- Identify points of agreement.
- Brainstorm multiple solutions for a problem.
- Evaluate the consequences of various options.
- Take accurate notes.
- Once it has been agreed upon, describe a clear win-win agreement in writing.

HEALTH SKILLS ACTIVITY

DECISION MAKING

When to Suggest a Mediator

Lisa, Tony, and Dave were all good friends until two weeks ago. After a serious argument, Tony and Dave stopped speaking to each other. Both are still speaking to Lisa, and each separately told Lisa his side of the conflict.

Dave told Lisa that Tony tries to copy Dave's school papers and tests. Dave explained that when he confronted Tony, Tony acted outraged and denied trying to copy anything. Later, Lisa listened to Tony's side of the story. Tony said that Dave is spreading lies about him, and that he will never be friends with Dave again. When Lisa suggested that Dave and Tony try to talk over their problem, Tony said, "Stay out of this! It's between Dave and me."

Lisa wonders if peer mediation would help settle their conflict. She thinks about suggesting it but is worried about Tony's warning. She decides to use the decision-making process to determine what she should do.

What Would You Do?

Apply the skills for decision making to Lisa's situation. Would you suggest mediation? Why or why not?

1. **STATE THE SITUATION.**
2. **LIST THE OPTIONS.**
3. **WEIGH THE POSSIBLE OUTCOMES.**
4. **CONSIDER VALUES.**
5. **MAKE A DECISION AND ACT.**
6. **EVALUATE THE DECISION.**

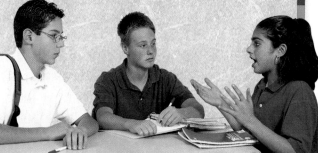

Lesson 2 Review

Using complete sentences, answer the following questions on a sheet of paper.

Reviewing Terms and Facts

1. **Vocabulary** Define *win-win solution.*
2. **Summarize** In your own words, summarize conflict resolution/mediation skills.
3. **Explain** What makes students effective mediators for their peers?

Thinking Critically

4. **Apply** Relate conflict resolution/mediation skills to personal situations: How have you used these skills in your life?
5. **Explain** How can a peer mediation program help make your school safer?

Applying Health Skills

6. **Conflict Resolution** With a partner, write a skit in which a conflict is resolved peacefully. Perform your skit for the class to demonstrate strategies for coping with problems related to conflict.

Avoiding and Preventing Violence

Quick Write

Write a short paragraph explaining why you think some young people resort to violence to settle differences.

LEARN ABOUT...

- factors that contribute to teen violence.
- policies to prevent violence in schools.
- ways to protect yourself from violence.

VOCABULARY

- violence
- homicide
- gang
- zero tolerance policy
- rape

Violence in Our Society

Hitting someone is clearly an example of violence, but what about *threatening* to hit or hurt someone? Is that violence? What about destroying property or yelling mean and hurtful words at someone? Is that violence? The answer is yes. **Violence** is *any act that causes physical or psychological harm to a person or damage to property.* **Homicide**, *the killing of one human being by another,* is violence at its worst. In recent years the numbers of homicides and other violent acts have declined in the United States. The rates are still unacceptably high, however, and homicide remains a leading cause of death among teens.

Various factors have been suggested as causes for the high rates of violence. Some people point to the violent acts shown on television and in movies as contributing factors. Others cite changes in family structure that tend to leave children unsupervised for hours at a time. Many also believe the availability of a variety of weapons, including guns, is a major cause of violence.

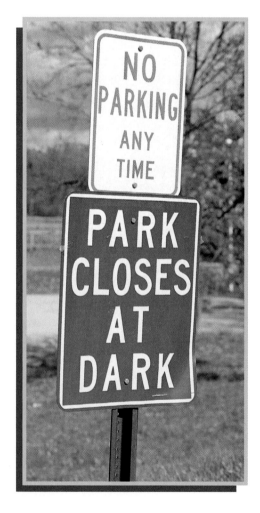

Incidents of violence have led communities to establish public curfews. *Analyze how this strategy can prevent the deliberate injuries that can result from violence.*

Violence and Teens

Much of the recent violence has involved teens. In 1998, about one-third of all victims of violent crime were ages 12 to 19. Teens are not just victims, however. Each year more than 120,000 youths are arrested for committing violent crimes. Teen violence often involves gangs, weapons, and drugs.

Gangs

Although gang activity was once associated with large cities, it is now a national problem. A **gang** is *a group of people who associate with one another to take part in criminal activity.* Typical gang activities include vandalism, graffiti, robbery, and drug dealing.

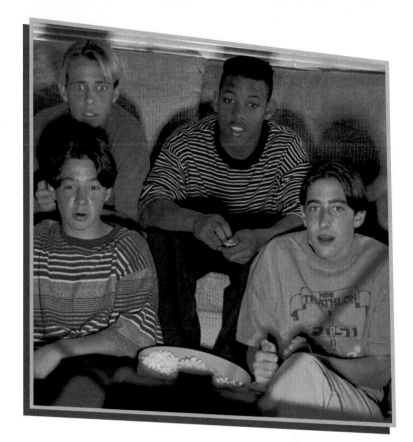

Violence is prevalent in the media. *How do you think the media's portrayal of violence influences individual and community health?*

Because gang members often carry weapons, they make an environment unsafe for everyone. In addition, some of their actions, such as random shootings, are unpredictable. As a result, innocent people are injured or killed. The presence of gangs in a school or community causes people to live in fear instead of in security.

Weapons

Firearm injuries are the second leading cause of death for young people ages 10 to 24. For every one person killed by a firearm, four are wounded. A survey of young people who had been shot revealed that 35 percent of them were carrying guns when they were wounded. Strategies to prevent firearm accidents include controlling gun ownership and installing safety devices on guns. Gun owners are advised to keep their firearms unloaded and to store ammunition in a separate locked place.

Drugs

Drugs and violence tend to go hand in hand. Drug users who are desperate for money to support their drug habit often turn to illegal and violent behavior. Drugs also affect a user's ability to think clearly and have good judgment. While under the influence of drugs, a person might shoplift, steal a car, or commit a violent crime.

Reading Check

Analyze word structure. Find the compound word in this list: *random, ammunition, ownership, firearms.* Locate other compound words on pages 172 and 173.

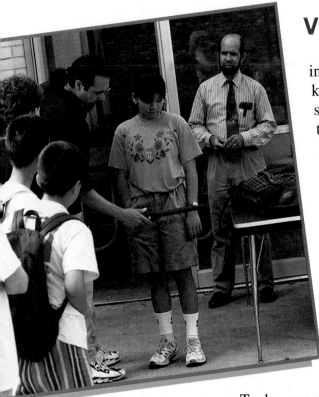

Violence in Schools

Incidents of violence in schools have led to increased security measures. Many schools now keep all or most doors to the school locked. In some schools, students must pass through metal detectors to enter the school. School officials may search lockers and students' belongings if they have reasonable suspicion that someone is planning a violent act.

To further increase safety, many schools have also adopted a zero tolerance policy for weapons or weapon look-alikes, drugs, and violent behavior. A **zero tolerance policy** is *a policy that makes no exceptions for anybody for any reason.* Any student found guilty of bringing any prohibited items to school, or of violent behavior, is automatically expelled.

To do your part to prevent school violence, follow the tips listed in the Health Skills Activity on this page. Understand and follow school rules related to health, including rules prohibiting the possession of weapons at school.

School violence gets a lot of publicity, but the vast majority of schools experience little or no violence. *Do you think most students feel safe in your school?*

HEALTH SKILLS ACTIVITY

ADVOCACY

Help Prevent School Violence

You can help prevent school violence by acting safely and by encouraging others to play their part. Here are some actions that you can take and advocate.

- Refuse to bring a weapon or weapon look-alike to school, to carry a weapon for another person, or to keep silent about those who carry weapons.
- Immediately report any violent incidents or threats of violence to school authorities or the police.

- Learn how to manage your own anger.
- Help others settle arguments peaceably.
- Welcome new students and get to know students who are often left out.
- Sign (or start) a Peace Pledge in which students promise to settle disagreements peaceably and to work toward a safe campus.

WITH A GROUP
Work with classmates to create a brochure that encourages all students to play their part in keeping the school safe.

FIGURE 7.4

Shield Yourself from Violence

Follow these precautions to protect yourself from violence. *What other strategies could you use to avoid violence, gangs, and weapons?*

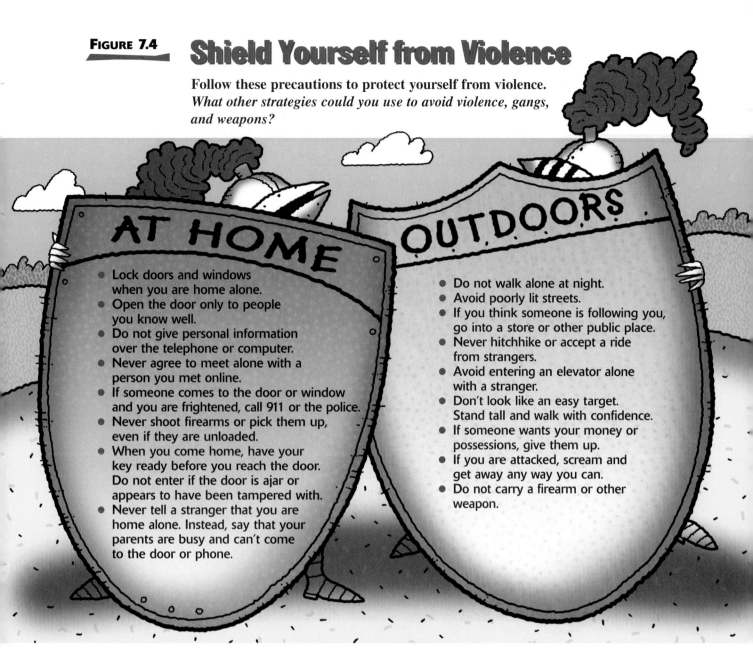

AT HOME

- Lock doors and windows when you are home alone.
- Open the door only to people you know well.
- Do not give personal information over the telephone or computer.
- Never agree to meet alone with a person you met online.
- If someone comes to the door or window and you are frightened, call 911 or the police.
- Never shoot firearms or pick them up, even if they are unloaded.
- When you come home, have your key ready before you reach the door. Do not enter if the door is ajar or appears to have been tampered with.
- Never tell a stranger that you are home alone. Instead, say that your parents are busy and can't come to the door or phone.

OUTDOORS

- Do not walk alone at night.
- Avoid poorly lit streets.
- If you think someone is following you, go into a store or other public place.
- Never hitchhike or accept a ride from strangers.
- Avoid entering an elevator alone with a stranger.
- Don't look like an easy target. Stand tall and walk with confidence.
- If someone wants your money or possessions, give them up.
- If you are attacked, scream and get away any way you can.
- Do not carry a firearm or other weapon.

Protecting Yourself from Violence

Protect yourself from violent crime by avoiding unsafe situations. Develop self-protection habits by being alert to what is going on around you and trusting your instincts. If a situation feels dangerous, it probably is. Be ready for threatening situations before they happen by planning ahead. With the adults in your family, identify some potential dangers. Figure out what you could do to get out of those situations safely. If you suspect or hear a student talking about violence, report it to school authorities.

Choosing your friends wisely is another way to protect yourself. Avoid people who have a low commitment to school, participate in illegal activities, or use alcohol or drugs. **Figure 7.4** suggests other ways to protect yourself from violence.

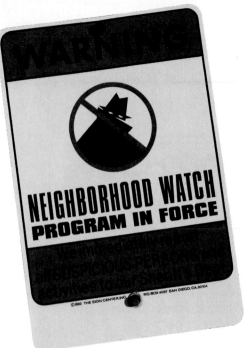

Protecting Yourself from Rape

Rape is *any kind of sexual intercourse against a person's will.* Over half of all rape victims know their attackers. Whenever a person is forced to have sex, whether with someone he or she knows or with a stranger, a rape has occurred. Rape is always an act of violence, and it is illegal. To protect yourself from rape, you need to recognize and avoid situations that might increase the risk of an attack. Here are some suggestions.

- If you go out alone with someone, make it clear that you're not interested in any sexual activity.
- Avoid secluded places.
- Don't drink alcohol or use other drugs or date people who do.
- Always carry money so you can call home or take a cab or bus if you feel unsafe.

Many communities have worked together with local law enforcement agencies to make their neighborhoods safer. *What is being done to protect your community?*

Preventing Violence

People across the nation are making an effort to reduce and prevent violence. Here are some of the actions they have taken:

- Holding stop-the-violence rallies
- Supporting stronger gun laws
- Installing lighting in parks and playgrounds
- Breaking up gang control of public parks
- Starting Neighborhood Watch programs
- Supporting teen curfews
- Teaching nonviolent conflict resolution
- Assigning more police to street patrols

Lesson 3 Review

Using complete sentences, answer the following questions on a sheet of paper.

Reviewing Terms and Facts

1. **Vocabulary** Define *violence* and *homicide.*
2. **Explain** What is the purpose of a zero tolerance policy?
3. **Identify** What are three basic ways you can protect yourself from violence?

Thinking Critically

4. **Explain** Why is it important to follow the rules prohibiting possession of weapons at school?

5. **Apply** What strategies could help teens in your community avoid violence and gangs?
6. **Analyze** Describe the dangers associated with weapons and strategies for avoiding weapons.

Applying Health Skills

7. **Practicing Healthful Behaviors** With a partner, write a skit in which a teen helps a peer avoid or cope with a potentially dangerous situation involving violence. Perform your skit for the class to demonstrate strategies for preventing deliberate injuries that may result from violence.

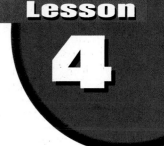
Preventing Abuse

Forms of Abuse

Abuse takes many forms and is a significant problem in the United States. In general, **abuse** can be defined as *the physical, emotional, or mental mistreatment of one person by another.* Abuse occurs among all ages, in all racial and ethnic populations, and in all economic groups. There is no situation in which abuse is okay. Abuse is damaging to everyone involved and is illegal.

Abuse occurs mostly in close relationships. Parents or guardians may abuse children, siblings may abuse each other, and friends may abuse friends. Many abusers are more powerful than their victims and try to make them feel that they deserve to be treated harshly. Abuse is not an acceptable form of discipline. No one ever deserves abuse, and it is never the victim's fault.

Physical Abuse

Physical abuse includes hitting, slapping, kicking, pushing, shoving, punching, choking, and other ways of doing physical harm to a person. An abuser could use a weapon, belt, or other item to harm the victim. Shaking is also abuse. Shaking a baby or young child is especially dangerous because it can cause brain damage. A legal term used to describe physical abuse is battery. **Battery** is *the beating, hitting, or kicking of another person.* Battery, like all other forms of abuse, is against the law.

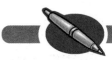

Quick Write

What does the term *abuse* mean to you? Who would you talk to if you thought a friend was being abused?

LEARN ABOUT...

- forms of abuse and their effects on victims.
- the cycle of abuse.
- ways to avoid abuse.
- where to get help if you are abused.

VOCABULARY

- abuse
- battery
- sexual harassment
- neglect
- cycle of abuse

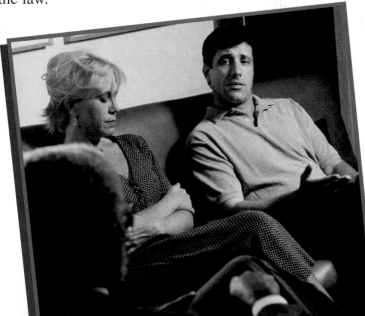

In most communities, help is available for victims of abuse and for those who abuse. *Where can students in your school report abuse?*

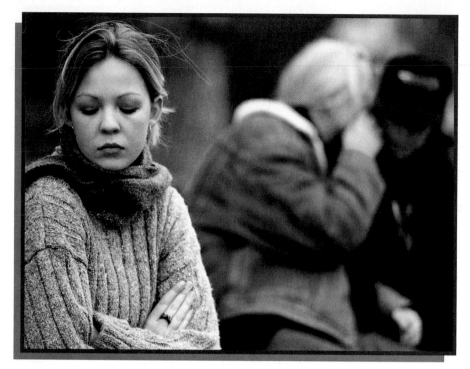

Emotional Abuse

Emotional abuse is the use of words or gestures to mistreat another person. It occurs when a person is made fun of, yelled at, bullied, and made to feel stupid, worthless, or helpless. Threats of physical violence are emotional abuse. If a male teen threatens his girlfriend when he sees her talking with another male teen, he is committing emotional abuse.

Emotional abuse can make a person feel isolated and unwanted. *How might you reach out to someone who needs help?*

Sexual Abuse

Sexual abuse occurs when a person is forced to participate in a sexual act against his or her will. It is sexual abuse any time an adult commits a sexual act with a child or young person below the age of consent. Often the sexual abuser of children and teens is an adult family member or friend. Sexual abusers don't always use physical force. Young people are often persuaded, bribed, tricked, or bullied into performing sexual acts. All sexual abuse is illegal.

One kind of sexual abuse that may happen at school is **sexual harassment**, which is *uninvited and unwelcome sexual conduct directed at another person.* Sexual harassment includes words, touching, jokes, looks, notes, or gestures with sexual meaning. When confronted, many people claim they meant it as a joke, but sexual harassment is not funny. It is illegal and must be reported to school personnel.

Neglect

People need love and encouragement, nourishing food, clothing, adequate housing, education, safety, and medical and dental care. Children, elderly people, and people with disabilities depend on other people to help them meet these needs. **Neglect** is *the failure to meet a person's basic physical and emotional needs.* Neglect causes physical and emotional harm. Children who are neglected may grow up feeling worthless and have difficulty setting and achieving goals. Neglect is a form of abuse and is against the law.

Effects of Abuse

The effects of abuse are long term and serious. In many cases, the mental and emotional effects remain long after any physical injuries have healed. Victims often blame themselves and are too afraid or too embarrassed to seek help. Yet if a person does not receive help, the effects of abuse can last a lifetime. Long-term effects of abuse include the following:

- Self-neglect or self-injury
- Depression, anxiety, panic attacks, and sleep disorders
- Violent and criminal behavior
- Chronic pain
- Abuse of alcohol and other drugs
- Eating disorders
- Inappropriate sexual conduct
- Suicide attempts
- Poor personal relationships

People who were abused as children are at risk of becoming abusers. *What can a person do to break the cycle of abuse?*

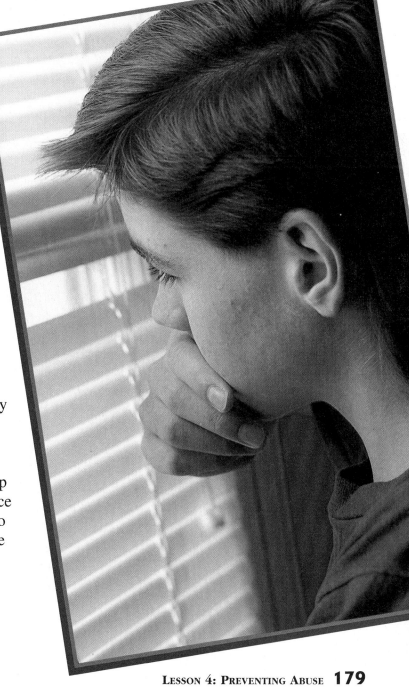

The Cycle of Abuse

A person who was abused as a child or who witnessed abuse of others may see abuse as a normal way of life. As adults, such people are more likely to abuse children. This *pattern of repeating abuse from one generation to the next* is known as the **cycle of abuse**. One key to stopping all forms of abuse is to break the cycle of abuse. That starts with getting help from someone you trust.

If you or someone you know is being abused, tell a parent, other family member, teacher, school nurse, doctor, or trusted adult. If you do not get the help you need from this adult, tell someone else. Abused people need help and so do abusers. Their past experience does not make it acceptable for them to abuse others. Abuse is never acceptable and is always illegal.

How to Avoid Abuse

To avoid abuse and to help prevent it, remember the three Rs:

- **Recognize.** Learn to recognize and avoid situations that can increase the risk of abuse.
- **Resist.** If someone tries to abuse you physically or sexually, resist. Fight back any way you can. Be assertive.
- **Report.** Tell someone about the incident as soon as you can.

Where to Get Help

Teens who are abused need help to get out of their situation. Asking for help is not a sign of weakness. Instead, it shows courage and a willingness to stand up for yourself. Seeking help can break the cycle of abuse.

Many helpful resources are available in your school and community. Ask a teacher or counselor about school resources for victims of abuse and abusers. Many religious organizations have counselors who can help with abuse problems. Also look for teen help lines, abuse hot lines, and crisis centers in your local phone

HEALTH SKILLS ACTIVITY

COMMUNICATION SKILLS

Helping a Victim of Abuse

When Alex noticed bruise marks on Lauren's arm, she said it happened when her boyfriend was just "goofing around." Later, Alex noticed other bruises, and one day Lauren came in with a black eye. Lauren's explanation of how she got it didn't make sense, and she seemed ashamed of the injury.

Alex thinks that Lauren might be in an abusive relationship. He knows that if Lauren is being abused, the one thing she needs most is for someone to hear and believe her. On the other hand, Lauren has brushed off Alex's questions before. Alex wants to talk to Lauren about her injuries, but he isn't sure how to handle the conversation. He decides to use the speaking and listening skills he has learned to help her cope with this dangerous situation.

WHAT WOULD YOU DO?

With a classmate, write and perform a skit to demonstrate how Alex could use the communication skills below to help his peer cope with this dangerous situation in a healthy way.

SPEAKING SKILLS

- "I" messages
- Clear, simple statements
- Honest thoughts and feelings
- Appropriate body language

LISTENING SKILLS

- Appropriate body language
- Conversation encouragers
- Mirror thoughts and feelings
- Ask questions

book. Most centers offer help for both the abused and the abuser. General resources are described below:

- **Police department.** Call here if someone is in immediate danger. In many communities the emergency number for the local police department is 911.
- **Hospital.** Hospitals provide emergency medical treatment.
- **Shelters.** Family members in danger of being abused can stay in shelters while they get help putting their lives in order.
- **Support or self-help groups.** In these groups, people have a chance to discuss their situation with others who have experienced similar problems.
- **Crisis hot lines.** These are telephone services that parents and abused children can call to get help. Hot line workers receive special training. All conversations are kept confidential, and the caller does not have to give his or her name.

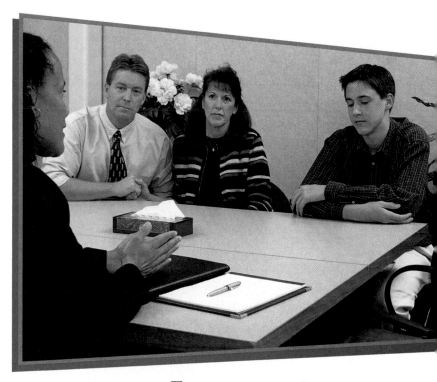

Families that experience abuse need the help of an experienced counselor. *Why must both the abuser and the victim get help?*

Lesson 4 Review

Using complete sentences, answer the following questions on a sheet of paper.

Reviewing Terms and Facts

1. **Vocabulary** Define *abuse* and use it in a sentence that shows that you understand its meaning.
2. **List** Give three examples of behaviors that could be viewed as sexual harassment.
3. **Explain** What is the *cycle of abuse?*
4. **Identify** What do the three Rs for avoiding abuse stand for?

Thinking Critically

5. **Explain** Why do you think some people are reluctant to report incidents of abuse?

6. **Evaluate** Analyze strategies for responding to deliberate injuries that may result from abuse. Which ones do you think would be the most effective? Why?

Applying Health Skills

7. **Advocacy** Identify several strategies for prevention and intervention of physical, emotional, and sexual abuse. Create a flyer that features these strategies and tells teens where they can go for help.

Stopping Violence Before It Starts

Teens are finding ways to make their classrooms safer.

Teen Brandon Boxler doesn't want anyone in his school to get hurt by violence—so he's doing something to prevent it. Brandon had heard that two of his classmates at Northern High in Durham, North Carolina, were moving from a war of words to physical fighting. So Brandon, president of his school's Students Against Violence Everywhere (SAVE) chapter, convinced the pair to participate in his group's peer-mediation program. Now, when the girls see each other in the hall, they just say hello and move on. "Everybody gets mad," Brandon says, "but how you deal with it is the difference between violence and a peaceful resolution."

Unfortunately, more students seem to be resorting to guns to solve problems. According to the National School Safety Center, there were 13 school shooting incidents during one recent school year—almost twice as many as the year before. Alarmed, school officials nationwide have started programs to help ensure safety.

Teens Stopping Crime

Palm Beach County, Florida, has had great success with its Student Crime Stoppers hot line. Over a five-month period, tips from young people led to 14 arrests—eight of which involved students with weapons. In Texas, each of Houston's 23 high schools has uniformed officers who patrol the halls and give metal detector tests to students in random classrooms. Violent crime in Houston schools dropped 20 percent. Nicole Vazquez, a student at Lamar High, is glad the officers are around: "[Their presence] prevents people from taking extreme actions."

Promoting School Safety

Many students aren't waiting for schools to make changes. Like Brandon and his fellow SAVE participants—80,000 total in 34 states—they're taking violence prevention into their own hands. Teen Monti Murphy and more than a dozen classmates started an antiviolence organization called Keep It Real at Woodrow Wilson Senior High in Washington state. After two

What Would You Do?

Take a look at the pie chart below to see how 5,000 teens responded to this question: If you suspected someone might commit a violent act, would you notify the school administration?

17% said no.

83% said yes.

students were shot following a fight at a school basketball game, Monti decided to try to stop the violence. Through the nonprofit group, 400 students have signed an antiviolence pledge. Now teen mentors talk to grade-school students about alternatives to fighting. Working with young people helps Monti understand the importance of nonviolence. "This eight-year-old girl told me about being scared to walk home, and we exchanged phone numbers. She calls me and we talk about her fear," Monti says. "We try to reach one person at a time."

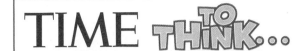

TIME TO THINK...

About Preventing School Violence

Study the pie chart above. About how many teens said that they would report a potential problem to the school administration? About how many said they'd keep the information to themselves? With your classmates, respond to the poll question on slips of paper. Your teacher will tally the results. How do they compare with the results above? As a class, discuss possible barriers to reporting potential violence and how these obstacles might be overcome.

WORKING THROUGH CONFLICTS

Model

Sophia and her brother Nathan often disagree over how to share household tasks. Read about how they compromised to resolve their conflict.

Sophia and Nathan are responsible for cleaning the house. Both teens prefer to vacuum. Neither likes to dust or clean the bathrooms. One Saturday, when Nathan rushed to get the vacuum first, Sophia became angry. She went for a bike ride to "cool off." When she returned, Sophia told Nathan she wanted to talk about their problem. She asked him to explain his side of the story.

Nathan said he thought cleaning the bathrooms was disgusting and dusting took too long. He liked to get his part of the cleaning done so he could do other things. Sophia said she didn't like cleaning the bathrooms either, but she would be willing to dust if Nathan would vacuum and clean the bathrooms. Nathan said that wasn't fair, since dusting didn't take as long as both of the other chores. He said that he would clean the bathrooms and vacuum most of the house if Sophia would dust the house and vacuum her bedroom. Sophia and Nathan agreed to try this solution.

Practice

Work with a partner to write a conversation based on one of the situations shown below. Each of you will take the part of one of the characters involved in the conflict. Have one partner begin the conversation by stating his or her character's point of view about the conflict. Pass the paper back and forth and take turns responding to each other's comments. Don't speak to each other or try to preplan your conversation. As you write, use the steps for conflict resolution to reach a win-win situation. When you're done, read your conversation to the class. Ask the other students to identify the T.A.L.K. steps that you used.

Elliot and Spencer share a bedroom. Elliot likes to listen to music while he studies. Spencer prefers peace and quiet when he's working.

Annabel wants to wear a new trendy outfit to a family celebration. Her father thinks it is entirely inappropriate for this event.

Kayla and Jeremy have been friends for a long time. This morning, Kayla heard from another friend that Jeremy was spreading rumors about her.

Apply/Assess

Write a story about two characters who are having a conflict. State the reason for their conflict and show how the characters use the T.A.L.K. steps to reach a win-win solution. You can use one of the ideas below or choose a situation that has created conflict for you or someone you know. When you are finished, read your story aloud to the class.

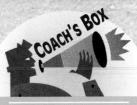

COACH'S BOX

Conflict Resolution

T Take a time out, at least 30 minutes.

A Allow each person to tell his or her side uninterrupted.

L Let each person ask questions.

K Keep brainstorming to find a solution.

Self-✓Check

- Does my story show how to use the T.A.L.K. steps to resolve conflict?
- Did I show a win-win solution?

CONFLICT: Someone approaches you when you're sitting on a school bench and tells you that this is his "turf."

CONFLICT: Another classmate pushes ahead of you in the cafeteria line.

CONFLICT: You and a friend like the same person as a girlfriend or boyfriend.

After You Read

Use your completed Foldable to review the information on the nature of conflict.

FOLDABLES™
Study Organizer

Reviewing Vocabulary and Concepts

On a sheet of paper, write the numbers 1–8. After each number, write the term from the list that best completes each statement.

- escalate
- compromise
- conflict
- win-win solution
- mediation
- prejudice
- peer mediation
- values

Lesson 1

1. A disagreement between people with opposing viewpoints, ideas, or goals is a(n) _____ .

2. The beliefs and ideals that you consider important are your _____ .

3. Poorly managed conflicts can _____ , or become more serious.

4. A negative and unjustly formed opinion, usually against people of a different racial, religious, or cultural group, is called _____ .

Lesson 2

5. A(n) _____ resolves a conflict by giving both parties something they want.

6. The process in which a third person helps those in conflict find a solution is called _____ .

7. In _____ , a student serves as the mediator for students involved in a conflict.

8. When you _____ , you give up something in order to reach a solution that satisfies everyone.

Lesson 3

On a sheet of paper, write the numbers 9–12. After each number, write the letter of the answer that best completes each statement.

9. A group of people who associate with one another to take part in criminal activity is a
   a. clique.
   b. gang.
   c. circle.
   d. club.

10. Any act that causes physical or psychological harm to a person or damages property is
   a. violence.
   b. battery.
   c. prejudice.
   d. cowardice.

11. A zero tolerance policy means that exceptions to school rules are made for
   a. good students.
   b. first-time offenders.
   c. no one.
   d. anyone.

12. Another word that means the killing of one human being by another is
   a. suicide.
   b. hate crime.
   c. battery.
   d. homicide.

Lesson 4

On a sheet of paper, write the numbers 13–15. Write *True* or *False* for each statement below. If the statement is false, change the underlined word or phrase to make it true.

13. A legal term used to describe physical abuse is <u>sexual harassment</u>.

14. The process of an abused child growing up and abusing his or her children is known as <u>bullying</u>.

15. The failure to meet a person's basic physical and emotional needs is <u>neglect</u>.

Thinking Critically

Using complete sentences, answer the following questions on a sheet of paper.

16. Identify List three healthy ways that peers can help each other avoid and cope with potentially dangerous situations involving violence or abuse.

17. Recognize Give two examples of how a teen might avoid situations that can increase the risk of abuse.

Career Corner

Professional Mediator Are you a good listener and able to see both sides of a disagreement? If so, then you may have what it takes to be a professional mediator. These professionals work in corporations, government agencies, and schools, helping people solve problems peacefully. To enter this career, you'll need a four-year college degree and training in mediation. If you think this career might match your skills, read more about it in Career Corner at health.glencoe.com.

Standardized Test Practice

Math

Read the paragraph below and then answer the questions.

Overcrowding can cause conflict to erupt. To minimize conflict, it is essential for each individual to have enough space to avoid the stress of overcrowding.

1. A school district determined that each student needs 12 square feet of space in a class. According to this guideline, how many students can occupy a classroom that measures 20 feet by 25 feet, if an area 5 feet by 25 feet is kept empty at the front of the room?

Ⓐ 25 students

Ⓑ 31 students

Ⓒ 41 students

Ⓓ 60 students

2. The classrooms in a certain school are different sizes. The numbers of students that can occupy the eighth-grade classrooms without being too crowded are 23, 30, 24, 21, 26, and 21. What is the mean of these numbers?

Ⓐ 21 students

Ⓑ 23 students

Ⓒ 24 students

Ⓓ 25 students

3. Explain why area instead of volume is used to determine the space needed to avoid overcrowding.

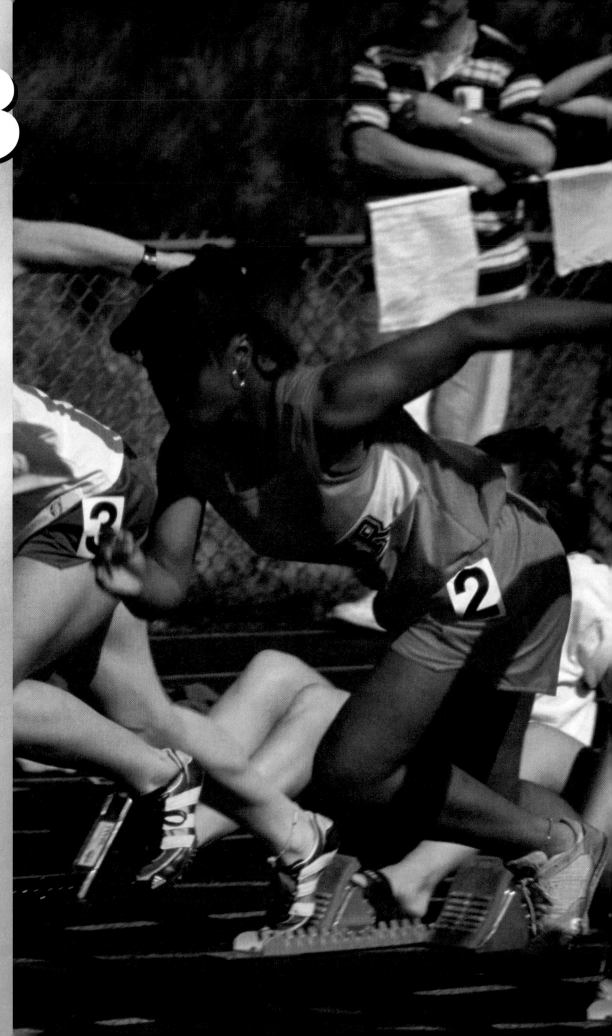

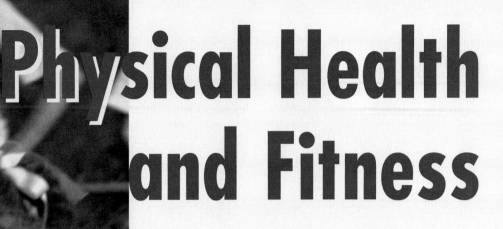

Physical Health and Fitness

HEALTH *in Action*

Choosing the right foods at every meal is just as important as staying active. Nutrition and physical activity work hand in hand to keep you alert, fit, and energetic. Healthy foods give you the fuel you need for your favorite sport, for a day at school, or for just hanging out with your friends. Daily physical activity is healthful, fun, and can keep you at the front of the pack, on or off the field. If you eat smart and keep moving, you'll always be on track!

How can eating breakfast get you to the finish line?

GRAPEFRUIT
89¢ lb.

Nutrition for Health

HEALTH *Online*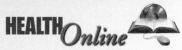

Do you practice healthy nutrition habits? Go to health.glencoe.com and take the Health Inventory for Chapter 8 to find out how you rate.

FOLDABLES™
Study Organizer

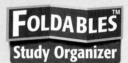

Before You Read

Make this Foldable to record what you learn in Lesson 1 about the body's need for nutrients. Begin with two plain sheets of 8½″ × 11″ paper.

Step 1

Collect two sheets of paper and place them 1″ apart.

Step 2

Fold up the bottom edges, stopping them 1″ from the top edges. This makes all tabs the same size.

Step 3

Crease the paper to hold the tabs in place. Staple along the fold.

Step 4

Turn and label the tabs as shown.

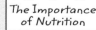

The Importance of Nutrition

Why You Need Nutritious Foods
Influences on Your Food Choices
Getting the Nutrients You Need

As You Read

Under the appropriate tab of your Foldable, define terms and record information on nutrients and influences on food choices.

The Importance of Nutrition

Quick Write

Write down six items that you've eaten recently, and list the factors that influenced your decision to eat each food. Determine the strongest influences on your food choices.

LEARN ABOUT...

- why your body needs nutritious food.
- what influences your food choices.
- the difference between appetite and hunger.
- getting the nutrients you need.

VOCABULARY

- calories
- nutrients
- nutrition
- appetite
- hunger
- nutrient deficiency

Why You Need Nutritious Food

When you drink a cold glass of milk or bite into a crisp apple, you probably are thinking about the taste and texture of the foods. Yet while you're enjoying the pleasures of eating, the foods you eat are influencing your overall health and wellness. When you make healthy choices about foods, you're more likely to look your best and perform at your peak.

One important reason you eat is to take in calories. **Calories** are *units of heat that measure the energy used by the body and the energy that foods supply to the body.* You need this energy for everything you do—from running laps to doing your homework. Food also provides **nutrients**, *substances in food that your body needs.* Nutrients have many important roles, including

- giving you energy.
- building new tissues and repairing cells.
- helping your body's processes and systems run smoothly.

Different foods contain different types and amounts of nutrients. You need a wide variety of healthful foods to get all the nutrients your body needs.

Nutrition is *the process of using food and its substances to help your body have energy, grow, develop, and work properly.* Good nutrition is one of the main factors in building and maintaining good health.

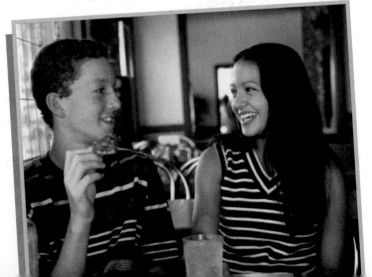

Eating also offers an opportunity to spend time with friends and family. *What types of food do you choose when you eat out with friends?*

FIGURE 8.1

FACTORS THAT INFLUENCE FOOD CHOICES

Factors	Description
Family and friends	You may prefer certain foods, like burritos or vegetable stir-fry, because you have grown up eating them at home. At the same time, your friends may persuade you to try new and different foods.
Cultural background	Different cultures have different traditions about what they eat, and perhaps where, how, and with whom they eat. For example, Mexican American families may eat beans, corn, and tortillas, while Italian American families may favor pasta dishes. Many Americans enjoy trying a variety of ethnic foods. What cultural foods are part of your eating pattern?
Food availability	Some foods are regional, growing only in certain areas. Some are seasonal and available only in certain months. Fresh blueberries, for example, are plentiful in summer but hard to find in the winter months. Still, modern transportation and growing methods have expanded the food supply. Many foods that were once regional or seasonal are now available in many areas year-round.
Time and money resources	Schedules and budgets affect a family's food choices. Eating fast foods or convenience foods often takes less time. Some families may look for bulk foods that provide more for the dollar.
Advertising	Have you ever tried a food because you heard about it from a television or magazine ad? Ads can influence our choices of certain brands and products and may persuade us to try new foods.
Knowledge of nutrition	The more you know about the nutrients in different foods, the better able you are to choose foods that supply the health benefits that you need.
Personal preferences	Your personal likes and dislikes and overall health goals contribute to your food choices. Some people have allergies or other medical conditions that affect their food choices. Among the foods that most often cause allergic reactions are milk, peanuts, wheat, and shellfish.

What Influences Your Food Choices?

What are your favorite foods? Do you know why you make these food choices? Chances are that you eat a variety of foods and that your food choices are influenced by many different factors. **Figure 8.1** describes some of these factors.

Appetite and Hunger

When you smell popcorn, do you want to try some? Does the sight of fresh strawberries make your mouth water? Do you love to crunch on fresh carrots? These are signs of your appetite at work. Your **appetite** is *the psychological desire for food*. It may be stimulated by the smell, sight, or texture of food.

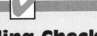

Reading Check

Build vocabulary. Write sentences using these words from the chapter: *calories, nutrients, appetite, hunger, nutrient deficiency.*

Appetite is different from hunger. **Hunger** is *the physical need for food.* When you are hungry, your brain sends a signal to find food. You may hear your stomach growl, or feel it contract. You may also feel tired or light-headed. These signs indicate that your body's supply of food energy and nutrients is running low.

When you eat, the hunger gradually goes away. Your stomach needs about 20 minutes to send a message back to the brain to turn off the hunger switch. Eating slowly allows time for your brain to receive the message. Many people overeat when they eat too fast.

Food and Emotions

Food can meet emotional needs too. Do certain foods that you associate with special events bring you happy memories? Perhaps you have favorite foods that comfort you when you are feeling ill or sad. Using food as a way of dealing with negative emotions is not a healthy way to respond to these feelings. People who eat to relieve stress or boredom need to develop more appropriate coping skills.

Getting the Nutrients You Need

Everyone needs the same nutrients to maintain good health, but the amount of nutrients needed depends on a person's age, gender, state of health, and level of activity. When you do not get enough of

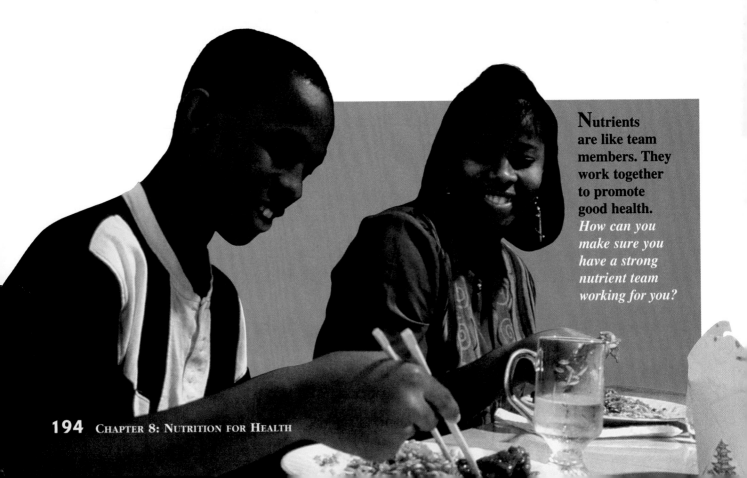

Nutrients are like team members. They work together to promote good health. *How can you make sure you have a strong nutrient team working for you?*

a particular nutrient, you could have a **nutrient deficiency**, *a shortage of a nutrient.*

As a teen, you need more calcium than you did before for building strong and growing bones. However, suppose you don't eat enough foods that supply calcium. Over time, the calcium deficiency could affect the strength of your teeth and bones. A food plan that includes calcium-rich foods helps prevent osteoporosis, a disease in which bones become brittle and more liable to break. You also need more iron because your body makes more red blood cells as you grow. A shortage of iron can lead to a blood disease called anemia. In general, teens need more of most nutrients to support growth and satisfy energy needs.

Most people in the United States get plenty of food, yet many still do not get the nutrients they need. This is partly the result of lifestyles that tend to encourage fast foods and promote foods that are high in fat and sugar. Eating low-nutrient, high-fat foods, along with overeating, can lead to long-term health problems such as obesity, heart disease, cancer, and diabetes. Your nutritional knowledge and healthful eating habits are your best defense against poor nutrition.

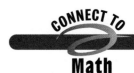
Math

UNIT PRICING
Calculating the unit prices of food products and comparing them can help you determine the most economical purchases. To compute the unit price, locate the weight or volume on a packaged food product. Divide the price of the product by its weight or volume. The result will be the unit price. *At the supermarket, find three sizes of the same packaged food. Calculate the unit price of each and compare to determine which product is the most economical purchase.*

Lesson 1 Review

Using complete sentences, answer the following questions on a sheet of paper.

Reviewing Terms and Facts

1. **Vocabulary** What are *calories?* What do they measure?
2. **Recall** What is *nutrition?* What is the relationship between nutrition and health?
3. **Compare** What is the difference between appetite and hunger?
4. **Explain** Why are calcium-rich foods an important part of a teen's food choices?

Thinking Critically

5. **Evaluate** Explain the role of media and technology in influencing food choices.

6. **Analyze** How is it possible to have plenty of food and yet be poorly nourished?

Applying Health Skills

7. **Analyzing Influences** Find an advertisement for a specific food product. Use critical-thinking skills to analyze the marketing and advertising techniques in the ad and their influence on food selection. Report your findings to the class.

Nutrients for Wellness

Quick Write

What's your idea of a healthful meal or snack? Create a menu for what you consider a day of healthful foods you would enjoy.

LEARN ABOUT...

- how your body uses different nutrients.
- the sources of different nutrients.
- the need for water and fiber in your meals and snacks.
- substances in food that should be limited.

VOCABULARY

- carbohydrates
- proteins
- amino acids
- saturated fats
- unsaturated fats
- vitamins
- minerals
- fiber

The Six Types of Nutrients

Food nourishes you with more than 40 different nutrients. These nutrients are grouped into six categories: carbohydrates, proteins, fats, vitamins, minerals, and water. Eating a variety of foods to provide these nutrients is essential to good health.

Carbohydrates

Carbohydrates are *the sugars and starches that provide your body with most of its energy.* Carbohydrates can be either simple or complex. Simple carbohydrates, or sugars, are found in fruit, milk, and honey. Sugar is also added to candy, cookies, and other foods. Complex carbohydrates, or starches, are found in breads, cereals, pasta, rice, potatoes, dry beans, corn, and other starchy vegetables. As your body digests complex carbohydrates, it breaks them down into simple sugars, which are absorbed into the bloodstream to provide energy. Nutritionists recommend that 45 to 65 percent of your daily calories come from carbohydrates.

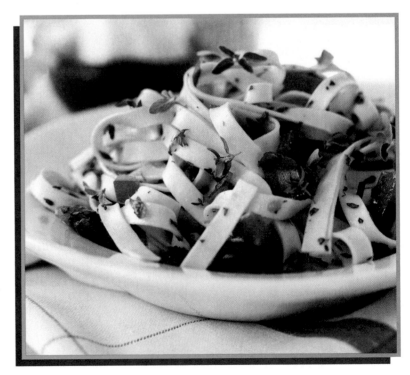

Most of your body's energy supply should come from carbohydrates. *What foods do you enjoy that are good sources of simple and complex carbohydrates?*

Proteins

Proteins are *nutrients your body uses to build, repair, and maintain cells and tissues.* They also help your body fight disease, and they provide energy when your body doesn't get enough from other sources.

Amino acids are *small units that make up protein.* Your body can produce most amino acids on its own. The remaining ones, called essential amino acids, must come from food you eat.

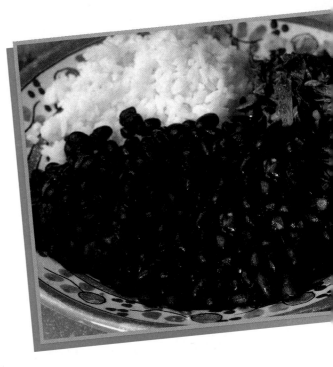

Foods from animal sources, such as meat, fish, poultry, eggs, milk, and yogurt, contain complete proteins. They provide all the essential amino acids. Foods from plant sources, such as soybeans, nuts, peas, and dry beans contain incomplete proteins. They lack one or more of the essential amino acids. Vegetarians can combine foods from plant sources to make complete proteins. Consuming a variety of plant foods, such as beans, rice, nuts, and peas, gives you complete protein and provides the essential amino acids. You don't need to eat these foods at the same meal to get the benefit. Just have a good variety throughout the whole day.

Meals that include a variety of plant-based foods can provide all the essential amino acids. *What are some of your favorite sources of protein?*

Fats

Fats are nutrients that provide energy and perform many functions for your body. They carry fat-soluble vitamins and promote healthy skin and normal growth. Foods that are high in fats tend to be high in calories. For this reason, health experts generally recommend that your eating plan include only moderate amounts of fat.

Saturated fats are *fats that are solid at room temperature.* They are found mostly in animal and dairy products, such as butter, some meats, cheese, and whole milk. An eating pattern that includes too many saturated fats can increase a person's risk of heart disease.

Unsaturated fats are *fats that remain liquid at room temperature.* They come mainly from plant sources. Foods containing mostly unsaturated fats include vegetable oils, nuts, avocados, and olives. Unsaturated fats lower cholesterol levels and are considered healthier than saturated fats. Trans fats are a type of fat produced when hydrogen atoms are added to unsaturated fats to make them solid. Trans fats have been linked to heart disease.

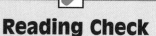

Reading Check

Study the words *saturated* and *unsaturated.* What difference does the prefix make in their meanings? What does the root mean?

Vitamins

Vitamins are *substances needed in small quantities to help regulate body functions.* Vitamins help your body fight infections, use other nutrients, and perform other tasks. Water-soluble vitamins, such as vitamin C and B vitamins, dissolve in water, cannot be stored in your body, and should be part of your daily eating pattern. Fat-soluble vitamins, including vitamins A, D, E, and K, dissolve in fat and can be stored in body fat until needed. See **Figure 8.2** for more information about functions and sources of selected vitamins.

FIGURE 8.2

VITAMINS AND MINERALS: FUNCTIONS AND SOURCES

Functions	Sources
Vitamin A Promotes healthy skin and normal vision	Dark green leafy vegetables (such as spinach); dairy products (such as milk); deep yellow-orange fruits and vegetables (such as carrots, winter squash, apricots); eggs; liver
B Vitamins Needed for a healthy nervous system; help in energy production	Poultry; eggs; meat; fish; whole-grain breads and cereals
Vitamin C Needed for healthy teeth, gums, and bones; helps heal wounds and fight infection	Citrus fruits (such as oranges and grapefruit); cantaloupe, strawberries, mangoes; tomatoes; cabbage and broccoli; potatoes
Vitamin D Promotes strong bones and teeth and the absorption of calcium	Fortified milk; fatty fish (such as salmon and mackerel); egg yolks; liver
Vitamin K Helps blood clot	Dark green leafy vegetables (such as spinach); egg yolks; liver; some cereals
Calcium Needed to build and maintain strong bones and teeth	Dairy products (such as milk, yogurt, cheese); dark green leafy vegetables (such as spinach); canned fish with edible bones (such as sardines)
Fluoride Promotes strong bones and teeth; prevents tooth decay	Fluoridated water; fish with edible bones
Iron Needed for hemoglobin in red blood cells	Red meat; poultry; dry beans (legumes); fortified breakfast cereal; nuts; eggs; dried fruits; dark green leafy vegetables
Potassium Helps regulate fluid balance in tissues; promotes proper nerve function	Fruits (such as bananas and oranges); dry beans and peas; dried fruits
Zinc Helps heal wounds; needed for cell reproduction	Meat; poultry; eggs; dry beans and peas; whole-grain breads and cereals

Minerals

Minerals are *elements needed in small quantities for forming healthy bones and teeth, and for regulating certain body processes.* Calcium, phosphorus, and magnesium help build strong bones and teeth. Iron plays a vital role in making red blood cells. See **Figure 8.2** for more information about functions and sources of selected minerals.

Water

Water is a nutrient that is vital to your life and health. It makes up over half of your body and serves many important functions. Water transports nutrients through your body, helps you digest food, lubricates your joints, removes wastes, and helps regulate body temperature.

You lose water every day in urine and sweat, and you need to replace it continually. Nutritionists generally recommend that you consume at least eight 8-ounce cups of fluids a day, and even more during hot weather. Choose liquids such as plain drinking water, fruit juices, milk, and soup. Beverages with caffeine or added sugar are not the best choices.

Other Substances in Food

Food contains many substances in addition to the major nutrients. Some of these substances, such as fiber, are important to your health and should be part of your everyday food choices. For good health, try to limit fats, cholesterol, added sugars, and salt. Go easy on drinks with caffeine, too.

Fiber

Fiber is *the part of fruits, vegetables, grains, and beans that your body cannot digest.* It helps move food particles through your digestive system. Including high-fiber foods in your eating plan may help lower your risk of certain types of cancer and reduce your risk of heart disease. Foods high in fiber include whole-grain breads and cereals, fruits and vegetables, and dry beans and peas.

Hidden Fats

Health experts recommend that no more than 35 percent of your daily calories come from fat. It's easy to cut down on the fats you can see. For example, put a smaller amount of butter on your baked potato, or trim fat from meat. Fats are often hidden in processed and prepared foods. It's harder to cut down on hidden fats, but it can be done. Go easy on fried foods and switch from whole to low-fat milk. Read the labels on packaged foods to check for fats and oils.

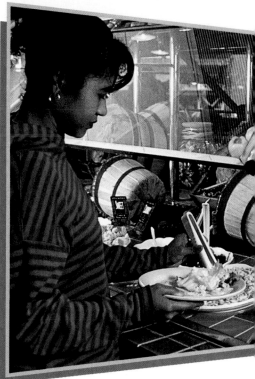

The fiber found in raw vegetables and fruit plays an important role in protecting your health. *What are some high-fiber foods that you like?*

Cholesterol

Cholesterol is a waxy substance used by the body to build cells and hormones and to protect nerve fibers. Most cholesterol is produced in your liver and circulates in the blood. Cholesterol is also found in foods of animal origin, including meats, chicken, egg yolks, and dairy products. Eating high-cholesterol foods can affect the levels of cholesterol in your blood. There are two types of cholesterol in your blood. Low-density cholesterol, or LDL, is a "bad" form that can leave deposits on the walls of your blood vessels. This buildup raises the risk of heart attack or stroke. High-density cholesterol, or HDL, is a "good" form that can help lower LDL levels. To help reduce LDL levels in your blood, limit your intake of foods that are high in fat and cholesterol. Regular physical activity also helps prevent LDL buildup.

Added Sugar

You may be surprised to learn that the average American eats about 100 pounds of sugar a year! Sugar occurs naturally in fruit

---

Hands-On Health

JARS OF SUGAR

Do you know how much sugar you consume when you grab a quick drink or snack? The following table lists the amount of sugar, in grams, that you might find in several popular foods.

Food	Grams of Sugar
Cola (12 oz.)	42
Fat-free, fruit yogurt (8 oz.)	35
Light popcorn (1 c.)	0
Fruit punch drink (8 oz.)	27
Sweetened breakfast cereal (¾ c.)	15
Three reduced-fat chocolate sandwich cookies	14
Chocolate candy bar (1.55 oz.)	40

WHAT YOU WILL NEED
- seven empty baby food jars
- container of sugar
- set of measuring spoons

WHAT YOU WILL DO
1. Note that 5 grams of sugar is equivalent to 1 level teaspoon of sugar; 1 gram is just under ¼ teaspoon; 2 grams is a little under ½ teaspoon.
2. Calculate how many teaspoons of sugar each listed product contains.
3. Using the spoons, measure the amount of sugar in each product. Place that amount in a jar and label the jar.

IN CONCLUSION
1. Evaluate your findings.
2. Take time out to determine the nutrient content of the foods in each list. Which foods offer the best nutritional value?

and milk, and it provides food energy. It is also added to many prepared foods, such as soft drinks, cookies, candy, breakfast cereal, and even spaghetti sauce. Sugar is not harmful in moderate amounts. However, you might develop health problems if you eat too many foods high in added sugar.

Added Salt

Sodium is a necessary nutrient that helps control the balance of fluids in the body. It occurs naturally in salt, in various foods, and in many prepared sauces. It is also used extensively in processed foods to flavor or preserve the food.

Most Americans eat too much salt. For some people, too much sodium may contribute to high blood pressure and fluid retention. You can lower your sodium intake by using spices instead of salt, and by using food labels as a guide.

Caffeine

Caffeine is a substance that stimulates the nervous system and can become habit-forming. It is an ingredient in "power drinks," cola, some other soft drinks, coffee, tea, and chocolate. Caffeine stimulates the heart rate and the appetite. It can perk you up, but then it makes you feel drowsy so that you want more. For this reason it's best to limit your intake of products containing caffeine.

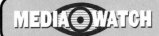

MEDIA WATCH

NUTRITION FACTS VS. FALLACIES

Not all information about the nutritional value of foods and food supplements is correct. Use critical-thinking skills to distinguish facts from fallacies concerning the nutritional value of foods and food supplements. *List claims you've heard about a food product or supplement, such as a multivitamin. Distinguish the claims that are true from those that are false.*

Lesson 2 Review

Using complete sentences, answer the following questions on a sheet of paper.

Reviewing Terms and Facts

1. **Vocabulary** Define *carbohydrates*. Give two examples of foods that contain simple carbohydrates and two examples of foods that contain complex carbohydrates.
2. **Explain** Why does your body need protein?
3. **Compare** What is the difference between saturated fats and unsaturated fats?
4. **Summarize** What kinds of foods contain added sugars?

Thinking Critically

5. **Hypothesize** Why do you think people tend to eat too much fat and too much sugar? What might be done to change this situation?

6. **Summarize** Select two of these four food substances: fiber, sodium, caffeine, and sugar. Explain whether or not they are components of your daily food and drink choices.

Applying Health Skills

7. **Accessing Information** Use reliable resources to determine when it might be appropriate to take a vitamin or mineral supplement. Develop and apply criteria for the selection or rejection of this health product. Report your criteria to the class.

Following Nutrition Guidelines

Quick Write

List the foods that you eat most often. Then describe why you choose them. Do you consider their nutritional value? How they look and taste? Their convenience?

LEARN ABOUT...

- resources that can help you make wise food choices.
- balancing the different foods you eat.
- using the nutrition information on food labels.

VOCABULARY

- Dietary Guidelines for Americans
- foodborne illness
- Food Guide Pyramid
- Percent Daily Value

Three Nutrition Guides

How do you know you're getting the nutrients you need? The U.S. government has developed three nutrition tools to help Americans make wise food choices. They are the Dietary Guidelines for Americans, the Food Guide Pyramid, and the Nutrition Facts panel.

The ABCs of Nutrition

The **Dietary Guidelines for Americans** are *recommendations about food choices for all healthy Americans age two and over.* The booklet has three sections, labeled A, B, and C: **A**im for fitness, **B**uild a healthy base, and **C**hoose sensibly.

Aim for Fitness

Fitness involves both healthful eating and regular physical activity. Follow these guidelines to keep healthy and fit.

- **Aim for a healthy weight.** Maintaining your weight helps you look and feel good. It also lowers your risk of heart disease, some cancers, and diabetes. Check with your health care provider to determine if you are at a healthy weight for your height and age.
- **Be physically active each day.** Physical activity can be almost any activity that keeps you moving. Try to include 60 minutes of moderate physical activity in your daily routine.

Build a Healthy Base

"Build a healthy base" refers to the base of the Food Guide Pyramid, which you'll learn more about later in the lesson. You'll learn that the foods located at the base of the Pyramid—grains, fruits, and vegetables—form the foundation of a healthful eating plan. Follow these guidelines to build a healthy base.

- **Let the Pyramid guide your food choices.** Eat the recommended number of servings from the five food groups.
- **Choose a variety of grains daily, especially whole grains.** You need the largest number of daily servings from the grains group. Whole-grain foods include whole-wheat bread, brown rice, and oatmeal.

- **Choose a variety of fruits and vegetables daily.** Eat all kinds and colors of fruits and vegetables to get the full range of vitamins and minerals, as well as fiber.
- **Keep food safe to eat.** Making sure that foods are safe from harmful bacteria and other contaminants will reduce the risk of **foodborne illness**, *a sickness that results from eating food that is not safe to eat.* Developing basic food-preparation skills, including sanitary food preparation and storage, will help keep food safe to eat. For example, wash your hands before and after handling foods, especially raw meat, poultry, and fish. Cook foods thoroughly and refrigerate perishable foods promptly.

Choose Sensibly

Sensible choices include foods that are low in fats, sugars, and salt. Follow these guidelines:

- **Choose foods that are low in saturated fat and cholesterol and moderate in total fat.** Foods high in saturated fats, such as butter and whole milk, raise blood cholesterol levels. Eat wisely by getting most of your calories from plant foods and by choosing nonfat or low-fat dairy products and lean meats.
- **Choose beverages and foods to moderate your intake of sugars.** Soft drinks provide many calories but few nutrients. They can also contribute to tooth decay. Limit your intake of drinks and foods containing added sugar. Check the ingredient list on packaged foods. If sucrose, corn syrup, honey, fructose, or other sweeteners are listed first or second, these foods are high in sugars.
- **Choose and prepare foods with less salt.** High salt or sodium intake can contribute to high blood pressure and cause calcium loss. Season foods with herbs or spices instead.

When shopping for foods, buy perishable foods last, take them straight home, and refrigerate them promptly. *List three sanitary food preparation and storage skills that can make food safe to eat.*

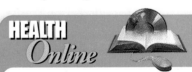

Topic: Food safety

For a link to more information on keeping foods safe, go to **health.glencoe.com**.

Activity: Using the information provided at this link, prepare a fact sheet on food safety.

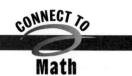
HEALTHY FOODS
ON A BUDGET
Use these effective
consumer skills to
purchase nutritious
foods within budget
constraints:
- Make a list so that
  you buy only what
  you need.
- Look for coupons
  for foods you buy
  regularly.
- Compute and com-
  pare unit prices
  (see Connect to
  Math on page 195).

The Food Guide Pyramid

The **Food Guide Pyramid** is *a guide for making healthful daily food choices.* **Figure 8.3** gives the sizes of the servings listed in **Figure 8.4**, the Food Guide Pyramid. The Food Guide Pyramid provides recommendations for the number of daily servings from each food group.

Following the Food Guide Pyramid is the easiest way to build a balanced eating plan. The following recommendations will help you follow advice from the Food Guide Pyramid and avoid overusing fat and added sugars.

- **Pay attention to serving sizes.** It is just as important to eat reasonable portions as it is to eat the right *number* of servings.
- **Keep meats lean.** Remove skin from poultry and visible fat from meat.
- **Read the labels on dairy products.** Choose nonfat or low-fat milk, cheese, and yogurt most of the time.
- **Use whole-grain or enriched grain products.** Check package labels and choose at least three servings of whole-grain breads and cereals each day. The rest should be enriched.
- **Cook it right.** Food preparation techniques make a difference. Baked or broiled foods have less fat than fried foods. Steamed vegetables retain more nutrients than vegetables cooked in water.

FIGURE 8.3

SAMPLE SERVING SIZES

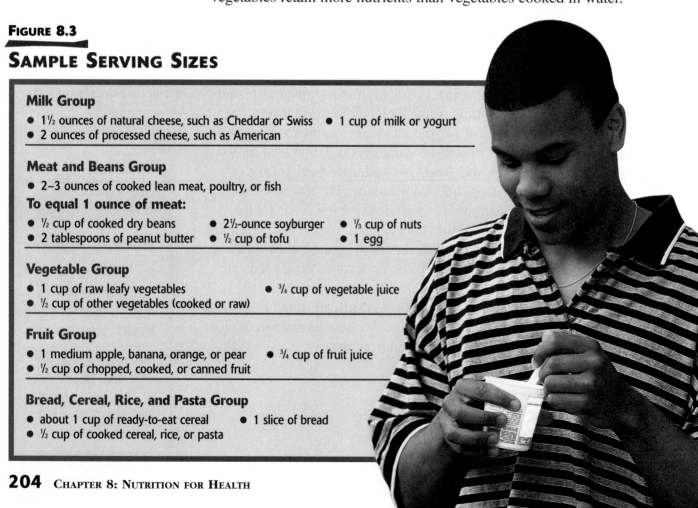

Milk Group
- 1½ ounces of natural cheese, such as Cheddar or Swiss
- 1 cup of milk or yogurt
- 2 ounces of processed cheese, such as American

Meat and Beans Group
- 2–3 ounces of cooked lean meat, poultry, or fish

To equal 1 ounce of meat:
- ½ cup of cooked dry beans
- 2½-ounce soyburger
- ⅓ cup of nuts
- 2 tablespoons of peanut butter
- ½ cup of tofu
- 1 egg

Vegetable Group
- 1 cup of raw leafy vegetables
- ¾ cup of vegetable juice
- ½ cup of other vegetables (cooked or raw)

Fruit Group
- 1 medium apple, banana, orange, or pear
- ¾ cup of fruit juice
- ½ cup of chopped, cooked, or canned fruit

Bread, Cereal, Rice, and Pasta Group
- about 1 cup of ready-to-eat cereal
- 1 slice of bread
- ½ cup of cooked cereal, rice, or pasta

FIGURE 8.4

THE FOOD GUIDE PYRAMID

By following the recommended number of daily servings and serving sizes from each group, you will have a balanced eating plan.

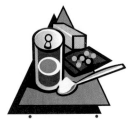

Fats, Oils, and Sweets
USE SPARINGLY

Foods: butter, salad dressing, sugar, candy, soft drinks

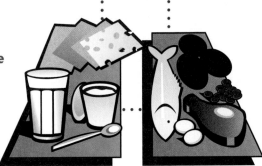

Milk, Yogurt, and Cheese Group (Milk Group)

3–4 servings for teens; 2–3 servings for adults

Foods: Milk, yogurt, cheese

Meat, Poultry, Fish, Dry Beans, Eggs, and Nuts Group (Meat and Beans Group)

2–3 servings

Foods: Beef, pork, veal, lamb, chicken, turkey, fish, shellfish, liver, eggs, beans, nuts, peanut butter

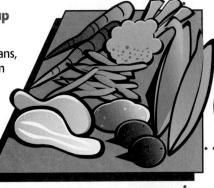

Vegetable Group
3–5 servings

Foods: Green beans, broccoli, dark green leafy vegetables, cabbage, carrots, corn, potatoes

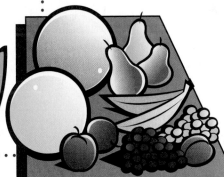

Fruit Group
2–4 servings

Foods: Citrus fruits, apples, bananas, peaches, pears

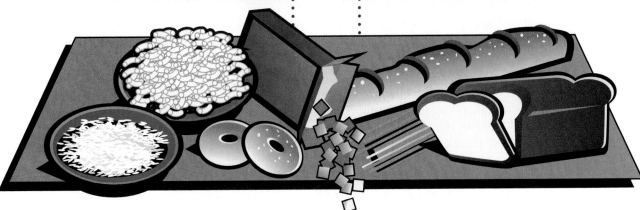

Bread, Cereal, Rice, and Pasta Group (Grains Group)
6–11 servings

Foods: Whole-grain or enriched breads, cereals, rice, pasta

Reading Check

Increase comprehension. Brainstorm the key concepts and ideas of this lesson. Jot down terms or phrases that you recall.

- **Consider nutritive values.** Choose foods that supply plenty of nutrients for the calories. Go easy on foods from the tip of the Pyramid, which have few or no nutrients, and on fatty and sugary foods within the five food groups.
- **Eat enough high-protein foods.** Sources include foods from the milk group and the meat and beans group.

Using Food Labels

Perhaps you have noticed that all packaged foods carry a label titled "Nutrition Facts." These labels provide valuable information for making healthful food choices. Food labels compare products to the **Percent Daily Value**. This figure is *the percent of the recommended daily amount of a nutrient provided in a serving of food.* The Percent Daily Value is based on an intake of 2,000 calories per day. Understanding how to read a food label, like the one shown in **Figure 8.5**, can help you select nutritious foods and balance your eating pattern.

HEALTH SKILLS ACTIVITY

ACCESSING INFORMATION

Reading a Food Label

The following information is provided on all Nutrition Facts panels. Use this information to compare foods and choose wisely.

- **SERVING SIZE.** The serving size is the portion that most people eat. Portion sizes allow for easy comparison of similar foods.
- **CALORIES.** Female teens should consume 2,200 calories per day, and male teens should have 3,000. Consider what percentage of this amount one serving of the food provides for you. Also consider how many of the calories in a serving come from fat.
- **NUTRIENTS.** Use the nutrient information to limit your intake of total fat, saturated fat, cholesterol, and sodium. Get enough dietary fiber, vitamins A and C, calcium, and iron.
- **PERCENT DAILY VALUE.** Determine how much the nutrients in a serving contribute

to your total daily eating plan. Use the "5–20 rule." Look for foods that provide 5 percent Daily Value or less of fat, cholesterol, and sodium. Choose foods that provide 20 percent Daily Value or more of dietary fiber, vitamins, and minerals.

1. How many grams of fat does one serving of the product contain? How much saturated fat does it have?
2. What percentage of your total daily sodium allowance does one serving contain?
3. What Percent Daily Value of vitamin A does one serving provide? Vitamin C? Is the product a good source of these vitamins?

ON YOUR OWN
Use the sample label in Figure 8.5 to help answer these questions. Assume that you take in about 2,500 calories a day.

FIGURE 8.5

WHAT THE FOOD LABEL TELLS YOU

Food labels provide important nutritional information that can help you make sensible food choices.

A The nutrient content of the food is calculated according to its serving size. The serving size on the food label may differ from sizes shown on the Food Guide Pyramid.

B The amount of total fat in one serving is listed, followed by the amount of saturated fat. The calories from fat are shown to the right of the total calories per serving.

C Major vitamins and minerals are shown, along with their Percent Daily Value.

Nutrition Facts
Serving Size 1/2 cup (114g)
Servings Per Container 4

Amount Per Serving	
Calories 90	Calories from Fat 30

	% Daily Value*
Total Fat 3g	**5%**
Saturated Fat 0g	0%
Cholesterol 0mg	**0%**
Sodium 300mg	**13%**
Total Carbohydrate 13g	**4%**
Dietary Fiber 3g	12%
Sugars 3g	
Protein 3g	

Vitamin A 80%	•	Vitamin C 60%
Calcium 4%	•	Iron 4%

* Percent Daily Values are based on a 2,000 calorie diet. Your daily values may be higher or lower depending on your calorie needs:

Calories	2,000	2,500
Total Fat	Less Than 65g	80g
Sat Fat	Less Than 20g	25g
Cholesterol	Less Than 300mg	300mg
Sodium	Less Than 2,400mg	2,400mg
Total Carbohydrate	300g	375g
Dietary Fiber	25g	30g

Calories per gram:
Fat 9 • Carbohydrate 4 • Protein 4

D Major nutrients are listed in milligrams (mg) or grams (g) and as a percentage of the recommended amount for a person consuming 2,000 calories per day.

E Dietary fiber and sugar are given under Total Carbohydrate.

F Information provided on the lower part of the Nutrition Facts panel is the same from product to product. It contains advice about the amounts of certain nutrients that should be eaten each day. Amounts are given for both a 2,000-calorie and a 2,500-calorie diet.

Lesson 3 Review

Using complete sentences, answer the following questions on a sheet of paper.

Reviewing Terms and Facts

1. **List** What are the three tools developed by the government to help Americans make wise food choices?
2. **Recall** What are the ABCs outlined in the Dietary Guidelines for Americans?
3. **Vocabulary** Define *foodborne illnesses.* How can foodborne illness be prevented?
4. **Give Examples** Name two foods in each of the five food groups that make up the Food Guide Pyramid.

Thinking Critically

5. **Analyze** Explain how the shape of the Food Guide Pyramid makes it easier to choose a balanced eating plan.

6. **Evaluate** Think about your own food choices. What food groups do you need to eat more from in your eating plan? What food groups do you need to cut down on?

Applying Health Skills

7. **Accessing Information** Use reliable resources to find out more about developing basic food-preparation skills, including sanitary food preparation and storage techniques that help prevent foodborne illness. Then, find recipes for a healthy breakfast and lunch that you would like to prepare. Write down the steps you would take to properly store the ingredients and prepare each meal safely.

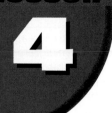

Planning Meals and Snacks

Plan Ahead

The Food Guide Pyramid is a great planning tool! Use it every day to plan your food choices and meet your goals for healthy eating. Remember that your daily food choices include not only regular meals but also snacks. The goal is to eat a variety of foods and to achieve the number of servings recommended by the Pyramid.

Start with Breakfast

You have probably heard people say that breakfast is the most important meal of the day. It's true! When you wake in the morning, you most likely haven't eaten for 10 to 12 hours. While you sleep, your body uses energy for breathing, keeping your heart beating, and growing and repairing cells. By morning, your body needs food to replenish its energy supply.

Studies have shown that eating breakfast regularly helps teens perform better in school. Teens who eat breakfast regularly tend to earn higher test scores and grades and have better school attendance. They are also more likely to maintain a healthy weight and have better muscle coordination.

Keep in mind that you can make breakfast quickly and take it with you. For example, you could grab a granola bar and an apple to eat at the bus stop.

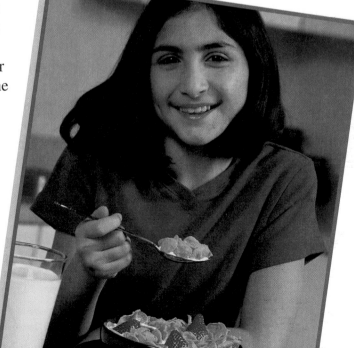

A healthful breakfast gives you energy to start the day. *What other benefits result from eating breakfast regularly?*

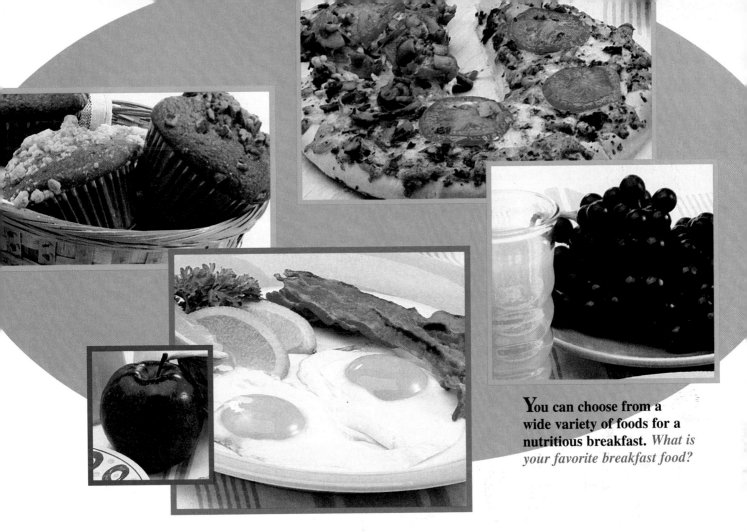

You can choose from a wide variety of foods for a nutritious breakfast. *What is your favorite breakfast food?*

Plan Meals Wisely

In any family, planning meals can be a challenge. Different people may have different needs. For example, you may be hungry for dinner before other family members get home. Try to work with your family to find an eating pattern that is right for you. Eating regular meals is important. When you eat regularly, you are less likely to get strong hunger pangs that can lead to overeating. You also maintain a balanced blood sugar level.

Choose Sensible Snacks

What do you think of when you hear the word *snack?* For many people, snacks mean candy bars, potato chips, and other foods with few nutrients. If you eat too many of these foods, you may consume excess calories, sodium, and fat.

As you learned earlier, the amount of energy that is available in foods is measured in calories. *Calories that come from foods that offer few, if any, nutrients* are called **empty calories**. They usually come from foods at the tip of the Food Guide Pyramid—fats, oils, and sweets.

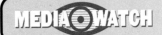

MEDIA WATCH

EXTRA-LARGE PORTIONS

Ads for extra-large portions may tell you about the value of bigger sizes. However, nutritional information is often omitted. *Use critical-thinking skills to analyze the influence of this advertising technique on food selection.*

Reading Check

Understand cause and effect. Complete this analogy: *Healthy snacks are to high nutrient density as _____ are to low nutrient density.*

How can you tell which snacks have a lot of nutrients and which provide only empty calories? One way is to compare their **nutrient density**, or *the amount of nutrients relative to the number of calories they provide.* A typical candy bar, for example, has low nutrient density. It provides about 250 calories but few nutrients. **Figure 8.6** provides suggestions for nutrient-dense snacks.

Eating Out, Eating Right

Eating out can present a challenge if you're trying to maintain a healthful eating plan. Many menu items are fried or served with butter, mayonnaise, gravy, or other high-fat toppings. By making wise choices, however, you can eat out but still eat healthful foods. Order food that is grilled, broiled, or baked, rather than fried. Ask for sauces and other toppings to be served on the side. Eat a sensible serving, and take the rest home to enjoy the next day.

HEALTH SKILLS ACTIVITY

DECISION MAKING

Choosing Healthful Snacks

Rosalie knew that she had developed some unhealthful eating habits. She often snacked on potato chips after school. On days when she had band practice, she would grab a candy bar. Rosalie snacked so much that she didn't eat all the nutrient-rich foods her parents provided for dinner.

Rosalie decided to change her eating habits and become more active. She began choosing nutrient-dense snacks like peanut butter on whole wheat crackers and carrot sticks. Rosalie also increased her physical activity by walking her dog every day and swimming several times a week.

Rosalie is proud of her healthier lifestyle. Now her friend Corey has called to suggest that they go to the movies with Josh and Molly. Rosalie wants to go, but her friends usually stop for fast food and ice cream after the movies. She wants to stick with her eating plan, but she's afraid of falling into old habits.

What Would You Do?

Apply the steps of the decision-making process to Rosalie's situation. With a partner, role-play a conversation in which Rosalie suggests some options to Corey.

1. **STATE THE SITUATION.**
2. **LIST THE OPTIONS.**
3. **WEIGH THE POSSIBLE OUTCOMES.**
4. **CONSIDER VALUES.**
5. **MAKE A DECISION AND ACT.**
6. **EVALUATE THE DECISION.**

FIGURE 8.6

Sensible Snacks

Sensible snacks, such as those shown and listed here, can be an important part of a healthful eating plan.

Meat, Poultry, Fish, Dry Beans, Eggs, and Nuts Group (Meat and Beans Group)
Slices of lean turkey, ham, or roast beef, hard-cooked egg, peanut butter, dry-roasted peanuts

Milk, Yogurt, and Cheese Group
Nonfat or low-fat milk, yogurt, cheese

Fruit Group
Any raw fruits, dried fruits such as raisins

Vegetable Group
Celery or carrot sticks, sliced peppers, broccoli or cauliflower spears, salad

Bread, Cereal, Rice, and Pasta Group
Air-popped popcorn without butter, graham crackers, plain bagel, instant oatmeal, rice cakes, tortillas

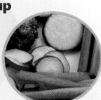

Lesson 4 Review

Using complete sentences, answer the following questions on a sheet of paper.

Reviewing Terms and Facts

1. **Recall** What are three benefits of eating a nutritious breakfast?
2. **Vocabulary** What are *empty calories?* What kinds of foods provide empty calories?
3. **Explain** How does knowledge of nutrient density help you choose sensible snacks?
4. **Give Examples** Suggest a healthful snack from each of the five food groups.

Thinking Critically

5. **Explain** Why might air-popped popcorn be a smarter snack choice than other types of popcorn?

6. **Analyze** David went to a fast-food restaurant for lunch. He ordered a cola drink; a taco with chicken, cheese, shredded lettuce, and tomato; and ice cream. Which of these items have high nutrient density? Which have low nutrient density?

Applying Health Skills

7. **Accessing Information** Find three recipes—one for a high-fat dish, one for a dish that calls for a large amount of salt, and one for a sugary dessert. Adapt each recipe to make it healthier by lowering the fat, salt, or sugar content and increasing the fiber content. Present your ideas to the class.

Teen Vegetarians

More kids are saying no to meat. Is this a healthy option?

Lauren Butts, a high-school student from Medford, Oregon, recalls the moment she became a vegetarian. At age 13, Lauren, a horse owner, accidentally ordered horsemeat at a restaurant in France. Although she avoided eating the burger, something clicked. "It made sense then," Lauren says. "There was no way I was going to eat the relatives of my horses."

Lauren is the author of *OK, So Now You're a Vegetarian*, the first vegetarian cookbook by a teen for teens. She is part of a small but fast-growing movement among young people ages 6 to 18 to cut out all meat. Inspired by everything from a love of animals to trendiness to a concern for the environment, young people are becoming vegetarians at higher rates than ever—often independent of their meat-eating parents.

Still, people who consider themselves vegetarians make up only about 6 percent of the population. Moreover, the definition of "vegetarian" can vary. (See "A Veggie Guide.") The number of those who just cut out red meat—or who refuse any animal products except eggs and dairy—is far greater than the number of strict vegans, who eat no animal products at all.

Whatever the definition, a recent poll found that 8- to 12-year-olds were signing on to vegetarianism at twice the rate of adults. "The jump among young people is clear," says Dennis Bier of the Children's Nutrition Research Center at Baylor College of Medicine in Houston, Texas. This raises an important question: Is vegetarianism a healthy choice? Bier says, "Concerns about proper growth and bone density should exist whether one's diet is vegetarian or not. However, there's no question that if it's well planned, a vegetarian diet is perfectly healthy for kids." A teen who is thinking about becoming a vegetarian should consult a doctor or a registered dietitian before changing his or her eating habits.

A Veggie Good Diet

Since beef, chicken, and fish are all good sources of protein and vitamins, nutritionists stress that a vegetarian diet requires research and careful meal planning. This is especially true during the growth spurts that occur in adolescence.

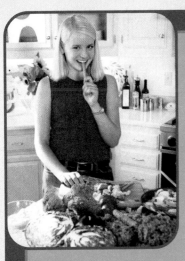

A Veggie Guide

Did you know that there are different kinds of vegetarians? Here are a few:

VEGAN: No animal products of any kind, including dairy products, eggs, and honey, are eaten. A vegan lifestyle often involves more than just avoiding all animal products; it's a philosophy that emphasizes reverence for all forms of life.
Keep in mind: Vegans need to eat foods that contain some fat (beans), iron (broccoli), calcium (fortified soy milk or orange juice), and zinc (whole grains). Vitamin B12, found only in foods of animal origin, can be taken in supplement form.

LACTO-OVO: These types of vegetarians don't eat meat, chicken, or fish, but do eat eggs and dairy products.
Keep in mind: Eggs, milk, yogurt, and cheese are all good sources of important nutrients, but contain a lot of fat and cholesterol. Lacto-ovo vegetarians should opt for low-fat products.

PESCO: The largest group of vegetarians, pesco-vegetarians eat fish, dairy products, and eggs but not chicken or red meat.
Keep in mind: The key nutrients are all there—pesco-vegetarians just need to make sure to include lots of fruits and vegetables in their dietary plan.

VEGGIE-LITE: This is an unofficial term that embraces pollo vegetarians (those who eat chicken) and others who eat meat occasionally but consider themselves vegetarians.
Keep in mind: Eat a variety of fruits and vegetables. Eating mostly pasta, pizza, and bagels will not provide the optimal amount of nutrients.

Strict vegans have to be very careful to make sure they get enough iron, zinc, calcium, and vitamin B12. (B12 is found only in animal products.) Yet most experts agree that a vegetarian eating style can be managed. Beans, tofu, peanut butter, broccoli, milk, eggs, and whole grains can provide protein, iron, calcium, and zinc.

Challenges of a New Lifestyle

Both parents and their children say the vegetarian lifestyle has its challenges. Eating out at restaurants, friends' houses, and school can be tricky. Worse, it sometimes encourages consumption of empty-calorie foods or even abstaining from eating. Meat-eating parents may disapprove of their child's new eating style, causing tension at mealtimes. Parents also worry about their children getting proper nutrition. "But kids need to watch what they're eating regardless," says Bier.

"Keep in mind, most Americans need to be eating more fruits and vegetables anyway. It's good stuff!" ∎

TIME TO THINK...

About Vegetarianism
Write down everything that you ate and drank yesterday. Now imagine that you are a vegan. (Use the information from this article and do your own research to find out more about what a vegan eating plan does and does not include.) How many things on your food list would you need to cross off if you were a vegan? Suppose you *had* subtracted those foods from what you ate that day: What vegan foods would you *add* to the list to ensure that you were getting the nutrients you need?

EATING FOR YOUR HEALTH

Model

An advocate is a person who takes a stand and tries to persuade others to change their behavior. Read about how Grace advocates healthful eating habits with her friend Caitlyn.

CAITLYN: What time will your dad pick me up for the track meet?

GRACE: Well, what time do you finish breakfast?

CAITLYN: I don't eat breakfast. I usually just drink a soda on the way.

GRACE: Are you nuts? I don't want my teammate running on empty. How are you supposed to function after a whole night without fuel?

CAITLYN: I do it all the time and it doesn't seem to affect me.

GRACE: You just don't realize how much better you'd perform if you ate first. There are even studies showing that eating breakfast improves your coordination.

CAITLYN: You sound like my mother.

GRACE: I sound like your friend who's looking out for you.

CAITLYN: Okay, okay. Pick me up after breakfast.

Practice

Read the following scenario about a teen who wants to help a relative. Answer the questions below on a sheet of paper.

Cody is concerned about his uncle Jack, who has high blood pressure. Jack's doctor told him he should change his eating habits. The doctor advised Jack to eat more fruits, vegetables, and whole-grain foods, and to avoid fried foods, fatty meats, and sugary desserts. Jack has not followed his doctor's advice. He doesn't understand what his food choices have to do with his health.

1. List three facts about nutrition that could help Jack understand why good food choices will improve his health.
2. Write three statements Cody could use to convince his uncle to improve his eating patterns.

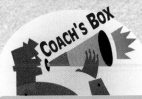

Apply/Assess

Work with a small group to create a cartoon that encourages teens to make healthful food choices. You may draw a single-panel cartoon or a comic strip with several panels. Use a combination of words and pictures to convince readers that they should eat a variety of foods each day. Support your position with facts about nutrition. Make your cartoon appealing and persuasive to teens. If you wish, you can tell a story or use humor to catch the reader's attention. Be prepared to share your cartoon with other students in your class.

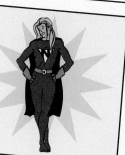

The Adventures of NUTRITIA
...bringing healthy foods to teens everywhere!

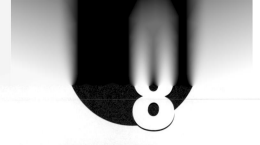

Use your completed Foldable to review the information on nutrients and influences on food choices. **FOLDABLES**™ Study Organizer

Reviewing Vocabulary and Concepts

On a sheet of paper, write the numbers 1–9. After each number, write the term from the list that best completes each sentence.

- amino acids
- fiber
- minerals
- nutrient deficiency
- nutrients
- vitamins
- appetite
- proteins
- hunger

Lesson 1

1. _____ are substances in food that your body needs.
2. The psychological desire for food is _____.
3. The physical need for food is called _____.
4. A person who doesn't eat enough foods that supply iron might have a(n) _____.

Lesson 2

5. _____ are nutrients your body uses to build, repair, and maintain cells and tissues.
6. Foods from animal sources provide all the essential _____.
7. _____ help your body fight infections, process nutrients, and perform other tasks.

8. Calcium and iron are examples of _____.
9. Although _____ is not a nutrient, it is essential for good digestion.

On a sheet of paper, write the numbers 10–18. Write *True* or *False* for each statement below. If the statement is false, change the underlined word or phrase to make it true.

Lesson 3

10. A diagram that helps you make daily food choices from the five food groups is the Food Triangle.
11. The Dietary Guidelines for Americans provide advice about food choices, such as "Aim for fitness," "Build a healthy base," and "Choose sensibly."
12. Eggs are included in the Milk, Yogurt, and Cheese Group.
13. The Percent Daily Value is based on recommendations for an eating plan of 2,000 calories.
14. One way to prevent foodborne illnesses is to wash your hands before and after handling foods.

Lesson 4

15. When you eat regularly, you are more likely to get strong hunger pangs that can lead to overeating.
16. Foods such as soft drinks and candy provide mostly empty calories with few nutrients.
17. A food's serving size is the amount of nutrients relative to the number of calories the food provides.
18. A wise choice when eating out is to choose foods that are served with butter, mayonnaise, gravy, or other high-fat toppings.

Thinking Critically

Using complete sentences, answer the following questions on a sheet of paper.

19. **Analyze** How might the nutritional needs of a teen differ from those of an adult?

20. **Explain** Describe the benefits of a high-fiber, low-fat eating plan.

21. **Apply** How could you use the Food Guide Pyramid to help you decide what to eat for an evening snack?

22. **Evaluate** Why might nutrient-dense foods be better for an eating program than other foods that are higher in fat but have the same number of calories?

Career Corner

Home Health Aide Home health aides provide an important service assisting elderly, disabled, and sick persons in their homes. In addition to caring for health needs, these professionals may shop for food and cook for their patients. Training for this career requires a one-year program at a community college or vocational/trade school. Find out more about this medical profession by clicking on Career Corner at health.glencoe.com.

Standardized Test Practice

Reading & Writing

Read the paragraphs below and then answer the questions.

When I was in the sixth grade, I decided to become a vegetarian. I thought about my decision carefully before I made it. I was convinced that a vegetarian diet was a healthy choice for me. I also knew that being a vegetarian in a meat-eating world was not going to be easy. Well, it has been more than two years now, and I believe that I made the right decision.

When I announced my decision to my family, my mother made it clear that she did not have the time to make special meals for me, and she didn't. She made sure that I had a basic understanding of nutrition and left the rest up to me. Soon I learned how to plan my meals, to combine plant foods to make sure I was getting enough protein, and to eat a well-balanced diet.

1. Which of these statements reflects the writer's attitude in the passage?

   (A) The writer thinks that everyone should become a vegetarian.

   (B) The writer is sure of her decision and wants others to understand it.

   (C) The writer is angry because others do not understand vegetarianism.

   (D) The writer is hoping that others will share her views on vegetarianism.

2. Which phrase from the passage represents an opinion?

   (A) I thought about my decision carefully.

   (B) I learned how to plan my meals.

   (C) I decided to become a vegetarian.

   (D) I believe that I made the right decision.

3. Write a paragraph identifying a healthy choice that you made and explaining why you made it.

218

Physical Activity and Fitness

HEALTH *Online*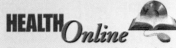

Do you get enough physical activity? Find out how you rate by taking the Health Inventory for Chapter 9 at health.glencoe.com.

FOLDABLES™ Study Organizer

Before You Read

Make this Foldable to help you organize the information on physical activity, exercise, and physical fitness presented in Lesson 1. Begin with a plain sheet of 11″ × 17″ paper.

Step 1

Fold the sheet of paper in half along the short axis, then fold in half again. This forms four columns.

Step 2

Open the paper and refold it in half along the long axis, then fold in half again. This forms four rows.

Step 3

Unfold and draw lines along the folds.

Step 4

Label the chart as shown.

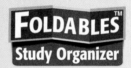

Chapter 9	Definition	Examples	Impact on my life
Physical Activity			
Exercise			
Physical Fitness			

As You Read

In the appropriate section of the chart, write down definitions and examples of physical activity, exercise, and physical fitness, as well as the impact each has on your daily life.

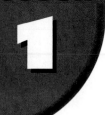
The Benefits of Physical Activity

Quick Write

Describe in a sentence or two what it means to be physically fit.

LEARN ABOUT...

- what it means to be physically fit.
- the benefits of physical activity.
- kinds of activities that will help you stay fit.

VOCABULARY

- physical activity
- exercise
- physical fitness
- balance
- coordination
- aerobic exercise
- anaerobic exercise

Physical Activity, Exercise, and Physical Fitness

The terms *physical activity, exercise,* and *fitness* are closely related, but each has a particular meaning. **Physical activity** refers to *any kind of movement that uses up energy.* Physical activity includes exercising and playing sports. It also includes the movements associated with an active lifestyle, such as biking to the store, raking leaves, and walking up and down the stairs. **Exercise** is *a specifically planned and organized session of physical activity that you do to improve or maintain your physical fitness.* By combining regular exercise with an active lifestyle and sound nutrition, you can be fit. **Physical fitness** is *the ability to handle the physical demands of everyday life without becoming overly tired.*

When you're physically fit, you have enough energy to do the things you want to do, plus energy in reserve for the unexpected.

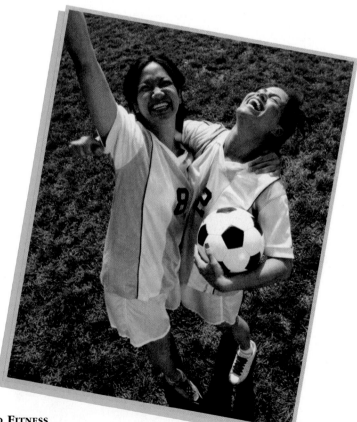

Some forms of physical activity let you enjoy the company of other people while helping you stay in shape. *What outdoor activities do you like?*

FIGURE 9.1

Benefits of Physical Activity

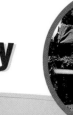

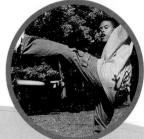

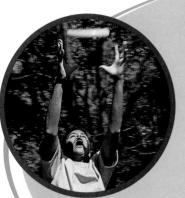

Mental/Emotional Benefits
- Feel more alert and energetic
- Reduce stress
- Learn new things
- Get a sense of accomplishment
- Lessen mental fatigue
- Build a positive self-image
- Increase self-confidence and self-esteem

Physical Benefits
- Strengthen heart and lungs
- Strengthen bones
- Manage weight
- Control blood sugar
- Control blood pressure
- Increase strength and stamina
- Improve flexibility and muscle tone
- Improve **balance**, the feeling of stability and control over your body
- Develop **coordination**, the smooth and effective working together of your muscles and bones
- Improve reaction time
- Increase body's defense against diseases
- Improve sleep

Social Benefits
- Engage in enjoyable activities
- Meet and interact with new people
- Work with others as a team
- Get support from friends
- Share goals and achievements with others

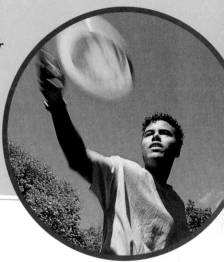

Benefits of an Active Lifestyle

Physical activity benefits you in both body and mind. Besides promoting your overall health, physical activity helps you look and feel better. Since many physical activities involve other people, you'll also get social benefits.

Physical activity provides mental and emotional benefits, too. Being active lets you clear your mind and "burn off" stress. In addition, the physical and social benefits that you get help you feel good about yourself as a person. **Figure 9.1** shows some of the mental/emotional, physical, and social benefits of physical activity.

Increasing Your Level of Fitness

How can you increase your level of physical fitness? The first step toward physical fitness is to recognize that physical activity is important to your lifelong health and well-being. The next step is to move more! Make physical activity part of your daily life.

Reading Check

Categorize words. Sort these words into categories: *biking, dancing, curl-ups, swimming, soccer, stretching, weightlifting, playing catch, tai chi, roller-blading.* Add more words to each list.

Becoming more active is as easy as seeing the opportunities for physical activity that are all around you. Instead of using elevators and escalators, take the stairs. Walk or ride a bike to the mall rather than asking your parents for a lift.

In addition to looking for everyday opportunities, plan regular sessions of exercise. Aim for at least three to five sessions a week. Start by exercising 10 to 15 minutes at a time and gradually work up to about 30 minutes or more. If you feel that you do not have time to spare, try breaking your physical activity down into smaller sessions during the day. Three 10-minute sessions provide the same benefit as one 30-minute activity.

Choosing the Right Activities

It is important to choose activities that give you the benefits you want. There are two main types of exercise: aerobic and anaerobic. **Aerobic exercise** is *rhythmic, nonstop, moderate to vigorous activity that requires large amounts of oxygen and works the heart.* Running, biking, and swimming are forms of aerobic exercise. **Anaerobic exercise** is *intense physical activity that requires little oxygen but uses short bursts of energy.* Sprinting and gymnastics are examples of anaerobic exercise.

Each type of exercise benefits the body in a particular way. You can combine both types of exercise to achieve optimum fitness. By choosing a variety of activities, you can receive the benefits of both types of exercise.

HEALTH SKILLS ACTIVITY

STRESS MANAGEMENT

Relaxation Exercises

Physical activity is an effective way to relieve stress and help you unwind. You might also do relaxation exercises to reduce feelings of stress. Here are some examples:

- **LIE ON YOUR BACK.** Make fists and tense your arms. Hold for a moment, then relax. In turn, tense and then relax your neck, shoulders, legs, feet, and abdomen.
- **LIE ON YOUR SIDE, WITH BOTH ARMS ABOVE YOUR HEAD.** Tense your whole body, then completely relax, letting your arms and legs fall where they may, as

though you were a rag doll. Turn to your other side and repeat.

- **SIT QUIETLY.** Close your eyes, take a slow, deep breath, and let it out slowly. Repeat two more times. Open your mouth, move your jaw to the right, and hold for a few seconds. Then move it to the left and hold. Repeat several times.

ON YOUR OWN

Try each of these exercises. Did they reduce your body tension? Which exercise had the greatest effect?

Stay Active: A Key to Fitness

Technology has made life simpler, easier, and more fun. As wonderful as technology is, though, it has a downside. It has replaced many of the physical activities that were once part of daily life. People ride instead of walk. They use machines to do the work that used to be done by hand. They sit at home, watching sports on TV, instead of playing ball in the park. They send e-mail instead of walking over to a friend's house.

Think about your own lifestyle. Estimate how many hours a week you watch television or sit at a computer screen. Now estimate the number of hours you spend doing something physically active. Compare the totals. Are you active most of the time or inactive? Because you know that physical activity and exercise are essential to fitness, this comparison may make you stop and think about how you spend your time.

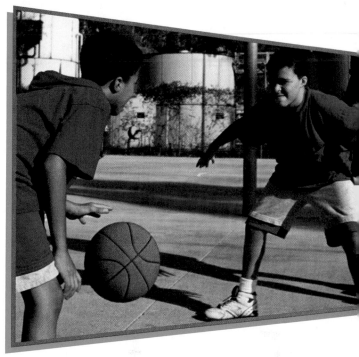

Playing basketball a few times a week is a good way to exercise and have fun at the same time. *How do you stay active?*

Lesson 1 Review

Using complete sentences, answer the following questions on a sheet of paper.

Reviewing Terms and Facts

1. **Vocabulary** Define *physical activity, exercise,* and *physical fitness.*
2. **Explain** Using your own words, tell what it means to be physically fit.
3. **Identify** Give three examples of the mental/emotional benefits of physical activity and three examples of the social benefits.
4. **Compare** What is the difference between aerobic exercise and anaerobic exercise?

Thinking Critically

5. **Analyze** Would you describe yourself as physically fit? Think back to last week and write down your physical activities. What do you conclude from your list?
6. **Explain** How might staying fit help you manage stress? How has physical activity provided you with an outlet for tension or anger?

Applying Health Skills

7. **Practicing Healthful Behaviors** Survey classmates, family members, and adult friends who are physically active. Ask each person why he or she maintains an active lifestyle. Write down the answers and compare them to the benefits shown in **Figure 9.1**. Present your survey findings to the class.

Endurance, Strength, and Flexibility

The Elements of Fitness

Exercise can be used to develop four elements of fitness: heart and lung endurance, muscle strength and endurance, body composition, and flexibility.

Heart and Lung Endurance

Endurance is your ability to engage in vigorous physical activity over time without tiring too easily or quickly. **Heart and lung endurance** refers to *how effectively your heart and lungs work when you exercise and how quickly they return to normal when you stop.* Heart and lung endurance is important in all kinds of exercise—biking, jumping rope, swimming, and playing ball. **Figure 9.2** shows one way to measure heart and lung endurance. Before performing the test in Figure 9.2, practice walking or jogging for six to eight weeks and learn to pace yourself so that you can walk or jog continuously.

The best way to build up heart and lung endurance is through sustained moderate to vigorous exercise lasting at least 20 to 30 minutes, three to five times a week. This kind of physical activity is called cardiovascular exercise because it raises your breathing rate and heartbeat and benefits your cardiovascular system.

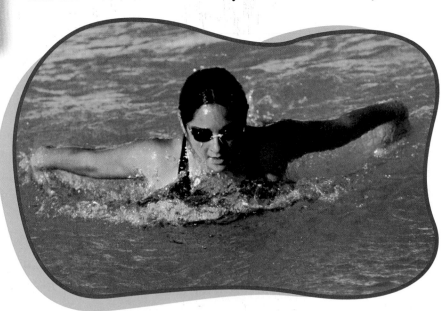

Swimming is an example of cardiovascular exercise.

FIGURE 9.2

DETERMINING HEART AND LUNG ENDURANCE

For this test, you'll see how far you can walk in 30 minutes or jog in 20 minutes.

1 Team up with a partner. Go to a track or running area with quarter-mile markers. Warm up with walking and gentle stretching exercises for 5 to 10 minutes.

2 Walk for 30 minutes or jog for 20 minutes. Have your partner record the distance that you cover. Cool down afterward by walking slowly and doing gentle stretching exercises.

3 Switch roles and repeat the exercise.

4 Caution: If you have a heart or lung disease, check with your doctor before attempting this test.

Scoring (miles)

If you score within the range given for your age and gender, your heart and lung endurance is acceptable. If not, continue to practice walking or jogging until you can score in the acceptable range.

Age	Females Walking	Jogging	Males Walking	Jogging
12	2–2.2	1.6–1.8	2.2–2.4	1.8–2.0
13	2–2.2	1.6–1.8	2.2–2.4	1.8–2.0
14	2–2.2	1.6–1.8	2.2–2.4	1.8–2.0
15	2–2.2	1.6–1.8	2.2–2.4	1.8–2.0

Source: Modified with permission from *Foundations of Personal Fitness: Any Body Can . . . Be Fit!*, by D. Rainey and T. Murray.

Some cardiovascular exercises are:

- **Walking/Jogging/Running.** Start off slowly, and then gradually increase your pace. Work up to a 30-minute walk, or alternate walking and jogging until you can jog or run for 20 minutes.
- **Swimming.** Swimming provides a total body workout. Gradually work up to 20 minutes of continuous swimming. Swim at a steady pace and vary your routine by using different strokes.
- **Jumping Rope.** As you jump, guard your joints against unnecessary strain by raising your feet just high enough to allow the rope to pass.

It's a good idea to vary your exercise routines. *Switching between different exercises* is known as **cross-training** and has benefits over doing one exercise all the time. Whatever exercise you choose, don't overdo it.

Muscle Strength and Endurance

The ability of your muscles to exert a force is called strength. **Muscle strength** measures *the most weight you can lift or the most force you can exert at one time.* **Muscle endurance** is *the ability of a muscle to repeatedly exert a force over a prolonged period of time.* The greater your muscle strength, the more force your muscles can exert. The greater your muscle endurance, the longer your muscles can exert their strength.

There are many ways to build and measure muscle strength (see **Figures 9.3** and **9.4**). Three basic strengthening exercises are push-ups, curl-ups, and step-ups.

- **Do push-ups to strengthen muscles in your arms and chest.** Lie facedown on the floor. Bend your arms and place your palms flat on the floor beneath your shoulders. Straighten your arms, pushing your entire body upward, and then lower your body to the floor. Repeat.
- **Do curl-ups to strengthen your abdominal muscles.** Lie on your back with your knees bent and your heels on the floor. Cross your arms over your chest. Curl your upper body forward so that both shoulder blades come off the floor. Uncurl and repeat.
- **Do step-ups to strengthen your leg muscles.** Step up onto a step with your left foot and then bring your right foot up. Step down with your left foot and bring the right foot down. Repeat, alternating between feet.

Many students your age become interested in weight training. Weight training is a good way to build muscle strength. Lift light weights multiple times, and make sure you learn from an expert, such as a fitness instructor.

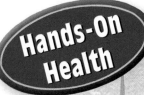
Hands-On Health

YOUR TARGET PULSE RATE

Exercise should increase your heartbeat to at least 50 percent of your maximum rate to provide a benefit for your heart and lungs. The heartbeat rate that will safely provide the greatest benefit is between 60 and 80 percent of your maximum rate. This is your target pulse rate (also known as target heart rate). In this activity, you will find your target pulse rate.

WHAT YOU WILL NEED
- watch with a second hand

WHAT YOU WILL DO
1. Determine your maximum heartbeat rate by subtracting your age from the number 220.
2. Multiply your maximum heartbeat rate by 60 percent and then by 80 percent.

Compare the range of your target pulse rate with those in the chart.
3. For the next two weeks, take your pulse while exercising. Write down the activity you are doing and your pulse rate.

IN CONCLUSION
Was your heartbeat rate generally within the range of your target pulse rate? Which activities produced the highest rate? The lowest?

AGE	MAXIMUM PULSE RATE	TARGET PULSE RATE
12	208	125–166
13	207	124–166
14	206	124–165
15	205	123–164

FIGURE 9.3

DETERMINING ABDOMINAL MUSCLE STRENGTH AND ENDURANCE

You can test the strength and endurance of your abdominal muscles by measuring your ability to do bent-knee curl-ups.

1 Team up with a partner.

2 Partner A lies on a mat with knees bent and feet flat on the floor. Partner B holds partner A's feet.

3 Partner A curls up slowly with arms crossed over the chest, and chin tucked to the chest so that the head never touches the mat. The curl-up is completed when partner A's shoulder blades return to the testing surface.

4 Partner A should do curl-ups at the rate of about 20 per minute, stopping when he or she can no longer continue, or has completed 60 curl-ups.

5 Partners A and B switch roles and repeat the exercise.

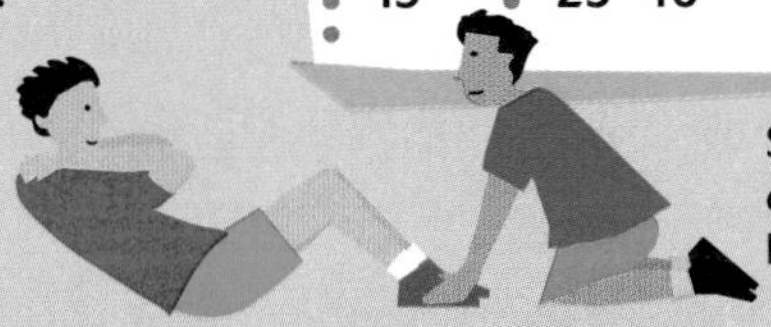

Scoring (number completed)

If you score within the range given for your age and gender, your abdominal strength and endurance is acceptable. If you do not score within the range, continue to practice your curl-ups until you can score in the acceptable range.

Age	Females	Males
12	20–35	25–40
13	25–40	30–45
14	25–40	30–45
15	25–40	30–45

Source: Modified with permission from *Foundations of Personal Fitness: Any Body Can . . . Be Fit!*, by D. Rainey and T. Murray.

FIGURE 9.4

DETERMINING UPPER BODY STRENGTH AND ENDURANCE

You can test your upper body strength and endurance by measuring the time you can hang from a bar with your chin above the bar.

1 Team up with a partner.

2 Partner A grasps horizontal bar with palms facing away, and raises body to position where chin is above bar, elbows are flexed, and chest is close to the bar. Partner B spots Partner A and stops Partner A from swinging.

3 Partner B starts stopwatch. Partner A remains in position for as long as possible.

4 Watch is stopped when Partner A's chin touches bar, head tilts backward, or chin falls below level of bar.

5 Partners A and B switch roles and repeat the exercise.

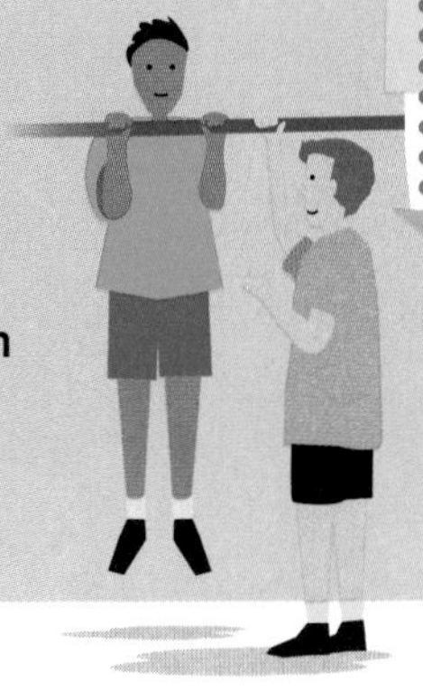

Scoring (seconds)

If you score within the range given for your age and gender, your upper body strength and endurance is acceptable. If you do not score within the range, continue to practice your static arm hang until you can score in the acceptable range.

Age	Females	Males
12	7–14	7–14
13	7–14	12–20
14	7–14	12–20
15	7–14	12–20

Source: Modified with permission from *Foundations of Personal Fitness: Any Body Can . . . Be Fit!*, by D. Rainey and T. Murray.

Personal responsibility and self-discipline go hand in hand. For example, when you take responsibility for becoming fit you need to discipline yourself to exercise regularly. *How have you recently shown self-discipline?*

Body Composition

A third element of fitness is body composition. **Body composition** is *the ratio of body fat to lean body tissue, such as bone, muscle, and fluid.* One way to measure body composition is to use the skinfold test. It involves pinching a fold of skin on your upper arm and on your calf. The fold is measured with an instrument called a skinfold caliper, and the two numbers are added together. Ask your fitness instructor about the skinfold test.

To maintain a healthy body composition, select nutritious, lower-calorie foods according to calculated energy expenditure (an estimate of how many calories your body burns), and participate in regular physical activity.

Flexibility

The fourth element of fitness, **flexibility**, is *the ability of your body's joints to move easily through a full range of motion.* When you have good flexibility, you can easily bend, turn, and stretch your body. People with limited flexibility may move stiffly or strain parts of their body. **Figure 9.5** shows how to measure the flexibility of muscles in your lower back and the backs of your legs.

FIGURE 9.5

DETERMINING FLEXIBILITY

Warm up with some light and easy stretches. When you take the test, move slowly and smoothly. Don't strain your muscles.

1. Remove shoes and sit down in front of 12-inch-high box. There should be a ruler on top with the "zero" end against the edge nearest you. Extend both legs with feet flat against box. Arms should extend over ruler with one hand on top of the other.

2. Reach forward with hands along the ruler four times. Hold position of the fourth reach for at least one second.

3. Record number of inches your fingers reach on the ruler.

Scoring

Females	Males	Rating
Reach beyond toes at least 1 inch	Reach beyond toes at least 1 inch	Acceptable flexibility
Cannot reach toes	Cannot reach toes	Low flexibility

Source: Modified with permission from *Foundations of Personal Fitness: Any Body Can . . . Be Fit!*, by D. Rainey and T. Murray.

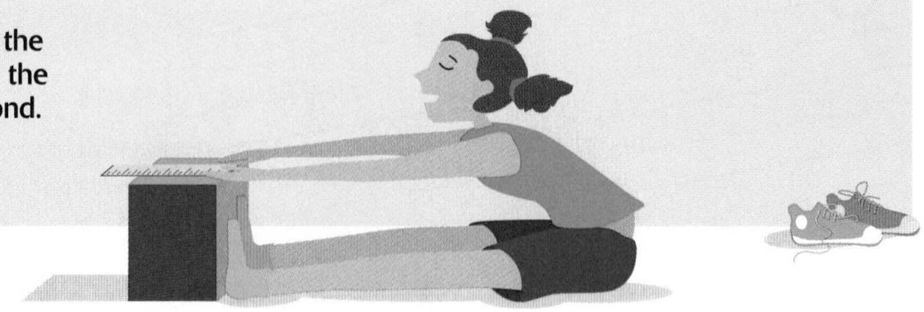

You can improve your flexibility through regular stretching, bending, and twisting exercises. Move slowly and gently, and improve the flexibility of different muscle groups gradually.

Your Fitness Level

After reading this lesson and completing the physical fitness tests described, you should have a clearer idea of your heart and lung endurance, muscle strength and endurance, body composition, and flexibility. Are you as physically fit as you should be? Are you as fit as you would like to be?

If you want to raise your level of physical fitness, you'll need to set goals for yourself and then decide how to achieve these goals. Remember to consider your limits, though. Some people improve faster than others, and some people have a higher fitness potential than others.

Heredity and overall health both play important roles in a person's physical abilities. For example, someone with asthma may become short of breath when exercising. A person with a physical impairment may not be able to participate in all activities. To develop a realistic plan that is right for you, check with your doctor before pursuing your fitness goals.

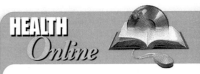

HEALTH *Online*

Topic: Fitness levels

For a link to more information on measuring fitness levels, go to **health.glencoe.com**.

Activity: Using the information provided at this link, set a fitness goal that will improve your health.

Lesson 2 Review

Using complete sentences, answer the following questions on a sheet of paper.

Reviewing Terms and Facts

1. **Vocabulary** Define *heart and lung endurance.* What is the best way to build heart and lung endurance?
2. **Compare** What is the difference between muscle strength and muscle endurance?
3. **Identify** Which part of your body is strengthened by curl-ups? By step-ups?
4. **Recall** What are the advantages of good flexibility?

Thinking Critically

5. **Apply** Your friend wants to improve her physical fitness. When she exercises, she rarely raises her heartbeat above 50 percent of her maximum heartbeat rate. What advice would you offer her? Why?
6. **Explain** How are strength, endurance, and flexibility related?

Applying Health Skills

7. **Advocacy** Look through magazines to find photos of people performing different types of physical activity or exercise. Cut them out and make a collage on a poster. Explain in captions how these activities contribute to these people's overall physical fitness. Share your poster with the class.

Setting Fitness Goals

Many people set out to improve their physical fitness through an exercise program. What factors might help to make an exercise program successful?

LEARN ABOUT...

- how to set and achieve fitness goals.
- writing an activity plan.
- the three stages of an exercise session.
- checking your fitness progress.

VOCABULARY

- warm-up
- cool-down

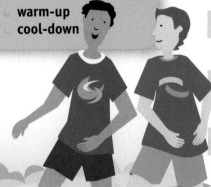

A Fitness Plan You Can Live With

Developing a fitness plan can be confusing. You may wonder which activities will best help you reach your fitness goals. Maybe you're not sure how to do an exercise. As a teen, you can turn to a fitness instructor, your physical education teacher, or a coach. Any of these experts can show you how to get started, what equipment to use, and how to exercise safely. An expert can also help you set fitness goals, stay motivated, and monitor your progress. **Figure 9.6** compares different types of activities.

FIGURE 9.6

RATING DIFFERENT ACTIVITIES

The ratings in this chart show the benefits of activities done for 30 minutes or more.

Exercise	Flexibility	Muscle Strength and Endurance	Heart and Lung Endurance
Handball	High	High	High
Swimming	High	Medium	High
Jogging	Medium	High	High
Bicycling	Medium	High	High
Tennis	High	Medium	Medium
Brisk walking	Medium	High	High
Slow walking	Low	Medium	Medium
Softball	Medium	Low	Low
Weight training	Low	High	Low

Being Active Every Day

Whatever your fitness goals may be, try to do one or more forms of physical activity or exercise each day. Include a mixture of activities during the week, and vary your routine in order to develop different parts of your body.

To become fit and stay fit, you need different types of physical activity. Here are some ideas for developing an active lifestyle.

- **Daily activity.** Look for opportunities to be active every day. Take the stairs instead of the elevator. Bike to a friend's home. Walk to the store. Rake leaves. Shovel snow. Wash and wax the car.
- **Aerobic exercise.** Aim to do at least 20 to 30 minutes of aerobic exercise 3 to 5 times a week. Swim laps. Join the track team. Take a brisk walk. Ride a stationary bike. Jump rope.
- **Sports, recreation, leisure activities.** Spend at least half an hour several times a week participating in activities that are fun and get your blood moving. Play soccer, racquetball, volleyball, or basketball. Hike a mountain trail. Take a dance class. Go skating or bowling.

HEALTH SKILLS ACTIVITY

PRACTICING HEALTHFUL BEHAVIORS

Activities for Fitness

You can achieve and maintain physical fitness by building a variety of activities into your lifestyle. When choosing the activities that work best for you, consider your options, interests, and the available facilities and equipment.

- **DAILY ACTIVITIES.** What aspects of your daily life can you change in order to add more activity? Think about your journey to school, your after-school activities, and the chores you do at home.
- **AEROBIC EXERCISE.** You need three to five sessions a week. Think of activities that you enjoy and that would keep you motivated.

- **SPORTS, RECREATION, AND LEISURE ACTIVITIES.** What are some fun ways to relax with your friends and be active at the same time? You may need to choose different activities for different seasons.

ON YOUR OWN

Divide a sheet of paper into three columns, one for each type of activity listed above. In each column, list at least two activities that interest you and that you might include in your personal fitness plan.

FIGURE 9.7

A SAMPLE WEEKLY ACTIVITY PLAN

A written plan will help you include a balance of activities in your weekly schedule.

Sunday	Monday	Tuesday	Wednesday	Thursday	Friday	Saturday
29	**30**	**31**	**1**	**2**	**3**	**4**
Bike ride 1 hr.	Gym class 30 min. Soccer practice 1 hr. Walk home from practice 20 min.	Basketball or jog after school 40 min. Karate class 1 hr.	Gym class 30 min. Soccer practice 1 hr.	Basketball or bike ride after school 40 min. Karate class 1 hr.	Gym class 30 min. Walk home from school 20 min.	Soccer game 50 min. Karate class 1 hr.
Total: 1 hour	Total: 1 hour 50 min.	Total: 1 hour 40 min.	Total: 1 hour 30 min.	Total: 1 hour 40 min.	Total: 50 min.	Total: 1 hour 50 min.

Preparing an Activity Plan

To achieve your fitness goals, you may find it helpful to make a weekly physical activity plan like the one in **Figure 9.7**. A written plan will keep you on track and help you exercise consistently. To develop your plan, first write down all scheduled physical activities or exercise sessions, such as gym periods, team practices, and dance classes. Next, pencil in a variety of physical activities and exercises.

Try to balance your schedule so that every day contains some activities but no single day is overloaded. Also, be flexible, and include some choices. For example, you might write, "Jog or bike ride," and then decide which activity you prefer when that day comes. Keep in mind that your activity plan should meet *your* personal fitness goals. Your friends' goals and activities may differ from yours.

Exercise Stages

Your exercise workouts should have three stages: the beginning warm-up, the workout itself, and then the cool-down. Each of these stages is discussed on the following pages. Because all three stages are important, it's wise not to skip any of them. Observing workout safety rules is a strategy for preventing accidental injuries during physical activities.

Warming Up

A **warm-up** is *a period of low to moderate exercise to prepare your body for more vigorous activity.* You should start every exercise session with a warm-up lasting about ten minutes. During this period, your heartbeat rate gradually increases, and your body temperature starts to rise. As the flow of blood to your muscles increases, they become more flexible, which makes them less prone to injury during exercise.

Begin a warm-up with gentle aerobic activities, such as a fast walk, followed by stretching exercises. When you stretch, move slowly and stretch the muscles little by little. Be careful not to overstretch or bounce as you stretch, which can damage body joints and tissues. **Figure 9.8** shows two typical stretching exercises. Some stretches are not good for your joints. Ask your fitness instructor for a good stretching routine.

Another way to warm up is to do the actual movements of your planned activity but at a slow and easy pace. For example, if you plan to play racquetball, you might warm up by gently hitting the ball back and forth with your opponent and then doing a variety of stretching exercises.

FIGURE 9.8

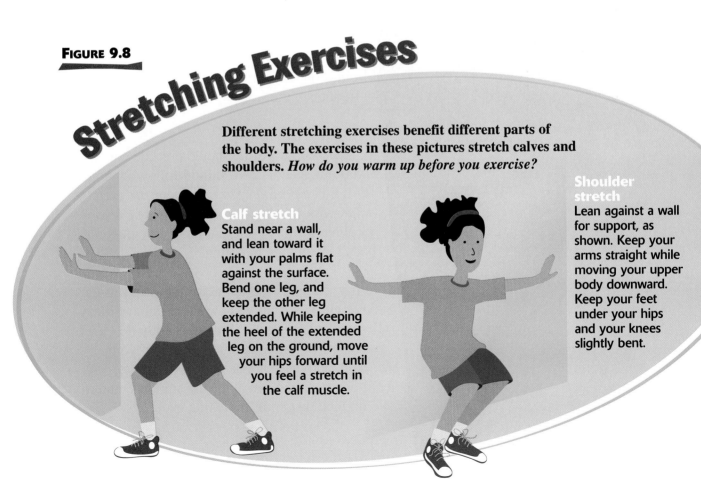

Stretching Exercises

Different stretching exercises benefit different parts of the body. The exercises in these pictures stretch calves and shoulders. *How do you warm up before you exercise?*

Calf stretch
Stand near a wall, and lean toward it with your palms flat against the surface. Bend one leg, and keep the other leg extended. While keeping the heel of the extended leg on the ground, move your hips forward until you feel a stretch in the calf muscle.

Shoulder stretch
Lean against a wall for support, as shown. Keep your arms straight while moving your upper body downward. Keep your feet under your hips and your knees slightly bent.

Working Out

Once you have warmed up, you're ready to work out. Your workouts should start off at a comfortable level of physical activity and build up gradually. Some guidelines for starting and increasing your workout program include:

- **Frequency.** Gradually increase the number of times you exercise per week. Start by exercising two or three times the first week and work your way up to exercising daily.
- **Intensity.** This refers to the difficulty of your physical activity or exercise session. The most common way of gauging intensity is in terms of heartbeat rate. You can usually increase intensity by speeding up—running faster, for example, or doing more sit-ups in less time. You can also increase intensity by making yourself work harder. For example, it's harder to bike up a hill than along a flat road.
- **Duration.** Limit your workout sessions to about 10 to 15 minutes at first. Gradually increase the time until you're exercising for about 30 to 45 minutes each session.
- **Order.** If you're doing both aerobic and strength-building exercises during a workout session, perform the aerobic exercise first. Your muscles will work more smoothly after aerobic activity.

As these teens' overall fitness levels have improved, they have increased the frequency and duration of their practice sessions. *What could they do to increase intensity?*

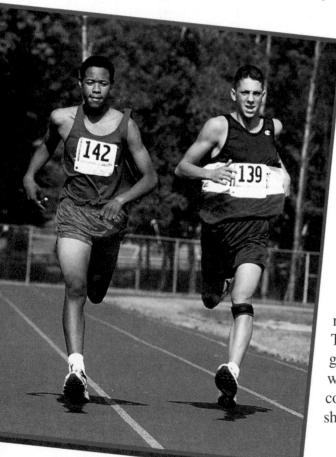

If you want to build on your workout, do it gradually. Change only one element at a time. For example, if you increase the duration of your workout, keep intensity and frequency the same.

Cooling Down

Just as a warm-up should precede your workout, a cool-down should follow it. A **cool-down** is *a period of low to moderate exercise to prepare your body to end a workout session.* Cooling down helps return blood circulation and body temperature to normal.

If you end a workout abruptly, your muscles may tighten up and you may feel faint or dizzy. To avoid such effects, slow your body down gradually. Continue the movements of your workout activity but at a slower, easier pace. A cool-down should last about ten minutes, and it should include gentle stretching exercises.

Monitoring Your Progress

As you work toward your fitness goals, you'll want to monitor your progress. Remember that change comes gradually. Don't expect to cut 30 seconds off your mile time after a week of working out. Here are some suggestions for monitoring your progress.

- Keep an exercise log or journal. Making performance notes after each workout will help you keep track of exercise sessions.
- After four to eight weeks of workouts, you should observe some improvement in your overall fitness. Depending on the exercises you've been doing, you should feel stronger, have more endurance, and have greater flexibility. You may also find that you feel better overall, look fitter, and have more energy.
- If you see no significant change after eight weeks, you need to evaluate the situation. Have you been exercising regularly? Do you need to modify your fitness goals?
- Another measure of fitness is your resting heartbeat rate, the number of times per minute your heart beats when your body is at rest. The average heartbeat rate ranges from 72 to 84 beats per minute. A resting heartbeat rate less than 72 is generally associated with physical fitness.
- Once you reach your fitness goals, consider setting new goals for yourself.

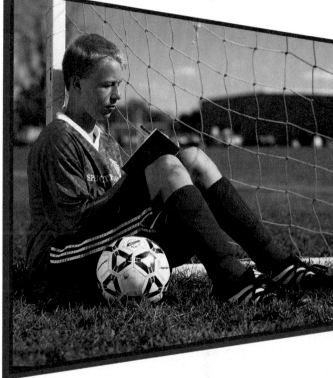

Recording your performance in an exercise log will help you assess your progress. *What system would you use to record your progress?*

Lesson 3 Review

Using complete sentences, answer the following questions on a sheet of paper.

Reviewing Terms and Facts

1. **Summarize** What should you keep in mind when preparing an activity plan?
2. **Recall** What are the three stages of an exercise workout?
3. **Vocabulary** Define *warm-up* and *cool-down*. What are their similarities and differences?
4. **Explain** Why would it be unwise to skip the cool-down stage?

Thinking Critically

5. **Apply** What adjustments do you need to make in frequency, intensity, and time to meet your personal workout needs?
6. **Explain** Why is it important to set fitness goals before starting an exercise program?

Applying Health Skills

7. **Practicing Healthful Behaviors** Make a weekly activity plan like the one shown in Figure 9.7 on page 232. Exchange plans with another student and offer suggestions to each other.

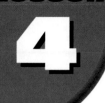
Staying Fit and Avoiding Injury

Quick Write

Some people love playing team sports. Others prefer to exercise on their own. Many enjoy doing both. Which group do you fit in? Explain your preference.

LEARN ABOUT...

- choosing sports activities that are right for you.
- preparing yourself to take part in sports.
- minimizing your risk of injury in sports.

VOCABULARY

- individual sports
- team sports
- sports conditioning
- dehydration
- anabolic steroids

Choosing Sports Activities

To choose the right sports for you, consider the kinds of activities you enjoy most. While both individual and team sports provide personal satisfaction and a way to stay active, one sport may suit your needs better than others. Of course, many teens take part in both individual *and* team sports.

Individual Sports

Individual sports are *physical activities that you can do on your own or with a friend.* You don't need to be part of a team to participate in individual sports. For example, biking, running, swimming, and skating are all sports you can do by yourself.

What are the advantages of individual sports? They are more flexible than team sports. You can do them whenever you feel like it, and you can do them for as long as you wish.

That's also one possible disadvantage to individual sports. You have to find the time and the motivation to take part in your chosen sport. Some people find it hard to stick to a plan if they have to do it on their own.

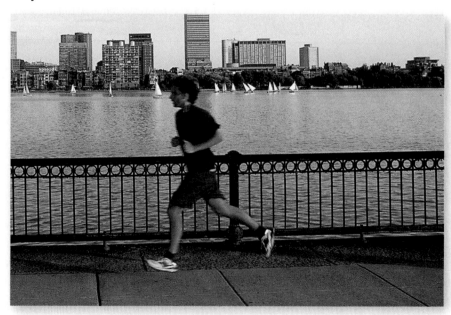

One advantage of individual sports is that you can set your own schedule. *What are other advantages?*

Team Sports

Many teens enjoy **team sports**—*organized physical activities with specific rules in which groups of people play together against other groups.* There are many different team sports to choose from, including baseball, soccer, basketball, volleyball, and football. Dual sports, requiring only two to four players, include tennis and racquetball. Team sports may be offered by

- schools.
- city or town recreation departments.
- community centers.
- teen clubs and organizations.
- sports and fitness centers.
- church and synagogue youth programs.

Playing on a team can be a positive and enjoyable experience. Many teens like the excitement of competition. Whether or not your team wins, you have the companionship and support of your teammates and coaches as you work together toward a common goal. Playing on a team also gives you an opportunity to develop communication and social skills. You learn about cooperation, compromise, and good sportsmanship.

Of course, team sports are not suitable for everyone. Some teens don't like having a set schedule, which typically requires them to attend several practices and games a week, after school and on weekends. Perhaps their family circumstances prevent them from committing themselves to a team. For these people, individual sports offer a better fitness alternative.

Developing Good Character

Sportsmanship

Being a good sport means treating others fairly and respectfully. It means playing by the rules and accepting both victory and defeat graciously. It can include helping a less-talented athlete by giving him or her pointers for a better game. *What real-life examples can you think of that show good sportsmanship?*

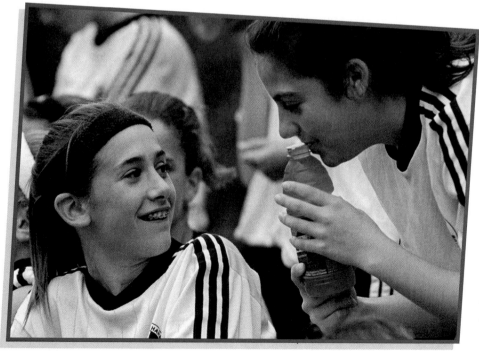

Team sports give you an opportunity to exercise, have fun, and make friends. *What are other benefits of team sports?*

Sports Conditioning

Whether you choose an individual sport or a team sport, you need to be physically fit to do your best. **Sports conditioning** is *regular physical activity or exercise to strengthen and condition muscles for a particular sport.* It takes time and effort. You'll also need to eat healthful foods, learn safety rules, and obtain appropriate equipment.

Sports and Nutrition

An important part of sports conditioning is eating a balanced, nutritious diet. Your choices should include a variety of foods from the different food groups and a limited amount of fat. Here are other guidelines.

- **Get enough carbohydrates.** Your body needs extra energy to play sports. Fruits, vegetables, pasta, and whole-grain breads provide carbohydrates, an excellent energy source.
- **Get enough vitamins and minerals.** These nutrients are essential to a balanced diet and to sports conditioning. Calcium, for example, strengthens bones, while iron helps provide muscles with oxygen during physical activity.
- **Don't eat too much protein.** Athletes need protein, but no more than anyone else, provided they are eating enough nutritious foods. Even though protein helps to build muscle tissue, it is only through exercise and training that you can develop your muscles.
- **Drink water!** If you play sports, your body will lose water through perspiration. To maintain fluid balance, drink a total of 9 to 13 glasses a day, especially when it is hot outside, and take a drink every 15 minutes. Your goal is to avoid **dehydration**, *excessive water loss from the body*, which can lead to dizziness, muscle cramps, and heatstroke.

These teens know the importance of avoiding dehydration. *How many glasses of water a day are recommended for athletes?*

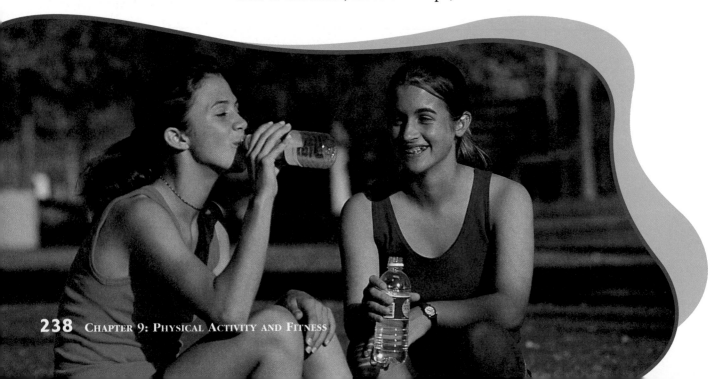

Safety First

Whenever you exercise or participate in sports, you increase your risk of injury. The three basic aspects of safety are safe behavior, safe and proper equipment, and knowing your limits.

Safe Behavior

Many sports-related injuries can be prevented by thinking ahead. Here are some tips.

- **Exercise where and when it's safe.** A soft, even surface is easier on your legs, knees, and feet than a hard or uneven surface. Exercise with another person and avoid deserted places. Protect yourself during hot weather by exercising in the cooler mornings or evenings. Remember to wear sunscreen outdoors.
- **Always warm up and cool down.** Gradually get your body ready to begin exercising. End your workout by cooling down.
- **Practice your sport regularly.** Team practices help you maintain your physical fitness levels and help you and your teammates learn to work together effectively and safely.
- **Learn the proper techniques and rules of the game.** Following the rules and regulations of a sport promotes both safety and good sportsmanship.
- **Keep your emotions under control.** Anger or frustration can lead to unsafe or unwise actions. Try to stay calm and relaxed.

Safe Equipment

What you wear when you exercise or play sports is important to your safety. Here are some clothing and equipment guidelines.

- **Wear loose-fitting or stretchable clothes.** For some sports, clothing that fits loosely gives you freedom of movement and helps you stay cooler. For other sports, tight, stretchable clothes are more appropriate.
- **If you exercise outdoors, make yourself visible.** Wear light-colored and reflective clothing so you'll be visible to drivers.
- **When exercising in cold weather, dress in layers.** You can easily add or remove layers as needed during your workout.
- **Wear protective equipment.** Different sports require protection for different parts of the body. Always wear the necessary gear.
- **Choose shoes carefully.** Shoes should fit properly, feel comfortable, provide adequate support, and be suitable for the activity you have chosen.
- **Select your equipment wisely.** Whether you're picking skates, a helmet, or a baseball glove, take the time to make a wise choice.

Reading Check

Investigate word parts. *Dehydration* uses the root word *hydrate,* the prefix *de-,* and the suffix *-tion.* Find each word part in a dictionary; then write your own definition.

Protective equipment that is properly sized and correctly worn helps prevent injury. *What protective gear is this hockey player wearing?*

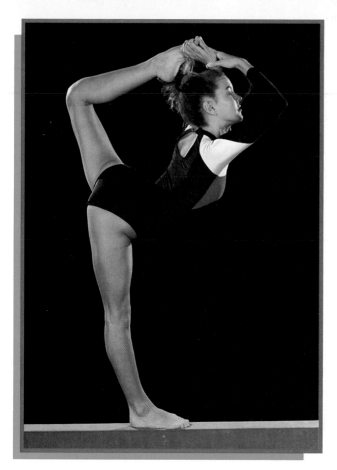

Know Your Limits

When exercising or playing sports, it's important to recognize your limits. Here are some suggestions that will help.

- **Listen to your body.** Exercise can cause discomfort, like mild breathlessness or tired muscles, but pain is not normal. If you're feeling pain, your body is telling you to slow down, rest, or stop completely. If pain persists, see a doctor.
- **Stop if you get injured or feel ill.** If you get hurt while exercising or while playing in a game, don't continue until someone checks you out. Consult a coach, fitness instructor, or doctor. Also, don't play sports if you're not feeling well.
- **Use the R.I.C.E. formula.** If you have a minor sports injury such as a sprained ankle, follow the Rest, Ice, Compression, Elevation formula. See Chapter 19 for details.

This teen was able to compete because she trained properly and knew her limits. *What strategies help you know your limits?*

HEALTH SKILLS ACTIVITY

REFUSAL SKILLS

Abstaining from Drugs

Ben enjoys being part of his school's traveling track team. In his last race, Ben came in second, a half step behind the lead runner. After the race, one of his teammates, Scott, came over and said, "You know, you could have won." When Ben asked what he meant, Scott smiled and held up a small bottle. "These pills will increase your speed like you won't believe!"

Ben wants to increase his speed, but he knows that taking a drug is not only cheating, it's also dangerous. He uses his refusal skills to let Scott know how he feels.

WHAT WOULD YOU DO?

Suppose you were Ben. Describe how you would apply the S.T.O.P. refusal skills in your conversation with Scott. With a partner, role-play the interaction between Ben and Scott.

SAY NO IN A FIRM VOICE.

TELL WHY NOT.

OFFER OTHER IDEAS.

PROMPTLY LEAVE.

Avoiding Harmful Substances

Anabolic steroids are *drugs that cause muscle tissue to develop at an abnormally fast rate.* Although steroids and certain other drugs may increase strength, the use of these drugs is both dangerous and illegal. Here are some of the side effects users may experience:

- Liver and brain cancers
- Weakening of tendons, leading to joint or tendon injuries
- Cardiovascular damage and high blood pressure, raising the risk of heart attack
- Mental and emotional effects, such as anxiety, severe mood swings, uncontrolled rage, and delusions
- Severe acne
- Trembling
- Bone damage
- Facial hair growth in females and breast development in males

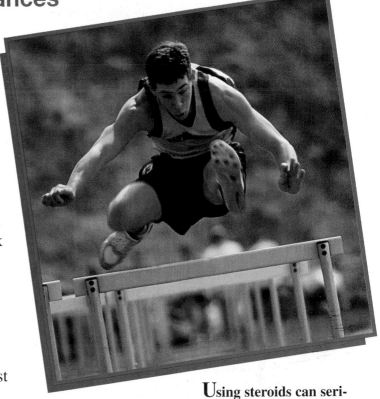

Using steroids can seriously damage a person's health, even later in life. Avoid harmful substances to perform well and stay healthy.

Anabolic steroids and other performance-enhancing drugs have no place in a healthy fitness plan. Besides damaging your body, they can destroy your athletic career.

Lesson 4 Review

Using complete sentences, answer the following questions on a sheet of paper.

Reviewing Terms and Facts

1. **Vocabulary** Explain the meaning of *sports conditioning.*
2. **Explain** What is *dehydration*? Why is it dangerous?
3. **Give Examples** List three ways to practice safe behavior in sports.
4. **Recall** What are the dangers of using anabolic steroids?

Thinking Critically

5. **Suggest** What advice would you give to a teammate who often misses practice or arrives late?

6. **Analyze** Carlton borrows his older brother's protective gear and his sports shoes, even though his brother is much bigger. How is he risking injury?

Applying Health Skills

7. **Accessing Information** With a partner, make a list of all the places in your community that provide opportunities to join a sports team. Include on your list information about the hours they are open and fees they charge. Share your list with your classmates.

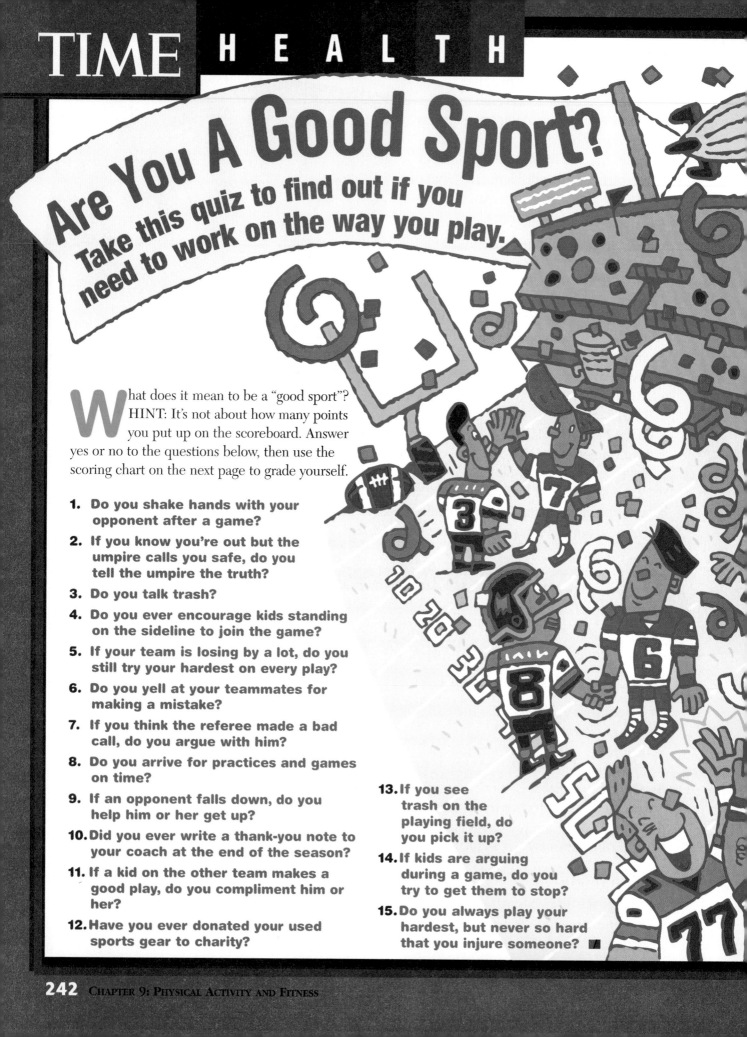

Are You A Good Sport?

Take this quiz to find out if you need to work on the way you play.

What does it mean to be a "good sport"? HINT: It's not about how many points you put up on the scoreboard. Answer yes or no to the questions below, then use the scoring chart on the next page to grade yourself.

1. Do you shake hands with your opponent after a game?

2. If you know you're out but the umpire calls you safe, do you tell the umpire the truth?

3. Do you talk trash?

4. Do you ever encourage kids standing on the sideline to join the game?

5. If your team is losing by a lot, do you still try your hardest on every play?

6. Do you yell at your teammates for making a mistake?

7. If you think the referee made a bad call, do you argue with him?

8. Do you arrive for practices and games on time?

9. If an opponent falls down, do you help him or her get up?

10. Did you ever write a thank-you note to your coach at the end of the season?

11. If a kid on the other team makes a good play, do you compliment him or her?

12. Have you ever donated your used sports gear to charity?

13. If you see trash on the playing field, do you pick it up?

14. If kids are arguing during a game, do you try to get them to stop?

15. Do you always play your hardest, but never so hard that you injure someone?

A Good Sport With a Great Idea!

Mark Guterman of Short Hills, New Jersey, celebrated his bar mitzvah recently. (At age 13, a Jewish boy often celebrates a bar mitzvah, a ceremony to commemorate the acceptance of religious duty and adult responsibility.)

To show that he was ready for his bar mitzvah, Mark did something to help other people: He sent letters to friends and relatives asking if they could donate used sports equipment to kids in need.

Mark and his family collected hundreds of pieces of equipment, such as in-line skates, baseball mitts, skateboards, tennis rackets, and footballs. Then they gave all the equipment to kids at a homeless shelter and a foster home.

"It lit up their faces. They were thrilled," says Mark. "It made me feel good to help. I wanted to give to people who are less fortunate than I am."

Scoring Chart

Give yourself 1 point for every "yes" answer that you gave to questions 1, 2, 4, 5, 8, 9, 10, 11, 12, 13, 14, and 15.

Give yourself 1 point for every "no" answer that you gave to questions 3, 6, and 7.

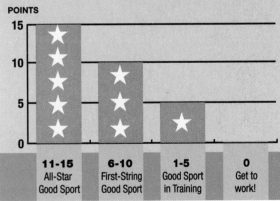

See how you scored by using the bar graph below.

POINTS			
11-15 All-Star Good Sport	6-10 First-String Good Sport	1-5 Good Sport in Training	0 Get to work!

TIME TO THINK...

About Being a Good Sport

Imagine that you're playing basketball. You take a shot and—wham! A player on the other team hits your arm so hard that you miss the shot. Amazingly, the referee does not call a foul. What would you do? Write down your thoughts in a brief paragraph. Then, as a class, discuss different options on what to do in this situation.

WARM UP! WORK OUT! COOL DOWN!

Model

Ryan and his twin sister Amber are getting ready to play in a neighborhood game of basketball. After their mom drops them off, Amber spends the first ten minutes warming up to prepare herself for exercise. She jogs slowly around the court a few times and then does some toe touches and other exercises to stretch her muscles. Ryan, however, is impatient to start playing. He grabs the basketball right away and starts dribbling it around the court. As he races toward the basket, Ryan suddenly clutches his left leg in pain; he has pulled his quadriceps and must sit out the game. Ryan promises himself he will be smarter next time.

Meanwhile, Amber has one of her best games. As she plays, she pays attention to her body's signals. She keeps herself working moderately hard, but she is careful not to push herself too far. After playing for half an hour, Amber takes another ten minutes to walk around the court while she waits for their mom to pick her and Ryan up. This cool-down helps her body come back to normal gradually.

Practice

Form groups of two or three. Tell the members of your group about your favorite way to work out. You may name more than one type of exercise if you wish. Write your choice or choices at the top of a sheet of paper. Then, as a group, discuss each of the exercises you have named. Try to think of appropriate ways to warm up for that type of exercise and to cool down afterward. Write down the group's ideas on your paper.

1. Did you think of at least one way to warm up and cool down for your favorite exercise?
2. Do you usually warm up and cool down when you do this activity? Why or why not?

Apply/Assess

Now that you know how to include warm-up and cool-down activities in a workout, use your knowledge to create your own workout plan. Use the chart below as a model. Fill in the activities you plan to do during each part of your workout. Include at least 10 minutes to warm up, 20 to 25 minutes to work out, and 10 minutes to cool down. If you include more than one type of activity in your workout, put aerobic activities before strength-building activities. Display your charts in the classroom.

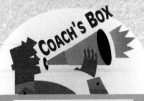

Warm Up	Work Out	Cool Down
Jog slowly 5 min. Stretch 5 min.	Run 15 min. Step-ups 5 min. Push-ups & Curls 5 min.	Jog slowly 5 min. Walk & Stretch 5 min.
Total: 10 min.	Total: 25 min.	Total: 10 min.

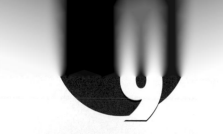

After You Read

Use your completed Foldable to review the information on physical activity, exercise, and physical fitness.

FOLDABLES™
Study Organizer

Reviewing Vocabulary and Concepts

On a sheet of paper, write the numbers 1–12. After each number, write the term from the list that best completes each sentence.

- heartbeat rate
- anaerobic
- muscle strength
- skinfold test
- intensity
- muscle endurance
- balance
- stretching exercises
- aerobic
- flexible
- coordination
- activity plan

Lesson 1

1. _____ is the feeling of stability and control over your body.
2. _____ is the smooth and effective working together of your muscles and bones.
3. _____ exercise works the heart.
4. Gymnastics is an example of _____ exercise.

Lesson 2

5. _____ measures the most weight you can lift or the most force you can exert at one time.
6. The greater your _____, the longer your muscles can exert their strength.
7. The _____ involves pinching and measuring folds of skin on your arm and calf.
8. The more _____ you are, the easier it is to bend, turn, and stretch your body.

Lesson 3

9. A weekly _____ can help you schedule your activities.
10. Warm-ups should start with light activity, followed by _____.
11. When developing an exercise program, consider the frequency, _____, duration, and order of your workouts.
12. The most common way to measure exercise intensity is by checking your _____.

Lesson 4

On a sheet of paper, write the numbers 13–15. After each number, write the letter of the answer that best completes each statement.

13. The advantage of individual sports is that
    a. it is more flexible than a team sport.
    b. you can do them whenever you wish.
    c. you can do them for as long as you wish.
    d. all of the above.
14. Good nutrition for athletes includes
    a. eating only high-protein foods.
    b. drinking a limited amount of water in order to prevent nausea.
    c. eating enough carbohydrates to give the body extra energy.
    d. cutting back on some minerals, especially calcium.
15. Many sports injuries can be prevented by
    a. becoming very emotional during competition so you don't build up anger.
    b. skipping some team practices so you don't overexert yourself.
    c. borrowing someone's safety gear.
    d. wearing shoes that are suitable for the activity or sport.

Thinking Critically

Using complete sentences, answer the following questions on a sheet of paper.

16. **Interpret** Explain how being fit can improve the quality of your everyday life.

17. **Apply** If you decided to raise your level of physical fitness, how would you proceed? What factors would you consider?

18. **Analyze** Participation in individual sports requires self-discipline. Do you think someone who doesn't have self-discipline can develop it? Why or why not?

19. **Explain** What actions can you take before, during, and after a game to protect yourself against a sports injury?

20. **Discuss** Your friend eats two steak sandwiches every day, claiming that protein develops muscles. What would you tell him?

Career Corner

Athletic Trainer Athletes often consult athletic trainers for advice on fitness programs. These professionals help athletes maintain their physical fitness by supervising nutrition and exercise. They also treat sports injuries. Athletic trainers need at least one to two years of community college, vocational/technical school, or an apprenticeship. Find out more about this and other health careers by clicking on Career Corner at health.glencoe.com.

Standardized Test Practice

Reading & Writing

Read the paragraphs below and then answer the questions.

Baseball, football, basketball—these sports were all invented in the United States, right? Wrong. Of these three, only basketball was invented and first played in the United States.

In 1891 a physical education teacher in Springfield, Massachusetts was asked to create a sport for students to play indoors during the cold New England winters. Using a soccer ball and two peach baskets attached to the balcony railing of the gym, he invented basketball. He wrote 13 rules for the game, taught them to his class, and the first game of basketball took place later that year. The new game required teamwork, quick reaction time, and endurance. Basketball caught on and was soon being played by YMCA, high-school, college, and professional teams across the United States. Today, it is the most popular indoor sport, with millions of fans crowding gyms and arenas to cheer their favorite teams. Millions more watch on television.

1. The author begins the passage with a question and answer in order to
   Ⓐ introduce the topic of basketball.
   Ⓑ inform readers about the rules of basketball.
   Ⓒ explain the difference between three sports.
   Ⓓ encourage readers to think about sports.

2. Which of the following best describes the organization of the second paragraph?
   Ⓐ presenting events in the order in which they occurred
   Ⓑ comparing sports as they developed
   Ⓒ explaining a problem and telling how to solve it
   Ⓓ ranking events in order of importance

3. Write a paragraph explaining the rules for playing a particular sport.

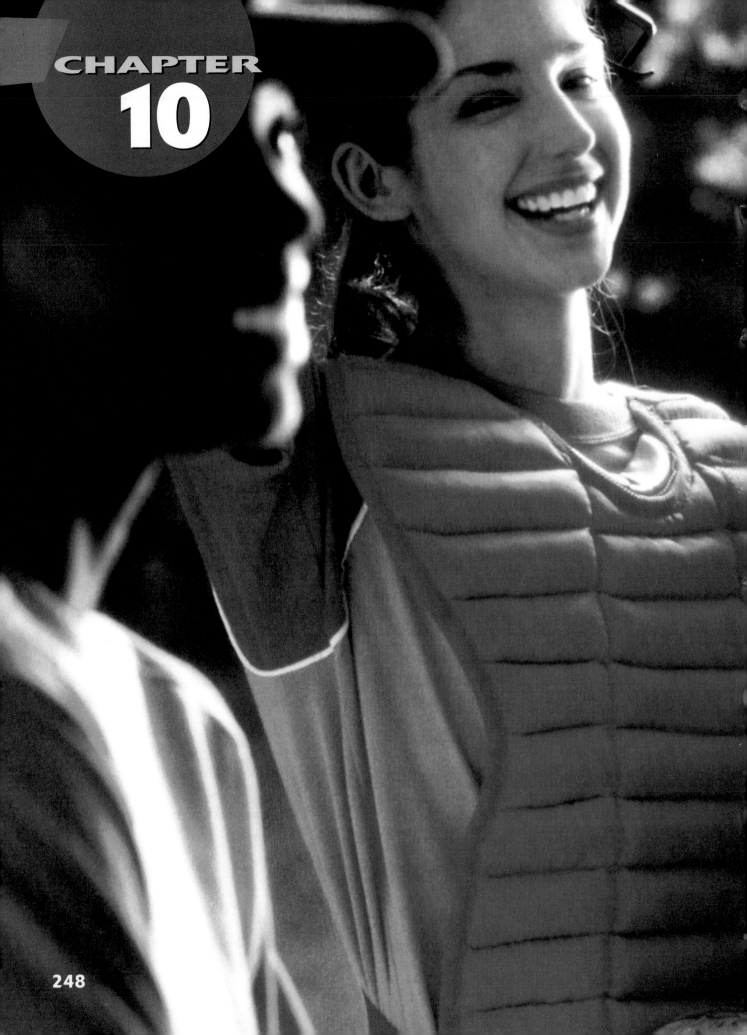

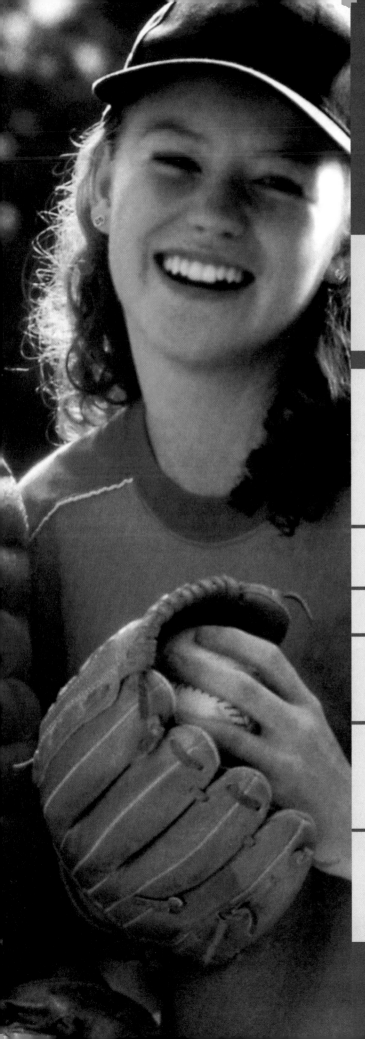

Your Body Image

HEALTH *Online*

Do you manage your weight in a healthy way? Find out by taking the Health Inventory for Chapter 10 at health.glencoe.com.

FOLDABLES™ Study Organizer

Before You Read

Make this Foldable to help you record what you learn about body weight in Lesson 1. Begin with a plain sheet of 8½″ × 11″ paper.

Step 1

Fold the sheet of paper in half along the long axis.

Step 2

Turn the paper and fold it into thirds.

Step 3

Unfold and cut the top layer along both fold lines. This makes three tabs.

Step 4

Turn the paper vertically and label the tabs as shown.

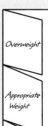

Overweight

Appropriate Weight

Underweight

As You Read

Under the appropriate tab of your Foldable, record definitions and take notes on each term relating to body weight.

1

Maintaining a Healthy Body

Quick Write

How are teens' body images portrayed in magazines and other media? Are they realistic? Write down your opinions on this issue.

LEARN ABOUT...

- the relationship between weight, growth, and health.
- how eating and physical activity habits affect weight.
- ways to maintain your healthy weight.

VOCABULARY

- body image
- appropriate weight
- Body Mass Index (BMI)
- overweight
- underweight

Body Image

How do you feel about your appearance? *The way you see yourself* is called your **body image**. A person who feels good about the way she or he looks is more likely to have a positive self-image.

Trying to look the same as a model, an athlete, or anyone else is not a healthy approach to body image. It's important to recognize and accept that there are differences in body type—no individual weight or body type is ideal at any age. Your body will grow and change throughout your teen years. A few extra pounds now, for example, could disappear in a few months as you grow. Someone who feels too skinny may fill out after he or she stops growing taller.

Your Appropriate Weight

Many factors influence your **appropriate weight**, or *the weight that is best for your body.* These factors include your gender, height, age, and body frame (small, medium, or large), and, during your teen years, your growth pattern. At your appropriate weight, you are more likely to feel good about yourself and have the energy you need for peak performance.

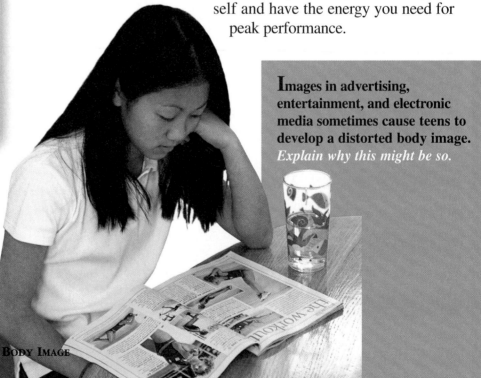

Images in advertising, entertainment, and electronic media sometimes cause teens to develop a distorted body image. *Explain why this might be so.*

FIGURE 10.1

Body Mass Index

To find your place on the chart, first calculate your BMI by following the formula given below. Then trace an imaginary line straight up from your age to the BMI you calculated. The point where your age and BMI meet tells you the approximate weight range you fall into. However, since people grow at different rates, this is only an estimate.

To calculate your BMI:

1 Multiply your weight in pounds by 0.45.

2 Multiply your height in inches by 0.025. Square the result.

3 Divide your answer to step 1 by your answer to step 2. The answer is your BMI.

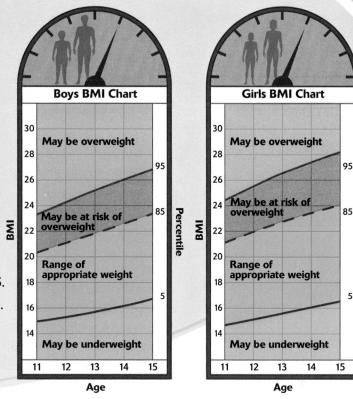

Boys BMI Chart

- May be overweight
- 95
- May be at risk of overweight — 85
- Range of appropriate weight
- 5
- May be underweight

BMI — Percentile — Age

Girls BMI Chart

- May be overweight
- 95
- May be at risk of overweight — 85
- Range of appropriate weight
- 5
- May be underweight

BMI — Percentile — Age

You can find out if your weight is appropriate by using the Body Mass Index chart in **Figure 10.1**. The **Body Mass Index (BMI)** is *a measurement that allows you to assess your body size, taking your height and weight into account.*

Weight Problems

Being overweight or underweight is unhealthy. People who are **overweight** are *more than the appropriate weight for gender, height, age, body frame, and growth pattern.* People who are **underweight** are *less than the appropriate weight for gender, height, age, body frame, and growth pattern.* Many teens are concerned that they have a weight problem. In reality, most teens don't need to lose or gain weight. In fact, unwise dieting can interfere with normal growth and development.

Overweight

Eating empty-calorie foods or eating more food than needed leads to weight gain. Busy teens on the run tend to grab food from fast-food places and convenience stores. Much of this food is high in fat and calories. Some food comes in extra-large portions, which attract consumers with a bargain price. Weight gain is also linked to a sedentary, or inactive, lifestyle. Many people spend their days sitting at desks. At home they may watch television, play video games, or use a computer. These activities burn fewer calories than those involving movement.

Reading Check

Identify the effects of being overweight. Then list the causes and effects of being underweight.

Excess weight puts strain on the heart and lungs. Overweight people have an increased risk of developing high blood pressure, diabetes, heart disease, cancer, and stroke. If you think that you are overweight, check with your health care professional. You may just be gaining a few pounds before getting taller. This is the body's way of storing up extra energy for growing.

Underweight

If you appear skinny during your teenage growth years, you are not necessarily underweight. You may simply be growing taller first. After reaching a certain height, your body may take time to catch up and add shape and muscle.

Some people are underweight because they do not consume enough nutrients. Others are underweight because of extreme dieting or excessive exercise. Both reasons pose serious health risks. People who are underweight may not have enough body fat to cushion the body's organs and bones. They may often feel tired due to insufficient food energy, and they have little body fat as an energy reserve. Underweight people are also more likely to develop disorders related to a low food intake, such as anemia.

Hands-On Health

CALCULATING FAT INTAKE

The Dietary Guidelines recommend that you receive no more than 35 percent of your calories from fat. In this activity, you will learn how to calculate the percentage of calories from fat in a given food.

WHAT YOU WILL NEED
- pencil and notebook
- calculator (optional)
- 3 Nutrition Facts food labels

WHAT YOU WILL DO
1. Choose one of your food labels. Divide the amount in the "calories from fat" category by the amount in the "total calories" category. For example, a 200-calorie granola bar might contain 80 calories from fat. Divide 80 by 200 and you get 0.4.

2. Multiply the result by 100 to express the figure as a percentage. 0.4 times 100 is 40. The granola bar derives 40 percent of its calories from fat.
3. Repeat this procedure with your other food labels and record the results.

IN CONCLUSION
1. Which, if any, of the foods provides over 35 percent of its calories from fat?
2. Save labels from as many foods you eat in a day as possible. Use the formula to determine the percentage of calories from fat of each.
3. How can you use the formula to make healthy choices about your daily food intake?

The Role of Calories

The calories you take in and use every day affect your weight. As you know, calories measure both the energy available in food and the energy your body uses. The more calories a food contains, the more energy it provides.

You consume calories whenever you eat. When you take in the same number of calories that your body burns, your weight remains the same. When your body burns more calories than you take in, you lose weight. When you take in more calories than your body burns, you gain weight. Your body stores the extra calories as fat. One pound is equal to 3,500 calories.

On average, teen females require 2,200 calories per day, and teen males require 3,000. Do not worry if you eat too much or too little in a given day. It is more important to focus on your average intake over the long term.

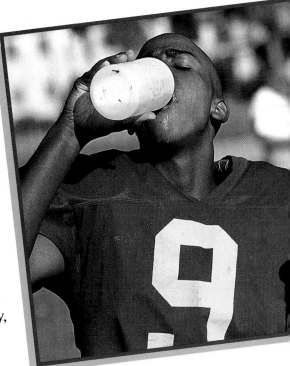

When you're thirsty, choose water instead of a soft drink. A 12-ounce can of cola may have 150 empty calories. *What are some other healthy beverage choices?*

Healthy weight management requires more than counting calories. You'll want to consider the nutrient value of the foods you eat. A healthful eating plan is based on foods with high nutrient density. These foods contain large amounts of nutrients relative to the number of calories they contain. The following are examples of foods with high nutrient density from each of the five food groups.

- **Grain Group:** whole-wheat pasta and breads, rice, tortillas, bagels
- **Fruit Group:** all fruits
- **Vegetable Group:** all vegetables
- **Meat and Beans Group:** tofu, chicken, lean beef, tuna, beans
- **Milk Group:** low-fat and fat-free milk, yogurt, cheese

Reaching Your Appropriate Weight

If you think that you might be above or under your appropriate weight, check with a health care professional. He or she can determine if you need to lose or gain weight while you are growing, and can suggest the best approach for you. Most successful weight change programs combine increased physical activity with a healthful eating plan, including mostly nutrient-dense foods.

Adjusting Calorie Intake

To reduce calorie intake, eat smaller servings. Instead of eating fried foods, choose foods that are broiled, baked, or steamed. Add flavor by using herbs and spices instead of oils or cream sauces. Drink fewer soft drinks and more water.

To increase calorie intake, eat more servings of lean and low-fat foods, including those with complex carbohydrates, such as breads, pastas, and vegetables. Whether you want to reduce or increase calorie intake, use the Food Guide Pyramid as a guide.

Increasing Physical Activity

Physical activity plays a key role in keeping a healthy weight. It helps tone muscle and reduce fat. You can also burn calories by increasing your level of activity. **Figure 10.2** lists some of the other benefits of regular physical activity.

Managing Weight Change

A person with an unrealistic body image may resort to unhealthy practices to alter his or her weight. Fad diets, diet pills, and other weight modification practices that promote quick results cannot replace informed choices. Use critical-thinking skills to analyze weight modification practices. Select appropriate practices to maintain, lose, or gain weight according to your individual needs and sound scientific research.

Most fad diets promote eating very few calories, eliminating certain healthful foods, or skipping meals. Most of these diets are ineffective and unsafe. They can lead to serious nutritional deficiencies. Fasting, or not eating for long periods of time, is also dangerous. Side effects can include loss of muscle tissue, heart damage, digestive problems, and stunted growth. Diet pills can be addictive and can have serious side effects. Body wraps cause water loss rather than loss of fat. With all these methods, any weight lost is usually regained.

FIGURE 10.2

PHYSICAL ACTIVITY AND YOUR WEIGHT

Physical activity helps you manage your weight and stay healthy. *How do you stay physically active?*

Physical Activity . . .

A Helps your heart and lungs work better.

B Can help strengthen and firm your muscles.

C Burns calories and helps you maintain a healthy weight.

D Helps you manage stress.

E Helps you feel good, have more energy, and develop higher self-esteem.

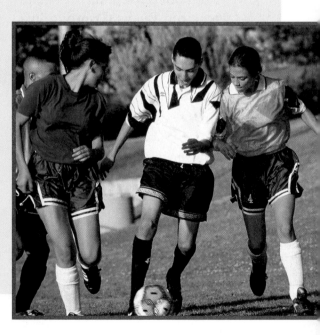

Recognize the Risks

These behaviors may put your health at risk:

- Following weight-loss programs that promise quick results
- Relying on special products or formulas
- Trying to lose more than ½ to 1 pound per week
- Eating fewer than 2,200 calories a day for a female, 3,000 for a male
- Skipping meals

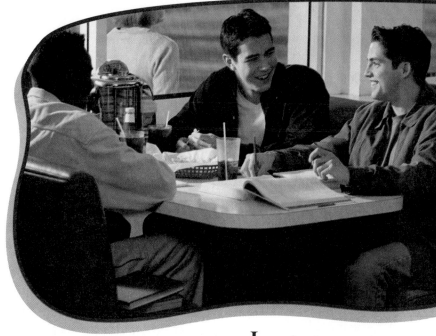

In moderate amounts, fast food can serve as part of a healthy food plan. *What do you choose when you eat out?*

Weight-Management Tips

To maintain a healthy weight, learn to eat smart and stay active for a lifetime. The following tips will help you manage your weight safely.

- Work with a health care professional to develop a safe weight-management program.
- Set realistic goals.
- Burn calories through fun physical activities, such as bike riding, dancing, skating, and swimming.
- Develop healthful eating habits; use the Food Guide Pyramid to help you select nutrient-dense foods.
- Plan your meals and snacks so that you take in the same number of calories as you burn.
- Watch your portion sizes so you know how much you're eating.

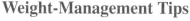

Lesson 1 Review

Using complete sentences, answer the following questions on a sheet of paper.

Reviewing Terms and Facts

1. **Vocabulary** Define *body image.* Use the term in an original sentence.
2. **Recall** What is the definition of *overweight?*
3. **Restate** Give two reasons why teens might become overweight.
4. **List** What are four tips for reaching and maintaining a healthy weight?

Thinking Critically

5. **Explain** Why are fad diets ineffective?
6. **Analyze** How can scientific research be used to select an appropriate weight-modification practice based on individual needs?

Applying Health Skills

7. **Goal Setting** Develop a plan to make healthful food choices and increase physical activity over the next three days.

Eating Disorders

Quick Write

Write down some of the things you have heard about eating disorders. After you read this lesson, add any new information that you learned.

LEARN ABOUT...

- why some people develop eating disorders.
- the health risks associated with eating disorders.
- where a teen with an eating disorder can get help.

VOCABULARY

- eating disorders
- anorexia nervosa
- malnutrition
- bulimia
- binge eating disorder

The Risks of Eating Disorders

Many teens spend a great deal of time worrying about their weight. Some even try to lose weight. Sometimes these worries and efforts get out of control. Obsession with food intake, coupled with mental and emotional problems, can lead to eating disorders. **Eating disorders** are *extreme and damaging eating behaviors that can lead to sickness and even death.*

Eating disorders can be triggered by many psychological factors, including low self-esteem, an unrealistic body image, and depression. Teens are at risk because of the normal stresses during the teen years and the natural growth patterns of their bodies. Eating disorders are serious; they can be fatal. People with eating disorders need to seek appropriate professional help.

Anorexia Nervosa

Anorexia nervosa is *an eating disorder characterized by self-starvation leading to extreme weight loss.* *Anorexia* means "without appetite," and *nervosa* means "of nervous origin." Most people who develop anorexia nervosa are teenage girls and young women. Men and teenage boys can also have the disorder, however. People with anorexia nervosa have a distorted body image. Most also have trouble coping with everyday stresses, such as high expectations, the need to achieve, or the need to be popular.

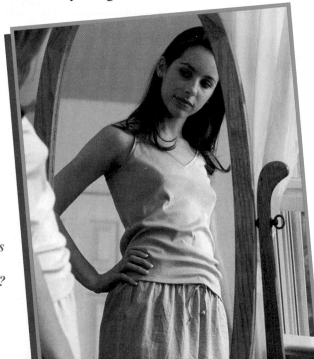

Even when they are very thin, people with anorexia nervosa see themselves as overweight. *Why does someone with such a distorted self-image need immediate medical help?*

Most people with anorexia nervosa eat very little. Some develop **malnutrition**, *a condition in which the body doesn't get the nutrients it needs to grow and function properly.* They may also develop shrunken organs, bone loss, low body temperature, low blood pressure, and a slowed metabolism. In some people with anorexia, an irregular heartbeat may lead to cardiac arrest.

Treatment for anorexia nervosa sometimes requires a stay at a hospital or clinic. There the person will get the nutrients needed to restore physical health. She or he will also receive counseling to address the underlying problems causing the disorder.

Bulimia

Another type of eating disorder is bulimia, or bulimia nervosa. **Bulimia** is *a condition in which a person eats large amounts of food and then tries to purge.* Many people with bulimia force themselves to vomit. Others take laxatives to force the food quickly through their body. Although bulimia is most common among young women and teenage girls, young men and teenage boys can also develop the disorder.

People with bulimia are extremely concerned about being thin and attractive. They have an overwhelming need to maintain control over their bodies. They might gorge on large amounts of food. Then, fearing that they are losing control of their bodies, they may take drastic steps to regain control. Some go on crash diets, including fasting, to try to make up for overeating. Others may exercise excessively.

Bulimia damages the body in many ways. Stomach acids from frequent vomiting can damage teeth and injure the mouth and throat. Vomiting can also cause the stomach to rupture. Repeated use of laxatives can damage the kidneys and liver, causing long-term health problems. Many people with bulimia suffer from malnutrition as a result of emptying the body of nutrients.

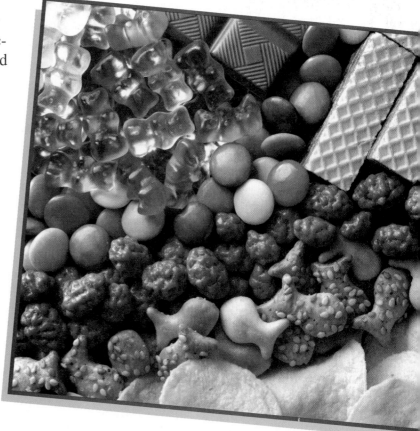

People with bulimia often eat large amounts of food high in calories and fat. Then they try to purge. *How does this eating pattern damage the body?*

Respect

It is important to value people for who they are on the inside, and to appreciate differences in body size and shape. If you are worried about the health of a friend, talk to a parent, a health professional, or a guidance counselor. However, be sure to do it with kindness and respect.

Binge Eating Disorder

Another eating disorder is **binge eating disorder**, or *compulsive overeating*. This disorder may be the most common eating disorder, affecting between 1 million and 2 million Americans. People with binge eating disorder eat unusually large amounts of food at a time. Unlike people with bulimia, though, they do not rid their bodies of the food. Afterward, they often feel a sense of guilt and shame.

People with binge eating disorder may use food as a way of coping with depression and other mental/emotional problems. However, the guilt and shame they feel after bingeing adds to the depression. This creates a cycle that can be difficult to break without professional help. Because binge eating disorder often leads to excess weight, it contributes to many health problems such as obesity, diabetes, and heart disease.

Help for People with Eating Disorders

People who have eating disorders usually need professional help. Sometimes this help can come from a counselor or psychologist. Help is also available through clinics and support groups such as Overeaters Anonymous, which are found in many communities. If a friend develops an eating disorder, you might want to speak to a school nurse or counselor. It is natural to want

HEALTH SKILLS ACTIVITY

DECISION MAKING

Helping a Friend

Recently, Jasmine has become concerned about her best friend Maria. At lunch, Maria barely touches her food. She doesn't have the energy for riding her bike anymore. She has become very thin. Yet when Jasmine and Maria went shopping recently, Maria complained about being fat, even though small-sized clothes were too big for her.

Jasmine is worried that Maria may have anorexia nervosa. Jasmine has tried to share her concerns with Maria, but Maria denies that she has a problem. Jasmine has thought about talking to Maria's mother, but she doesn't want to make Maria angry by going behind her back.

WHAT WOULD YOU DO?

Apply the decision-making process to Jasmine's situation. With a classmate, role-play a conversation in which Jasmine expresses her concerns to Maria. Then role-play a conversation between Jasmine and Maria's mother. What other options does Jasmine have?

1. **STATE THE SITUATION.**
2. **LIST THE OPTIONS.**
3. **WEIGH THE POSSIBLE OUTCOMES.**
4. **CONSIDER VALUES.**
5. **MAKE A DECISION AND ACT.**
6. **EVALUATE THE DECISION.**

to solve your friend's problem by yourself. However, you can help most by showing support and guiding him or her to a health professional.

Family and friends can also provide much-needed support for a person with an eating disorder. Often their role is to encourage the person to seek help. **Figure 10.3** takes a closer look at the role that family and friends can play.

FIGURE 10.3

HELPING SOMEONE WITH AN EATING DISORDER

Someone you know may have an eating disorder. Following these steps may enable you to help him or her.

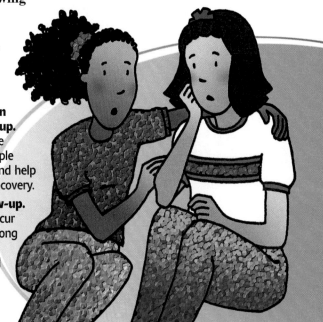

A **Encourage the person to seek help.**
A person with an eating disorder may not be aware of the seriousness of the condition. The person may also deny that the problem exists and may not want to be helped.

B **Tell an adult.**
You can talk to your parent or guardian, the school nurse, a counselor, or another trusted adult to see if they can help the person.

C **Get professional help.**
Psychological problems are usually the cause of eating disorders. The person with the disorder requires professional help. Sometimes family members are also encouraged to meet with the counselor.

D **Encourage the person to join a support group.**
Support groups provide encouragement to people with eating disorders and help them on the road to recovery.

E **Recommend a follow-up.**
Eating disorders can recur and could become lifelong problems. Follow-up visits to counselors and support groups are an important part of the recovery process.

 Lesson 2 Review

Using complete sentences, answer the following questions on a sheet of paper.

Reviewing Terms and Facts

1. **Vocabulary** What is an *eating disorder?*
2. **List** Name four ways in which anorexia and bulimia can harm the body.
3. **Recall** Identify and describe the three types of eating disorders.
4. **Give Examples** What kinds of people can help a person with an eating disorder?

Thinking Critically

5. **Hypothesize** Why are many people with eating disorders unwilling to seek help?

Applying Health Skills

6. **Analyzing Influences** Find a magazine article or book about someone with bulimia or anorexia nervosa. Read the article or book and write a brief summary of it. What influences or pressures contributed to the disorder? Were the influences internal or external?

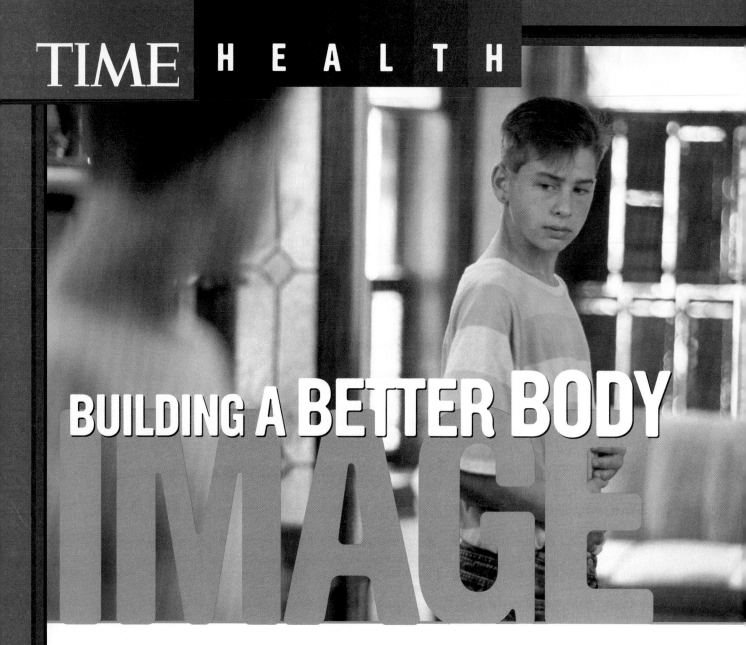

BUILDING A BETTER BODY IMAGE

Making positive life changes can boost how people think about themselves. Here are a few ideas.

1. Remind yourself that you're a work in progress.

The more you know about puberty and how your body is growing (read books, pay attention in health class, ask your doctor questions), the more you'll understand that it's a time of tremendous change. For instance, even though it's normal to experience about a 25 to 30 percent weight gain during puberty, that doesn't mean you need to prepare for a lifetime of sudden weight gain. "The body you have at fourteen is not necessarily the body you will have at nineteen," says Dr. L. Kris Gowen, an expert in adolescent body image at Stanford School of Education. "Your body is a long-term project," she adds. "Think of puberty as the first-draft phase of writing a term paper."

2. Be good to your body.

It works hard for you, so be sure to take time out to pamper your body. You don't have to do anything complicated. Sometimes the tiniest thing can make you feel better about yourself, such as using a new shampoo, going for a walk after school with a friend, or taking time out to relax. The most harmful thing you can do to your body is hate it, Dr. Gowen says.

3. Learn to love being healthy.

"People who are healthy feel good and look good," says Dr. Gowen. "Being beautiful isn't necessarily about being thin or buff." To get on the right track, try to eat sensibly, make physical activity a habit, and get plenty of sleep. Avoid any extreme behaviors (such as crash diets or working out to the point of injury), which are always unhealthy.

4. Compare yourself with...you.

Competing with the entire world is exhausting and destructive—though understandable. "Our culture encourages us not to be satisfied with what we have—especially girls, who are considered stuck up if they regard themselves as beautiful," says Dr. Gowen. "As a result, everyone is insecure—even the person you think you want to look like." Your goal should be like a runner who's trying to achieve a personal best instead of trying to beat the pack.

5. Practice zero tolerance toward teasing.

The amount of teasing that goes on in locker rooms and school hallways has reached destructive levels. Stick up for yourself and stick up for each other when you hear your friends or classmates making petty comments about the way someone looks.

6. Spend time on activities that have nothing to do with appearance. Do more of what you excel at and love.

You'll be reminded that there's more to you—and others—than mere looks. Sing, play guitar, hike, paint, design a Web site, or write a poem. Challenge yourself with new projects. Do them with other people if you can. Not only will you appreciate your own talents, regardless of your appearance, but you'll also begin to appreciate, value, and possibly learn from others.

Stay Positive!

If you're a teen and you've got a body, you might have very mixed feelings about it. Too often these feelings are negative, as you can see from the answers to the poll question below. After you check out the results (based on the responses of 4,000 young people), think about ways you might put a more positive spin on the way you think about your body.

Which of the following makes you unhappy with the way you look?

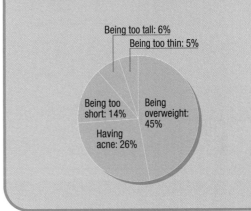

Being too tall: 6%
Being too thin: 5%
Being too short: 14%
Being overweight: 45%
Having acne: 26%

7. Recognize serious body-image problems.

Teens might try to cope with their body-image problems by engaging in harmful behaviors such as overexercising, binge eating, smoking, or drug and alcohol abuse. Destructive behaviors such as these require immediate professional help. If you're hurting, talk to an experienced professional about what you're going through and the way you're feeling. ◼

TIME TO THINK...

About Body Image

With the poll results above in mind, create a pamphlet entitled "Five Ways to Feel Better about Your Body." What are the top five tips you would offer your readers? What practical ways can you suggest to make it easy for the reader to use each tip in his or her life? Share the completed pamphlet with the rest of the class.

SHARPEN YOUR BODY IMAGE

Model

Blair is a teen who feels good about her body. As you read about her, notice the influences on her body image.

Blair knows that many girls her age feel uncomfortable with their bodies. Some believe they are unattractive, while others are afraid that people will tease or reject them because of their weight. Teens may also want to look like the superthin women they see in magazines, on TV, and in films. This attitude may lead them to develop eating disorders or to harm their health with fad diets or pills. Blair promises herself she will never let this happen to her. She knows that she is growing and changing as she goes through adolescence, and that these changes are normal. She understands enough about health to know that her body weight is healthy. By showing that she likes the way she looks, she makes it easier for her friends to accept themselves.

Practice

Read the following scenario and answer the questions below.

Kirk is dissatisfied with his body. All his friends seem to be growing faster than he is, and he is now the shortest boy in his class. He also thinks his muscles are not big enough. Kirk wishes he could look like his older brother, who is on the high school football team and is very popular. Sometimes Kirk watches sports events on TV and imagines himself looking like the star athletes he sees.

1. What influences affect Kirk's body image?
2. What could help Kirk feel better about how he looks?

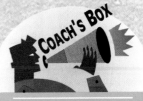

COACH'S BOX

Analyzing Influences

Influences on your body image may include

Internal
- knowledge.
- values.
- desires.
- fears.

External
- family and friends.
- media and culture.
- role models.

Apply/Assess

What influences your body image? Copy the list in the Coach's Box onto a separate sheet of paper. Then think of ways that each item influences your body image. For example, if one of your role models is someone with a healthy, but not "perfect," body, you could write this down under "role models." If you do not believe that a factor influences you in any way, write down "not an influence" under that factor.

When you are finished, look at each item on your list. If it describes something that makes you feel good about your body, write "+" next to the statement. If it describes something that makes you feel bad about your body, write "-." Identify the factor that has the most positive influence on your body image and the one that has the most negative influence. Then, at the bottom of your paper, write a statement about what you could do to improve your body image.

Self-√ Check

- Did I identify influences on my body image?
- Did I show the most positive and the most negative influences on my body image?
- Did I describe how to improve my body image?

After You Read

Use your completed Foldable to review the information on body weight.

FOLDABLES
Study Organizer

Reviewing Vocabulary and Concepts

On a sheet of paper, write the numbers 1–9. After each number, write the term from the list that best completes each sentence.

- appropriate weight
- nutrient density
- Body Mass Index
- body image
- calories
- Food Guide Pyramid
- extra-large
- overweight
- underweight

Lesson 1

1. When you have a positive _____, you feel good about the way you look.
2. Your _____ is influenced by your gender, height, age, body frame, and growth pattern.
3. You can use the _____ chart to determine if you are at an appropriate weight.
4. _____ is a condition in which people weigh more than their appropriate weight.
5. Someone who is _____ is less than the appropriate weight for his or her gender, height, age, body frame, and growth pattern.
6. When you take in the same number of _____ that your body burns, your weight remains the same.
7. A healthful eating plan is based on foods with high _____.
8. Foods with _____ portions may contribute to weight problems.
9. Using the _____ will help you develop healthful eating habits.

Lesson 2

On a sheet of paper, write the numbers 10–14. After each number, write the letter of the answer that best completes each statement.

10. Anorexia nervosa is an eating disorder characterized by
    a. overeating.
    b. binge eating.
    c. self-starvation.
    d. laxative abuse.
11. Which of the following best describes the disorder of a person who eats huge amounts of food but does not purge?
    a. anorexia nervosa
    b. binge eating disorder
    c. bulimia
    d. malnutrition
12. A condition in which the body does not get the nutrients it needs to grow and function properly is called
    a. overnourishment.
    b. malnutrition.
    c. obesity.
    d. low blood pressure.
13. Which of the following usually involves vomiting and abuse of laxatives?
    a. anorexia nervosa
    b. binge eating disorder
    c. bulimia
    d. obesity
14. You can help a person with an eating disorder by
    a. encouraging the person to seek help.
    b. telling a trusted adult that you believe the person needs help.
    c. encouraging the friend to join a support group.
    d. all of the above.

Thinking Critically

Using complete sentences, answer the following questions on a sheet of paper.

15. Evaluate Why should people who want to manage their weight be aware of the nutrient value of foods?

16. Hypothesize Why do you think magazines feature very thin models even though extreme thinness is unhealthy?

17. Explain Why is physical activity an important part of weight management?

18. Suggest Why might an athlete such as a gymnast develop an eating disorder?

Career Corner

Psychologist Are you fascinated by how the mind works? Do you wonder why people behave the way they do? Then consider a career as a psychologist. Psychologists study human behavior. In practice, they help people understand and improve their behaviors. A doctoral degree in psychology is required to enter this profession. Find out more about this and other health careers by visiting the Career Corner at health.glencoe.com.

Standardized Test Practice

Reading & Writing

Read the paragraphs below and then answer the questions.

I urge you to support the school uniform proposal. I believe that it will benefit everyone at school if uniforms are worn here. Wearing uniforms will save money, improve students' grades and behavior, and reduce competition among students.

Uniforms will save money because they are less expensive than regular clothing. Students who are not distracted by what they or others are wearing can focus more on their schoolwork and behavior. Fewer behavior problems will make learning easier for students; better grades will improve the school's reputation. Uniforms will also reduce the stress of competition among students. If everyone wears a uniform, students will not feel that they have to have certain clothes or wear something different each day.

1. Which sentence expresses an opinion?

(A) I believe that it will benefit everyone at school if uniforms are worn here.

(B) I urge you to support the school uniform proposal.

(C) Uniforms will also reduce the stress of competition among students.

(D) Fewer behavior problems will make learning easier for students.

2. Which sentence in the speech best summarizes the speaker's argument?

(A) I believe that it will benefit everyone at school if uniforms are worn here.

(B) I urge you to support the school uniform proposal.

(C) Fewer behavior problems will make learning easier for students.

(D) Wearing uniforms will save money, improve students' grades and behavior, and reduce competition among students.

3. Write a paragraph that features your views on the issue of school uniforms and give reasons for your opinion.

UNIT 4

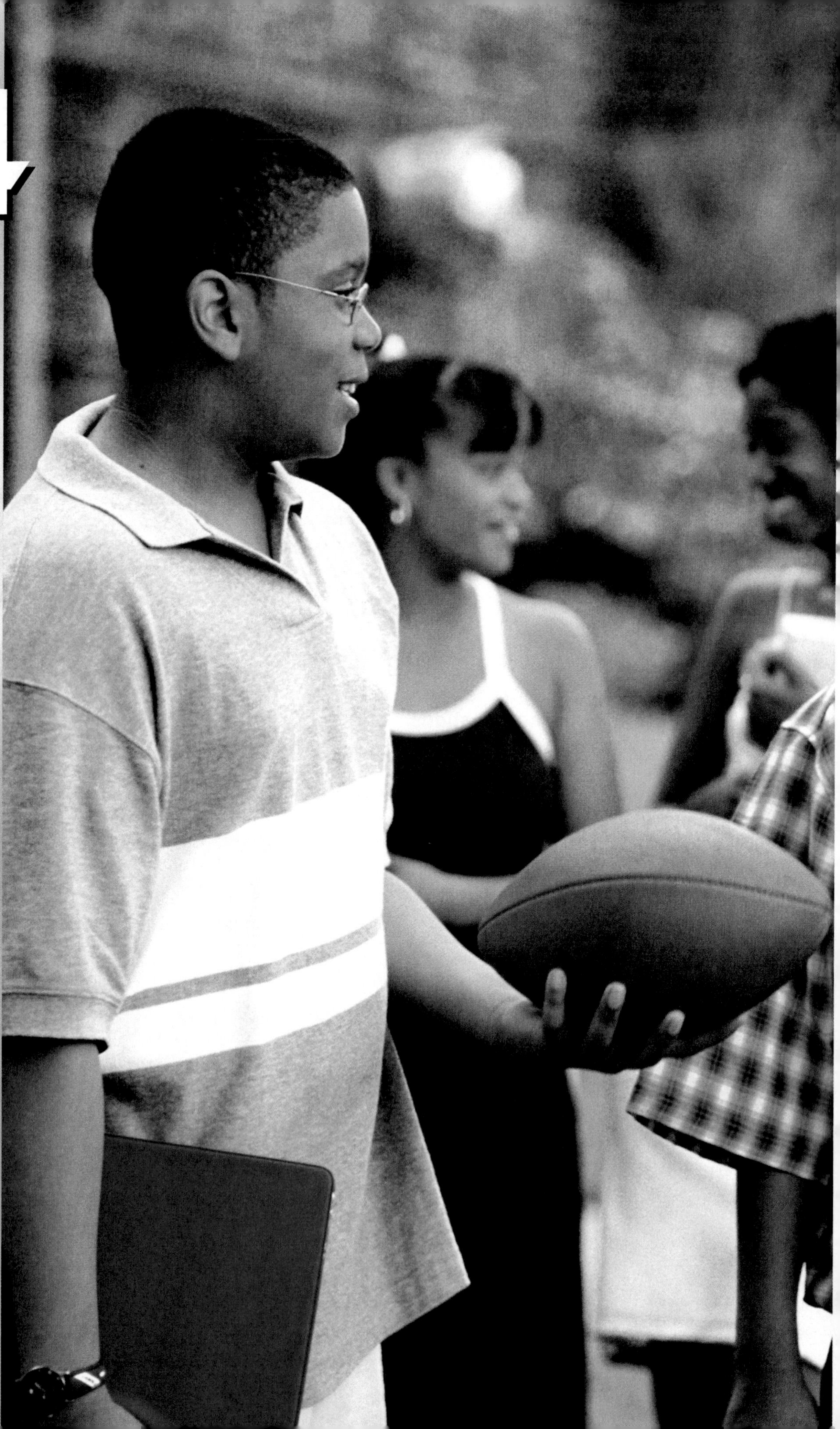

Making Safe and Drug-Free Decisions

HEALTH in Action

Whether you're planning a pick-up football game or planning your future, avoiding tobacco, alcohol, and other drugs will ensure that you'll be able to follow through on those plans. By following your doctor's orders with regard to prescriptions and being careful with over-the-counter medications, you can maintain the physical, mental/emotional, and social health you need to set and meet your goals.

How does staying drug free help you plan?

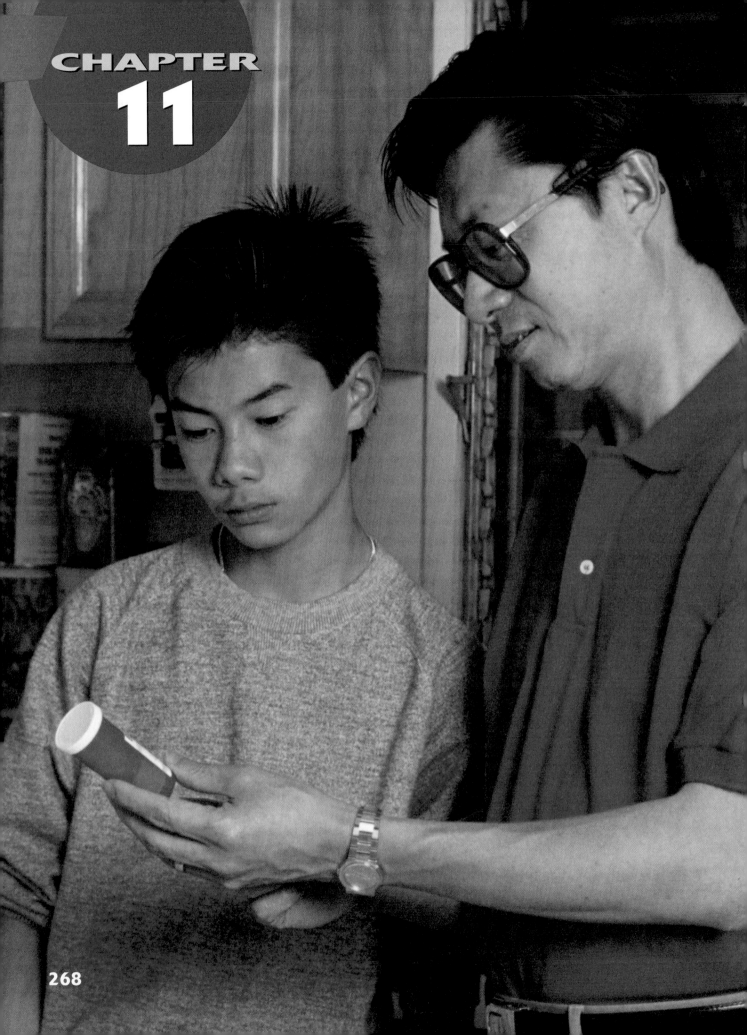

Medicines and Drugs

HEALTH *Online*

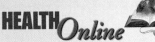

Before you begin the chapter, assess your knowledge, behavior, and attitudes concerning medicines and drugs. Take the Chapter 11 Health Inventory at health.glencoe.com.

FOLDABLES™
Study Organizer

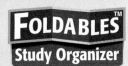

Before You Read

Make this Foldable to help you organize the information on medicines and drugs in Lesson 1. Begin with a sheet of notebook paper.

Step 1

Fold the sheet of notebook paper in half along the long axis.

Step 2

On the top layer, cut every third line. This will form 10 tabs.

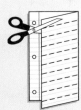

Step 3

Label the tabs as shown.

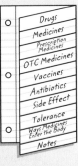

Drugs
Medicines
Prescription Medicines
OTC Medicines
Vaccines
Antibiotics
Side Effect
Tolerance
Ways Medicines Enter the Body
Notes

As You Read

Under the appropriate tab of your Foldable, write notes and define terms related to medicines and drugs.

269

Using Medicines Wisely

Medicines and Drugs

What do you think of when you hear the words *medicines* and *drugs?* Many people use the terms interchangeably. However, there is a difference. **Drugs** are *substances other than food that change the structure or function of the body or mind.* **Medicines** are *drugs that are used to treat or prevent diseases and other conditions.* All medicines are drugs, but not all drugs are medicines.

Medicine Safety

In the United States, the Food and Drug Administration (FDA) is responsible for ensuring that all medicines are safe and effective. The FDA approval process includes the following steps.

1. A potential new medicine is discovered.
2. Researchers conduct experiments to help decide how the new medicine might be used to treat an illness. Early testing is conducted on animals to determine if the medicine has any harmful effects.
3. The FDA reviews the preliminary research and test results. If approved, the new medicine is studied in humans.
4. If the FDA decides that the medicine is safe and effective for its intended use, the FDA approves it.
5. Once approved, the medicine can be made available for physicians to prescribe or for consumers to purchase.

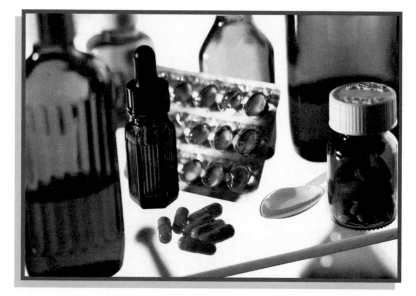

Medicines come in many different forms. *What medicine did you take the last time you had a cold?*

FIGURE 11.1

PRESCRIPTION MEDICINE LABEL

Medicine labels provide important information. *How many times can this prescription be refilled?*

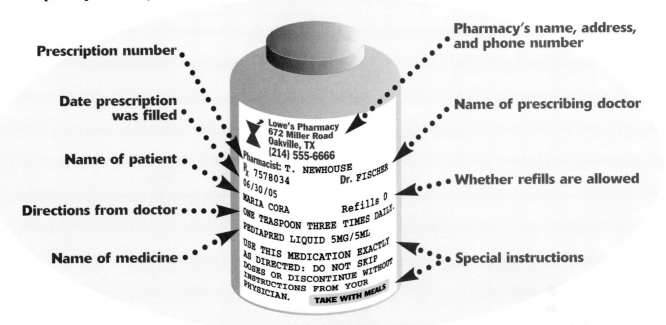

Prescription number

Date prescription was filled

Name of patient

Directions from doctor

Name of medicine

Pharmacy's name, address, and phone number

Name of prescribing doctor

Whether refills are allowed

Special instructions

Lowe's Pharmacy
672 Miller Road
Oakville, TX
(214) 555-6666
Pharmacist: T. NEWHOUSE
℞ 7578034   Dr. FISCHER
06/30/05
MARIA CORA   Refills 0
ONE TEASPOON THREE TIMES DAILY.
PEDIAPRED LIQUID 5MG/5ML
USE THIS MEDICATION EXACTLY
AS DIRECTED: DO NOT SKIP
DOSES OR DISCONTINUE WITHOUT
INSTRUCTIONS FROM YOUR
PHYSICIAN.
TAKE WITH MEALS

Prescription Medicines

Some medicines are very strong and potentially harmful, so doctors must write special orders for them. These **prescription medicines** are *medicines that can be sold only with a written order from a physician.* **Figure 11.1** shows the information that must appear on all prescription medicine labels. Before you take a prescription medicine, read the label carefully and make sure that you are interpreting the instructions correctly.

Over-the-Counter (OTC) Medicines

Have you ever used cough syrup or nasal spray when you had a cold? These **over-the-counter (OTC) medicines** are *medicines that are safe enough to be taken without a written order from a physician.* OTC medicines may cause harm if not used as directed.

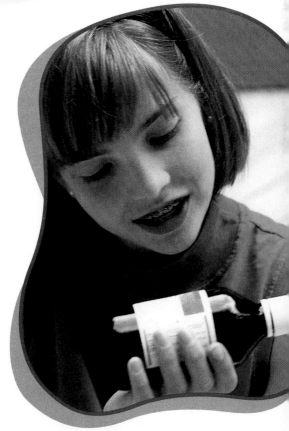

Potential side effects are listed on medicine container labels. *Why should you read the label carefully before taking any medication?*

OTC medicines are available at pharmacies, supermarkets, and other stores that sell medicine. Always check with an adult before using any OTC or other medicine. Be sure to read and interpret correctly the information provided on an OTC medicine container label.

Types of Medicines

There are different types of medicines, and each type affects the body in specific ways. The most common uses for medicines are preventing disease, fighting infection, and relieving pain.

Medicines to Prevent Diseases

Some medicines, known as vaccines, prevent a disease from developing. A **vaccine** is *a preparation of dead or weakened germs that causes the immune system to produce antibodies.* Antibodies are proteins that attack and kill or disable specific germs that cause disease.

Medicines are used to prevent disease, fight infection, and relieve pain. *Why are some medicines available only by prescription?*

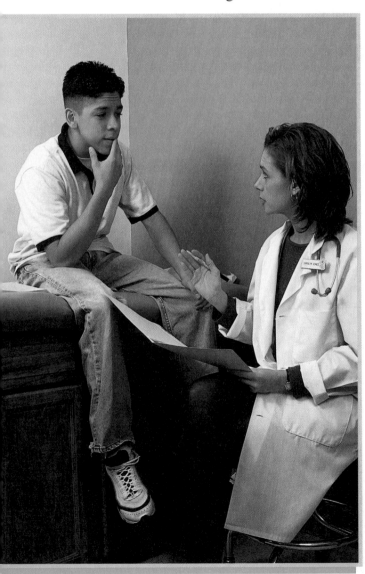

Common vaccines given today include those that protect you from communicable diseases (those that can spread), such as diphtheria, whooping cough, measles, mumps, rubella, chicken pox, pneumonia, and hepatitis A and B. These vaccines provide long-lasting protection. Others, such as the flu vaccine, must be administered periodically.

Medicines to Fight Infection

Many communicable diseases cannot be prevented with vaccines. Instead, certain medicines are used to restore health. **Antibiotics** (an·ti·by·AH·tiks) are *medicines that reduce or kill harmful bacteria in the body.* Each type of antibiotic fights only certain types of bacteria. For example, penicillin (pen·uh·SI·luhn) is highly effective in killing the bacteria that cause strep throat and pneumonia.

Medicines to Relieve Pain

Many people take medicines to relieve pain. When the body feels pain, such as that from a headache or toothache, pain messages travel along the nerves and spinal cord to the brain. Pain medicines block these pain messages or lessen their effect.

Aspirin is one of the most commonly used medicines for treating minor pain. Aspirin substitutes such as acetaminophen and ibuprofen are also popular. These pain medicines are widely available and do not require a doctor's prescription. Occasionally a serious illness or a chronic disease will cause serious pain. In this case a doctor may prescribe stronger medicines such as codeine or morphine.

Other Medicines

A variety of medicines is available to treat people with certain health problems or conditions. Specific medicines are used by people with chronic conditions including heart and blood pressure problems, diabetes, and allergies.

Medicine in the Body

The effects of a medicine in the body depend on the type and amount of medicine taken. The way a medicine is taken will also affect how quickly it begins to work in the body. **Figure 11.2** illustrates the four main ways in which medicines can enter the body.

Medicines will affect each person differently. That is why it is important for medicine to be used only as prescribed or directed, and only by the person who needs the medicine.

✓ **Reading Check**

Investigate word parts. Analyze the words *injection* and *ingestion*. What does the prefix *in-* mean? What is the root of each word? What do the roots mean?

FIGURE 11.2

HOW MEDICINES ENTER THE BODY

The way medicines enter the body depends on their form.

Ingestion
Medicine in the form of pills, tablets, capsules, and liquids is ingested, or swallowed. The medicine moves through the stomach and small intestine and is absorbed into the bloodstream and circulated throughout the body. You can take cold medicines this way.

Injection
Medicine given through injection goes directly into the blood. Some injections are given in a vein, others under the skin or into a muscle. If you have diabetes, you may need to give yourself daily injections.

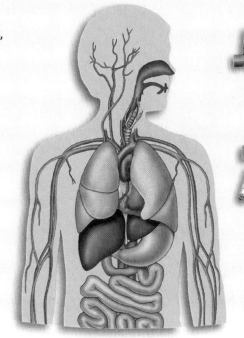

Inhalation
When a liquid medicine is changed into a fine mist, it can be inhaled, or breathed in. If you have asthma, you may need an inhaler.

Absorption
Creams and ointments are applied to the skin or scalp and absorbed by the body. Skin patches are applied to the skin and release medicine over time. If you have a cold, you may rub ointment on your chest to clear your lungs.

Side Effects

In addition to the intended effect, some medicines also cause one or more side effects. A **side effect** is *any effect of a medicine other than the one intended.* Common side effects include headaches, an upset stomach, and drowsiness. If you have side effects with a medicine, talk to your doctor, nurse, or pharmacist. Some side effects, such as kidney failure, can be serious. Others may stop after the body adjusts to the medicine. Some people may be allergic to certain medicines and may need to see a doctor about a replacement.

Tolerance

When used over a long period of time, certain medicines can cause a person to develop a tolerance. **Tolerance** is *a condition in which a person's body becomes used to the effect of a medicine and needs greater and greater amounts of it in order for it to be effective.* In some cases, the medicine ceases to be effective and the doctor must prescribe a different type of medicine.

HEALTH SKILLS ACTIVITY

PRACTICING HEALTHFUL BEHAVIORS

Medicine Safety in the Home

How much do you know about medicine safety? Follow these tips to store, use, and dispose of medicines safely.

- Store medicines in a cool, dry place.
- Keep medicines safely sealed in childproof containers, and keep them out of the reach of children.

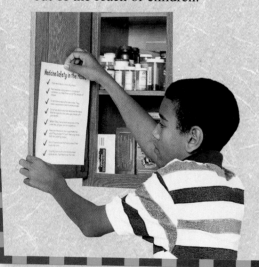

- Do not share prescription medicines. They could cause serious harm to someone else.
- Do not use nonprescription medicines for more than ten days at a time unless you check with your doctor.
- Before taking two or more medicines at the same time, get your doctor's approval.
- Know what medicines are in your home and what they are used to treat. Keep only those that are currently needed.
- Do not use medicines that have passed their expiration date.
- To safely dispose of outdated or unused liquids or pills, flush them down the toilet.

WITH A GROUP
Create a "Medicine Safety Checklist" suitable for home use. Review the completed checklist with your family. Post the list in an appropriate place in your home.

Overuse of Medicines

If medicines are overused, they can lose their ability to fight diseases. For example, the use of penicillin became widespread in the 1940s. Within just a few years, new strains of bacteria had developed. The new bacteria were resistant to penicillin. The more often antibiotics are used, the more likely it is that bacteria will develop a resistance to them. This is another reason why medicines must always be used wisely and in moderation.

Mixing Medicines

When two or more medicines are taken at the same time, the combined effects may be dangerous. The following reactions are possible.

- Each medicine may have a stronger effect than it would have if taken alone.
- The medicines may combine to produce unexpected effects.
- One medicine may cancel out the expected effects of the other.

Because mixing medicines can produce unpredictable and sometimes even deadly results, it is vital to let your physician know about all medicines you are presently taking.

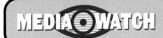

MEDIA WATCH

MEDICINE ADS

Find several magazine ads for medicines. Look for common information in the ads. *Use critical-thinking skills to interpret the ads' messages. What conclusions can you draw about the legal requirements for medicine ads?*

Lesson 1 Review

Using complete sentences, answer the following questions on a sheet of paper.

Reviewing Terms and Facts

1. **List** Give three reasons people take medicines.
2. **Relate** How can medicines be used to prevent or treat communicable disease?
3. **Vocabulary** What is a *side effect?*
4. **Give Examples** List the three possible reactions that can result from taking more than one medicine at the same time.

Thinking Critically

5. **Contrast** Explain the difference between prescription medicines and over-the-counter medicines.

6. **Draw Conclusions** Every day, Rose took the same dose of the same medicine to manage her arthritis pain. After taking the medicine for two years, it no longer helped. What might have happened?

Applying Health Skills

7. **Advocacy** Write a letter to the editor of your school or community newspaper promoting the responsible use of antibiotics. Be sure to mention the problems caused by overuse of antibiotics.

Narcotics, Stimulants, and Depressants

Quick Write

Why do you think some drugs are illegal?

LEARN ABOUT...

- the difference between drug misuse and drug abuse.
- how narcotics affect the body.
- the effects of stimulants on the body.
- what depressants do to the body.

VOCABULARY

- narcotics
- addiction
- stimulants
- amphetamine
- methamphetamine
- depressants

Drug Misuse and Abuse

People can harm themselves by not using drugs properly. Drug misusers take legal drugs in an improper way. Drug abusers take substances that are against the law or are not supposed to be taken into the human body. They may also use legal drugs for nonmedical purposes. The following are forms of drug misuse and drug abuse.

Drug Misuse

- Using a drug without following the directions
- Combining medicines without a physician's advice
- Taking more of a drug than the doctor ordered
- Using a drug prescribed for someone else
- Giving your prescription to someone else
- Using a drug for longer than a physician advises

Drug Abuse

- Using any illegal drug
- Using a medicine when you do not need it
- Taking a substance that was not meant to enter the body
- Using a drug for purposes other than medical treatment
- Faking health problems to obtain or renew a prescription

Teens who use illegal drugs face serious consequences. Getting dropped from the school team is an immediate one. *What might be some longer-term consequences of drug abuse?*

Narcotics

Narcotics are *specific drugs that are obtainable only by prescription and are used to relieve pain.* Doctors may prescribe the narcotics morphine or codeine, for example, to treat extreme pain. Narcotics can be safe when taken under a physician's supervision, but they are so addictive that their sale and use is controlled by law. People with an **addiction** have a *physical or psychological need for a drug.* Another name for drug addiction is chemical dependency. Pharmacists must keep records of all sales of narcotics.

Heroin

Heroin (HEHR·uh·win) is an illegal narcotic that is made from morphine. It is the most commonly abused narcotic and is highly addictive. When users do not get the heroin they need, they feel severe pain. Heroin depresses the central nervous system and can lead to coma or death.

Because drug users often share dirty needles, users of heroin and other injected drugs are at increased risk of contracting HIV. According to recent CDC data, half of all new infections with HIV occur among abusers of injected drugs.

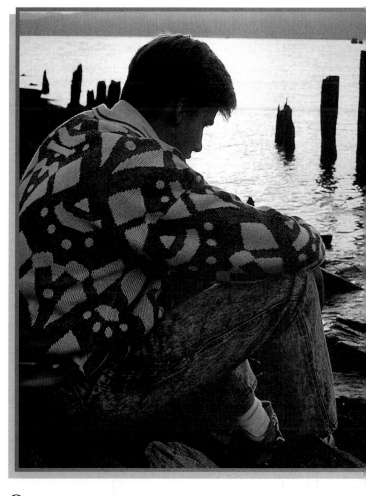

Once a person develops an addiction, he or she constantly needs to find and use more of the drug. *Explain how chemical dependency and addiction to a drug might impact a person's life.*

Stimulants

Stimulants (STIM·yuh·luhnts) are *substances that speed up the body's functions.* Stimulants make the heart beat faster, increase breathing rate, and raise blood pressure. The effects of some stimulants are so mild that people may not even realize they are using a drug. Caffeine is a stimulant found in cocoa, coffee, tea, and many soft drinks.

Some stimulants may be prescribed to help people with certain physical or emotional problems. Stimulant abuse can be very dangerous, however. High doses of strong stimulants may cause blurred vision, dizziness, anxiety, loss of coordination, or collapse. Stimulants such as amphetamine, cocaine, and crack can also become habit-forming, and users can become addicted quickly. **Figure 11.3** on the next page describes some common stimulants and their harmful effects.

Reading Check

Three paragraphs on this page present a definition of a term, followed by characteristics of it. For each term, write the definition followed by at least one of its characteristics.

FIGURE 11.3

EFFECTS OF STIMULANTS

Stimulants come in a variety of forms, all of which can be very dangerous if abused.

Substance	Other Names	Forms	Methods of Use	Harmful Effects
Amphetamine	Crystal, ice, glass, crank, speed, uppers	Pills, powder, chunky crystals	Swallowed, snorted up the nose, smoked, injected	Uneven heartbeat, rise in blood pressure, physical collapse, stroke, heart attack, and death
Methamphetamine	Meth, crank, speed, ice	Pills, powder, crystals	Swallowed, snorted up the nose, smoked, injected	Memory loss, damage to heart and nervous system, seizures, death
Cocaine	Coke, dust, snow, flake, blow, girl	White powder	Snorted up the nose, injected	Damage to nose lining, liver, and heart; heart attack, seizures, stroke, and death
Crack	Crack, freebase rocks, rock	Off-white rocks or chunks	Smoked, injected	Damage to lungs if smoked, seizures, heart attack, and death

Developing Good Character

Citizenship

Find out about organizations in your school or community that promote a drug-free environment and sponsor drug-free events. Identify the organizations' goals and how students can participate. *Which organization would you be interested in joining? Why?*

Amphetamine

Amphetamine (am·FE·tuh·meen) is *a drug that stimulates the central nervous system.* Doctors may prescribe amphetamines to treat hyperactive children. Amphetamines are highly addictive, however. People who use or abuse amphetamines can develop a dependence on the drugs, needing larger and larger doses to get the desired effect.

Methamphetamine

Methamphetamine is *a stimulant similar to amphetamine.* Doctors prescribe methamphetamines to treat diseases such as narcolepsy, Parkinson's disease, and obesity. In recent years, methamphetamines have appeared in "club drugs"—dangerous, illegal substances available at dance clubs and all-night parties.

Cocaine

Cocaine is a powerful, illegal stimulant. Its abuse has become a major health problem in the United States. Among teens, cocaine abuse increased during the 1990s. However, studies showed a significant drop in teen cocaine use in 1999.

Some people use cocaine because it makes them feel happy and energetic. This feeling is short-lived, however, and is followed by depression as the drug wears off. Users often take more cocaine to relieve the depression, thus forming an addiction to it. Cocaine is a dangerous drug, and an overdose can be fatal.

Crack

Crack is a concentrated form of cocaine that can be smoked. Smoking crack has the same effects on the body as using cocaine, only stronger. Crack reaches the brain within seconds and produces an intense high. The high lasts only for a few minutes, though, and is followed by an equally intense low. The user then craves more of the drug to relieve the intense bad feelings. For these reasons, crack is one of the most addictive and dangerous drugs used in the United States today.

Depressants

Depressants are *substances that slow down the body's functions and reactions.* These substances, which are often called sedatives, lower blood pressure and slow down heart rate and breathing. Doctors sometimes prescribe depressants for relief of anxiety, tension, nervousness, and sleeplessness. There are three main kinds of depressants.

- **Tranquilizers** (TRAN·kwuh·ly·zerz), when used as prescribed by a physician, can help reduce anxiety and relax muscles.
- **Barbiturates** (bar·BI·chuh·ruhts) are powerful sedatives that produce a feeling of relaxation.
- **Hypnotics** (hip·NAH·tiks) are very strong drugs that bring on sleep.

A teen with strong values will choose healthful behaviors and avoid the use of drugs.

MEDIA WATCH

ANTIDRUG ADS

Collect newspaper and magazine ads that advocate against drug abuse. As a group, develop evaluation criteria for the ads and then evaluate them. *Is the media message suitable for the intended audience? How effective is the message?*

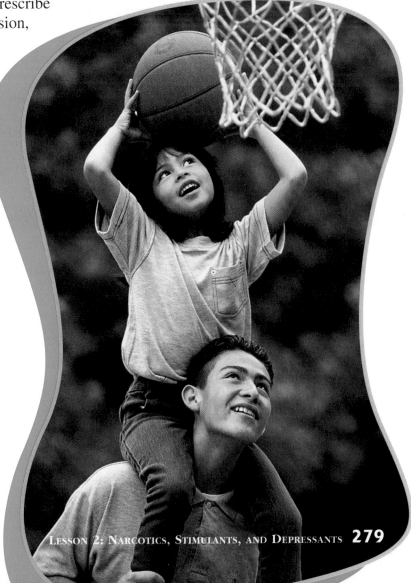

Depressants should be taken only under a doctor's supervision. If taken over an extended period, they can cause dependence and a need for more and more of the drug.

Depressants produce effects similar to those produced by alcohol, which itself is a form of depressant. When depressants are combined with alcohol, the effects increase and the risks multiply. The results can be deadly. **Figure 11.4** provides more information about depressants and their effects on the body.

FIGURE 11.4

EFFECTS OF DEPRESSANTS

If abused, depressants can have many harmful effects on the body, up to and including death.

Substance	Other Names	Forms	Methods of Use	Harmful Effects
Tranquilizer	Valium, Librium, Xanax	Pills or capsules	Swallowed	Anxiety; reduced coordination and attention span. Withdrawal can cause tremors and lead to coma or death.
Barbiturate	Downers, barbs, yellow jackets, reds	Pills or capsules	Swallowed	Causes mood changes and excessive sleep. Can lead to coma.
Hypnotic	Quaaludes, Ludes, Sopor	Pills or capsules	Swallowed	Impaired coordination and judgment. High doses may cause internal bleeding, coma, or death.

Lesson 2 Review

Using complete sentences, answer the following questions on a sheet of paper.

Reviewing Terms and Facts

1. **Recall** What are three forms of drug misuse and three forms of drug abuse?
2. **Vocabulary** What is *addiction?* Use it in a complete sentence.
3. **Explain** How is heroin use related to the spread of HIV?
4. **Give Examples** List two types of stimulants, and describe their effects on the body.

Thinking Critically

5. **Contrast** How do the effects of stimulants differ from those of depressants?
6. **Apply** How would you refuse an offer to try crack?

Applying Health Skills

7. **Stress Management** Some people use illegal drugs because they think that drugs will help them manage stress. Write down five examples of healthful ways to manage stress without using drugs.

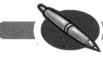

Lesson 3

Marijuana and Other Illegal Drugs

Street Drugs

Companies that manufacture drugs sold as medicines must follow strict government regulations. These laws ensure that the medicines are pure and consistent in strength, known risks, and side effects.

Any drug that is made or sold outside of these laws is considered a street drug. Street drugs include illegally made, packaged, or sold legal drugs, such as amphetamines. Street drugs also include illegal drugs, such as heroin and marijuana. There are no laws to protect the purity and content of street drugs. People who use them don't know how much of the drug they are taking. As a result, they risk being poisoned and dying of accidental overdose.

Marijuana

Marijuana is the most commonly used street drug. The main active chemical in marijuana is THC (tetrahydrocannabinol), which affects the brain. Hashish, which is made from the same plant, is much stronger than marijuana because it contains more THC. **Figure 11.5** lists the effects of marijuana.

Quick Write
List at least two dangers of illegal drug use.

LEARN ABOUT...

the risks of using marijuana.
the dangers of hallucinogens.
how inhalants affect the body.
what club drugs and steroids do to the body.

VOCABULARY

hallucinogens
psychological dependence
inhalant
physical dependence

FIGURE 11.5

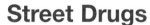

EFFECTS OF MARIJUANA

Common street names for marijuana include pot, grass, weed, joint, and herb.

- Reduces memory, reaction time, and coordination, and impairs judgment
- Reduces initiative and ambition
- Increases heart rate and appetite and lowers body temperature

- Damages heart and lungs
- Interferes with normal body development in teens by changing hormone levels
- May cause addiction

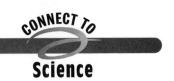
Although some users mix marijuana with food and eat it, most choose to smoke it. As a result, marijuana smokers experience many of the same lung problems as tobacco smokers. These include persistent coughing, bronchitis symptoms, and frequent colds. Marijuana smoke contains three to five times the amount of tar and other cancer-causing substances found in tobacco smoke.

Hallucinogens

Hallucinogens (huh·LOO·suhn·uh·jenz) are *drugs that distort moods, thoughts, and senses.* Physical effects of hallucinogens include increased heart rate and blood pressure and lack of muscle coordination. Hallucinogens can also cause decreased sensitivity to pain, which can result in serious self-injury.

Taking a hallucinogen may cause the user to hallucinate, or see things that are not really there. Sometimes it can trigger uncontrolled, violent behavior. Hallucinogens also cause people to lose their sense of direction, distance, and time. These effects often lead to misjudgments that result in serious injuries and death.

PCP

Phencyclidine (fen·SI·kluh·deen), commonly called PCP, is a powerful and dangerous hallucinogen whose effects last a long time. PCP produces strange, destructive behavior, which causes many users to end up in hospital emergency rooms. PCP use often leads to **psychological dependence**, *an addiction in which the mind sends the body a message that it needs more of a drug.* **Figure 11.6** provides more information about PCP.

LSD

LSD is an abbreviation for lysergic (luh·SER·jik) acid diethylamide (dy·e·thuh·LA·myd), another powerful hallucinogen. Use of LSD often produces rapid mood swings and hallucinations. Some users have terrifying thoughts and feelings, such as fear that they are dying or going crazy. Many LSD users experience flashbacks. During a flashback, the effects of LSD may recur days, months, or years after the drug was taken. **Figure 11.6** gives additional information about LSD.

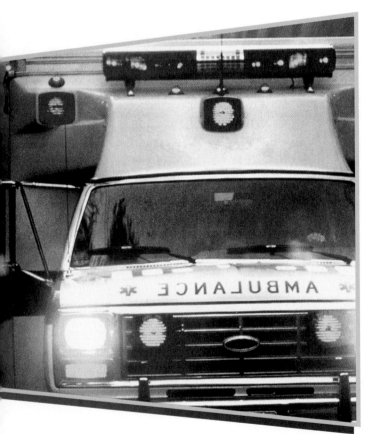

People cannot always predict how their bodies might react to drugs. *How might drug use and the abuse of medicines lead to health problems in later life and other adverse consequences?*

FIGURE 11.6

EFFECTS OF HALLUCINOGENS

Hallucinogens can have many harmful effects on the body, up to and including death.

Substance	Other Names	Forms	Methods of Use	Harmful Effects
PCP	Angel dust, supergrass, killer weed, rocket fuel	White powder; liquid	Applied to leafy materials and smoked	Loss of coordination; increase in heart rate, blood pressure, and body temperature; convulsions, heart and lung failure, or broken blood vessels; bizarre or violent behavior; temporary psychosis; false feeling of having super powers.
LSD	Acid, blotter, microdot, white lightning	Tablets; squares soaked on paper	Eaten or licked	Increase in blood pressure, heart rate, and body temperature; chills, nausea, tremors, and sleeplessness; unpredictable behavior; flashbacks; false feeling of having super powers.

Inhalants

Any substance whose fumes are sniffed and inhaled to produce mind-altering sensations is considered an **inhalant**. Household products that come in aerosol spray cans are commonly used as inhalants. These products include spray paint, cleaning fluid, lighter fluid, hair spray, nail polish remover, and other harmful substances. These substances are not meant to be taken into the body and can be very dangerous.

When inhalants are breathed in, their harmful fumes go directly to the brain. These fumes commonly cause headache, nausea, vomiting, and loss of coordination. A single use can result in sudden death. Inhalant use can lead to **physical dependence**, *a type of addiction in which the body itself feels a direct need for a drug.* Long-term inhalant use can damage the liver, kidneys, and brain.

Club Drugs

Club drugs are drugs that are associated with nightclubs, concerts, and all-night dance parties called raves. Other terms for drugs associated with these activities are designer drugs and look-alike drugs. The term *designer drug* often refers to a synthetic version of a natural drug. Look-alike drugs are drugs that resemble and are passed off as another drug.

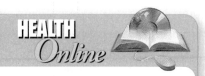

HEALTH
Online

Topic: Dangers of drugs

For a link to more information on how drugs harm the body, go to health.glencoe.com.

Activity: Using the information provided at this link, list some harmful effects of three different drugs.

Some club drugs are colorless, tasteless, and odorless. These properties have led to the dangerous practice of drug slipping. Drug slipping occurs when a drug is placed in someone's food or beverage without that person's knowledge. Because drug slipping has been used to aid in committing rape, some club drugs are sometimes called date rape drugs. Commonly used club drugs include:

- **Ecstasy**, also called E, X, and XTC, is a stimulant and a hallucinogen in pill form. Users may experience confusion, depression, anxiety, nausea, faintness, chills, or sweating. Ecstasy can cause permanent brain damage.
- **GHB** is a depressant, and its street names include Liquid Ecstasy, Liquid X, Georgia Home Boy, and Grievous Bodily Harm. Available in powder and liquid form, GHB is especially dangerous when taken with alcohol or other drugs. The combination may result in sleep, coma, and death.
- **Rohypnol** is a powerful sedative. It's also called the date rape drug, Roofies, and R-2. Rohypnol is typically a small white tablet which, when dissolved in liquid, has no taste or odor. The drug's short-term effect is a sleepy, relaxed feeling that lasts two to eight hours. The user might also black out.
- **Ketamine** is an anesthetic used for medical purposes, mostly in treating animals. Misused as a club drug, ketamine is often sold as a white powder to be snorted, like cocaine, or injected. The drug is also smoked with marijuana or tobacco products. Ketamine causes hallucinations and dreamlike states. Its use may result in death through respiratory failure.

HEALTH SKILLS ACTIVITY

REFUSAL SKILLS

Refusing Drugs

Megan is thrilled when Nina invites her to "join the crowd" at her home after school. It isn't often that a junior like Nina would even talk to Megan, a freshman.

When Megan gets to Nina's house, she sees that there are five or six girls from school but no adults. Nina brings out a little bag of tablets and tells the girls that the pills are a cool new club drug. She says that all the kids are taking the pills at dance parties. She starts to pass the pills around. Megan sits frozen in her chair.

WHAT WOULD YOU DO?

Apply refusal skills to Megan's situation. With a classmate, role-play a scenario in which Megan used S.T.O.P. to refuse Nina's offer of a club drug.

SAY NO IN A FIRM VOICE.
TELL WHY NOT.
OFFER OTHER IDEAS.
PROMPTLY LEAVE.

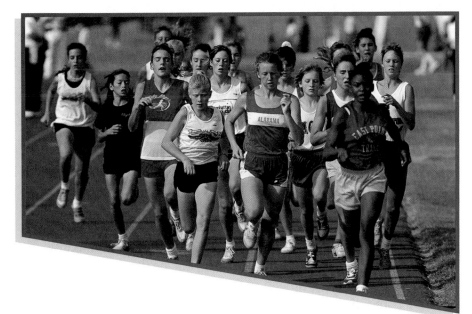

The best way to improve your athletic performance is to practice. *How could drug use ruin, rather than help, an athlete's career?*

Anabolic Steroids

Some athletes mistakenly believe that drugs will improve their performance. They may start using steroids, which bulk up muscle at an abnormally fast rate. In time, the harmful effects of steroids become obvious. They include acne, mood swings, nausea, liver damage, brain cancers, and shorter adult height when taken by children and teens. Athletes are routinely tested for illegal drugs. If they have been using steroids or other drugs, they face stiff penalties and may lose their right to compete.

Lesson 3 Review

Using complete sentences, answer the following questions on a sheet of paper.

Reviewing Terms and Facts

1. **Vocabulary** Define the terms *hallucinogen* and *inhalant*. Explain the relationship between the two terms.
2. **List** Name two hallucinogens known by their initials.
3. **Compare** What is the difference between *psychological dependence* and *physical dependence?*
4. **Explain** Why are club drugs especially dangerous?

Thinking Critically

5. **Apply** Explain the impact of chemical dependency and addiction to illegal drugs and other substances.
6. **Analyze** Why are teens more likely than adults to abuse inhalants?

Applying Health Skills

7. **Accessing Information** Use reliable resources to research marijuana's harmful effects on body systems. Report your findings to the class.

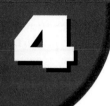
Staying Drug Free

Avoiding Drugs

You have the responsibility to be the healthiest person you can be. The best way to meet that responsibility is to make wise choices that have a positive effect on your health. One of the most important decisions you can make is to be drug free. **Figure 11.7** shows some of the many advantages of avoiding drugs. What can you add to the list?

FIGURE 11.7

Reasons to Be Drug Free

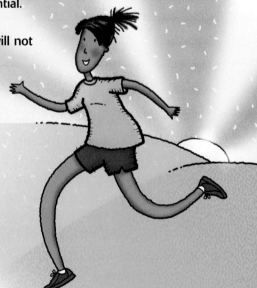

- You will not be breaking the law.
- You will have better concentration and memory.
- You will make wiser decisions.
- You will be able to focus on improving your talents and enjoying your interests.
- You will have more natural energy.
- You can reach your full growth potential.
- You can be as healthy as possible.
- You will look better because drugs will not ruin your appearance.
- You will have better control of your feelings and actions.
- You will not regret foolish actions caused by drug-impaired judgment.
- You will not waste money on drugs.
- You will have better relationships with family members.
- You will respect yourself for taking care of your body and mind.
- You will be able to succeed in education.
- Your mental and emotional development will be on time, not delayed.

Kicking the Habit

Kicking the drug habit once it has been established is much harder than resisting the pressure to start. The first step is for the drug user to recognize that a problem exists. The next step is to start the recovery process.

If the person has become physically or psychologically addicted to a drug, then the recovery process involves withdrawal. **Withdrawal** includes *the physical and psychological symptoms that occur when someone stops using an addictive substance.* Withdrawal symptoms vary depending on the drug used, but may include vomiting, headaches, chills, and hallucinations.

Withdrawal is often a painful process, and medications are usually given to ease the withdrawal symptoms. In addition to ridding one's body of the addictive substance, the recovering drug user must change his or her thinking and the habits that led to the drug use. Although withdrawing from drugs is difficult, the benefits of becoming drug free are well worth the effort.

Reading Check

Build vocabulary. Search for key terms in blue print throughout the chapter. Create flashcards for each term.

Getting Help

Drug users need help to recover from their addiction. Most communities offer support groups and treatment programs for drug addiction. A support group is a group of people who share a common problem and work together to help one another cope and recover. Common support groups for drug addiction include Narcotics Anonymous and Cocaine Anonymous. Nar-Anon provides help for those who have been affected by someone else's drug use.

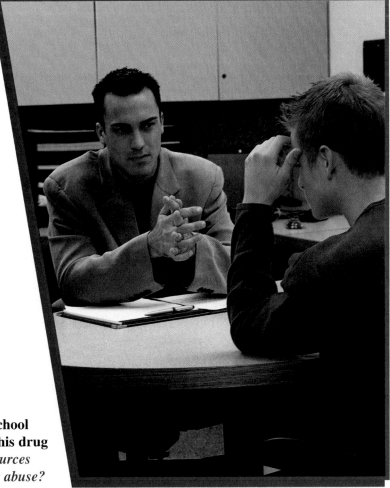

This teen is talking to a school counselor to get help for his drug problem. *What other resources offer support against drug abuse?*

A good drug treatment program has trained experts who provide education and support, and who can help the user through the withdrawal period. Withdrawal often requires **detoxification** (dee·tahk·si·fi·KAY·shuhn), *the physical process of freeing the body of an addictive substance.* "Detox" also involves helping the user overcome psychological dependence on the substance and regain health. A variety of treatment centers are available to help people recover from drug abuse.

- **Detox units** are usually part of a hospital or other treatment center. Addicts remain under a doctor's care while going through detoxification.
- **Inpatient treatment centers** are places where people stay for a month or more to fully concentrate on recovery.
- **Outpatient treatment centers** are places where people get treatment for a few hours each day. Then they return to their homes and regular surroundings.

Hands-On Health

DRUG-FREE CAMPAIGN

Kicking a drug habit is much harder than resisting the pressure to start using drugs. You can help spread this important message to young people. Work with a small group of classmates to create an advertising campaign that promotes staying drug free. Design your campaign to reach younger students.

WHAT YOU WILL NEED
- art supplies and paper
- computer access, if possible

WHAT YOU WILL DO
1. Decide what media you will include in your campaign. For example, you might create a poster or a Web page for the school Web site.
2. Choose an advertising technique to use. You might create an informational, persuasive, or sensational ad.
3. Brainstorm ideas for an effective ad. Then divide the work so that each group member has a task to complete.

4. Post your ads in the classroom, in the school newspaper, or on the school Web site, as appropriate.

IN CONCLUSION
1. As a class, evaluate the effectiveness of each group's ad campaign. How well was the message conveyed?
2. What are some other ways to encourage younger students to stay drug free?

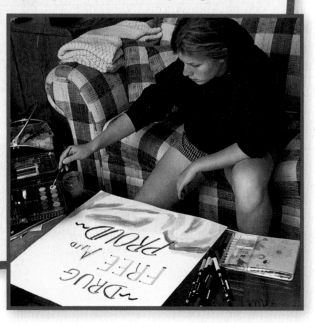

Living Drug Free

There are many healthy alternatives to drug use. Here are some strategies for counteracting risk factors:

If you feel lonely, depressed, or bored:

- Learn a new sport, hobby, or join a club.
- Start a regular physical activity routine.
- Volunteer to help people in your community.
- Identify and participate in positive alternative activities, such as drug-free events. Encourage your peers to attend as well.

If you need help solving personal problems:

- Talk to an adult you trust.
- Contact a hot line or support group.

If you are tense and anxious:

- Learn to relax by taking deep breaths.
- Get enough rest and physical activity.
- Use time management skills to avoid overscheduling your time.

If peers pressure you to use drugs:

- Recognize this as a negative social influence.
- Avoid situations in which this pressure may occur.
- Respond by using refusal skills.
- Obtain help from a trusted adult if necessary.

Choosing to stay drug free gives teens the opportunity to enjoy life. *How do you show your commitment to staying drug free?*

Lesson 4 Review

Using complete sentences, answer the following questions on a sheet of paper.

Reviewing Terms and Facts

1. **Identify** List five reasons to be drug free that are most important to you.
2. **Vocabulary** Define the term *withdrawal.*
3. **Recall** In your own words, describe what *detoxification* does.
4. **List** Name the three types of drug treatment programs.

Thinking Critically

5. **Hypothesize** Why do you think more and more teens are deciding to stay drug free?
6. **Explain** Why is it important to follow the rules prohibiting the possession of drugs?

Applying Health Skills

7. **Communication Skills** Identify ways that a teen could use effective communication skills to obtain help in resisting pressure to use drugs. Share your ideas with the class.

Marijuana Myths

Despite what some people may think, marijuana is a dangerous drug. Here's the truth behind a few common myths.

Marijuana by the Numbers

Match the numbers at the bottom with the correct description.

1. **The number of cigarettes a person has to smoke to do the kind of damage to his or her lungs that smoking one joint does.**

2. **The approximate percentage of teens who have used marijuana at least once in the past year.**

3. **The number of times more potent today's marijuana is than it was a few decades ago. (Newer, stronger types of marijuana are being grown, so it's more harmful to your body and brain than ever before.)**

A. 30   B. 20   C. 5

Answers: 1. C.; 2. A.; 3. B.

MYTH "Marijuana is not addictive—users can stop whenever they want."

FACT Marijuana *is* an addictive drug. Some people claim that they only use marijuana when they're stressed or depressed. Martha Gagné, director of the American Council for Drug Education, says that even occasional use can lead to a bad situation: "Suddenly, when people want to escape their problems, or even to feel good about themselves, they need to use marijuana." That's called a psychological addiction. Worse, marijuana might also be physically addictive. After a marijuana user hasn't smoked it in a while, he or she may experience such withdrawal symptoms as sweating, jitteriness, and nausea. One recent study has shown that marijuana has the same addictive effect on the brain as heroin.

MYTH "Marijuana is natural—it can't harm the body."

FACT Wrong! In males, heavy marijuana smoking can delay the onset of puberty, decrease sperm count, and make sperm abnormal. In girls, marijuana use can disturb menstrual cycles and decrease fertility. It may also raise levels of the hormone testosterone, which can increase the growth of facial and body hair and cause acne. Also, when people smoke marijuana, their responses are slower and they can't think as clearly, which can lead to serious, or even fatal, accidents.

MYTH "Smoking marijuana is safer than using other drugs."

FACT There's no way to tell if the marijuana is laced with another drug, such as cocaine, crack, or heroin. So a marijuana smoker might sample another dangerous drug without knowing it and become physically addicted to it.

MYTH "Getting caught with marijuana is no big deal."

FACT Marijuana is illegal. If someone gets caught using the drug, he or she can go to jail. Depending on the state where they live, marijuana users risk landing themselves sentences ranging from probation to something more severe—like time at a residential drug-treatment center or a juvenile detention center. ◢

TIME TO THINK...

About Marijuana's Harmful Effects

Review the information presented in this article and in the sidebar. Then, create several bumper stickers that feature antimarijuana slogans. Each slogan should focus on a different harmful effect of the drug. Slogans should be brief, as well as catchy and thought provoking.

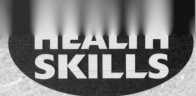

SAYING NO TO DRUGS

Model

Advocating healthful behaviors to another person is one way to make a difference. Read about how a teen named Steve uses the advocacy skill to express his concern for his younger brother J.R.

STEVE: J.R., I'd like to talk to you about something.

J.R.: Sure, what's up?

STEVE: It's about your new friend Lucas. I know he's your friend, but I'm kind of worried about you hanging out with him.

J.R.: What, just because he smokes a little grass?

STEVE: You sound like you think that's no big deal. Let me tell you something: that stuff really messes you up. I know a guy who started using it and it was like he stopped caring about everything. His grades got really bad and finally he just stopped going to school.

J.R.: What happened to him?

STEVE: His parents found out and put him in a rehab program. You see, I don't want that kind of thing to happen to you.

STEVE: Don't worry. I won't do anything that stupid. Maybe I should talk to Lucas—he probably doesn't know how dangerous it is.

Practice

Read the scenario below about a teen named Marnie who wants to advocate avoiding drugs to her friends. What are some of the ways Marnie could take a stand on this issue? What approach do you think would be most effective? Write a dialogue in which Marnie shares her views with her friends. Show how she uses advocacy skills to take a clear position and be convincing.

> *Marnie is having lunch with some friends. A few of the other girls start talking about a party they went to where some people were using drugs. They are talking about it as if they think it's normal. Marnie is worried about her friends. She wants to make sure they understand about the dangers of using drugs.*

Apply/Assess

Work with a group to create an illustrated brochure that will convince other teens to remain drug free. Use three or four blank sheets of unlined paper. On them, provide information about how drug use can harm physical, mental/emotional, and social health. Your brochure should also include information about the many benefits of a drug-free lifestyle. Use design features such as color, highlighting, and bulleted lists to make your main points stand out. Illustrate your brochure with your own drawings or with photographs cut out of magazines and newspapers. Finally, make an attractive cover for your brochure and give it a catchy, health-promoting title.

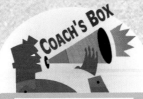

COACH'S BOX

Advocacy

Using the skill of advocacy means you
- take a clear stand on an issue.
- persuade others to make healthy choices.
- are convincing.

Self-√Check

- Did our brochure take a clear stand against drugs?
- Did we give reasons for avoiding drugs?
- Would our message persuade others to stay drug free?

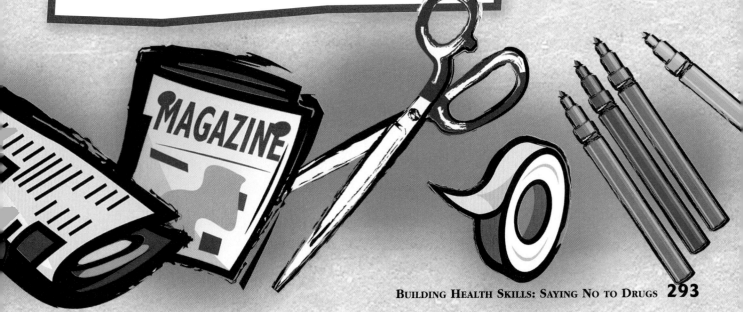

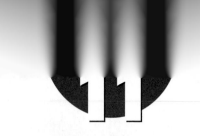

After You Read

Use your completed Foldable to review the information on medicines and drugs.

FOLDABLES
Study Organizer

Reviewing Vocabulary and Concepts

On a sheet of paper, write the numbers 1–6. After each number, write the term from the list that best completes each sentence.

- medicines
- over-the-counter (OTC) medicine
- prescription medicine
- drugs
- tolerance
- vaccines

Lesson 1

1. _____ change the structure or function of the body or mind.
2. _____ cause the immune system to produce antibodies.
3. A type of medicine that requires a physician's written order is _____.
4. To treat or prevent diseases, you might take _____.
5. _____ occurs when a person's body becomes used to the effects of a substance.
6. Medicine that is safe enough to be taken without a written order from a physician is _____.

Lesson 2

On a sheet of paper, write the numbers 7–10. Write *True* or *False* for each statement below. If the statement is false, change the underlined word or phrase to make it true.

7. Substances that speed up body functions are called <u>depressants</u>.
8. <u>Stimulants</u> are substances that slow down the body's functions and reactions.
9. Physicians may prescribe <u>narcotics</u> such as morphine to treat extreme pain.
10. <u>Hypnotics</u> are very strong drugs that bring on sleep.

On a sheet of paper, write the numbers 11–15. After each number, write the letter of the answer that best completes each statement.

Lesson 3

11. PCP and LSD are examples of
    a. narcotics.
    b. hallucinogens.
    c. inhalants.
    d. stimulants.
12. An addiction in which the body feels a direct need for a drug is
    a. physical addiction.
    b. abusive addiction.
    c. psychological addiction.
    d. dependent addiction.
13. Which is associated with club drugs?
    a. bulking up muscles
    b. inhaling harmful fumes
    c. increased acne
    d. drug slipping

Lesson 4

14. Someone who stops using an addictive substance may experience symptoms such as
    a. hallucinations.
    b. vomiting.
    c. chills.
    d. all of the above.
15. The physical process of freeing the body of an addictive substance is called
    a. withdrawal.
    b. quitting.
    c. kicking the habit.
    d. detoxification.

Thinking Critically

Using complete sentences, answer the following questions on a sheet of paper.

16. **Suggest** Give three examples to show how reading the label of an OTC medicine and interpreting the instructions correctly can help you use it safely.

17. **Evaluate** Why would it be dangerous to ride in a car with a driver who has been smoking marijuana?

18. **Apply** How could a teen use positive peer pressure to help counteract the negative effects of living in an environment where drug abuse exists?

Career Corner

Medical Record Technician If you like managing information, consider a career as a medical record technician. These professionals maintain patients' records in hospitals, clinics, and doctor's offices. They track health information to ensure that patients receive the right treatments and medications.

A medical record technician has an associate's degree in information management. Find out more about this and other health careers by clicking on Career Corner at health.glencoe.com.

Standardized Test Practice

Math

Read the paragraph below and then answer the questions.

Over-the-counter medicines have an expiration date printed on them. These dates tell you the last date that you can assume that the medicine is safe to use. Prescription medicines have a date printed on the label. This is the date that the prescription was filled. According to the instructions of how much to take and for how long, the medication will be fresh for the length of time of its use.

1. Gina had a bacterial infection and was given 30 antibiotic tablets to take. She is to take one pill three times a day. The date on the prescription bottle is April 23, 2005. What is the last date she should use the medication?

   (A) April 30, 2005
   (B) May 2, 2005
   (C) May 23, 2005
   (D) May 30, 2005

2. Marcus bought some cough syrup dated January 14, 2005. He is to take two teaspoons twice a day and expects to take the medicine for a week. What is the last day he should use this cough syrup?

   (A) January 7, 2005
   (B) January 14, 2005
   (C) January 21, 2005
   (D) January 28, 2005

3. Kai bought some prescription eye drops for his allergies on August 12. They had an expiration date on the label of November 28 of the same year. There are enough drops in the bottle to last for 100 days. Identify the date that Kai should use to determine when he should stop using the drops.

 TH05_C3.glencoe.com/quiz

CHAPTER 12

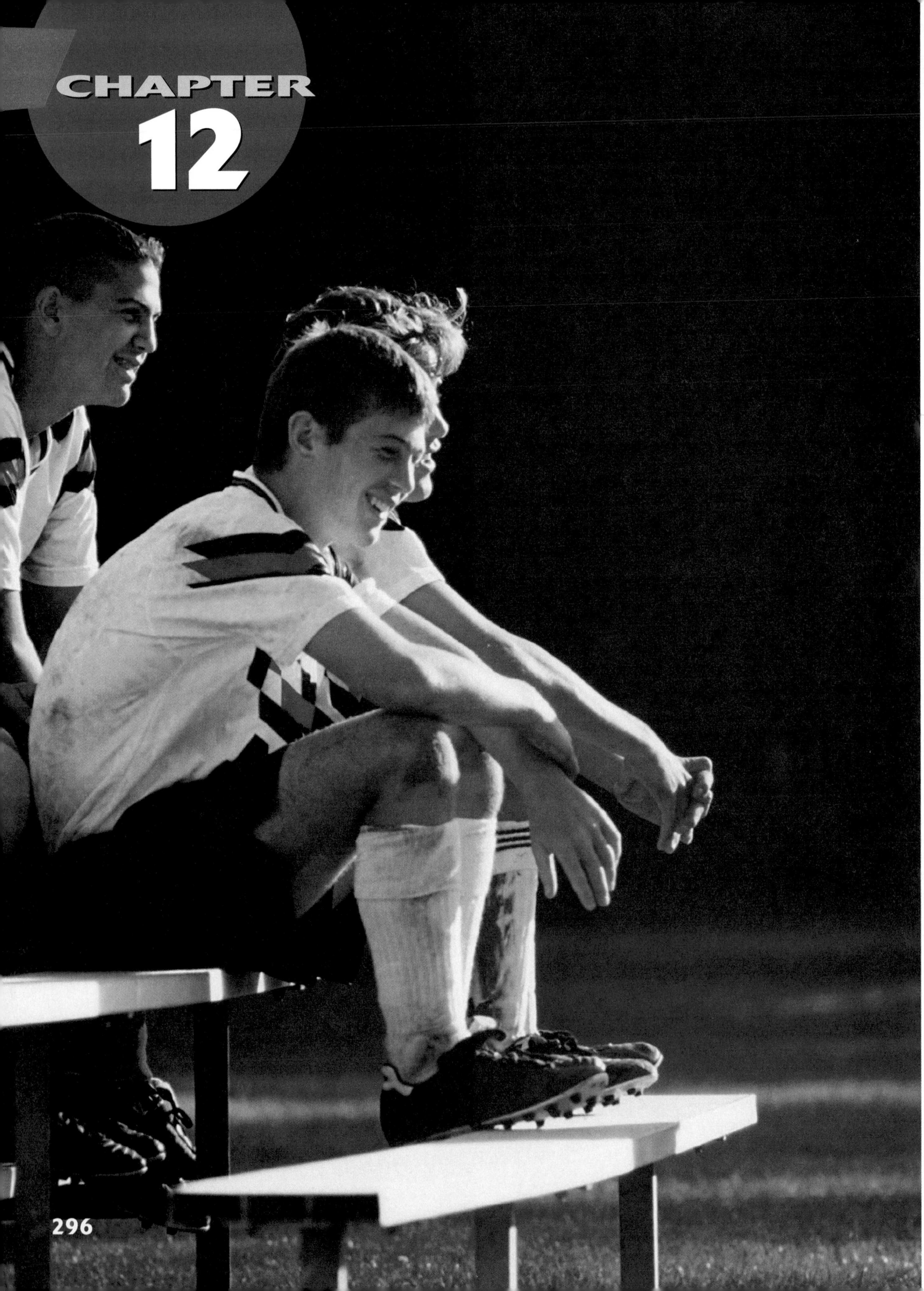

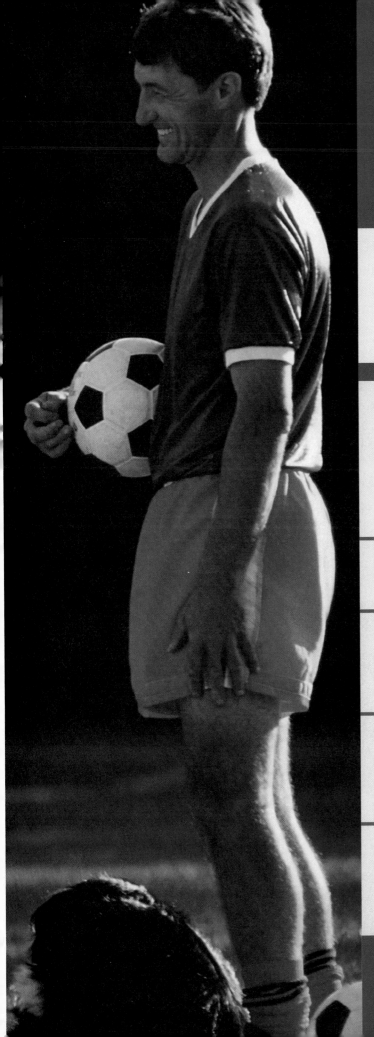

Tobacco

HEALTH *Online*

Do you know the truth about how tobacco damages lifelong health? To find out, take the Health Inventory for Chapter 12 at health.glencoe.com.

FOLDABLES™
Study Organizer

Before You Read

Make this Foldable to record what you learn in Lesson 1 about tobacco's harmful effects. Begin with a plain sheet of 8½" × 11" paper.

Step 1

Fold a sheet of paper in half along the short axis.

Step 2

Open and fold the bottom edge up to form a pocket. Glue the edges.

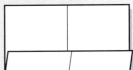

Step 3

Label the front of the booklet as shown. Label the pockets "Tobacco Products" and "Harmful Effects." Place an index card or quarter sheet of notebook paper into each pocket.

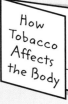

How Tobacco Affects the Body

As You Read

On index cards or quarter sheets of notebook paper, take notes on the different types of tobacco products and how they harm the body. Store these cards in the appropriate pocket of your Foldable.

How Tobacco Affects the Body

Quick Write

Tobacco use is hard to hide. List telltale signs that help you identify a person who smokes or chews tobacco.

LEARN ABOUT...

- the different forms in which tobacco is sold and consumed.
- the harmful substances in all forms of tobacco.
- the damage tobacco does to body systems.
- the negative effects that tobacco may have on appearance.

VOCABULARY

- nicotine
- addictive
- tar
- cilia
- carbon monoxide

What Is Tobacco?

Tobacco is a plant that grows best in warm, humid climates. The leaves of a tobacco plant are dried, aged for two or three years, mixed with chemicals, and then used to make various products for smoking or chewing.

Tobacco contains a powerful drug that changes the brain's chemistry. This change makes the tobacco user want more and more tobacco. Tobacco use is harmful to people's health and is a major cause of early and preventable death. Nonetheless, many people use some form of tobacco on a regular basis.

Different Tobacco Products

Tobacco products come in many different forms, including cigarettes, cigars, and smokeless tobacco. Regardless of the form, all tobacco products are harmful. That's why there are laws to control the advertising and sale of tobacco products.

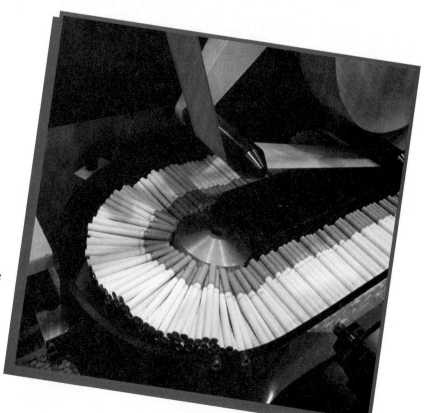

Despite the fact that tobacco use is harmful, tobacco companies continue to produce billions of tobacco products every year. *What creates the demand for tobacco products?*

Cigarettes

Cigarettes are the most common form of tobacco. In the United States, millions of people smoke cigarettes. Cigarettes put smokers at risk for emphysema and other lung and heart diseases, cancer, infertility, and stroke. Each year more than 430,000 people in the U.S. die from diseases caused by cigarette smoking.

Cigars and Pipes

Cigars contain the same dangerous substances as cigarettes but in much larger quantities. One large cigar can contain as much tobacco as a pack of cigarettes. Cigar smokers are four to ten times more likely to contract cancer of the mouth, larynx, and esophagus than nonsmokers, and they have a greater risk of dying from heart disease.

Some people smoke pipes, using loose tobacco. Pipe smokers usually inhale less than cigarette smokers, but they still increase their risk of cancer. Cancers of the lip, mouth, and throat are common among pipe smokers.

Smokeless Tobacco

Smokeless tobacco is tobacco that is chewed or sniffed. Common names for it are spit, chew, and snuff. Many people believe that smokeless tobacco is safer than other tobacco products because the user doesn't inhale tobacco smoke. This is not true. Users of smokeless tobacco still absorb poisonous substances through the mouth or nose. Smokeless tobacco has been linked to cancers of the mouth, esophagus, larynx, stomach, and pancreas. Chewing tobacco also stains the teeth and causes tooth loss and gum disease. Moreover, tobacco chewers need to spit out tobacco juice from time to time—a habit that many people find offensive.

Specialty Cigarettes

The use of bidis and cloves has increased in the United States. Bidis are flavored, unfiltered cigarettes from India. Clove cigarettes, which are made in Indonesia, contain tobacco and ground cloves. Bidis and cloves are often sold in health food stores, which may give people the impression that they are safe to smoke. These specialty cigarettes can, however, be even more dangerous than regular cigarettes. Some bidis contain pure tobacco with seven times as much nicotine and twice as much tar as regular cigarettes.

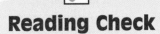

Reading Check

Synonyms are words that have similar meanings. Identify synonyms for the following words: *smokeless tobacco, cigarette.*

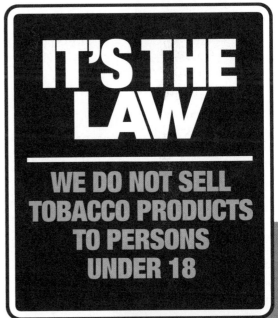

IT'S THE LAW

WE DO NOT SELL TOBACCO PRODUCTS TO PERSONS UNDER 18

State governments have strict laws to keep tobacco out of the hands of anyone under 18. *Why do states specifically regulate teen smoking?*

What Is in Tobacco?

Tobacco and tobacco smoke contain approximately 4,000 chemicals. Over 200 of them are known to be dangerous to humans, especially nicotine, tar, and carbon monoxide.

Nicotine is *an addictive drug found in tobacco leaves and in all tobacco products.* An **addictive** drug is one that is *capable of causing a user to develop intense cravings for it.* When smoked or chewed, nicotine takes less than 7 seconds to reach the brain, where it creates a feeling of stimulation. About 30 minutes later, when the chemicals have left the brain, the user begins to feel discomfort. The desire to recapture the feeling and avoid the feeling of discomfort causes the user to crave more tobacco. The user is chemically dependent on the nicotine in tobacco.

Tar is *a dark, thick, sticky liquid that forms when tobacco burns.* When smokers inhale, tar gets into their lungs. It leaves a residue that destroys **cilia**, the *tiny, hairlike structures that protect the lungs.* Over time, it also destroys the air sacs in the lungs. The presence of tar can make breathing difficult. It is known to cause emphysema, lung cancer, and other lung diseases.

Carbon monoxide is *a colorless, odorless, poisonous gas that is produced when tobacco burns.* The carbon monoxide in smoke passes through the lungs into the bloodstream. There it reduces the amount of oxygen the blood cells can carry. A reduced oxygen supply weakens muscles and blood vessels, which, in turn, may lead to heart attacks and stroke.

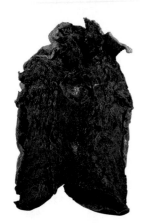

To understand the damage that smoking can do, compare the healthy lung (top) with the diseased lung (bottom).

HEALTH SKILLS ACTIVITY

REFUSAL SKILLS

Choose to Refuse Tobacco

Elena, an eighth grader, attends a school that includes grades seven through twelve. One day Phoebe, a popular junior, stops to talk to her on the way home from school. Elena feels flattered by the older girl's attention. Her good mood turns to alarm, however, when Phoebe offers her a bidi.

Elena's health class has just finished a unit on tobacco, and she knows that bidis are harmful. She decides to use the S.T.O.P. refusal skills to deal with the situation.

WHAT WOULD YOU DO?

Apply the S.T.O.P. refusal skills to Elena's situation. With a classmate, role-play a conversation between Elena and Phoebe. Reverse roles and do the role-play again. Were you comfortable using the S.T.O.P. refusal skills? Why or why not?

SAY NO IN A FIRM VOICE.
TELL WHY NOT.
OFFER OTHER IDEAS.
PROMPTLY LEAVE.

How Tobacco Affects the User's Body

The chemicals in tobacco and tobacco smoke cause damage to most of the body's systems. Tobacco use is particularly damaging to teens because their bodies are still growing and developing. Some of the effects of tobacco use are evident almost immediately. Others become apparent over time. **Figure 12.1** shows both the short-term and the long-term harmful effects of tobacco use on body systems.

FIGURE 12.1

SHORT-TERM AND LONG-TERM EFFECTS OF TOBACCO USE

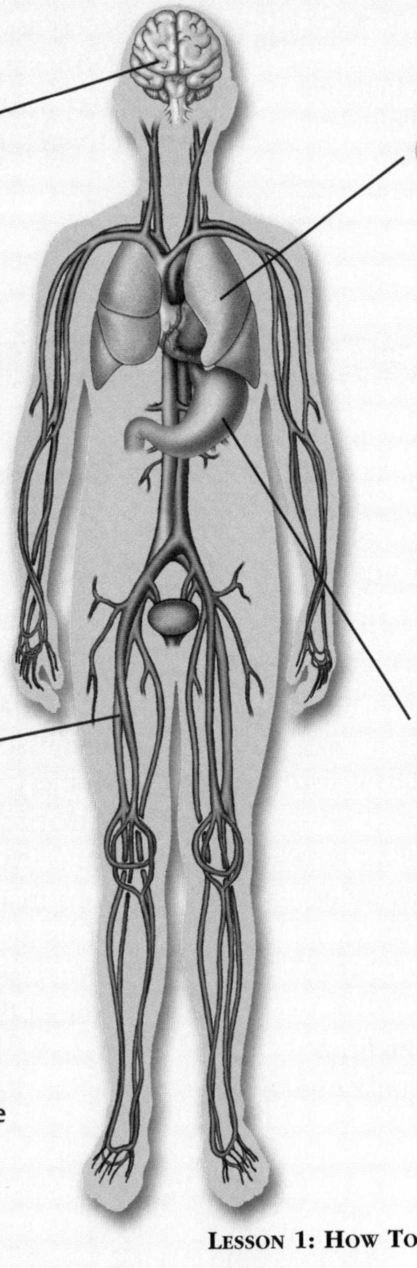

A Nervous System

Short-term effects: Changes take place in brain chemistry. Withdrawal symptoms (nervousness, shakes, headaches) may occur as soon as 30 minutes after the last cigarette. The heart rate and blood pressure increase.

Long-term effects: There is an increased risk of stroke due to decreased flow of oxygen to the brain.

C Respiratory System

Short-term effects: User has bad breath, shortness of breath, reduced energy, coughing, and more phlegm (mucus). Colds and flu are more frequent. Allergies and asthma problems increase. Bronchitis and other serious respiratory illnesses increase.

Long-term effects: Risk of lung cancer, emphysema, and other lung diseases increases.

B Circulatory System

Short-term effects: Heart rate is increased. Energy is reduced because less oxygen gets to body tissues.

Long-term effects: Blood vessels are weakened and narrowed. Cholesterol levels increase. Blood vessels are clogged due to fatty buildup. Oxygen flow to heart is reduced. Risk of heart disease and stroke is greater.

D Digestive System

Short-term effects: User has upset stomach, bad breath, stained teeth, dulled taste buds, and tooth decay.

Long-term effects: Risk of cancer of the mouth and throat, gum and tooth disease, stomach ulcers, and bladder cancer increases.

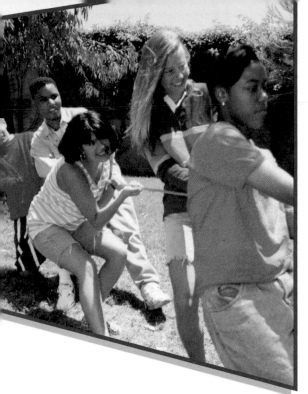

Tobacco and Appearance

Most of the damage caused by tobacco use occurs inside the body. However, tobacco use also harms a person's outer appearance. Every time a person uses a tobacco product, the smell of tobacco lingers on his or her hands, breath, hair, and clothing.

Over time, tobacco use can lead to stained teeth and fingers. Tobacco users often look older more quickly because their skin wrinkles. With shortness of breath and frequent coughing, smokers are generally less physically fit than nonsmokers. Smokeless tobacco users often develop cracked lips, inflamed gums, and sores in their mouths.

A tobacco user's appearance can affect his or her social relationships. Many people are offended by a tobacco user's smelly breath, hair, and clothing, and they don't want to get close to him or her.

The benefits of healthy habits that you develop in your teen years will last a lifetime. *How does staying tobacco free help you maintain a healthy appearance?*

Lesson 1 Review

Using complete sentences, answer the following questions on a sheet of paper.

Reviewing Terms and Facts

1. **Recall** Name five forms of tobacco.
2. **Explain** Why is smoking cigars or using smokeless tobacco just as harmful as smoking cigarettes?
3. **Vocabulary** Define the terms *nicotine* and *addictive*.
4. **Restate** Describe some long-term effects that tobacco has on the respiratory system and the digestive system.

Thinking Critically

5. **Hypothesize** Why do you think cigarettes are more commonly used than other forms of tobacco?

6. **Synthesize** Explain why tobacco use can negatively affect a person's social relationships.

Applying Health Skills

7. **Advocacy** Demonstrate ways to use health information to help others: Find a local chapter of the American Cancer Society, American Heart Association, American Dental Association, or American Lung Association on the Internet. Request information about the effects of smoking or using smokeless tobacco. Use this information to prepare a display for the school library or nurse's office on what tobacco does to the body.

Tobacco and Society

Who Buys Tobacco?

Tobacco is a big business in the United States. In one year, tobacco companies spend over $6.8 billion on marketing and advertising campaigns. That's more than $18.5 million every day! In spite of all this advertising, tobacco use among adults has declined over 40 percent since 1965. Today, the majority of adults—about 75 percent—don't use tobacco.

Tobacco companies want to attract new users to replace those who have either quit or died. In the eyes of the tobacco industry, children and teens represent the most profitable market. People who become addicted to nicotine as teens are likely to spend thousands of dollars on tobacco products in their lifetime. As a result of lawsuits settled in 1998, tobacco companies have agreed not to use cartoon characters and other advertising methods that might attract children and teens. Nevertheless, the industry continues to find ways to lure young smokers.

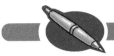

Quick Write

What can be done to reduce the number of people in your community who use tobacco?

LEARN ABOUT...

- why people become addicted to tobacco.
- how tobacco use harms other people.
- the costs to society of tobacco use.

VOCABULARY

- addiction
- physical dependence
- psychological dependence
- withdrawal
- secondhand smoke
- mainstream smoke
- sidestream smoke

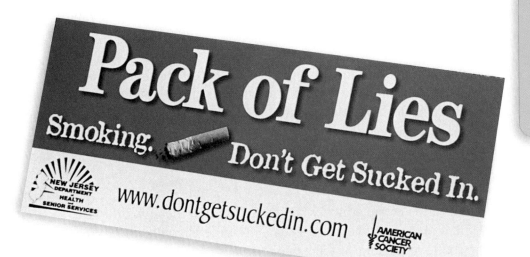

Antitobacco advertisements tell another side to the tobacco story. *Explain how billboards like this one can positively influence individual and community health.*

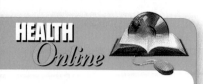

Topic: Tobacco

For a link to more information on tobacco use, go to health.glencoe.com.

Activity: Using the information provided at this link, prepare an oral report that includes statistics on tobacco use. Make sure you emphasize the importance of a tobacco-free lifestyle.

An Expensive Habit

Tobacco use is not only an unhealthy habit but also an expensive one. People who use tobacco frequently pay higher health insurance rates. They generally have more doctor and dental bills because of tobacco-related illnesses. There is also the cost of the tobacco product itself. A pack of cigarettes costs around $3.25. At that rate, smokers who smoke a pack a day will spend over $1,100 each year just on cigarettes.

Tobacco Addiction

Despite the high personal costs and health risks of tobacco use, a number of people continue to smoke or chew tobacco. They may want to stop but find it difficult or frustrating. This is because they have formed a chemical dependency on, or addiction to, the nicotine in tobacco. An **addiction** is *a physical or psychological need for a drug.* Addiction develops from regular use of a drug. Nicotine addiction can occur in a short amount of time. Nicotine causes two types of addiction.

- **Physical dependence** is *a type of addiction in which the body itself feels a direct need for a drug.* Nicotine affects body temperature, heart rate, digestion, and muscle tone. Once the nicotine level drops or the nicotine leaves the body's systems, the body craves more. Tobacco users don't feel normal unless their bodies are under the influence of nicotine.
- **Psychological dependence** is *an addiction in which the mind sends the body a message that it needs more of a drug.* Certain events, situations, and habits trigger a desire to use tobacco. Teens might think they need to smoke a cigarette to help them relax at a party or to help them be more alert before a test. Many smokers feel the need for a cigarette every time they talk on the telephone or finish a meal.

According to the Centers for Disease Control and Prevention, nicotine addiction is the most common form of drug addiction in the United States. Nicotine is more addictive than heroin or cocaine. Teens are more likely to develop a severe level of addiction than people who begin to use tobacco at a later age.

You Can Quit!

Two-thirds of the adults who smoke say that they would like to quit, and teen smokers are as eager to quit as adults are. In the year 2000, 70 percent of teen smokers said they regretted having started. Despite the difficulties associated with quitting, approximately 44 million American adults are now former smokers. **Figure 12.2** shows the number of former smokers in the United States population between 1970 and 1998.

Withdrawal

In order to quit, tobacco users have to go through **withdrawal**, *the physical and psychological symptoms that occur when someone stops using an addictive substance.* Physical symptoms of nicotine withdrawal include the craving to use nicotine, headaches, shakiness, fatigue, increased appetite, and nausea. Psychological symptoms include feeling irritable, nervous, anxious, and sad. People going through withdrawal may have trouble thinking during the day and sleeping during the night. The intensity of withdrawal symptoms and the length of time they last vary from person to person. An inability or reluctance to cope with withdrawal is often the main obstacle to quitting tobacco use.

FIGURE 12.2

LOOK WHO'S NOT SMOKING

The number of Americans who don't smoke, either because they never started or because they quit, has been rising steadily.

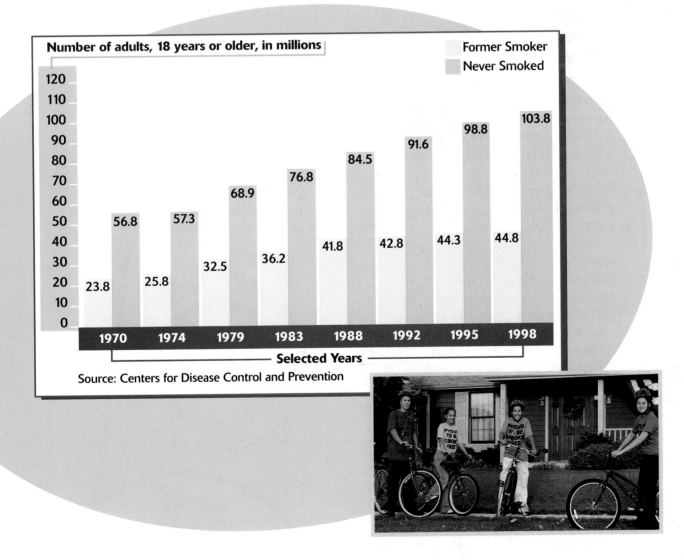

Number of adults, 18 years or older, in millions

Former Smoker
Never Smoked

	1970	1974	1979	1983	1988	1992	1995	1998
Former Smoker	23.8	25.8	32.5	36.2	41.8	42.8	44.3	44.8
Never Smoked	56.8	57.3	68.9	76.8	84.5	91.6	98.8	103.8

Selected Years

Source: Centers for Disease Control and Prevention

The Costs to Society

Individuals who use tobacco are not the only ones harmed by its effects. Smoke from cigarettes, cigars, and pipes also threatens the health of nonsmokers. In addition, the harm tobacco causes adds up to serious costs for families and society.

Secondhand Smoke

Secondhand smoke is *air that has been contaminated by tobacco smoke.* There are two kinds of secondhand smoke. **Mainstream smoke** is *smoke that a smoker inhales and then exhales.* **Sidestream smoke** is *smoke given off by the burning end of a cigarette, cigar, or pipe.* Sidestream smoke contains twice as much tar and nicotine as mainstream smoke.

Hands-On Health

TOBACCO FACTS PAMPHLETS

Antitobacco programs in schools have been very successful in reducing tobacco use among young people. In this activity you will use your health knowledge to help other teens stay away from tobacco.

WHAT YOU WILL NEED
- sheet of paper
- pen and colored markers

WHAT YOU WILL DO
1. Think of a group to whom you would like to deliver an antitobacco message. It should be a group you know well, such as your scout troop, your soccer teammates, or friends in your community.
2. Fold a sheet of paper into thirds to make a six-page pamphlet.
3. Put a catchy title for your pamphlet on the cover.
4. Use the other pages to list facts that may persuade the group to stay tobacco free.
5. Illustrate your pamphlet with antitobacco drawings, cartoons, or logos.
6. Photocopy your pamphlet so you have enough copies for everyone in the group.

IN CONCLUSION
Give your pamphlet to the members of the group. Ask them to share the pamphlet with other groups of teens.

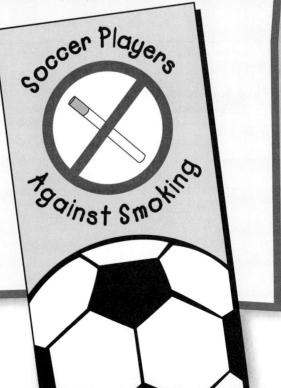

Nonsmokers can develop respiratory illnesses such as pneumonia and bronchitis as a result of secondhand smoke. Infants and young children who are constantly exposed to secondhand smoke have more colds, ear infections, allergies, and asthma than children who grow up in smoke-free homes. Secondhand smoke can also lead to lung disease, heart disease, and cancer in nonsmokers.

Public Health Costs

Tobacco-related illnesses increase the cost of medical care for everyone. Consumers must pay higher rates for health care insurance in order to cover these costs. Taxpayers must also pay the medical bills of patients who lack health insurance.

Costs to the Nation's Economy

People who miss work because of tobacco-related illnesses produce fewer goods and services. As a result, companies earn less money. Productive time is also lost when tobacco users leave their workstations to have a cigarette. Tobacco use costs the United States almost $100 billion each year in health care costs and lost productivity.

Pregnancy and Tobacco

Females who smoke during pregnancy increase their risk of having a low birth weight baby and a premature delivery. Nicotine and carbon monoxide keep needed nutrients and oxygen from the fetus. The incidence of Sudden Infant Death Syndrome (SIDS) is also higher in homes where parents smoke.

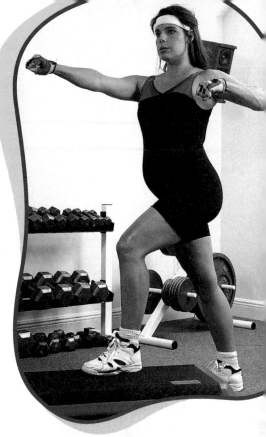

Because smoking can harm a fetus and a young baby, pregnant females should never smoke. *What other healthful behaviors can pregnant females practice?*

Lesson 2 Review

Using complete sentences, answer the following questions on a sheet of paper.

Reviewing Terms and Facts

1. **Vocabulary** Define the term *addiction.* Use it in an original sentence.
2. **Contrast** How do physical dependence and psychological dependence differ?
3. **Recall** What are three symptoms of nicotine withdrawal?
4. **Describe** Identify the two types of smoke that nonsmokers might inhale.

Thinking Critically

5. **Apply** Explain the impact of chemical dependency and addiction to tobacco.
6. **Summarize** Why are pregnant women advised not to smoke?

Applying Health Skills

7. **Advocacy** Make a poster showing the effects of secondhand smoke on non-smokers. Your poster should express a point of view about the rights of non-smokers. Be sure to include the facts to support your point of view. Display your poster in the classroom.

Choosing to Be Tobacco Free

Quick Write

Why do some teens begin using tobacco? List all the reasons you can think of.

LEARN ABOUT...

- reasons some teens start using tobacco.
- strategies for avoiding tobacco use.
- ways to quit using tobacco.

VOCABULARY

- cold turkey
- nicotine patch

Why Some Teens Start to Use Tobacco

The good news is that the majority of young teens—about 65 percent—don't smoke. In addition, smoking among high school students began to decline in 1998. The bad news is that each day, 4,800 teens smoke their first cigarette. Of this group, 2,000 will become regular smokers. One-third of these will eventually die of smoking-related illnesses.

Internal Influences

Teens may start using tobacco because of internal influences.

- **Stress.** Teens may think that tobacco will help them relax and cope with stress. They don't realize that the symptoms of withdrawal from nicotine, which occur as often as every 30 minutes, will add to their daily stresses.
- **Weight.** Some teens wrongly believe that using tobacco will help them maintain a healthy weight. In reality, its use reduces a person's capacity for aerobic exercise and sports.
- **Image.** Using cigarette lighters and blowing smoke makes some teens feel grown up. Teens who are really mature know that they don't want to give up lifelong health just to look "cool."

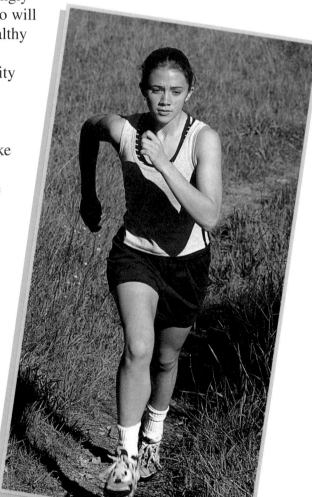

The best way to maintain a healthy weight is to stay active and eat a healthful diet. *Why doesn't tobacco fit into a healthy weight-management plan?*

- **Independence.** Tobacco use may seem to be a sign of independence. However, it's really just the opposite. Tobacco users become dependent on their unhealthy and costly habit.
- **Peer acceptance.** Teens may think they need to smoke in order to fit in with their peer group. However, most teens today don't want anything to do with tobacco users.

External Influences

External influences may also cause teens to start smoking.

- **Role models.** Some teens want to be like a friend, a celebrity, or some other role model who uses tobacco. They don't realize that their role models wish they could quit their tobacco habit.
- **Peers.** Peers, siblings, and friends are powerful influences. Many teens try their first cigarette with a friend who already smokes.
- **Media.** Movies and television shows often portray tobacco use in ways that appeal to teens. Tobacco companies pay millions of dollars to have their products featured in movies.
- **Advertising.** There is strong evidence that tobacco advertising influences teens. One study found that 86 percent of kids who smoke prefer the three most heavily advertised brands.
- **Family members and other adults.** Some teens see their parents and other adults using tobacco and think that it's all right for them to use it, too.

Reading Check

Analyze the internal and external influences listed here and write an *If . . . , then . . .* statement for each. For example: *If you use tobacco, then you may become dependent on it.*

HEALTH SKILLS ACTIVITY

ANALYZING INFLUENCES

Be Prepared

When you can recognize internal and external influences on your personal health behavior, you'll be ready to handle them. Here are some examples of people, events, and situations that might tempt teens to use tobacco.

- A stressful day at school.
- Constantly being exposed to ads for tobacco products on the Internet or in a convenience store.
- Curiosity about what it would feel like to smoke.

- Discovering that a highly respected person used tobacco.
- Seeing a tobacco ad that features young adults having fun.
- Hearing that smoking helps keep weight down.

ON YOUR OWN

Draw up your own list of internal and external influences that might pressure you to start using tobacco. Make a plan showing how you would deal with each one.

TRUTH IN ADVERTISING?

Think about the tobacco ads you've seen in stores or in magazines and newspapers. *Use your critical-thinking skills to analyze and interpret the media messages in these ads: How do the ads portray tobacco use? How do the messages compare with the facts about tobacco?*

How Not to Start

The best way to lead a tobacco-free life is never to start using tobacco products. About 90 percent of adult smokers began smoking before the age of 21, and half of them had become regular smokers by age 18. If you avoid using tobacco during middle school or high school, there's a good chance you'll never start.

Resisting peer pressure to use tobacco can be difficult. However, you can use several strategies to help you.

- **Choose friends who don't use tobacco.** If your friends don't use tobacco, you won't be pressured to use it yourself.
- **Avoid situations where tobacco may be used.** You may be invited to a party where you know your peers will be using tobacco. Give your reasons for not going and then enjoy an alternative activity with your tobacco-free friends instead.
- **Use refusal skills.** If tobacco users urge you to try tobacco, you can respond by saying no. If the pressure continues, however, you can explain your reasons for avoiding tobacco products. **Figure 12.3** shows some ways to refuse tobacco. Remember to be assertive. If your peers continue to pressure you, leave. If necessary, obtain help from a trusted adult.

FIGURE 12.3

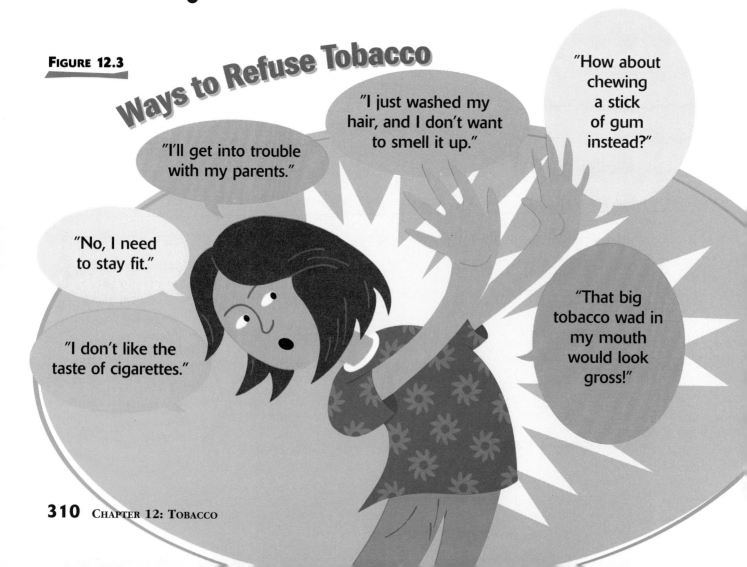

Ways to Refuse Tobacco

"No, I need to stay fit."

"I'll get into trouble with my parents."

"I just washed my hair, and I don't want to smell it up."

"How about chewing a stick of gum instead?"

"I don't like the taste of cigarettes."

"That big tobacco wad in my mouth would look gross!"

Strategies for Quitting

A variety of strategies are available to help someone break the tobacco habit. One way is to quit gradually by reducing the number of cigarettes smoked or the frequency of using chew over a period of time. Another way to quit is **cold turkey**, or *stopping all at once.* Cold turkey is thought to be more effective than trying to quit gradually.

Tobacco users, no matter what age, may need products such as a nicotine patch or nicotine gum to help them through withdrawal. The **nicotine patch** is *a medication that allows tobacco users to give up tobacco right away while gradually cutting down on nicotine.* The patch is available both by prescription and over the counter. Nicotine gum is available over the counter, and it works in a similar way as the patch.

Tobacco users who want to quit may seek help from local support groups and organized programs or from professional counselors. The American Lung Association, the American Heart Association, and the American Cancer Society, as well as hospitals and health groups, offer programs to help tobacco users quit. Identify and participate in any tobacco-free events that are taking place in your community.

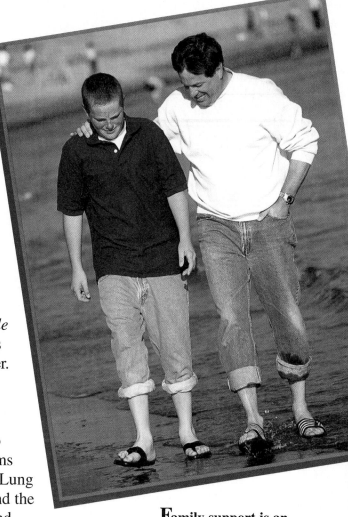

Family support is an important factor in quitting the use of tobacco successfully.

Lesson 3 Review

Using complete sentences, answer the following questions on a sheet of paper.

Reviewing Terms and Facts

1. **Restate** List internal and external influences that affect tobacco use.
2. **Recall** What are three strategies for resisting peer pressure to use tobacco?
3. **Vocabulary** What does it mean to quit *cold turkey?*
4. **Describe** What resources are available to help tobacco users quit?

Thinking Critically

5. **Explain** Why are efforts to prevent teens from using tobacco so important?

Applying Health Skills

6. **Accessing Information** Research and identify tobacco-free events that are taking place in your community. Choose one event to participate in and encourage your peers to get involved as well.

Smoke Signals

How much do you know about the dangers of smoking cigarettes? Take this quiz and find out.

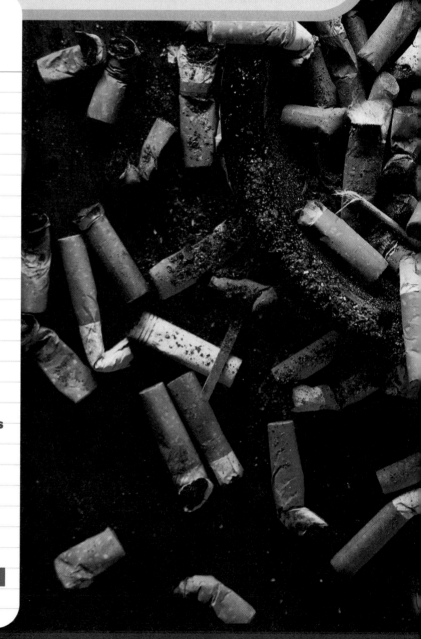

Quiz

1. How long does it take before smoking starts to affect your health?
   a. Within days
   b. Two weeks
   c. A year
   d. Three years

2. How many cigarettes do you have to smoke until you're likely to become addicted?
   a. One
   b. Three
   c. A pack
   d. Five packs

3. Smoking is as addictive as harder drugs, such as cocaine and heroin.
   a. True   b. False

4. If you've been smoking for less than a year, quitting is easy.
   a. True   b. False

5. How many fewer years can a long-term smoker be expected to live?
   a. 3   b. 5   c. 10   d. 12

Answers: 1.a. 2.b. 3.a. 4.b. 5.d.

Check out the explanations on the next page!

Explanations

1. **Damage to the lungs, heart, and circulation occurs within days after a person starts smoking,** says Jack Fincham, Ph.D., of the University of Kansas. That's because cigarette smoke contains a lethal list of toxins: cyanide, methanol (wood alcohol), ammonia, and poisonous gases like carbon monoxide. In addition, check out this scary statistic: The younger a person is when he or she starts smoking, the more likely lung growth will be stunted for life.

2. According to Fincham, nearly 50 percent of all previous nonsmokers who smoke more than two cigarettes go on to become regular smokers within a year. **What's more, of those new smokers, nearly 90 percent are under age 21.** (Most smokers start their habit between the ages of 10 and 18.)

3. As surprising as it may sound, **cigarettes are considered as addictive as drugs like cocaine and even heroin,** according to Saul Shiffman, Ph.D., of the Smoking Research Group at the University of Pittsburgh. That's because nicotine, which occurs naturally in tobacco, is very addictive. Also, cigarette smoking is associated with other drug use. According to a recent Surgeon General's report, teens who smoke are three times more likely to use alcohol, eight times more likely to use marijuana, and 22 times more likely to use cocaine than teens who don't smoke.

4. According to the Centers for Disease Control and Prevention (CDC), **teens often underestimate the addictiveness of nicotine.** Seventy-five percent of people who were daily smokers in high school but planned to quit were still smoking six years later. Also, even after quitting, former smokers have a permanent physical tolerance to nicotine. That means even one cigarette smoked years later could be enough to get a person hooked again.

5. **According to reports by the CDC, lifelong smokers who die from a smoking-related disease have probably lost about 12 years of their typical life span.** The upside: Fifteen years after smokers quit, their life expectancy reverts to nearly the same as that of lifelong nonsmokers. ∎

New Names, Same Danger

Are "herbal" cigarettes just as dangerous as regular cigarettes? You bet. Here are the facts:

BIDIS: These small, unfiltered cigarettes are imported from India. Aside from added flavorings, they're nothing more than tobacco leaves rolled in a cigar-like casing. They have three times the nicotine of regular cigarettes and, because they have no filter, a lot more of the tar that causes lung damage.

CLOVES: These are typically two-thirds tobacco and one-third ground cloves. When people inhale, an ingredient deadens sensation in the throat, allowing them to inhale more deeply and hold the smoke in for a longer period. This makes clove cigarettes especially harmful to the lungs.

TIME TO THINK...

About the Dangers of Smoking

Brainstorm with your classmates to create an original antismoking ad campaign. What new angle can you take? Use reliable online and print resources to research the subject and to find statistics and facts that will enhance your campaign. Use images from the Internet or from newspapers and magazines to increase the impact of your message. With your teacher's permission, create posters and flyers and distribute them throughout your school.

STEER CLEAR OF TOBACCO

Model

Jackson is an ambitious teen. One of his goals is to start his own business walking dogs in his neighborhood. This is a long-term goal that will require a lot of effort to achieve.

Jackson knows that using tobacco will make it much more difficult for him to achieve his goal. Chemicals in tobacco could harm his health, making it harder for him to find the energy he needs to walk the dogs. Using tobacco would also cost him a lot of money that he could be spending to promote his business. So Jackson has made avoiding tobacco one of the steps in his plan to achieve his long-term goal. He makes a conscious effort, not only to be tobacco free himself, but also to avoid secondhand smoke. He politely asks others not to smoke near him when they are in a car or any other enclosed space. With his worries about tobacco out of the way, Jackson can move on to the other steps in his plan to get his business started.

Practice

Teens often have many different goals for their future. Below is a list of short-term and long-term goals a teen might have. With a small group, brainstorm a list of ways that tobacco use could interfere with these goals. Write your ideas on a sheet of paper. When you are done, share your ideas with the class.

Goals for Teens

- having fun with friends
- being part of a sports team
- being part of a musical group
- improving physical fitness
- forming mature relationships
- going to college

Apply/Assess

How can being tobacco free help you achieve your goals? Think about some of the short-term and long-term goals you have set for yourself. Choose one goal that you think will be easier to reach if you remain tobacco free. Write this goal on a sheet of paper and explain in one or two sentences why tobacco would interfere with your ability to reach the goal. Remember that tobacco use has short-term and long-term effects. Then use the goal-setting steps to develop a strategy for achieving your goal. Include avoiding tobacco as one of the steps in your plan.

Share your plan with your classmates. As a class, brainstorm a list of situations in which you could be exposed to tobacco smoke or pressured to use tobacco products. Then identify ways, such as alternative activities, you could avoid tobacco in each of those situations. Add these strategies to your goal-setting plan.

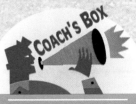

COACH'S BOX

Goal Setting

1. Identify a specific goal.
2. List the steps you will take.
3. Get help and support from others.
4. Set up checkpoints.
5. Reward yourself.

Self-√Check

- Have I explained why tobacco will interfere with my goal?
- Have I used the goal-setting steps to create a plan?
- Have I included strategies for avoiding tobacco in my plan?

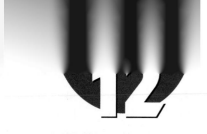

After You Read

Use your completed Foldable to review the information on the harmful effects of tobacco.

FOLDABLES Study Organizer

Reviewing Vocabulary and Concepts

On a sheet of paper, write the numbers 1–5. After each number, write the term from the list that best completes each sentence.

- nicotine
- chew
- tar
- bidis
- carbon monoxide

Lesson 1

1. Although _____ may be sold at health food stores, they can be even more dangerous than regular cigarettes.

2. _____ is a powerful, addictive drug found in tobacco leaves and all tobacco products.

3. Over time, the _____ that gets into a user's lungs can make breathing difficult and lead to lung diseases and cancer.

4. Once it passes from the lungs to the bloodstream, _____ reduces the amount of oxygen the blood cells can carry.

5. Another name for smokeless tobacco is _____.

Lesson 2

On a sheet of paper, write the numbers 6–10. Write *True* or *False* for each statement below. If the statement is false, change the underlined word or phrase to make it true.

6. A physical or psychological need for a drug or other substance is called <u>withdrawal</u>.

7. Headaches, nausea, and fatigue are all <u>physical</u> symptoms of nicotine withdrawal.

8. People who reach for some form of tobacco when they begin certain activities have a <u>physical dependence</u>.

9. <u>Sidestream smoke</u> is smoke that is exhaled from the lungs of smokers.

10. <u>Mainstream smoke</u> is smoke that comes from the burning tip of a cigarette.

Lesson 3

On a sheet of paper, write the numbers 11–14. After each number, write the letter of the answer that best completes each statement.

11. Cold turkey is a
    a. withdrawal symptom.
    b. way of quitting tobacco use.
    c. chemical in tobacco.
    d. type of drug.

12. Nicotine patches and gums are
    a. types of candy cigarettes.
    b. ingredients in pipe tobacco.
    c. medications that help tobacco users quit.
    d. types of spit tobacco.

13. An example of an external influence to start smoking is
    a. advertising.
    b. concerns about weight.
    c. stress.
    d. independence.

14. One strategy to avoid starting to use tobacco is to
    a. wear a nicotine patch.
    b. use refusal skills.
    c. listen to negative peer pressure.
    d. choose friends who use smokeless tobacco.

Thinking Critically

Using complete sentences, answer the following questions on a sheet of paper.

15. **Hypothesize** Smoking filtered or low nicotine cigarettes is as dangerous as smoking regular cigarettes. Explain why.

16. **Cause and Effect** Many experts believe that teens who use tobacco are more likely to use alcohol and other drugs. Why do you think this might be so?

17. **Evaluate** How can using positive peer pressure help counteract the negative effects of living in an environment where tobacco dependency exists?

Career Corner

Respiratory Therapist Smokers who develop serious lung damage may need the help of a respiratory therapist. These professionals evaluate, treat, and care for patients with such breathing disorders as emphysema. Respiratory therapists can become registered after attending a two-year program at a community college or vocational school. Learn more about this and other health careers by clicking on Career Corner at health.glencoe.com.

Standardized Test Practice

Reading & Writing

Read the paragraphs below and then answer the questions.

We are here today to urge the City Council to vote in favor of a ban on smoking in restaurants in our city. Smoking is banned inside public buildings, schools, and stores; and we feel that restaurants should be protected in the same way.

Cigarette smoking does not just harm smokers. Nonsmokers exposed to second-hand smoke are also in danger. Sidestream smoke, the smoke coming from the burning tip of another person's cigarette, contains twice as much tar and nicotine as does the smoke that smokers inhale. We believe that nonsmokers have the right to eat out without being affected by sidestream smoke.

Please vote in favor of the smoking ban.

1. Which sentence in the second paragraph represents an opinion?

   (A) Cigarette smoking does not just harm smokers.

   (B) Nonsmokers exposed to secondhand smoke are also in danger.

   (C) Please vote in favor of the smoking ban.

   (D) We believe that nonsmokers have the right to eat out without being affected by sidestream smoke.

2. What is paragraph two mainly about?

   (A) eating in restaurants

   (B) the unhealthy aspects of sidestream smoke

   (C) the dangers of smokeless tobacco

   (D) smokers who quit

3. Write a paragraph developing your own argument for banning smoke in restaurants or another public place.

 TH05_C3.glencoe.com/quiz

School
Play
Sponsored by
Teens
Against
Alcohol

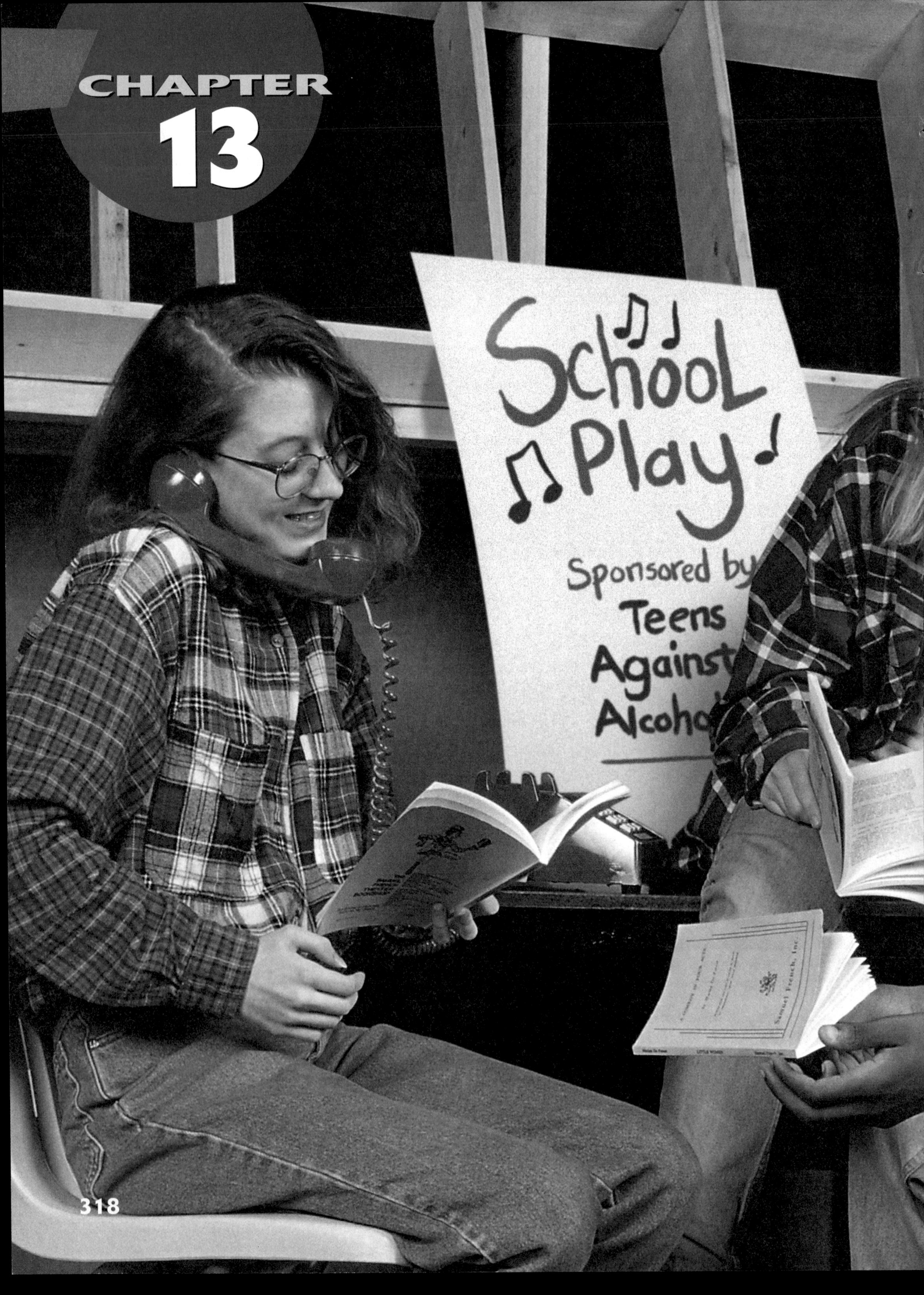

Alcohol

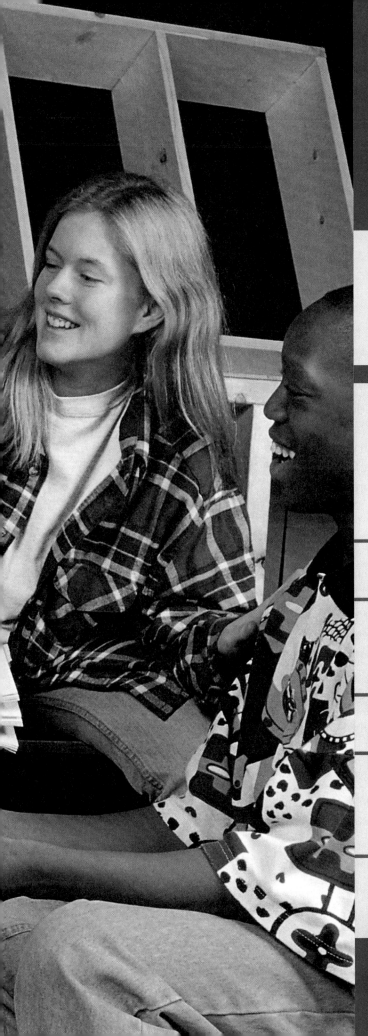

HEALTH Online
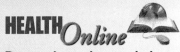

Do you know how to help someone who has a problem with alcohol? You can find out more by taking the Chapter 13 Health Inventory at health.glencoe.com.

FOLDABLES™
Study Organizer

Before You Read

Make this Foldable to organize the information in Lesson 1 on alcohol and its effects on the body. Begin with a plain sheet of 11″ × 17″ paper.

Step 1

Fold the sheet of paper into thirds along the short axis. This forms three columns.

Step 2

Open the paper and refold into thirds along the long axis, then fold in half lengthwise. This forms six rows.

Step 3

Unfold and draw lines along the folds.

Step 4

Label the chart as shown.

Effects	Short Term	Long Term
Mouth and Esophagus		
Heart and Blood Vessels		
Brain and Nervous System		
Liver		
Stomach and Pancreas		

As You Read

In the appropriate section of the chart, take notes on the short- and long-term effects of drinking alcohol.

319

1

What Alcohol Does to the Body

Quick Write

List two or three ways that you think alcohol negatively affects the body.

LEARN ABOUT...

- the effects of alcohol on the body.
- why alcohol affects each individual differently.
- the effects of alcohol on a fetus.
- the problems alcohol causes in teens.

VOCABULARY

- alcohol
- cirrhosis
- blood alcohol concentration (BAC)
- intoxicated
- binge drinking
- fetal alcohol syndrome (FAS)

Alcohol and the Body

Alcohol is *a drug that is produced by a chemical reaction in fruits, vegetables, and grains.* It is a depressant that has powerful effects on the body. In the United States, the law prohibits alcohol use by minors. Adults, however, can choose whether or not to drink alcohol. To make responsible decisions about alcohol use, people need to understand how alcohol affects the body.

Alcohol, like other depressant drugs, slows down the functions of the brain and other parts of the nervous system. It also affects the digestive and urinary systems. Excessive use of alcohol over a long period can damage almost every organ in the body. **Figure 13.1** shows some of the short-term and long-term effects of alcohol consumption.

Avoiding alcohol will help you concentrate and stay focused.
What day-to-day activities in your life require precision and skill?

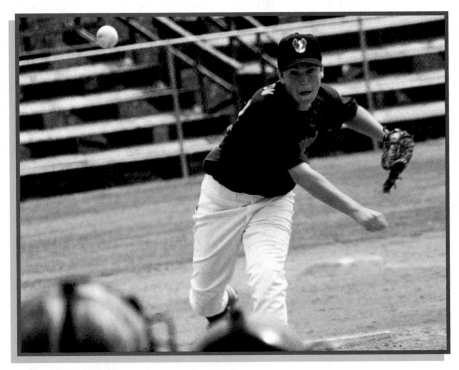

FIGURE 13.1

EFFECTS OF ALCOHOL ON THE BODY

Short-term effects occur within minutes of drinking alcohol. Long-term effects develop over time.

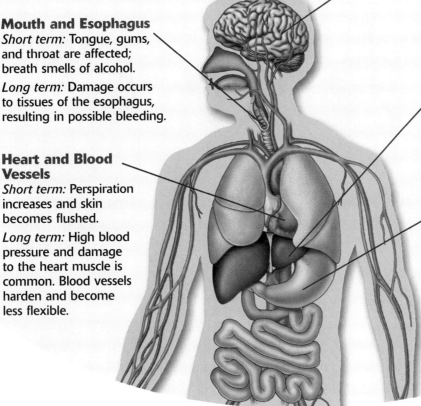

Mouth and Esophagus

Short term: Tongue, gums, and throat are affected; breath smells of alcohol.

Long term: Damage occurs to tissues of the esophagus, resulting in possible bleeding.

Heart and Blood Vessels

Short term: Perspiration increases and skin becomes flushed.

Long term: High blood pressure and damage to the heart muscle is common. Blood vessels harden and become less flexible.

Brain and Nervous System

Short term: Speech is slurred and vision is blurred. Drinker has difficulty walking.

Long term: Brain cells, many of which cannot be replaced, are destroyed. Damage occurs to nerves throughout the body, resulting in numbness in the hands and feet.

Liver

Short term: Liver changes alcohol into water and carbon dioxide.

Long term: Liver is damaged, possibly resulting in **cirrhosis** (suh·ROH·sis), *scarring and destruction of the liver.*

Stomach and Pancreas

Short term: Stomach acids increase, which often results in nausea and vomiting.

Long term: Irritation occurs in the stomach lining, causing open sores called ulcers. Pancreas becomes inflamed.

Alcohol and the Individual

The effect that alcohol has on a person is influenced by a number of factors, including:

- **Body size.** The same amount of alcohol has a greater effect on a small person than it does on a larger person.
- **Gender.** In general, alcohol moves into the bloodstream faster in females.
- **Time frame.** A person who drinks a lot in a short period of time is more likely to become intoxicated. Rapid drinking overwhelms the liver's ability to break down the alcohol.
- **Amount.** Drinking a large quantity of alcohol causes alcohol levels in the bloodstream to rise. If the levels become too high, alcohol poisoning can occur. **Figure 13.2** on the next page shows the alcohol content of some common alcoholic beverages.
- **Food.** Food in the stomach slows down the passage of alcohol into the bloodstream.
- **Medicine.** Alcohol can interfere with the effects of medicines, and medicines can intensify the effects of alcohol.

FIGURE 13.2

ALCOHOL CONTENT OF DIFFERENT DRINKS

Each of the following contains the same amount of alcohol—0.5 oz. of pure alcohol. Beer and wine contain a lower percentage of alcohol by volume than distilled liquors such as vodka or whiskey.

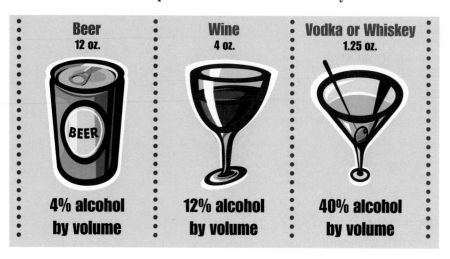

Beer 12 oz. — 4% alcohol by volume
Wine 4 oz. — 12% alcohol by volume
Vodka or Whiskey 1.25 oz. — 40% alcohol by volume

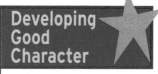

Developing Good Character

Responsibility

One sign of responsibility is thinking before you act. For example, never put yourself in danger by riding with a driver who has been drinking. Instead, look for a safe alternative for getting home. You might prepare a list of people you could call for a ride.

Blood Alcohol Concentration

The amount of alcohol in a person's bloodstream is referred to as the **blood alcohol concentration (BAC)**. BAC is expressed as a percentage of total blood volume. For example, if a person's BAC is 0.1 percent, then 1/10 of 1 percent of the fluid volume of his or her blood is actually alcohol. A person's BAC depends on the amount of alcohol consumed as well as body size and the other factors discussed on page 321.

A person with a BAC of 0.1 percent—or in some states, 0.08 percent—is considered legally **intoxicated**, or *physically and mentally impaired by the use of alcohol*. Driving while intoxicated can result in a jail term and, in some states, loss of driver's license. For anyone under 21, a BAC above 0 percent is illegal.

Binge drinking—*the consumption of several alcoholic drinks in a very short period of time*—is especially dangerous. Because alcohol is a depressant, it slows body systems down. If the BAC of a binge drinker rises sharply enough, the person will stop breathing and will die.

Fetal Alcohol Syndrome

When a pregnant female drinks alcohol, it passes from her body into her developing baby's bloodstream. A fetus exposed to alcohol in this way may be born with fetal alcohol syndrome.

Fetal alcohol syndrome (FAS) is *a group of alcohol-related birth defects that include both physical and mental problems.*

FAS is the leading known cause of mental retardation in the United States. The good news is that it is entirely preventable. Since even small amounts of alcohol can harm a fetus, the only safe decision for a pregnant female is not to drink any alcohol at all.

Alcohol and Teens

Alcohol can interfere with a teen's growth process. Studies show that teens who abuse alcohol have poorer language skills than other teens. New research also suggests that exposure to alcohol during the teen years reduces levels of certain hormones essential to normal development. It may also delay the onset of the menstrual cycle and affect other aspects of sexual maturity.

Teen alcohol use also has many other adverse consequences:

- Up to two-thirds of suicides on college campuses involve alcohol.
- Almost one-half of all traffic deaths of people under age 25 involve alcohol.
- Nearly a quarter of all violent crimes committed by teens involve alcohol.
- Between one-third and two-thirds of date rape cases among teens and college students involve alcohol.

☑
Reading Check
Build your vocabulary. Consider what the term *alcohol* means to you. Relate as many details as you can.

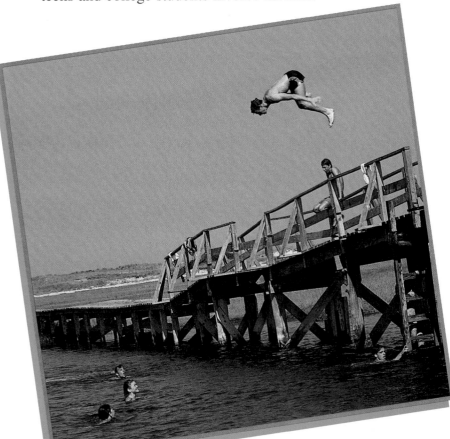

Avoiding alcohol helps prevent injuries and builds a better foundation for life. *How might alcohol use contribute to a drowning accident?*

LESSON 1: WHAT ALCOHOL DOES TO THE BODY **323**

COMMUNICATION SKILLS

Helping a Friend Stay Safe

Leah and Becky both read the open invitation to an end-of-school party tacked up in the locker room. Becky asks Leah if she wants a ride. Leah hesitates before answering. She had heard the party's host, Mike, say that his parents would be out of town. He bragged about his father's bar.

Leah does not want to go to Mike's party—it seems like trouble. Leah wants to help Becky change her mind about going to the party. What could she say to Becky?

What Would You Do?

Apply the skills for good communication to this situation. With a classmate, role-play a conversation between Leah and Becky.

The teen taking the part of Leah should state facts that Becky should consider before making her decision.

Speaking Skills

- Use "I" messages.
- Make clear, simple statements.
- Be honest with thoughts and feelings.
- Use appropriate body language.

Listening Skills

- Use appropriate body language.
- Use conversation encouragers.
- Mirror thoughts and feelings.
- Ask questions.

Lesson 1 Review

Using complete sentences, answer the following questions on a sheet of paper.

Reviewing Terms and Facts

1. **Vocabulary** Define the term *alcohol*. Use it in an original sentence.
2. **Recall** What kind of drug is alcohol? How does it affect the nervous system?
3. **Give Examples** List three factors that will influence the way an individual is affected by alcohol.
4. **Vocabulary** What is *BAC* short for? What does it measure?

Thinking Critically

5. **Apply** Why is a small female who drinks the same amount of alcohol as a large male more likely to experience a stronger effect from the alcohol?
6. **Explain** Why are pregnant females generally advised to avoid all alcohol during their pregnancies?

Applying Health Skills

7. **Advocacy** Do your part to advocate against binge drinking. Prepare a public service announcement in which you emphasize the extreme dangers of binge drinking by teens. If possible, record your announcement and arrange to have it played at school.

Alcohol and Society

Alcohol: A Threat to Everyone

Alcohol use is widespread in American society. Nearly 14 million adult Americans have physical, social, and psychological problems related to alcohol use. It causes premature death from a variety of diseases. It also contributes to unnecessary deaths and injuries on the roads and in the home.

Drinking and Injuries

Drinking and driving are a dangerous, and potentially deadly, combination. Drinking alcohol impairs a person's vision, reaction time, and physical coordination. Consequently, a person who has been drinking should never get behind the wheel of a car.

Alcohol causes other kinds of unintentional injuries as well. It impairs a person's ability to ride a bicycle, skateboard, or scooter. About one-third of all bicyclists and pedestrians who die in motor vehicle collisions have been drinking. Alcohol is also linked to about one-third of all drowning deaths and about half of all deaths by fire.

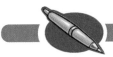

Quick Write

Write a short note to an older person, over 21, persuading him or her not to drink and drive.

LEARN ABOUT...

- the dangers of drinking.
- the disease called alcoholism.
- how alcoholics can recover.
- sources of help for alcohol addiction.

VOCABULARY

- alcoholism
- recovery
- detoxification
- sobriety

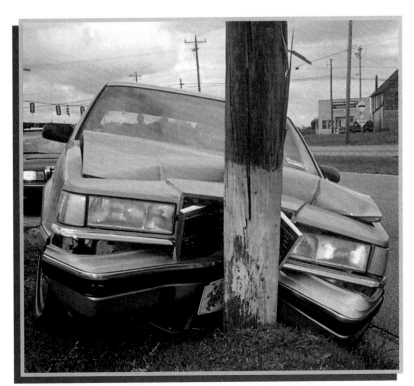

More than half of the drivers killed in nighttime automobile collisions are legally drunk. *What could be done to prevent drunk driving in your community?*

Alcoholism

Alcohol can become addictive. **Alcoholism** is *a progressive, chronic disease involving a mental and physical need for alcohol.* People with this disease are called alcoholics. Alcoholics cannot control their drinking. They drink even when they know they are harming their health and hurting others.

A chemical dependency, or addiction to, alcohol is both psychological and physical. With psychological addiction, the mind sends the body a message that it needs more and more alcohol. With physical addiction, the body develops a direct need for the drug. Either way, an alcoholic feels very uncomfortable when alcohol is withheld for even a brief period.

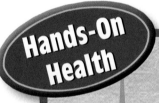

DRUNK-DRIVING STATISTICS

You probably have seen public service announcements about drunk driving on television and billboards. Find out whether these campaigns help reduce alcohol-related collisions.

WHAT YOU WILL NEED
- pencil
- ruler
- sheet of graph paper

WHAT YOU WILL DO
Study the following statistics from the National Highway Traffic Safety Administration. The statistics show the percentage of people killed in traffic accidents involving a person who was legally drunk, out of the total number of people killed in all traffic accidents.

Create a line graph to examine the data. Divide the horizontal x-axis into ten one-year segments, and label each year from 1990 to 1999. Label the vertical y-axis with percent values in increments of 5, ranging from 25 percent at the bottom to 45 percent at the top. Graph the data. Then answer the questions that follow.

YEAR	PEOPLE KILLED IN ALCOHOL-RELATED ACCIDENTS
1990	39.6 percent
1991	38.4 percent
1992	36.3 percent
1993	34.9 percent
1994	32.2 percent
1995	32.5 percent
1996	32.0 percent
1997	30.3 percent
1998	30.0 percent
1999	30.0 percent

IN CONCLUSION
Examine your graph and determine how the data changed over a ten-year period. Did alcohol-related fatalities increase, decrease, or stay the same? What factors may have caused a change in the rate of alcohol-related fatal collisions?

Stages of Alcoholism

Alcoholism develops in three stages. These stages develop over time and are not the same for each alcoholic.

- **Stage 1.** A person starts using alcohol to relieve stress or to relax. Soon the person needs alcohol to cope with daily life. He or she begins to lie or make excuses about drinking.
- **Stage 2.** As the person continues to drink, the body develops a need for more and more alcohol. The drinker may be absent from school or work but continues to deny that there is a problem.
- **Stage 3.** In the final stage of alcoholism, the problem is clear to other people. The drinker's body is strongly addicted, and the drinking is now out of control.

Help for the Dependent Person

A person who is addicted to alcohol is dependent on it. The addiction can be treated, however. *The process of learning to live an alcohol-free life* is called **recovery**. The steps of recovery are shown in **Figure 13.3**.

Recovering from alcoholism is difficult, but it can be done. Many alcoholics join support groups to help them be successful. One of the best known is Alcoholics Anonymous (AA). AA is an organization of recovering alcoholics who know firsthand the difficulty of beating alcohol addiction. Maintaining **sobriety**, which is *living without alcohol,* is a lifelong struggle.

FIGURE 13.3

STEPS TO RECOVERY

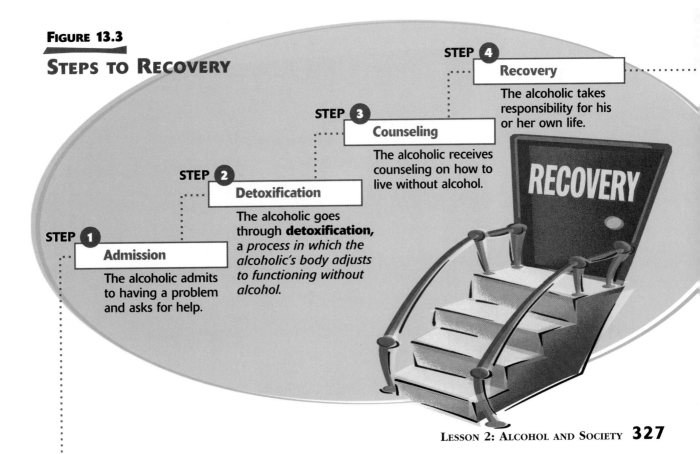

STEP 1 Admission
The alcoholic admits to having a problem and asks for help.

STEP 2 Detoxification
The alcoholic goes through **detoxification,** *a process in which the alcoholic's body adjusts to functioning without alcohol.*

STEP 3 Counseling
The alcoholic receives counseling on how to live without alcohol.

STEP 4 Recovery
The alcoholic takes responsibility for his or her own life.

RECOVERY

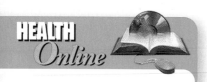

Topic: Alcohol

For a link to more information on the dangers of alcohol use, go to health.glencoe.com.

Activity: Using the information provided at this link, create a flyer that encourages teens to avoid alcohol.

Help for the Family

The harmful effects of alcohol do not affect only the drinker. The drinker's family members and friends suffer as well. One in four families in the United States is affected by alcoholism. Alcohol abuse is a factor in the breakup of many families. Many cases of spousal abuse and child abuse involve someone who has been drinking.

A growing number of young people are living with a person who is addicted to alcohol. These teens may not realize that they need help for themselves as well as for the problem drinkers in their lives. The first step to take is to admit that the problem exists. The second is to reach out for help.

Many alcohol treatment centers offer help to family members of the alcoholic. These programs teach family members about alcoholism and provide individual and family therapy. Some family members join support groups where they can talk with other people who have faced the same problems. Two of these support groups are described here.

- **Al-Anon** helps family members and friends of alcoholics. Al-Anon members learn how to help themselves as well as the person dependent on alcohol.
- **Alateen** helps young people cope with having a family member or friend who is an alcoholic. Its members share their experiences and work together to improve their lives.

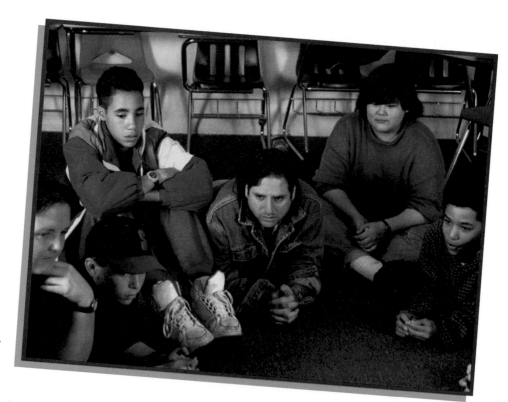

Support groups can help teens who have an alcoholic in their family. *What are the benefits of joining a support group?*

How You Can Help

If a friend or family member has a problem with alcohol, he or she needs help. Always remember, however, that your most important responsibility is to yourself. If you are close to an alcoholic, try not to let that person's drinking problem change your own behaviors and attitudes. Here are some ways you may be able to help an alcoholic.

- When the drinker is sober, talk calmly with him or her about the harm that alcohol does.
- Tell the drinker how concerned you are, and encourage her or him to seek help. Let the person know that the drinking worries you.
- Help the drinker feel good about quitting, and provide information about groups that can help.

Using positive peer pressure may help counteract the negative effects of living in an environment where alcohol abuse exists.

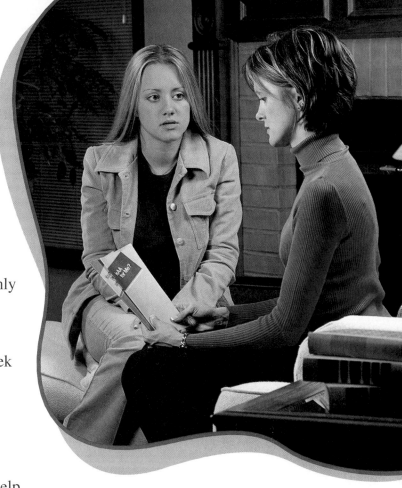

Gathering information is a good way to help someone with a drinking problem. *Where would you find information in your community?*

Lesson 2 Review

Using complete sentences, answer the following questions on a sheet of paper.

Reviewing Terms and Facts

1. **Explain** In what ways does alcohol impair a person's ability to drive?
2. **Vocabulary** Define the term *alcoholism.* Use it in an original sentence.
3. **Recall** Name the two kinds of addiction involved in alcoholism.
4. **Describe** What happens during the first stage of alcoholism?

Thinking Critically

5. **Suggest** What could be done to reduce the number of collisions resulting from drinking and driving?

6. **Apply** Explain the impact of chemical dependency and addiction to alcohol.

Applying Health Skills

7. **Advocacy** Play your part to stamp out drunk driving. Check out the Web site for Students Against Destructive Decisions (SADD). Use some of the information and ideas you find there to prepare your personal campaign to advocate against drinking and driving.

Lesson 3

Choosing to Be Alcohol Free

Quick Write

Write a refusal statement that you can use to avoid the pressure to use alcohol.

LEARN ABOUT...

- the reasons some teens use alcohol.
- the reasons to avoid alcohol use.
- how the media influence our view of alcohol.
- alternatives to alcohol for fun and relaxation.

VOCABULARY

- alternatives

Why Some Teens Drink Alcohol

You have learned that alcohol will harm your physical and mental/emotional health, and that drinking alcohol is against the law for teens. Why, then, do some young people experiment with alcohol? Here are some statements teens may give, followed by what they should know about alcohol.

What Teens May Say	What Teens Should Know
• "I'll look more grown-up with a drink in my hand."	• You won't look mature getting in trouble for illegal underage drinking.
• "If I drink, I'll be able to forget my problems."	• The problems will still be there when the effects of the alcohol wear off.
• "I'm stressed out about this test. A drink will help me relax."	• Alcohol does not relieve stress; it disrupts sleep and can create more stress.
• "My friends keep pressuring me to try alcohol."	• Real friends won't pressure you to do something harmful.
• "The ads make drinking look like fun."	• Alcohol companies want people to spend money on their products.

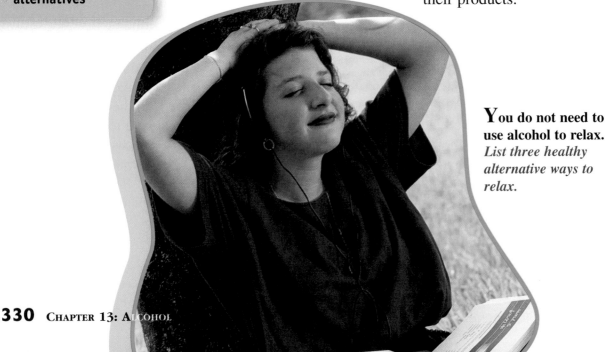

You do not need to use alcohol to relax. *List three healthy alternative ways to relax.*

Reasons to Refuse Alcohol

At least one-third of Americans do not drink alcohol at all, and many who used to drink have stopped. As people become aware of the physical and emotional damage that drinking can cause, fewer choose to start drinking. More and more young people are choosing not to drink also. Here are some of their reasons:

- **It is illegal.** Drinking is against the law for anyone under age 21. Obeying the law makes your life easier and safer.
- **It interferes with your activities.** As a teen, your life is full of activities. You go to school, and you have family responsibilities and friendships. Teens who choose not to drink will be better able to meet these challenges.
- **It promotes foolish behaviors.** Drinking can make people sick. It can also cause them to embarrass or endanger themselves.
- **It is not smart.** Smart teens know that drinking does not enhance popularity. Drinking does not make a person more mature. Acting responsibly is a sign of maturity.
- **It disappoints those who care about you.** Teens who drink alcohol have to hide their behavior. Many young people would rather not have to be dishonest with people they care about.
- **It harms your health.** Drinking alcohol harms body organs, particularly the liver, and increases the chance for injuries.

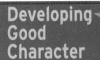

Developing Good Character

Responsibility

As you grow up, you make more and more choices for yourself. Knowing the facts about an issue and making choices based on those facts show responsibility. Make a list of the facts in this chapter that are the most meaningful factors in your decision not to drink alcohol.

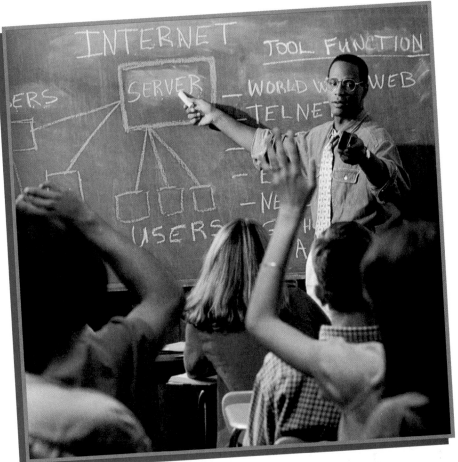

Refusing alcohol is one of the healthiest decisions you can make. *Predict three positive consequences of refusing to use alcohol.*

Reading Check

Increase comprehension. Research the meaning and history of the word *alcohol*.

Seeing Through Media Messages

Television, magazines, newspapers, and billboards often show attractive, healthy people drinking alcohol. Beer advertisements often link drinking with sporting events, fast cars, popularity, and fun. If you were to believe the hidden messages, you might think that it is normal, smart, and sophisticated to drink. You might also notice that the models often look very young. Why do you think that the beer manufacturers might want that young look?

Keep in mind that alcohol companies spend billions of dollars each year promoting their products. Their advertisements focus on people's activities while using these products, rather than on the products themselves.

When you see ads for alcohol, use critical thinking to analyze the messages in these ads. Will an alcoholic drink really make you more attractive or more popular? Will your relationships be successful as a result of drinking? The negative impact of alcohol use on individual and community health is not shown by alcohol manufacturers. You must dig deeper to find the facts.

HEALTH SKILLS ACTIVITY

REFUSAL SKILLS

Saying No to a Drink

Antonio has just transferred to a new school. He loves living in a bigger city, but does not know many people. One day, he and a classmate named Noel start talking about computer games. They both love to play, and they begin to spend a lot of time at Noel's house after school.

Antonio feels great about his new friend. He becomes uneasy, however, when Noel goes to the refrigerator and offers Antonio a beer. Antonio wants to avoid this negative social influence and refuse, but does not want to risk ruining the friendship. What should he say?

What Would You Do?

Write down three responses that Antonio can make to Noel using the S.T.O.P. guidelines. Share them with your classmates and decide which seem most effective.

SAY NO IN A FIRM VOICE.
TELL WHY NOT.
OFFER ANOTHER IDEA.
PROMPTLY LEAVE.

Alternatives to Drinking Alcohol

Why do some teens give in to the pressure to drink alcohol? One reason is that they have not thought about alternatives. **Alternatives** are *other ways of thinking or acting*. Below are some positive alternatives to drinking:

- **Become good at something that requires concentration.** Assemble a model airplane, play a video game, or paint a picture. Then congratulate yourself—a person whose senses are dulled by alcohol could not accomplish what you have.
- **Join other teens for alcohol-free fun.** Plan an alcohol-free event or outing. Make sure that all invited know that alcohol use will not be tolerated. Identify and participate in alcohol-free events taking place within your community.
- **Volunteer to help others.** Volunteer at a hospital or nursing home, or lend a hand to a community improvement organization such as Habitat for Humanity.
- **Learn something new.** You might learn a musical instrument, computer program, or foreign language. Learn a sport you have never tried before, such as karate or kickboxing.
- **Advocate.** Volunteer to speak to an elementary school class about the dangers of alcohol and the benefits of remaining alcohol free. Younger children look up to teens like you as role models.

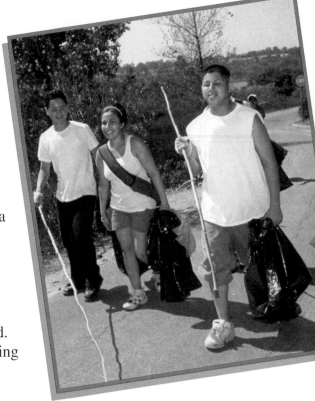

Volunteering to help others is a healthy and productive way to spend your free time. *Learn more about organizations in your area that need teen volunteers.*

Lesson 3 Review

Using complete sentences, answer the following questions on a sheet of paper.

Reviewing Terms and Facts

1. **List** Name three factors that might influence a teen to drink alcohol.
2. **Explain** Why is it a bad idea to use alcohol to relieve stress?
3. **Vocabulary** Define the term *alternatives.* Use it in an original sentence.
4. **Identify** Which alternative to drinking makes you a positive role model to younger students?

Thinking Critically

5. **Identify** What are two ways to obtain help to resist peer pressure to use alcohol?
6. **Suggest** Identify four ways to prevent the use of alcohol.

Applying Health Skills

7. **Practicing Healthful Behaviors** List all the reasons you can think of for not drinking alcohol. Organize your list into three parts to correspond to the three sides of your health triangle: physical, mental/emotional, and social.

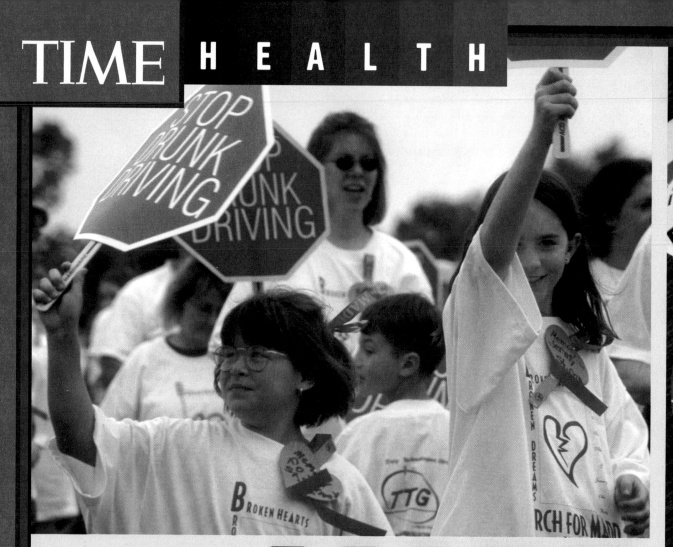

Getting **MADD**

Here's what one teen, Matt Oppenheimer, had to say about his experience with MADD **(Mothers Against Drunk Driving).**

" Did you know that underage drinking kills more young people in the United States than all illegal drugs combined? That's why I joined 435 other high-school students from around the country to tackle underage drinking—and especially drunk driving—during Mothers Against Drunk Driving's National Youth Summit.

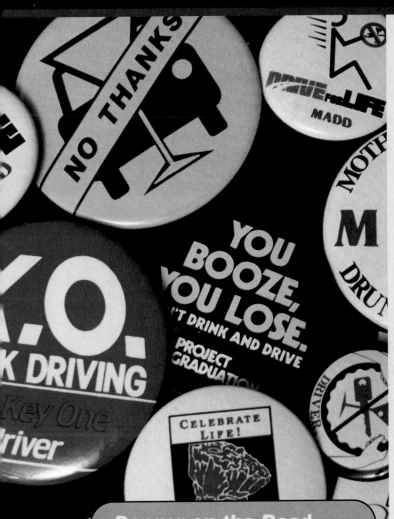

"First we learned about the overall drinking and driving issue and how each of us could make a difference back home. These messages came from leaders like former attorney general Janet Reno. We also broke into smaller workshops to brainstorm possible solutions for reducing teen drinking. At the end of the conference, we recommended that Congress increase the tax on alcoholic beverages and use that money to fund youth substance-abuse awareness and prevention programs. We also suggested that the federal government lower the blood-alcohol limit while driving from .10 percent to .08 percent.

"What I'll remember most are the stories many attendees shared about why they got involved. Cody Cowan, a teen delegate from Murray, Utah, joined MADD after a drunk driver severely injured one of his friends and killed two others. '[At first], I fell into a deep depression,' Cody said. Later, on a friend's advice, Cody said, 'I took all my negative energy and turned it into positive. I focused on changing the community and helping them realize that we really do have a problem with drinking.'

"Cody's story—and those of many others— reminded me of what might happen if I don't stand up and express my beliefs. Without my voice, underage drinking really could endanger the lives of people I care about. That would be something I couldn't live with."

Danger on the Road

As the statistics show, drinking and driving don't mix.

- **In 2002, car crashes killed 42,850 people; 42% of those who died were involved in alcohol-related crashes.**
- **Almost a third of all Americans will be in a traffic accident that involves alcohol.**
- **In 2002, 30% of 15- to 20-year-old drivers who were killed in car crashes had been drinking.**

Alcohol causes more problems than just auto accidents. In the United States, drinking alcohol is a factor in
- **40% of all suicide attempts.**
- **50% of all boating accidents.**
- **54% of all violent crimes.**
- **80% of all domestic disputes.**

Source: MADD

TIME TO THINK...

About Alcohol's Harmful Effects

Using reliable sources on the Internet and in your school's media center, conduct research to learn more about alcohol's effects on a person's perception, judgment, coordination, reaction time, and balance. Then, make a list of five common activities (for example, riding a bike or walking down stairs) and describe how drinking alcohol might negatively affect the performance of those activities, sometimes dangerously so. Share your findings with the class.

HELPING SOMEONE GET HELP

Model

Carly is worried about her friend Sandy. Sandy's grades have gone down and she has recently dropped out of all school activities. When Carly tries to make plans to study with Sandy, Sandy says she's too tired or has too much to do at home. Carly has seen Sandy hanging out with a group of older teens known for their drinking parties. She's concerned that Sandy might be drinking too. Carly wants to help Sandy but doesn't want her to stop being her friend. She uses the decision-making process to decide what to do.

1. STATE THE SITUATION
I'm worried that my friend is developing a drinking problem.

2. LIST THE OPTIONS
I could say nothing.
I could confront Sandy with my concerns.
I could talk to Sandy's parents.

3. WEIGH THE POSSIBLE OUTCOMES
If I say nothing, Sandy could get worse. If I confront her, she might get angry and not be my friend anymore.

4. CONSIDER VALUES
Sandy is my friend; sometimes you have to tell friends things they don't want to hear.

5. MAKE A DECISION AND ACT
I will tell Sandy my concerns and let her know there are many people who can help.

6. EVALUATE YOUR DECISION
Sandy and I had a long talk; she will see the school counselor on Monday; I think I made a good decision.

Practice

Using the decision-making process, write a paragraph in response to Drew's situation.

One day Drew goes to visit his older sister Stacey, who has a baby. When Drew lets himself into the apartment, he sees the baby crying in the crib and Stacey asleep on the couch. There are several empty beer bottles on the counter. Drew has long suspected that his sister has a drinking problem. He is worried for his sister and his little niece. What could he say or do?

Apply/Assess

In groups, develop two scenarios involving teens and alcohol use. Write them on index cards. The scenarios will be collected by your teacher and distributed to other groups to role-play for the class. Your scenario should have at least two characters and should describe a realistic situation involving a teen who must decide how to help someone who may have an alcohol problem.

When your group receives the scenario description, rehearse your role-play and perform it in front of the class.

COACH'S BOX

Decision Making

1. State the situation.
2. List the options.
3. Weigh the possible outcomes.
4. Consider values.
5. Make a decision and act.
6. Evaluate your decision.

Self-√ Check

- Did our role-play correctly use the steps for decision making?
- Did we show several options?
- Did we identify the consequences of each option?
- Did we reach a healthy decision?

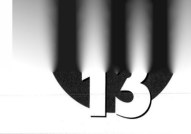

After You Read

Use your completed Foldable to review the information on the harmful effects of alcohol.

FOLDABLES
Study Organizer

Reviewing Vocabulary and Concepts

On a sheet of paper, write the numbers 1–12. After each number, write the term from the list that best completes each sentence.

- addiction
- alcohol
- alcoholism
- blood alcohol concentration (BAC)
- cirrhosis
- detoxification
- fetal alcohol syndrome (FAS)
- liver
- recovery
- sobriety
- intoxicated
- Alateen

Lesson 1

1. _____ is a depressant drug produced by a chemical reaction in fruits, vegetables, or grains.
2. Over time, excessive alcohol consumption damages the _____, the organ that chemically breaks down alcohol.
3. Children born with _____ have a set of mental and physical birth defects due to alcohol exposure.
4. _____ depends on several factors, such as gender, body size, and amount of alcohol consumed.
5. In the disease _____, scarring and destruction of liver tissue may result from alcohol consumption.
6. In some states, a person with a blood alcohol concentration of .08 is legally _____.

Lesson 2

7. _____ to alcohol is both physical and psychological.
8. _____ is a progressive, chronic disease that involves a need for alcohol.
9. During _____, the alcoholic's body adjusts to functioning without alcohol.
10. _____ involves living without alcohol.
11. _____, the process of becoming well after alcoholism, generally has three steps.
12. _____ is a support group for young people who have a friend or family member addicted to alcohol.

Lesson 3

On a sheet of paper, write the numbers 13–18. Write *True* or *False* for each statement below. If the statement is false, change the underlined word or phrase to make it true.

13. <u>Few</u> teens choose to abstain from alcohol.
14. Consumption of alcohol by teens is <u>illegal</u> in the United States.
15. Underage drinking <u>impresses</u> those who care for you.
16. Many people who used to drink alcohol are <u>giving it up</u> for a combination of health reasons and practical reasons.
17. Some healthful alternatives to alcohol use include <u>volunteering and learning a new sport</u>.
18. Alcohol advertisements often use <u>obvious</u> messages that are designed to influence people to buy their products.

Thinking Critically

Using complete sentences, answer the following questions on a sheet of paper.

19. **Relate** How can alcohol use cause health problems in later life and other adverse consequences?

20. **Evaluate** What is wrong with this statement: "A 4-ounce glass of liquor will have the same effect as a 4-ounce glass of beer"?

21. **Analyze** How might having an alcoholic in your life influence your attitudes toward alcohol?

22. **Compare and Contrast** Discuss some ways in which alcoholism is similar to an addiction to illegal drugs. Discuss some ways in which it differs.

Career Corner

Alcohol Abuse Counselor Alcohol abuse counselors help alcoholics recover from their addictions. These professionals give emotional support and counsel patients on how to stay alcohol free. To pursue this career, you need at least a two-year degree in substance abuse counseling from a community college. Find out more about this and other health careers by clicking on Career Corner at health.glencoe.com.

Standardized Test Practice

Reading & Writing

Read the paragraphs below and then answer the questions.

Today we have, as a guest, a volunteer from MADD—Mothers Against Drunk Driving.

What do MADD volunteers do? They guide victims of drunk-driving accidents through the legal process. They also develop youth programs, such as alcohol-free proms.

Has MADD been successful? MADD's activism has resulted in a number of federal and state laws to control drunk driving. The most well-known of these is the 1984 federal law requiring states to increase the legal drinking age or lose highway funding. Since MADD's beginnings, alcohol-related traffic fatalities have declined 43 percent. MADD will not close its doors until drunk drivers stop taking lives.

1. Telling MADD's story in an interview helps the reader understand
   - **A** exactly what MADD volunteers do.
   - **B** how to become a volunteer.
   - **C** how MADD started.
   - **D** how MADD has failed to reduce drunk-driving fatalities.

2. Which sentence in the interview best shows the reader that the volunteers at MADD are very serious about their work?
   - **A** They also develop youth programs, such as alcohol-free proms.
   - **B** MADD's activism has resulted in a number of federal and state laws to control drunk driving.
   - **C** Since MADD's beginnings, alcohol-related traffic fatalities have declined 43 percent.
   - **D** MADD will not close its doors until drunk drivers stop taking lives.

3. Write a paragraph containing additional questions that you would like to ask a MADD volunteer.

UNIT

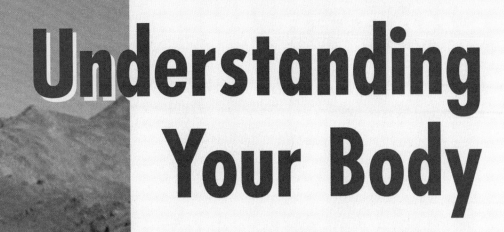

Understanding Your Body

How can taking care of your body systems be a breeze?

Staying well and looking your best don't just happen automatically—they're the rewards for practicing healthy habits. Taking care of your teeth, skin, nails, and hair not only enhances your appearance, but also contributes to your overall well-being. Eating healthy foods, staying active, and getting enough sleep will keep your body systems in tip-top shape. Once you know what to do to stay healthy, taking care of your body is a breeze!

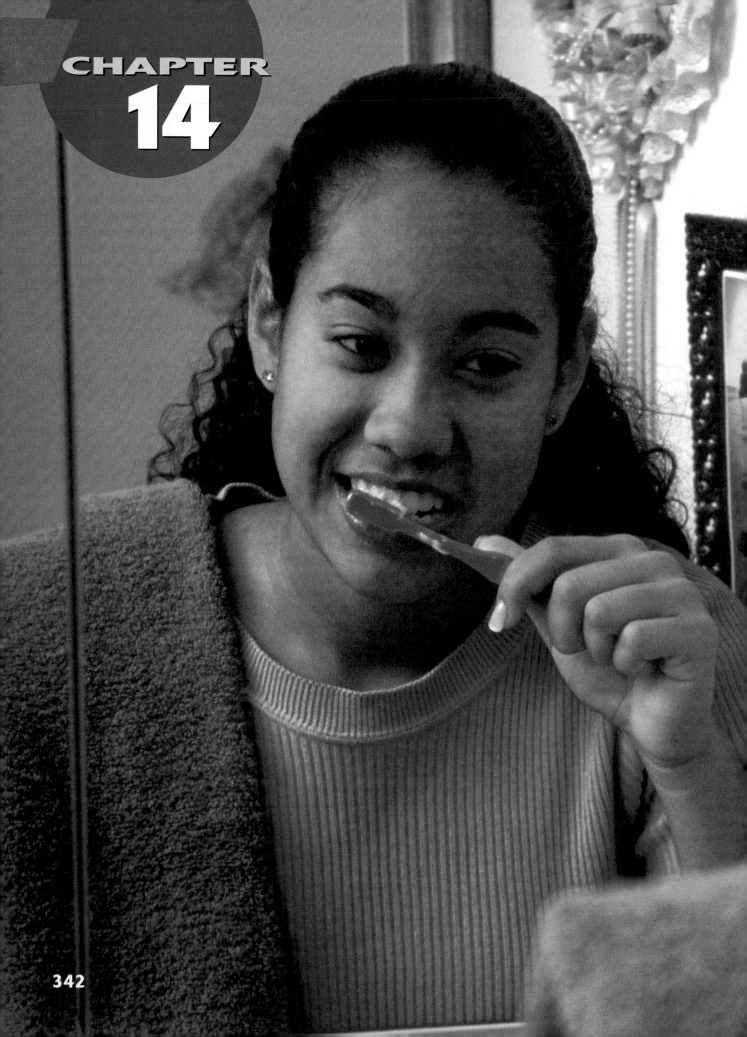

Personal Care

FOLDABLES™
Study Organizer

Before You Read

Make this Foldable to record the main ideas on healthy skin presented in Lesson 1. Begin with a plain sheet of 8½″ × 11″ paper.

Step 1

Fold the sheet of paper along the long axis, leaving a 2″ tab along the side.

Step 2

Turn the paper and fold it into thirds.

Step 3

Unfold and cut the top layer along both fold lines. This makes three tabs.

Step 4

Label the tabs as shown.

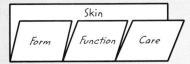

Skin | Form | Function | Care

As You Read

Under the appropriate tab, define terms and write down what you learn about the form, function, and care of the skin.

Healthy Skin, Hair, and Nails

Healthy Skin

Your skin is the largest organ of your body. Unlike other organs, such as your heart and lungs, your skin can be seen, making it an important part of your appearance. It also performs several other functions. **Figure 14.1** describes these functions.

Parts of the Skin

The visible and outermost layer of the skin is called the **epidermis** (e·puh·DER·mis). Beneath the epidermis is *a thick inner layer of skin,* called the **dermis**. Below the dermis is *a layer of fat* called the **subcutaneous** (suhb·kyoo·TAY·nee·uhs) **layer**, which connects your skin to bones and muscles.

Blood vessels, nerve endings, hair follicles, and glands are all found in the dermis. Oil glands make oils that keep the skin soft and waterproof. Sweat glands secrete perspiration, which is released through tiny holes in the skin called pores. This is the way your body cools itself.

Taking Care of Your Skin

Proper skin care can be a part of your daily routine. Here are some ways to keep your skin healthy.

- **Keep your skin clean.** Bathing or showering every day with mild soap will rid your skin of bacteria and excess oils. If you use makeup, use nongreasy products and remove them before you go to bed.
- **Protect your skin from the sun.** The sun's rays can cause premature aging and, more seriously, skin cancer. Wear sunscreen and protective clothing when in the sun. Avoid sunlight or use extra sunscreen protection between 10:00 A.M. and 4:00 P.M.
- **Treat your skin gently.** Harsh scrubbing, squeezing, or picking blemishes can result in scars. Administer appropriate first aid to cuts, scrapes, and burns.

FIGURE 14.1

The Skin's Functions

The skin is a barrier against water. Like a formfitting raincoat, your skin keeps out water when you swim or take a bath.

The skin helps control body temperature. When you're hot, sweat glands in your skin release perspiration to cool your body down. When you're cold, blood circulation slows to conserve body heat.

The skin is a sense organ. Nerve endings in your skin let you know when something touches your body. They allow you to feel textures. They also let you know if something is hot, cold, or painful.

The skin is the first line of defense against pathogens. This is why you need to care for any cuts or burns.

Dealing with Acne

Many teens experience a skin problem called acne. During puberty, hormones can overstimulate oil glands in the face, chest, neck, and back, resulting in clogged hair follicles, or pores. Bacteria in clogged pores release chemicals that irritate the skin and cause bumps on the skin's surface, as shown in **Figure 14.2**.

Minor cases of acne can be treated with over-the-counter products and good hygiene. If the condition is serious, you might want to see a **dermatologist** (DER·muh·TAHL·uh·jist), *a physician who treats skin disorders.*

FIGURE 14.2

FORMS OF ACNE

Whiteheads, blackheads, and pimples are three common forms of acne.

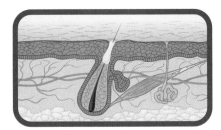

A whitehead is a pore that is clogged with an oily substance called sebum, which is produced inside the skin.

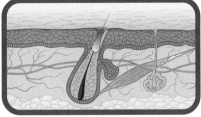

A blackhead is a pore that is clogged with sebum that has darkened after being exposed to the air.

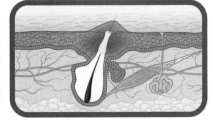

A pimple is a clogged pore that has filled with pus. The skin may be red at the base of the pimple.

Follow these tips to care for acne.

- Gently wash the infected area with mild soap and warm water every morning and evening. Do not scrub the skin.
- Choose oil-free cosmetics and haircare products.
- Use acne-fighting preparations prescribed by your doctor.
- Keep your hands and hair away from the infected area.
- Protect your skin from the sun.

Other Skin Problems

Other skin problems teens may experience include:

- **Cold sores.** These blisters or small sores near or on the lips are caused by the herpes simplex 1 virus. They usually go away in 10 to 14 days, but they can spread if you scratch them. The sores are contagious. Do not let anyone touch the sores, and always wash your hands after touching them yourself to prevent the spread of the virus.
- **Warts.** These small growths on the skin are caused by a virus and can be spread to others by touch. Over-the-counter medicine might help over time, or the wart may go away on its own. If the wart does not go away, see a doctor about treatment.

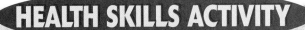

HEALTH SKILLS ACTIVITY

PRACTICING HEALTHFUL BEHAVIORS

Protect Yourself from the Sun

Protecting your skin during your teen years reduces your risk of developing skin cancer later in life. The Centers for Disease Control and Prevention (CDC) has developed a program called "Choose Your Cover." It suggests this five-step approach.

- **SEEK SHADE.** This is especially important between 10:00 A.M. and 4:00 P.M., when the sun's rays can do the most damage.
- **COVER UP.** Cover exposed skin with clothing.
- **GET A HAT.** A wide brim will shade your face, neck, and ears.
- **GRAB SHADES.** Sunglasses protect your eyes from sun damage. Try to get sunglasses rated "special purpose" or "general purpose" by the American National Standards Institute.
- **RUB ON SUNSCREEN.** Look for one that has an SPF of 15 or higher and that provides protection against UVA *and* UVB rays. Protect the tops of ears, hands, and feet.

ON YOUR OWN
Pretend you are preparing for a day at the beach. Make a list of items to include in your beach bag.

FIGURE 14.3

Taking Care of Your Hair

Keep your hair healthy by giving it daily attention. *What is your daily hair care routine?*

A Wash your hair frequently with a gentle shampoo.

B Let your hair air dry. The heat from blow dryers can rob your hair of oils and make hair ends rough and dry.

C Brush or comb your hair a few times each day to remove dirt.

D Avoid dyes, permanents, and hair spray that can damage hair. Some styling gels and conditioners can build up on your hair, making it look and feel greasy. Avoid preparations that contain alcohol, which can dry out your hair.

The Sun and Your Skin

Sunburn, caused by the ultraviolet (UV) rays in sunshine, is a sign of damaged skin. UVB rays are the primary cause of sunburn, while UVA rays contribute to skin aging and can also cause sunburn. Both types of UV rays can cause skin cancer, and both cause the skin to wrinkle and age faster than normal.

The best ways to protect your skin from cancer, and from other harmful effects of the sun, are to cover your skin with clothing and to use a sunscreen with an SPF (sun protection factor) of 15 or higher. Avoid sun lamps and tanning salons. Tanning devices can actually expose your skin to higher doses of UVA rays and can be more damaging than sunbathing. Remember that protecting your skin during the teen years will help you look and feel better for years to come.

Tattoos and Body Piercing

Any time the skin is punctured, you risk infection because pathogens can enter your body. Even if a tattoo or piercing is performed under sterile conditions, the skin is open to germs until it heals.

Healthy Hair

The same hormones that contribute to acne can also affect your hair. An oil gland is attached to each strand of hair. Normally, the oils make hair shiny and attractive. During puberty, however, the oil glands can secrete too much oil, making the hair look and feel greasy. **Figure 14.3** provides tips on taking care of your hair.

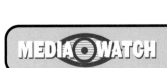

MEDIA WATCH

UV FORECASTS

The National Weather Service predicts the next day's solar-hazard ratings in the Ultraviolet (UV) Index Forecast. This daily rating ranges from 0 (minimal health risk) to 15 (serious health risk). *How can the UV Index Forecast help you protect your skin?*

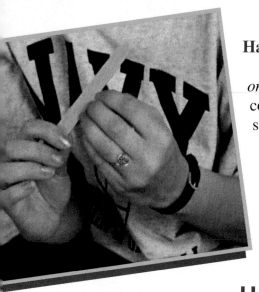

Hair and Scalp Problems

Dandruff, *a flaking of the outer layer of dead skin cells on the scalp,* is usually caused by a dry scalp. It can often be controlled with a special shampoo, but if the problem persists, see a doctor. You may have a skin infection or scalp condition.

An itchy scalp may be caused by head lice. These tiny insects live in hair and are spread easily from person to person. That is why you should avoid sharing combs, brushes, and hats. To get rid of head lice, use a medicated shampoo and wash all items that have touched your head, such as bedding, towels, and hats.

Use an emery board or nail file to smooth out the rough edges of your nails. Use a nail clipper to cut your nails. *How do you usually trim your nails?*

Healthy Nails

Fingernails and toenails grow out of the skin's dermis. Around the base of each nail is *a fold of epidermis* called the **cuticle** (KYOO·ti·kuhl). Taking care of your nails and cuticles is important for your appearance and for your health.

Some minor problems can affect nails. A **hangnail** is *a split in the cuticle along the edge of a fingernail.* If you carefully cut away the broken skin, the cuticle should heal in a few days. An **ingrown toenail** is *a condition in which the nail pushes into the skin on the side of the toe.* This can happen if you cut your toenails in a curve rather than straight across, or if you wear shoes that are too tight. If the toe becomes inflamed and sore, see a doctor because it may be infected.

Lesson 1 Review

Using complete sentences, answer the following questions on a sheet of paper.

Reviewing Terms and Facts

1. **List** Name the three layers of skin.
2. **Recall** What are two harmful effects that the sun's UV rays can have on skin?
3. **Describe** What are the two main ways you can protect your skin from the sun?
4. **Explain** How can you avoid getting an ingrown toenail?

Thinking Critically

5. **Apply** Your friend Kelly is thinking about getting his eyebrow pierced at the mall. Based on the information in this lesson, what advice would you give him?
6. **Suggest** What advice would you give teens who spend long hours in the sun working on a tan?

Applying Health Skills

7. **Analyzing Influences** Look through teen magazines for advertisements and articles that promote tanning, tattoos, or body piercing. Bring the articles to school and discuss how these media messages might influence teen decisions.

Healthy Mouth and Teeth

Your Mouth and Teeth

Your mouth, teeth, and tongue play important roles in your health and appearance. They allow you to taste and digest food, to speak, and to make a positive impression on others. The list below explains these roles:

- **Tasting.** When food touches sensitive regions of your tongue called taste buds, a signal goes to your brain. The brain tells you whether the food is sweet, sour, salty, or bitter.
- **Digesting.** Digestion begins in your mouth. Your teeth and tongue break the food into smaller pieces. Saliva in your mouth moistens the food and starts to change it chemically.
- **Speaking.** All the consonant and vowel sounds you make are formed by precise placements of the tongue, lips, teeth, and other parts of your mouth.
- **Appearance.** Your teeth and mouth say a lot about who you are. Healthy and clean teeth tell others that you care about yourself and your appearance.

Quick Write

Write down at least three health benefits of brushing and flossing your teeth daily.

LEARN ABOUT...

- the functions of the mouth and teeth.
- the causes of tooth decay and gum disease.
- caring for your teeth and gums.

VOCABULARY

- periodontium
- plaque
- tartar
- orthodontist
- gingivitis
- periodontal disease

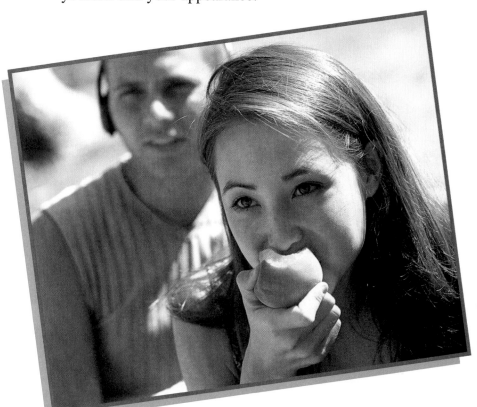

Your teeth and mouth allow you to bite, chew, and taste all kinds of food. *How do your taste buds help you enjoy food?*

Reading Check

Increase comprehension. Identify the causes and effects of tooth decay.

Your Teeth

Different types of teeth perform various functions. The incisors in the front of your mouth, for example, cut and tear food. The molars at the back do the major work of chewing.

As you can see in **Figure 14.4**, each tooth has three main parts: a crown, a neck, and a root. Each tooth is also made up of enamel, dentin, pulp, and cementum. The area around a tooth is called the **periodontium** (per·ee·oh·DAHN·shee·um), *a structure made up of the jawbone, the gums, and connectors called ligaments.* This structure supports the teeth.

Causes of Tooth Decay

Tooth decay is the gradual wearing away of a tooth's enamel and dentin layers. If you don't clean the food off your teeth after eating, bacteria in your mouth convert the sugars in the food into acids. Even though tooth enamel is one of the hardest substances in your body, acids can eat holes in it. **Figure 14.5** shows how tooth decay occurs.

Although tooth decay is widespread, it is one of the most preventable diseases in the United States. Some dental problems are inherited, but good habits and regular dental checkups can usually overcome them. You can make a big difference in the health and appearance of your teeth later in life by taking care of them now.

FIGURE 14.4

PARTS OF THE TOOTH

Each tooth is made up of many parts.

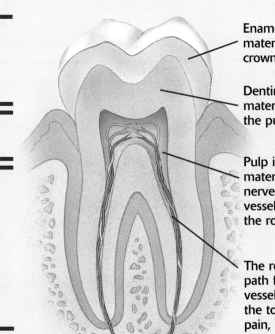

The crown is the part of the top surface of the tooth that you see.

The neck is the part of the tooth between the crown and the root.

The root is the part of the tooth inside the gum.

Enamel is the hard material that covers the crown of a tooth.

Dentin is bonelike material surrounding the pulp of a tooth.

Pulp is soft, sensitive material containing nerves and blood vessels deep within the root of a tooth.

The root canal provides a path for nerves and blood vessels. The nerves allow the tooth to feel pressure, pain, heat, and cold.

FIGURE 14.5

THE PROCESS OF TOOTH DECAY

When teeth are not cared for properly, tooth decay results.
What regular habits can help you prevent tooth decay?

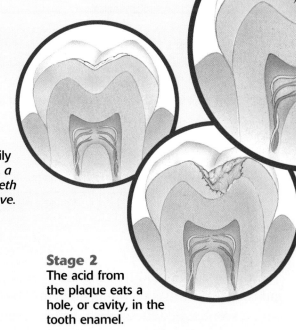

Stage 1
Food and saliva form **plaque** (PLAK), *a soft, colorless, sticky film containing bacteria that coats your teeth.* The bacteria combine with sugary foods to form an acid. Plaque that is not removed daily can harden into **tartar**, *a hard coating on the teeth that is difficult to remove.*

Stage 2
The acid from the plaque eats a hole, or cavity, in the tooth enamel.

Stage 3
The decay spreads to the dentin. When it reaches the pulp, it exposes a nerve. Air hitting the exposed nerve causes your tooth to hurt.

Taking Care of Your Teeth

You can have healthy teeth and gums for years to come if you practice sensible dental care. Here's what you need to do.

- **Brush and floss your teeth after eating and before bedtime.** Bacteria work rapidly, so it's important to remove food particles after eating. If you can't brush after a meal, rinse your mouth.
- **Choose snacks wisely.** Raw vegetables, plain yogurt, and fruits are good choices. Avoid snacks that are high in sugar or that remain in the mouth for a long time, such as soft drinks and hard or sticky candies.
- **Protect your teeth when you play contact sports.** Use a mouth guard to prevent your teeth from being chipped or knocked out during sports.
- **Get regular dental screenings.** A dentist or dental hygienist can clean your teeth and treat tooth decay and gum disease before they become serious problems.

Developing Good Character

Responsibility

Learning how to brush and floss properly can help you avoid pain and expense in later life. Schedule regular exams with your dentist, and ask the hygienist for tips on how to care for your teeth. Cooperate with any recommendations dental professionals give you.

FIGURE 14.6

HOW TO BRUSH AND FLOSS YOUR TEETH

Regular brushing and flossing will prevent tooth decay and gum disease

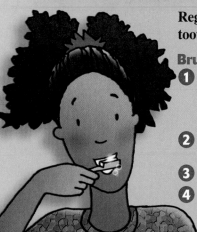

Brushing

1. Brush the outer surfaces of your teeth, using small circular or side-to-side strokes.
2. Brush the chewing surfaces.
3. Brush the inside surfaces.
4. Brush your tongue and rinse with mouthwash or water.

Flossing

1. Wrap about 18 inches of floss around the middle finger of each hand.
2. Grip the floss tightly between thumb and forefinger.
3. Slide the floss back and forth between teeth toward the gumline until it touches your gumline.
4. Forming a C with the floss around each tooth, slide the floss back and forth as you move it up and down the side of the tooth. Do the same for all of your teeth.

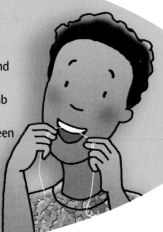

Brushing and Flossing

Daily brushing and flossing are essential for healthy teeth and gums. Most dentists recommend gently brushing gums and teeth with a soft-bristled toothbrush, using a fluoride toothpaste, for at least two minutes. **Figure 14.6** lists the correct methods for brushing and flossing. Replace your toothbrush every two or three months, or after an illness.

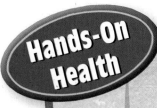

Hands-On Health

PLAQUE ATTACK

This activity will show how effective you are at fighting plaque.

WHAT YOU WILL NEED
- toothbrush
- toothpaste
- dental floss
- plaque-disclosing tablets or food coloring and water
- mirror

WHAT YOU WILL DO
1. Brush and floss your teeth the way you normally do.
2. Follow the manufacturer's instructions for using the disclosing tablets, or mix two drops of food coloring in a glass of water. Swish the colored water around your mouth and spit it out.
3. Examine your teeth in the mirror. The places where color sticks to your teeth did not get clean.
4. Brush and floss again, concentrating on the parts you missed last time. Check the results with a disclosing tablet or food coloring. Repeat if necessary.

IN CONCLUSION
What did you learn about your ability to remove plaque from your teeth? What can you do to improve your brushing and flossing?

Orthodontics

For many adolescents, the teen years are the time when braces are applied to correct crooked or poorly aligned teeth. The main cause of these problems is heredity, but thumb sucking and tooth loss can also cause the teeth not to line up properly.

An **orthodontist** (or·thuh·DAHN·tist) is *a dentist who prevents or corrects problems with the alignment or spacing of teeth.* Orthodontists often recommend braces, which provide steady pressure on the teeth to gently move them into the desired positions.

Other Dental Problems

Some problems of the mouth and teeth result from poor dental hygiene. Bad breath, for example, is often caused by failing to clean the teeth adequately. Other causes of bad breath are tooth decay, use of tobacco, and upset stomach. Tongue brushing and mouthwash use are important for controlling bad breath.

Gingivitis (jin·juh·VY·tis) is *a common disorder in which the gums are red and sore and bleed easily.* Gingivitis is the first stage of gum disease, and it can be cured with good oral hygiene. Left untreated, gum disease can result in receding gums and tooth loss. *Advanced gum disease, in which the periodontium is infected with bacteria,* is called **periodontal** (per·ee·oh·DAHNT·uhl) **disease**. Most adult tooth loss is the result of periodontal disease.

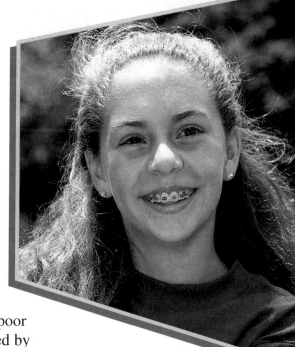

Colored braces are a popular option for dental patients. *Why is it important for teens to feel good about the way their braces look?*

Lesson 2 Review

Using complete sentences, answer the following questions on a sheet of paper.

Reviewing Terms and Facts

1. **Vocabulary** Define *plaque*. What does plaque harden into if it is not removed?
2. **Recall** How does tooth decay occur?
3. **Explain** What kinds of snacks are most harmful to your teeth?
4. **Identify** What are four possible causes of bad breath?

Thinking Critically

5. **Evaluate** Your friend Ellis brushes his teeth "in record time." You notice that he brushes only the outer surfaces of his teeth. He says that he brushes after every meal so he doesn't have to brush more carefully. What would you recommend to him?

6. **Analyze** Explain the role of regular dental checkups in the prevention and treatment of disease.

Applying Health Skills

7. **Accessing Information** Use the Web to access information about fluoride. Find out why dentists recommend fluoride tooth-paste. Prepare a brief presentation of your findings, including statistics to back up the case for fluoride use.

Healthy Eyes and Ears

Quick Write

List the actions you take to protect your eyes and ears from damage.

LEARN ABOUT...

- how your eyes work and how to protect them.
- how your ears work and how to protect them.

VOCABULARY

- cornea
- iris
- pupil
- lens
- retina
- optometrist
- ophthalmologist
- eustachian tube
- decibel

The Structure of the Eye

Your eyes are your windows to the world. They enable you to distinguish shapes, colors, movement, and light. It is through your eyes that you gain most of your knowledge! Although they are independent of one another, your eyes work together. **Figure 14.7** shows the main parts of the eye.

FIGURE 14.7

PARTS OF THE EYE

Each part of the eye has a specific function.

A The **cornea** is *a clear protective structure that lets in light.*

B The aqueous (AY·kwee·uhs) humor is the watery fluid in between the cornea and lens. It helps maintain pressure in the eye.

C The **iris** is *the colored part of the eye.* It controls the size of the pupil.

D The **pupil** is *a dark opening in the center of the iris.* The pupil controls the amount of light that enters the eye.

E The **lens** is *a clear flexible structure that focuses light on the retina.*

F The **retina** (RE·tin·uh) is *a thin layer of nerve cells that absorb light.* It covers the interior back of the eye.

G The optic nerve is a cord of nerve fibers that carries messages from the retina to the brain.

H The sclera (SKLEHR·uh) is the white of the eye. It protects the eyeball and gives it its shape.

FIGURE 14.8

HOW THE EYE SEES

The eye requires light in order to see. *What happens to your vision when you enter a dark room?*

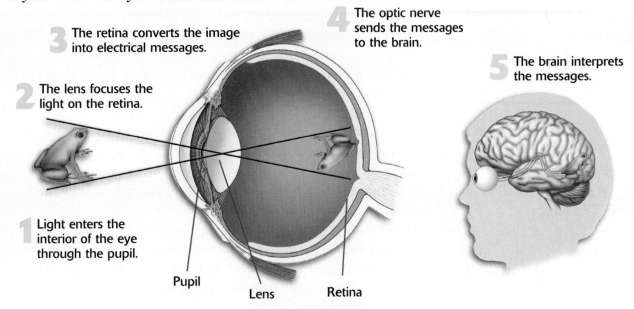

3 The retina converts the image into electrical messages.

4 The optic nerve sends the messages to the brain.

5 The brain interprets the messages.

2 The lens focuses the light on the retina.

1 Light enters the interior of the eye through the pupil.

Pupil   Lens   Retina

Your Eyes

The human eye is similar to a camera. It has an opening that lets in different amounts of light. As **Figure 14.8** shows, light passes through the cornea, aqueous humor, pupil, and lens to the retina. The lens can change shape to focus on objects that are close or far away.

Color Vision

Within the retina are millions of nerve endings. Some of the nerve endings distinguish objects in shades of black, white, and gray. These nerve endings are known as rods, and your eyes use them in dim light. Other nerve endings, called cones, distinguish the colors red, blue, and green. When information about these three colors is mixed, you are able to see all possible colors. Cones help you see sharp, color images in bright light. Both rods and cones send messages to the brain, which interprets the information.

A person who is missing one or more kinds of cones is unable to distinguish certain colors, an inherited condition called color blindness. In the most common form of color blindness, the person is unable to distinguish between red and green. Color blindness occurs in about 1 in 10 males and very rarely in women.

In this circle, a number is printed in another color. *A person who cannot distinguish between the colors has what condition?*

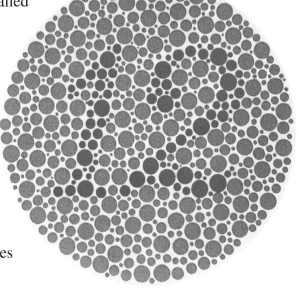

Protecting Your Eyes

Protecting your eyes from injury, dust, and overexposure to sunlight is a positive health habit. Here are some guidelines.

- **Wear protective sunglasses and avoid exposing your eyes to bright light.** A day in intense sun can burn your cornea. Over time, sunlight can damage the lens, retina, and cornea, as well as give you cataracts. Never look directly into the sun.
- **Wear protective eyewear when participating in an activity that could injure your eyes.** Special eye protection is available for different sports, hobbies, and work activities.
- **Read, watch television, and use the computer in a well-lighted room.** Position the computer screen about two feet from your eyes. Prevent eyestrain by taking a ten-minute break from the computer once every hour. Take breaks while reading and watching television, as well.
- **Avoid rubbing your eyes.** Rubbing irritates your eyes. Itchy eyes may be a sign of infection or foreign objects in your eyes.
- **Avoid touching your eyeball when applying makeup.** Also, do not use old makeup or makeup that has been used by another person. After a few months, eye makeup starts to grow bacteria.

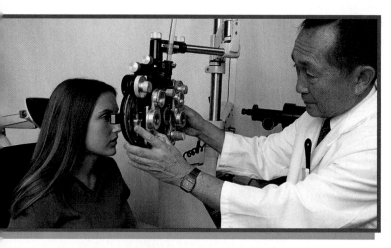

Your vision and the health of your eyes are checked during an eye examination. *When was the last time you had an eye checkup?*

Getting Your Eyes Checked

Two kinds of professionals provide eye checkups. An **optometrist** (ahp·TAHM·uh·trist) is *a professional who checks your vision and prescribes corrective lenses.* An **ophthalmologist** (ahf·thuhl·MAHL·uh·jist) is *a medical doctor who specializes in medical and surgical treatment of the eyes, and who prescribes corrective lenses.*

If you wear glasses or contact lenses, have your eyes checked once a year. If you do not wear corrective lenses and can see properly, every two years is sufficient. Your eye doctor may also test for glaucoma and cataracts during an examination. Common vision problems include:

- **Farsightedness.** A person can see distant objects clearly, but nearby objects appear blurred.
- **Nearsightedness.** A person can see nearby objects clearly, but distant objects appear blurred.
- **Astigmatism** (uh·STIG·muh·tiz·uhm). Images are distorted or blurred because of an irregularly shaped lens or cornea.

Treating Vision Problems

Most vision problems can be corrected with eyeglasses and contact lenses. Eyeglasses are a more common choice because they are often less expensive than contacts and require fewer visits to the optometrist. Moreover, eyeglasses do not require special cleaning and storage procedures.

Many Americans wear contact lenses. Soft lenses are usually more comfortable than hard lenses, but they are more difficult to clean. Extended wear contact lenses can be worn for a week at a time but increase the risk of eye infection or cornea damage.

Some vision problems can be corrected with laser surgery. This kind of surgery may eliminate the need for glasses or contact lenses. However, it is not recommended for teens because their eyes are still changing.

The Structure of the Ear

You might think of your ears as external to your head, but in fact they go deep into your skull. **Figure 14.9** shows the different parts of the ear.

HEALTH *Online*

Topic: The eye

For links to more information on the eye, go to **health.glencoe.com**.

Activity: Using the information provided at these links, write down five facts you learned about the eye and vision.

FIGURE 14.9

PARTS OF THE EAR

The ear has three main parts: the outer ear, the middle ear, and the inner ear.

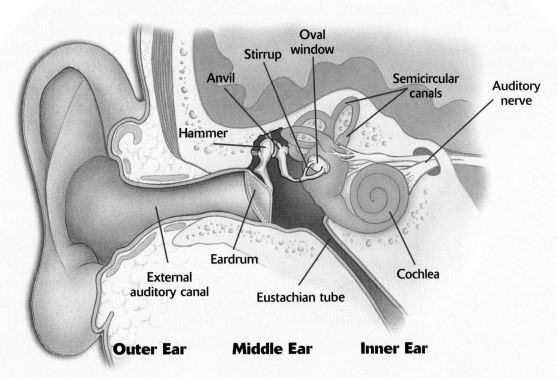

Oval window
Stirrup
Anvil
Semicircular canals
Auditory nerve
Hammer
External auditory canal
Eardrum
Eustachian tube
Cochlea

Outer Ear   **Middle Ear**   **Inner Ear**

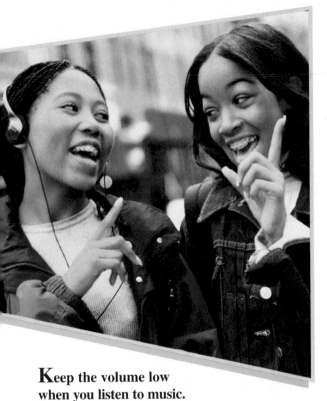

Keep the volume low when you listen to music. *What other ways can you protect your ears?*

Reading Check

Memorize. Make a word web to organize and remember facts about the ear.

How Your Ears Work

Hearing involves a fairly complicated chain of events. First, the outer ear—the part we can see—guides sound waves deep into the ear. These sound waves travel through the external auditory canal to the middle ear, where they cause the eardrum to vibrate. This vibration moves three tiny bones—the hammer, the anvil, and the stirrup—in the middle ear.

The hammer, the anvil, and the stirrup then transmit the vibration to the oval window in the inner ear. The oval window causes fluid in the cochlea to move. The movement of this fluid sets tiny hair cells inside the cochlea into motion. The hair cells produce electrical messages that travel through the auditory nerve to the brain, which interprets the messages, enabling you to identify the sound.

In order for you to hear properly, the pressure on both sides of the eardrum must be equal. The **eustachian** (yoo·STAY·shuhn) **tube** is *the part of the ear that allows air to pass from the nose to the middle ear so the air pressure is equal on both sides of the eardrum.* The eustachian tube runs from the throat to the middle ear.

Ears and Balance

The semicircular canals in the inner ear control your balance. Fluid and tiny hair cells inside the canals send messages to your brain when you move or change your position. The brain interprets the messages and tells your body how to adjust or change to meet the new situation. Sometimes the canals send too many or too few messages to the brain, which can result in balance problems. Two common balance problems are dizziness and motion sickness.

Protecting Your Ears

Over time, loud noises can cause permanent hearing loss. A **decibel** is *a measure of the loudness of sound.* The softest sound a person with normal hearing can hear is set at 0 decibels. A normal conversation is usually about 60 decibels. Any noise level above 85 decibels can harm your hearing over time. Just one short exposure to a noise above 125 decibels can cause serious damage. A ringing sound in your ears may signal damage. Tinnitus (TIN·uh·tuhs) is a condition in which a constant ringing sound is heard in the ear. The most common cause of tinnitus is overexposure to loud noises. Generally, if you have to shout to talk over a noise, it's too loud.

Here are some ways you can protect your ears.

- Cover your ears with earmuffs, a hat, or a scarf in cold weather.
- Keep foreign objects such as sharp objects and even cotton swabs out of your ears.
- Wear hearing protection such as earplugs when you are exposed to loud noises at a concert or indoor sporting event.

HEALTH SKILLS ACTIVITY

ADVOCACY

Reducing Noise Levels

Did you know that listening to loud music for as little as 15 minutes can damage your hearing? Over time, exposure to loud sounds can cause permanent hearing loss. The list below gives you some examples of how many decibels typical sounds have.

- **60–95 DECIBELS**—hair dryer, alarm clock, ringing telephone, television.
- **110–120 DECIBELS**—rock concert, busy video arcade, football game.
- **140–150 DECIBELS**—firecracker, airplane taking off.

WITH A GROUP
Prepare a campaign to inform other students about hearing loss. Include ways to reduce noise levels and protect hearing. Be sure to include specific strategies to reduce noise levels and protect hearing.

Lesson 3 Review

Using complete sentences, answer the following questions on a sheet of paper.

Reviewing Terms and Facts

1. **Vocabulary** Define the terms *pupil* and *iris*. Use them in an original sentence.
2. **Recall** What are rods and cones? What do they enable you to do?
3. **Explain** What is the difference between farsightedness and nearsightedness?
4. **Recall** What is tinnitus? What causes it?

Thinking Critically

5. **Analyze** Your friend Magda never wears sunglasses, even when she is at the beach.

She says the sun does not hurt her eyes. How might you help her better protect her health?

6. **Explain** Why is the process of hearing described as a chain of events?

Applying Health Skills

7. **Practicing Healthful Behaviors** Look for examples of loud noise levels at home. Perhaps you have a noisy vacuum cleaner. Perhaps a family member turns the volume on the television or stereo up high. List the examples you find, and then discuss with family members what can be done to reduce noise levels in your home.

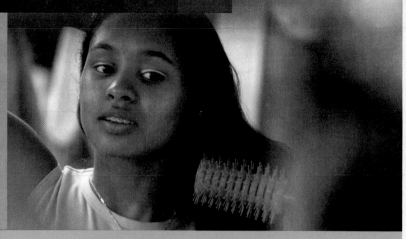

The Truth Behind Popular Health Tips

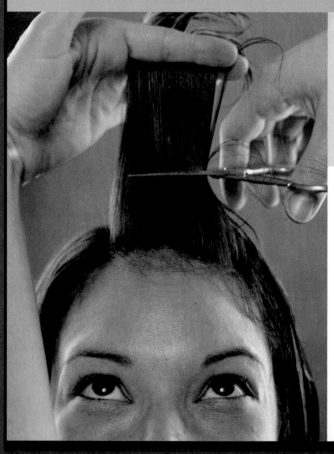

Take a look at a few common health tips, and discover what's fact and what's fiction.

1. "Cutting your hair will make it grow faster."

FACT: That won't cut it. "Your hair isn't like a lawn or a rosebush, where cutting can stimulate fresh growth," says Philip Kingsley, a hair and scalp expert in New York City. The length of your hair is genetically predetermined—when it reaches a certain length, it stops growing. When you trim the ends of your hair, you're merely cutting off dead split ends. This can make hair look healthier, but it won't help it grow any faster. Gently massaging your scalp may stimulate some growth by increasing blood flow and oxygen to the area. Besides, it feels good.

2. "Baby oil is a good substitute for suntan lotion."

FACT: This slippery advice comes from the fact that the mineral oil found in baby oil decreases your skin's refractive index, says Cincinnati dermatologist Brett Coldiron, M.D. Translation: Oil makes your skin absorb more light instead of reflecting it off your skin. "Oils will tan or burn your skin faster. You're basically marinating your skin so it soaks up more sun," says Dr. Coldiron. "That is, without a doubt, the worst thing you can do for your skin." The best thing you can do for your skin is to apply a sunscreen with a sun protection factor (SPF) of *at least* 15 to all exposed areas before going outdoors.

3. "Sitting too close to the TV will make you go blind."

FACT: This isn't even close to being true. Planting yourself in front of the tube might make your eyes or your head hurt, but it won't take away your sight, says Kerry Beebe, an optometrist with the American Optometric Association. "You should sit about 8 to 10 feet from the screen, because the closer you sit to the television, the harder your eyes strain to focus," Beebe says. If you have to sit any closer, this could be a sign that you're nearsighted (which means you have trouble seeing at a distance). See an eye doctor for a vision screening to determine whether you need corrective lenses.

4. "Brushing your hair 100 strokes a day will keep it shiny and clean."

FACT: This idea is hardly a stroke of genius—and, according to Kingsley, the practice is actually bad for your hair. "If you brushed a wool sweater repeatedly, you would wear a hole in it," he says. "Likewise, your hair can get worn out." Besides: All the brushing does is spread natural oils over your hair. These can act as a dirt magnet, which will only weigh down your 'do.

5. "Chewing on ice can damage the enamel on your teeth."

FACT: This one's true. Think of it this way: If you knock two rocks together, chances are good that one of the rocks will chip. The same goes for your teeth, says Matthew Messina, D.D.S., a

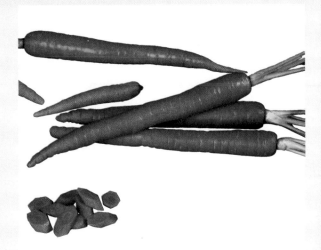

consumer adviser with the American Dental Association. "Tooth enamel is a crystal, and so is ice. When you push one against the other, one of them has to break," says Messina. This just goes to show that chewing on ice isn't all it's cracked up to be.

6. "Eating lots of carrots will make you see better in the dark."

FACT: You could see it that way. Many brightly colored fruits and veggies—including carrots, apricots, and broccoli—contain beta-carotene, a substance that the body converts to vitamin A. This vitamin *can* improve night vision, but only if your body is lacking it to begin with, says Carl Kupfer, M.D., director of the National Eye Institute at the National Institutes of Health. "Most of us get enough vitamin A in our diet, so eating lots of carrots won't change anything," says Dr. Kupfer. ◼

TIME TO THINK...

About Good Health Advice

Where do you get your health tips? Magazines? Friends? Older siblings? Create a "My Top Five List of Health Advice Sources," putting the source you rely on the most at number one. Now, evaluate your sources. How reliable is each one? Create a new list called "My Top Five List of Most Reliable Health Advice Sources." How do the two lists compare?

SEEING BEYOND THE PERFECT LOOK

Model

As a teen, the way you feel about your personal appearance may be influenced by the images of teens you see in movies, television, or magazines. Read about a teen named Jennifer and how she learned the truth about media images.

When Jennifer looks through teen magazines, she can't help but notice how perfect the girls in the advertisements look. Their hair is never out of place, their skin never has a blemish, and their teeth are always perfect.

Jennifer used to worry that she needed to try to look just like these teens. Then her mother explained that these girls are models who are assisted by hairstylists, makeup artists, and fashion experts. The photographers even use computers to make the pictures look perfect.

Jennifer's mother, a pediatrician, said she would be happy to speak in Jennifer's health class about the importance of respecting physical differences and not believing media messages about how everyone is "supposed" to look.

Practice

Ads use "picture perfect" models to influence teens to purchase certain products or services. In small groups, look through magazines and, using scissors, cut out what the media portray as pictures of health to influence teens to use a particular personal care product. For example, cut out examples of "healthy hair," "healthy skin," and "healthy teeth." Glue or tape them to poster board.

Answer the questions below to analyze the health information in these ads. Explain your answers to the class.

1. What products are advertised with these images?
2. What messages do they contain?
3. How do they try to influence teens?
4. Do you think these messages affect the choices teens make?

Apply/Assess

Imagine that your group is responsible for writing an advice column for teens. Read the following letter and prepare a response. Base your responses on the questions in the Practice activity. Explain the role of the media in influencing individual and community health.

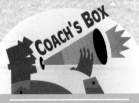

COACH'S BOX

Analyzing Influences

When analyzing media messages that may affect your health, you need to consider
- the source of the information.
- the purpose of the message.
- how the message tries to influence people.

Self-√Check
- Did my letter explain how advertisements often portray unrealistic images of healthy people?
- Did I emphasize sound health practices?
- Did I describe how media messages affect health choices?

Dear Teen Adviser:

I'm writing because I am so frustrated. Every time I open a magazine, I see pictures of perfect teens and I want to be like them. I do all the right things to take care of my skin, my hair, and my teeth. I usually eat healthy foods, and I do some kind of physical activity almost every day. My friends tell me that I'm in great shape. However, I really want to look more like these models I see in the ads.

Some of the ads sell nutritional supplements that are supposed to make me look "picture perfect." The supplements are too expensive, and I'm afraid that they may be harmful. Please advise.

Damien

After You Read

Use your completed Foldable to review the information on the form, function, and care of the skin.

FOLDABLES™
Study Organizer

Reviewing Vocabulary and Concepts

On a sheet of paper, write the numbers 1–11. After each number write the term from the list that best completes each sentence.

- dandruff
- epidermis
- periodontal disease
- tartar
- dermatologist
- periodontium
- hangnail
- enamel
- orthodontist
- plaque
- ingrown toenail

Lesson 1

1. The outermost layer of skin is the _____.

2. A(n) _____ is a physician who treats skin disorders.

3. _____ is a flaking of the outer layer of dead skin cells from the scalp.

4. A(n) _____ is a split in the cuticle along the edge of a fingernail.

5. A(n) _____ can result from wearing tight shoes.

Lesson 2

6. The _____ is a structure made up of the jawbone, the gums, and connectors called ligaments.

7. A tooth cavity is the result of acid eating a hole in the tooth's _____.

8. _____ is a sticky film on your teeth that is formed by food and saliva.

9. Hardened plaque that is difficult to remove is called _____.

10. A dentist who prevents or corrects problems with the alignment or spacing of teeth is called a(n) _____.

11. Most adult tooth loss is the result of _____.

Lesson 3

On a sheet of paper, write the numbers 12–16. After each number, write the letter of the answer that best completes each statement.

12. People who can see nearby objects clearly, but for whom faraway objects appear blurred, have
    a. astigmatism.
    b. nearsightedness.
    c. farsightedness.
    d. glaucoma.

13. The thin layer of nerve cells covering the interior back of the eye is the
    a. cornea.
    b. retina.
    c. iris.
    d. pupil.

14. The amount of light that enters the eye is controlled by the
    a. retina.
    b. pupil.
    c. lens.
    d. cornea.

15. The loudness of sound is measured in
    a. degrees.
    b. decibels.
    c. watts.
    d. amps.

16. The part of the ear that allows air to pass from the nose to the middle ear is the
    a. eustachian tube.
    b. anvil.
    c. eardrum.
    d. ear canal.

Thinking Critically

Using complete sentences, answer the following questions on a sheet of paper.

17. **Analyze** Give at least two reasons for flossing your teeth every day even if you brush after every meal.

18. **Explain** What are the health risks associated with tattoos and body piercing?

19. **Recommend** What recommendations would you make to encourage your peers to protect themselves from hearing loss?

20. **Synthesize** Create a list of healthful habits that will help prevent vision problems as well as eye diseases and injuries.

Career Corner

Speech Therapist Students interested in how people communicate might want to consider a career as a speech therapist. These professionals work with people who have hearing and speech impairments to find possible causes and treatments. They also help patients improve their speaking skills. Speech therapists need a master's degree in audiology or speech therapy. Read more about this and other health careers by clicking on Career Corner at health.glencoe.com.

Standardized Test Practice

Reading & Writing

Read the paragraphs below and then answer the questions.

Having long nails and wearing nail polish are recent trends, right? Wrong. The idea of coloring nails began thousands of years ago. Gold manicure tools that have been found in Egyptian tombs and ancient Egyptian writings tell us that Egyptian women painted their fingernails. Long nails were a privilege reserved for those of high status because they showed that these women had servants to do the labor in their homes. In fact, Queen Nefertiti decreed that nail color could be worn only by the nobility.

Centuries later, in the United States, glamorous Hollywood stars of the 1930s made nail polish popular. Women all over the country started painting their nails. False nails, made out of plastic, also became fashionable. These were glued to nails and then polished.

Nail polish and false nails continue to be popular today.

1. What is the first paragraph mainly about?
   - **A** how nail coloring was invented in ancient Egypt
   - **B** the use of nail coloring in ancient Egypt
   - **C** the rules for wearing nail coloring in ancient Egypt
   - **D** how nail coloring has developed over the years.

2. From the information in the second paragraph, the reader can conclude that
   - **A** people continue to use nail polish.
   - **B** most people who use polish are rich.
   - **C** nail polish is no longer popular.
   - **D** nail polish should not be worn.

3. Think of a current trend. Write a paragraph explaining why you think this trend is popular.

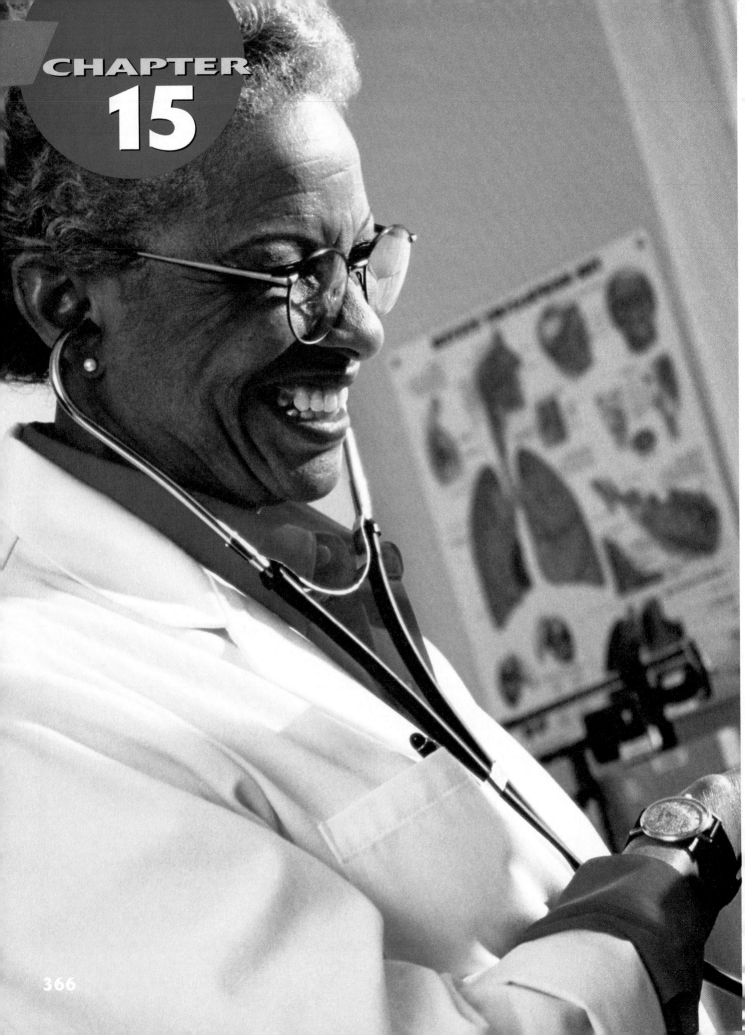

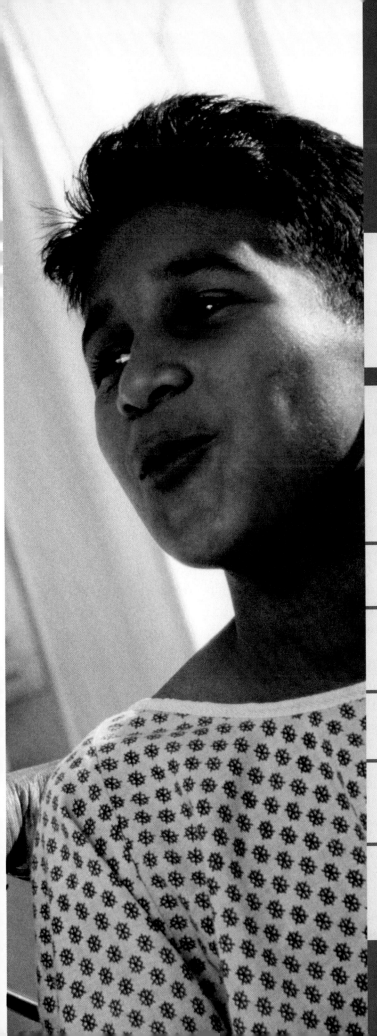

Your Body Systems

HEALTH *Online*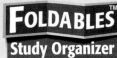

How much do you know about behaviors that keep your body systems healthy? You can rate your habits by taking the Chapter 15 Health Inventory at health.glencoe.com.

FOLDABLES™
Study Organizer

Before You Read

Make this Foldable to organize what you learn about the skeletal system in Lesson 1. Begin with two plain sheets of 8½″ × 11″ paper.

Step 1

Collect two sheets of paper, and place them 1″ apart.

Step 2

Fold up the bottom edges of the paper, stopping them 1″ from the top edges. This makes all tabs the same size.

Step 3

Crease the paper to hold the tabs in place. Staple along the fold.

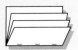

Step 4

Turn and label the tabs as shown.

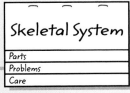

Skeletal System

Parts

Problems

Care

As You Read

Under the appropriate tab, record main ideas and supporting facts about the parts, problems, and care of the skeletal system.

Your Skeletal System

Quick Write

Make a list of words or phrases that describe the different functions of bones.

LEARN ABOUT...

- the different functions of the skeletal system.
- how joints allow different types of movement.
- how to keep your skeletal system healthy.

VOCABULARY

- skeletal system
- marrow
- joints
- cartilage
- ligaments
- tendons

Your Body's Framework

All structures need some sort of framework to give them strength and shape. Your body's framework, which is called the **skeletal system**, is *an internal system made up of bones, joints, and connective tissue.* See **Figure 15.1**.

Bones

The 206 bones that shape your skeleton are living tissue, composed of cells. Besides providing a framework for your body, bones perform many other important functions:

- **Allow movement.** Bones provide points of attachment for different muscles. Body parts, such as your arms and your legs, move when muscles pull on bones.
- **Provide support.** Your backbone is made up of 24 bones called vertebrae (VER·tuh·bray). Together, these bones support your head and upper body and also protect your spinal cord.
- **Protect other parts of your body.** Your bones provide a framework that supports your body's internal organs. Your skull protects your brain. Your ribs protect your lungs and heart from injury.
- **Form new blood cells.** Bones play a role in your circulatory system, too. Red and white blood cells are formed by **marrow**, *a tissue in the center of some bones.*
- **Store minerals.** Bones store minerals such as calcium and phosphorus for use when needed by the body.

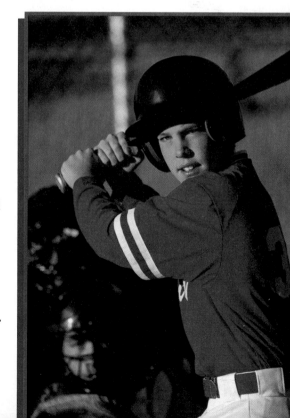

Your bones give your body shape and provide a framework for its other systems. *Which bones protect your heart and lungs?*

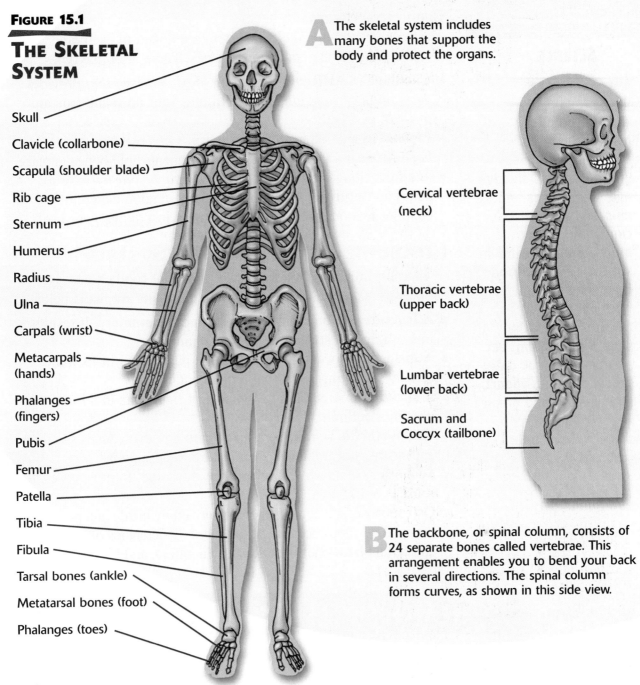

FIGURE 15.1

THE SKELETAL SYSTEM

A The skeletal system includes many bones that support the body and protect the organs.

Skull

Clavicle (collarbone)

Scapula (shoulder blade)

Rib cage

Sternum

Humerus

Radius

Ulna

Carpals (wrist)

Metacarpals (hands)

Phalanges (fingers)

Pubis

Femur

Patella

Tibia

Fibula

Tarsal bones (ankle)

Metatarsal bones (foot)

Phalanges (toes)

Cervical vertebrae (neck)

Thoracic vertebrae (upper back)

Lumbar vertebrae (lower back)

Sacrum and Coccyx (tailbone)

B The backbone, or spinal column, consists of 24 separate bones called vertebrae. This arrangement enables you to bend your back in several directions. The spinal column forms curves, as shown in this side view.

Joints

Joints are *the points at which bones meet.* Joints differ from one another in the type of movement they allow. Some joints allow movement in one direction only; others have a more open range of motion. The different types of joints are explained below.

- **Hinge joints** (elbows and knees) move in one direction only.
- **Gliding joints** (wrists and ankles) enable bones to slide over one another.
- **The pivot joint** (between the neck and head) moves from side to side and up and down and allows for limited rotation.
- **Ball-and-socket joints** (hips and shoulders) move in all directions, allowing complete rotation.

Connective Tissues

The bones in your skeletal system are linked to each other and to muscles by strong connective tissues. There are three types:

- **Cartilage** (KAHR·tuhl·ij). *Strong, flexible tissue that provides cushioning at your joints* is **cartilage**. Your nose and ears are made of cartilage.
- **Ligaments** (LI·guh·ments). *Strong cords of tissue that connect the bones in each joint* are **ligaments**. Ligaments hold bones in place.
- **Tendons.** *Tough bands of tissue that attach your muscles to bones* are **tendons**. You can feel a large tendon called the Achilles tendon on the back of your leg just above your heel.

Problems of the Skeletal System

Injuries, infections, poor posture, and poor food choices can damage the skeletal system. Common problems are listed below.

- **A fracture** is a break in a bone caused by an injury. It results in swelling and sometimes extreme pain.
- **A dislocation** occurs when a bone is pushed out of its joint, usually stretching or tearing a ligament.
- **A sprain** is a stretching or twisting of ligaments in a joint, causing swelling.
- **Osteoarthritis** is a breakdown of cartilage that causes swelling and stiffness of joints. It is caused by wear and tear.
- **Scoliosis** is a sideways curvature of the spine. In most cases, the cause is not known.
- **Osteoporosis** is a condition characterized by brittle and porous bones. It develops because of long-term deficiencies of calcium and certain hormones, insufficient vitamin D, and lack of exercise.

HEALTH SKILLS ACTIVITY

ACCESSING INFORMATION

Scoliosis Screening

Scoliosis is a disorder in which the spine curves to one side of the body. When viewed from behind, the spine appears to have a slight S- or C-shaped curve. In more severe cases of scoliosis, the spine actually rotates, causing the ribs to spread out or move closer on different sides of the body. Here are some facts about scoliosis.

- It is usually painless, but it can cause back pain and difficulty with breathing.
- It affects about 2 percent of Americans, mostly children.

WITH A GROUP
Gather information about screening programs for scoliosis from your library and from reliable sources on the Internet. Present your findings to the class.

Care of the Skeletal System

You can add to your bone mass only while you are still growing, so now is an important time to focus on building healthy bones. Following healthful habits will help protect and strengthen your skeletal system now and for years to come.

- **Be physically active.** Regular physical activity—especially weight-bearing exercise such as walking and jogging—increases bone mass. Weight training is also good, even for older adults.
- **Eat foods high in calcium and phosphorus.** Calcium is essential for building and maintaining strong bones, especially during the teen years. Phosphorus, another vital mineral, combines with calcium to give bones rigidity. Phosphorus can be found in dairy products, beans, liver, and whole grains.
- **Sit, stand, and walk with straight posture.** Straight, upright posture keeps your spine healthy and protects your spinal cord.
- **Pay attention to your shoes.** Shoes should provide correct arch support and be long enough so you can wiggle your toes. Properly fitting shoes provide support for the bones of the feet.

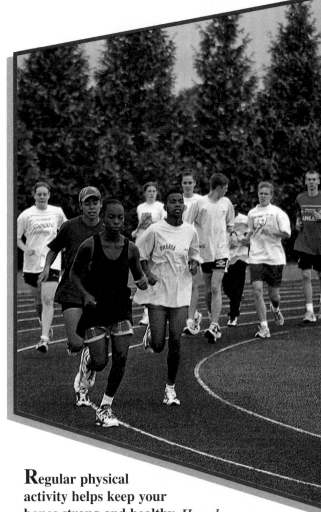

Regular physical activity helps keep your bones strong and healthy. *How do you protect and strengthen your bones?*

Lesson 1 Review

Using complete sentences, answer the following questions on a sheet of paper.

Reviewing Terms and Facts

1. **Vocabulary** Name the three components that make up the *skeletal system.*
2. **List** Name the different types of joints in your body. Describe how each allows bones to move.
3. **Compare** What is the difference between *ligaments* and *tendons?*
4. **Explain** In what way does physical activity contribute to the health of the skeletal system?

Thinking Critically

5. **Suggest** What are some ways that you can act now to prevent osteoporosis later in life?
6. **Apply** Maura is choosing new shoes and has asked your advice about qualities to look for. What would you advise, based on what you have learned about shoes and the skeletal system?

Applying Health Skills

7. **Practicing Healthful Behaviors** Create a lunch menu for one week that includes at least two calcium-rich foods every day. How do you meet your calcium requirements and enjoy a variety of choices?

Your Muscular System

Muscles and Movement

Muscles give you the power to lift weights or pet your cat, and the endurance to run 5 miles or do 15 push-ups. Your **muscular system** is *the group of structures that make your body parts move.*

You control the muscles that move your body. However, your muscular system also includes muscles that you do not control. Many organs, such as your stomach and intestines, are lined with muscles that move without your being aware of them. The most important muscle is your heart, which contracts on its own about 100,000 times a day.

How Muscles Work

Muscles are stimulated by nerves and work by contracting and relaxing. Many of your skeletal muscles work in pairs. When one muscle in the pair contracts, or shortens, the other muscle extends, or lengthens. This teamwork produces movement at a joint, as shown in **Figure 15.2**.

FIGURE 15.2

HOW MUSCLES WORK

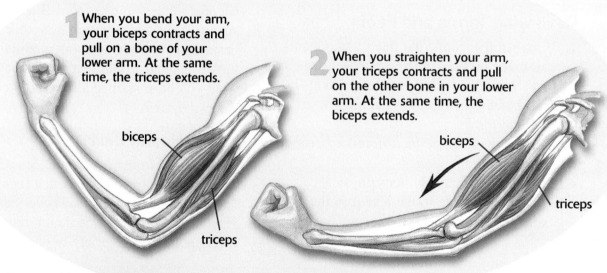

1 When you bend your arm, your biceps contracts and pull on a bone of your lower arm. At the same time, the triceps extends.

biceps

triceps

2 When you straighten your arm, your triceps contracts and pull on the other bone in your lower arm. At the same time, the biceps extends.

biceps

triceps

Your body has three different types of muscle tissue: skeletal muscle, smooth muscle, and cardiac muscle. **Skeletal muscle** is *muscle attached to bones that enables you to move your body.* Because you can control skeletal muscles, they are called voluntary muscles. **Smooth muscle** is *muscle found in organs and in blood vessels and glands.* You do not consciously control the contraction of the smooth muscles. These are involuntary muscles. **Cardiac muscle**, also involuntary, is *muscle found only in the walls of your heart.* Contracting and relaxing continually, cardiac muscle enables your heart to pump blood throughout your body. **Figure 15.3** shows the major skeletal muscles of your body.

FIGURE 15.3

THE MUSCULAR SYSTEM

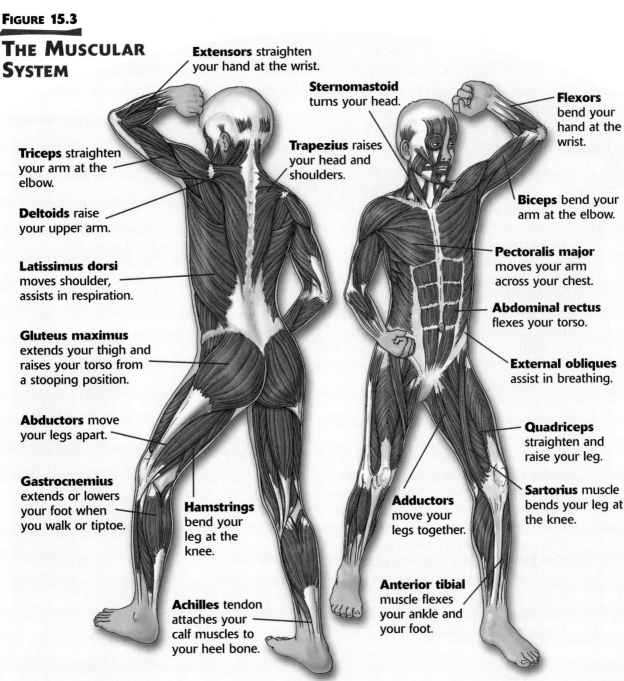

Extensors straighten your hand at the wrist.

Sternomastoid turns your head.

Trapezius raises your head and shoulders.

Flexors bend your hand at the wrist.

Triceps straighten your arm at the elbow.

Deltoids raise your upper arm.

Latissimus dorsi moves shoulder, assists in respiration.

Gluteus maximus extends your thigh and raises your torso from a stooping position.

Abductors move your legs apart.

Gastrocnemius extends or lowers your foot when you walk or tiptoe.

Hamstrings bend your leg at the knee.

Achilles tendon attaches your calf muscles to your heel bone.

Biceps bend your arm at the elbow.

Pectoralis major moves your arm across your chest.

Abdominal rectus flexes your torso.

External obliques assist in breathing.

Quadriceps straighten and raise your leg.

Sartorius muscle bends your leg at the knee.

Adductors move your legs together.

Anterior tibial muscle flexes your ankle and your foot.

Problems of the Muscular System

You may have experienced sore muscles a day or two after heavy exercise or strenuous physical activity. This soreness is caused by a buildup of acid in your muscles, and it is usually temporary. Some muscular conditions, however, are chronic, meaning that they last for long periods. Muscular problems include the following.

- **A pulled or torn muscle** has been torn away from the bone or has been damaged within itself.
- **Muscle strain** is any type of soreness that develops in a muscle because of overuse. It is caused by small tears to the muscle or tendon.
- **A cramped muscle** remains contracted rather than extending, or relaxing. It typically feels tight and sore, and is usually a sign to drink more water.
- **Muscular dystrophy** is a disorder that is usually inherited. It causes gradual weakening of the skeletal muscles, eventually resulting in an inability to walk or stand.

Hands-On Health

STRETCH OUT

Any warm-up routine should include gentle stretches. Stretching lengthens tendons, warms up ligaments, and prepares joints for activity. Stretching also improves muscle flexibility and coordination, and relieves tension and tightness. Here are some basic stretching exercises you can try.

WHAT YOU WILL NEED
- space to do the stretches

WHAT YOU WILL DO
1. **Back Scratch Stretch.** Raise right hand in the air with palm facing back. Bend elbow and place palm of hand between shoulders. Bring left hand behind back and try to touch right hand. Hold for 10 to 30 seconds. Repeat twice on each side.
2. **Calf Stretch.** Lean against wall. Put right leg behind you. With right heel on floor, slightly bend right knee. Lean forward and hold for 10 to 30 seconds. Repeat twice with each leg.

3. **Thigh Stretch.** Stand and grasp left foot behind you with right hand. Slowly pull leg back so that knee moves away from body. Hold for 10 to 30 seconds. Repeat twice with each leg.

IN CONCLUSION
1. Did you notice a difference in the way your body felt after performing the stretches?
2. Make these stretching exercises part of your warm-up routine whenever you engage in physical activity.

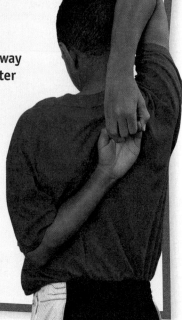

Care of the Muscular System

Your muscles need proper care to stay healthy and work properly. You also need to maintain muscle tone—the natural tension in the fibers of muscles. Below are some guidelines for keeping your muscles healthy.

- **Engage in regular physical activity.** The more you use your muscles, the stronger and more efficient they will become. Regular physical activity strengthens the heart muscle as well.
- **Warm up before physical activity.** A program that includes warm-up and stretching, followed by a cool-down exercise and light stretching, helps prevent muscle injury and increases muscle flexibility.
- **Eat foods containing carbohydrates and protein.** Carbohydrates are a source of energy. Protein is needed for the growth and regeneration of muscle cells.
- **Maintain a healthy weight.** Extra body weight can strain the muscles in your back. Healthful eating and regular physical activity will help you reach and maintain your appropriate weight.
- **Learn to lift properly.** The correct way to lift a heavy object is to bend your knees, keep your back straight, and use your leg muscles to do the lifting. Keep the load close to your body.

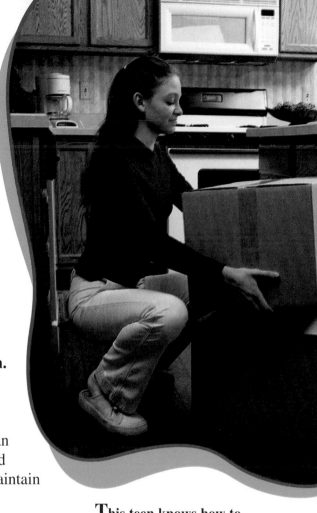

This teen knows how to protect her back by using her legs to lift a heavy box. *Name two other behaviors that protect your muscles.*

Lesson 2 Review

Using complete sentences, answer the following questions on a sheet of paper.

Reviewing Terms and Facts

1. **Vocabulary** What is the body's *muscular system,* and what three types of muscles does it include?
2. **Explain** How do skeletal muscles work together to make movement possible?
3. **List** What are four problems that occur in muscles? Which of these is typically inherited?
4. **Name** What are three practices you can follow to keep your muscles healthy?

Thinking Critically

5. **Apply** Are any activities that you engage in likely to result in muscle damage? If so, what can you do to prevent the damage?
6. **Explain** Why is it important to warm up and stretch before physical activity and to cool down and stretch afterward?

Applying Health Skills

7. **Practicing Healthful Behaviors** List your favorite activities that strengthen and tone your muscles. Share your list with classmates.

Your Circulatory System

Quick Write

Your heart pumps blood throughout your body 24 hours a day. What behaviors might help keep your heart healthy?

LEARN ABOUT...

- what your circulatory system does.
- the different parts of your circulatory system.
- keeping your circulatory system healthy.

VOCABULARY

- circulatory system
- cardiovascular system
- pulmonary circulation
- systemic circulation
- arteries
- veins
- capillaries

The Body's Transport System

The **circulatory** (SER·kyuh·luh·tohr·ee) **system** consists of *organs and tissues that transport essential materials to body cells and remove their waste products.* This body system is also known as the **cardiovascular** (KAR·dee·oh·VAS·kyoo·ler) **system**.

Pumped by your heart, your blood is moved through a vast circulatory network. Different organs serve as transfer stations. At some stations, blood picks up needed nutrients and other materials and delivers them to the cells. Blood also picks up waste products and carries them to other transfer stations, where they are removed from the body. See **Figure 15.4**.

FIGURE 15.4

HOW THE CIRCULATORY SYSTEM WORKS

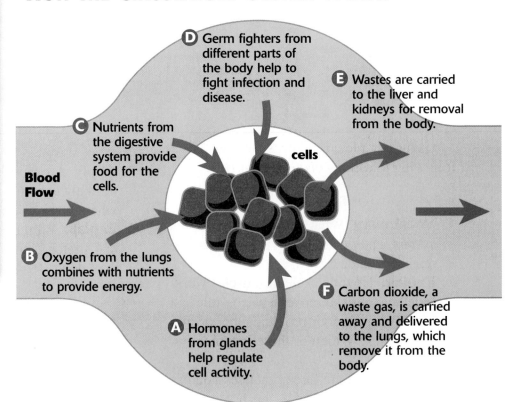

D Germ fighters from different parts of the body help to fight infection and disease.

E Wastes are carried to the liver and kidneys for removal from the body.

C Nutrients from the digestive system provide food for the cells.

cells

Blood Flow

B Oxygen from the lungs combines with nutrients to provide energy.

A Hormones from glands help regulate cell activity.

F Carbon dioxide, a waste gas, is carried away and delivered to the lungs, which remove it from the body.

Parts of the Circulatory System

Your circulatory system includes your heart, blood vessels, and blood (see **Figure 15.5**). Your heart pumps blood through two major pathways. **Pulmonary circulation** is *the flow of blood from the heart to the lungs and back to the heart.* **Systemic circulation** is *the flow of blood to all the body tissues except the lungs.*

FIGURE 15.5

THE CIRCULATORY SYSTEM

In these drawings, red represents oxygen-rich blood, and blue represents blood containing carbon dioxide.

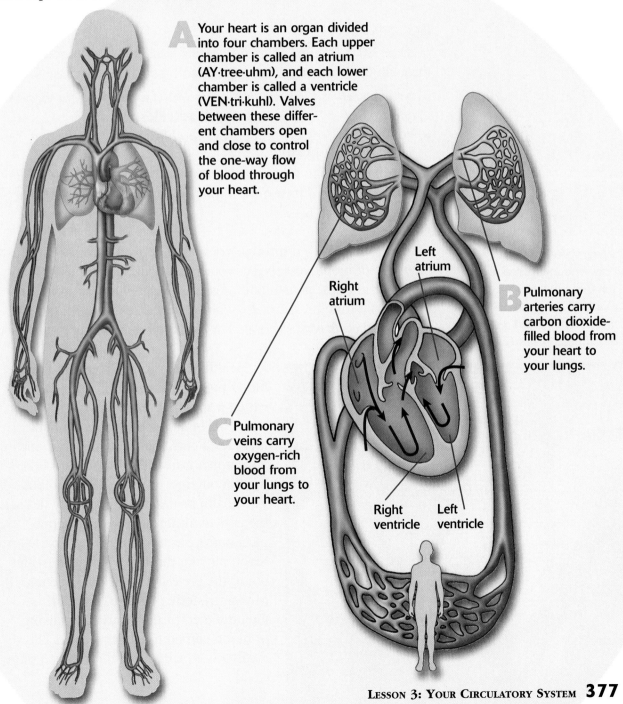

A Your heart is an organ divided into four chambers. Each upper chamber is called an atrium (AY·tree·uhm), and each lower chamber is called a ventricle (VEN·tri·kuhl). Valves between these different chambers open and close to control the one-way flow of blood through your heart.

B Pulmonary arteries carry carbon dioxide-filled blood from your heart to your lungs.

C Pulmonary veins carry oxygen-rich blood from your lungs to your heart.

Right atrium

Left atrium

Right ventricle

Left ventricle

✓ **Reading Check**

The word *circulatory* comes from a Latin word meaning "to go around." Use a dictionary to find other words stemming from the same root, *circul.*

Blood

Blood is a mixture of solids in a large amount of liquid called plasma (PLAZ·muh). The different solid components of blood are red blood cells, white blood cells, and platelets.

- **Plasma** is about 92 percent water. It transports blood solids, nutrients, hormones, and other materials.
- **Red blood cells** carry oxygen to cells and carbon dioxide away from them.
- **White blood cells** help fight disease and infection by attacking germs that enter the body.
- **Platelets** help blood form a clot at the site of a wound. A clot seals a cut and prevents excessive blood loss.

Blood Vessels

Over 80,000 miles of blood vessels transport your blood throughout your body. There are three types of blood vessels.

- **Arteries.** *Blood vessels that carry blood away from the heart to other parts of the body* are called **arteries**.
- **Veins.** *Blood vessels that carry blood from the body back to the heart* are called **veins**.
- **Capillaries.** *Tiny tubes that carry blood from the arteries to the body's cells, and then back to the veins* are called **capillaries**.

Blood Pressure

As blood is moved through your body, it exerts pressure against the walls of blood vessels. As your heart contracts to push blood into your arteries, your blood pressure is at its highest point. This is called systolic pressure. As your heart relaxes to refill, blood pressure is at its lowest point. This is called diastolic pressure.

Having your blood pressure measured is a normal part of a physical exam. *What pressure measurements are taken during this procedure?*

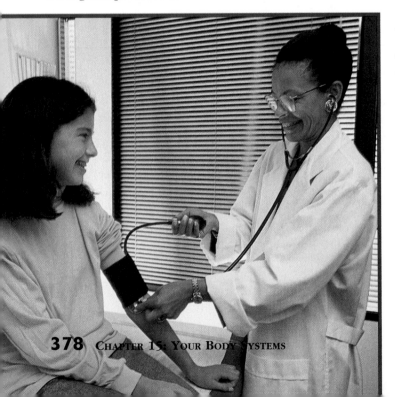

Health professionals measure your blood pressure using an instrument called a sphygmomanometer (sfig·mo·muh·NAH·muh·ter). This instrument includes a cuff that is wrapped around your upper arm and inflated until it is tight enough to stop the flow of blood. The health professional gradually deflates the cuff until, through a stethoscope placed on your arm, she or he first hears blood pulsing through your arm. At this point, the pressure in the cuff is equal to your systolic pressure. The cuff is then deflated further, until the pulsing of blood can no longer be heard. This reading is equal to your diastolic pressure.

Blood Types

There are four different blood types—A, B, AB, and O. These blood types are determined by the presence or absence of certain substances. Type A blood has substance A, type B has substance B, type AB has both A and B, and type O has neither. Blood may also carry another substance—the Rh factor. Most people are Rh positive, which is written as Rh+.

Knowing a person's blood type is essential if the person needs a blood transfusion. Mixing certain blood types can cause dangerous immune responses such as fevers, difficulty in breathing, and possibly death. To avoid these responses, health professionals check the recipient's blood type and match it with a blood type that is compatible. People with type O-negative blood are called universal donors because their blood is compatible with all blood types.

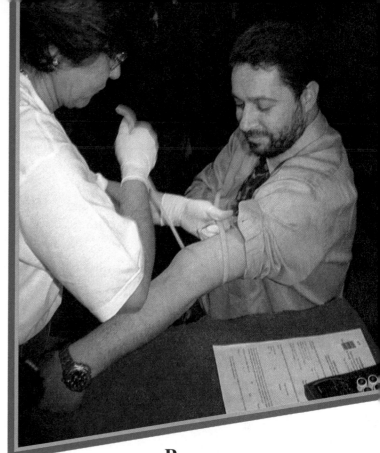

People who are between the ages of 17 and 70 and in good health can give the gift of life—their blood.

Giving and Receiving Blood

People who are between the ages of 17 and 70 and in good health can give blood to the Red Cross or to other charitable organizations. The blood is frozen or refrigerated and stored in blood banks for later use by hospitals. United States regulations make it very safe to give and receive blood. A new needle is used every time blood is taken or received. All donated blood is tested for diseases such as HIV, anemia, and hepatitis. Blood that fails any test is discarded.

Problems of the Circulatory System

Some problems of the circulatory system affect the heart and blood vessels. Others affect the blood itself.

- **Hypertension** is a condition in which blood pressure is consistently higher than normal, which can lead to heart attack, stroke, or kidney failure.
- **Stroke** usually results from blood clots that block vessels in the brain, or from the rupture of a blood vessel.
- **Heart attack** is blockage of the flow of blood to the heart.
- **Arteriosclerosis** is a condition in which arteries harden, reducing the amount of blood that can flow through them.

Science

ANEMIA AND YOUR FOOD
Anemia is a condition in which red blood cells cannot carry sufficient amounts of oxygen to other cells in the body. The most common type of anemia is iron-deficiency anemia. You can increase the iron levels in your diet by eating iron-fortified cereal, green leafy vegetables, dried beans, and raisins.

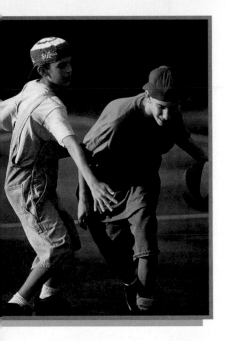

- **Anemia** is an abnormally low level of hemoglobin, a protein that binds to oxygen in red blood cells.
- **Leukemia** is a disease in which extra white blood cells are produced.
- **Hemophilia** is a disease in which the blood plasma does not contain substances that help the blood to clot.

Care of the Circulatory System

Keeping your heart strong and healthy will help you feel better now and may also enable you to live a longer, healthier life.

- **Limit fat in your foods.** Dietary fat can cause fatty deposits to form on the inner walls of arteries, narrowing them and increasing blood pressure. Then your heart must work harder to circulate blood.
- **Get regular physical activity.** Regular activity strengthens your heart muscle, allowing it to pump more blood with each beat.
- **Avoid tobacco.** Tobacco products contain the drug nicotine. Nicotine narrows arteries, requiring blood pressure to be higher to circulate blood through the body.
- **Manage stress.** When you are under stress, your body secretes adrenaline, a substance that increases blood pressure. High blood pressure strains the entire cardiovascular system.

Learning to manage stress by taking time to relax and get exercise will help keep your cardiovascular system healthy. *How can stress affect blood pressure?*

Lesson 3 Review

Using complete sentences, answer the following questions on a sheet of paper.

Reviewing Terms and Facts

1. **Vocabulary** Define the term *circulatory system*. What is another name for it?
2. **Recall** Identify the three solids that make up blood. What is the liquid portion of blood called?
3. **Review** What are *arteries, veins,* and *capillaries?* Explain how they are different.
4. **List** What steps are taken in the United States to make sure that donated blood is safe?

Thinking Critically

5. **Compare and Contrast** What are *systemic circulation* and *pulmonary circulation?* Which one carries newly oxygenated blood?
6. **Analyze** Your friend Colleen has been looking tired and pale. Which circulatory disorder might she have? What can you suggest to help?

Applying Health Skills

7. **Accessing Information** Learn more about how one of the following substances affects your circulatory system: *salt, fats, cholesterol.* Prepare a brief presentation for your classmates.

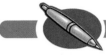
Your Respiratory System

The Need for Air

Air contains oxygen, a gas the body needs to maintain life. In fact, a person can live only a few minutes without air. Breathing—inhaling and exhaling—is carried out by the **respiratory system**. This system consists of *the organs that provide the body with a continuous supply of oxygen and rid the body of carbon dioxide.* **Figure 15.6** on page 382 shows the parts of the respiratory system.

How the Respiratory System Works

The respiratory system has two important jobs. First, it supplies oxygen to the blood—oxygen that is then carried to all the cells of the body. In the cells, oxygen combines with nutrients to provide energy that the cells can use. When oxygen is used to produce energy in the cells, carbon dioxide—a waste gas—is produced. The second job of the respiratory system is to remove carbon dioxide from the blood and release it outside the body.

Quick Write

List at least three conditions or situations that can affect the health of your lungs.

LEARN ABOUT...

- the parts of your respiratory system.
- how your body uses the air that you breathe.
- keeping your respiratory system healthy.

VOCABULARY

- respiratory system
- epiglottis
- larynx
- trachea
- bronchi
- diaphragm
- alveoli

The carbon dioxide that you breathe out is absorbed by plants and converted back into oxygen. *Why do you need oxygen?*

LESSON 4: YOUR RESPIRATORY SYSTEM **381**

FIGURE 15.6

THE RESPIRATORY SYSTEM

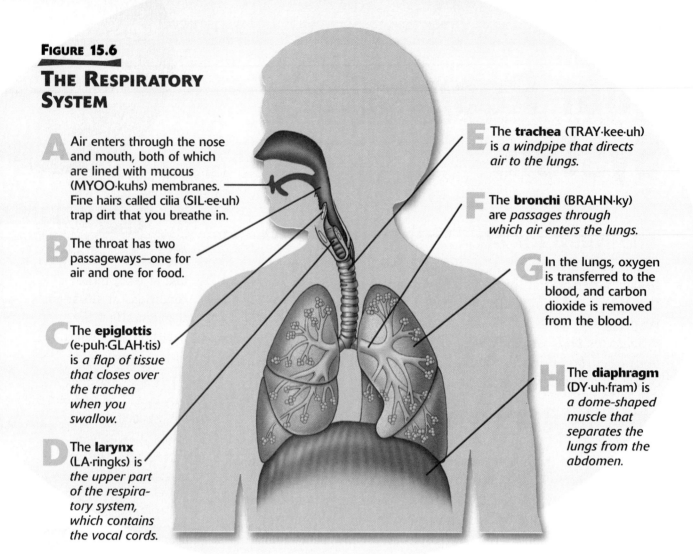

A Air enters through the nose and mouth, both of which are lined with mucous (MYOO·kuhs) membranes. Fine hairs called cilia (SIL·ee·uh) trap dirt that you breathe in.

B The throat has two passageways—one for air and one for food.

C The **epiglottis** (e·puh·GLAH·tis) is *a flap of tissue that closes over the trachea when you swallow.*

D The **larynx** (LA·ringks) is *the upper part of the respiratory system, which contains the vocal cords.*

E The **trachea** (TRAY·kee·uh) is *a windpipe that directs air to the lungs.*

F The **bronchi** (BRAHN·ky) are *passages through which air enters the lungs.*

G In the lungs, oxygen is transferred to the blood, and carbon dioxide is removed from the blood.

H The **diaphragm** (DY·uh·fram) is *a dome-shaped muscle that separates the lungs from the abdomen.*

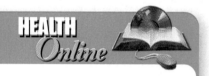

Topic: The respiratory system

For a link to more information on the parts of the respiratory system, go to **health.glencoe.com**.

Activity: Using the information provided at this link, create your own word search puzzle that features respiratory system terms.

Inhaling and Exhaling

When you inhale, you bring air into your body from outside. When you exhale, you release air to the outside. In this process, oxygen is exchanged with carbon dioxide inside your lungs. This continual exchange of gases helps maintain a constant supply of oxygen in your cells. **Figure 15.7** describes the process of inhaling and exhaling.

Exchanging Oxygen and Carbon Dioxide

The air that you exhale contains more carbon dioxide and less oxygen than the air that you inhale. Carbon dioxide–containing blood is pumped from the heart to the lungs through the pulmonary arteries and capillaries. Carbon dioxide passes from the blood into bronchioles, which are smaller bronchial tubes, and then into **alveoli** (al·VEE·uh·ly), *microscopic air sacs in the lungs,* where it is exchanged with oxygen. Oxygen passes from the alveoli to the capillaries and into the blood.

Problems of the Respiratory System

Problems of the respiratory system include the following.

- **Influenza** and colds are caused by viruses. The symptoms include coughing, runny nose, aches, and fever.
- **Bronchitis** is swelling of bronchi—the lungs' air passages— due to infection. It causes coughing, fever, and chest tightness.
- **Allergies** are immune responses to foreign substances in the environment. They can cause sneezing, itchy eyes, runny nose, and hives.
- **Asthma** is an inflammatory disease that causes the bronchi to become blocked or narrowed. Its symptoms are wheezing, shortness of breath, and coughing.
- **Pneumonia** is a lung infection caused by viruses or bacteria. It can lead to fever, chest pain, and breathing difficulties.
- **Emphysema** is a disease in which the alveoli are damaged or destroyed. Strongly linked to smoking, it causes serious breathing difficulties.
- **Tuberculosis** is a bacterial lung infection that causes a dry cough in early stages and chest pain later on.
- **Lung cancer** is a disease in which tissues of the lung are destroyed by the growth of a tumor. The cause in most cases is smoking or secondhand smoke.

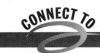

CONNECT TO
Performing Arts

SELF-CARE FOR SINGERS
Professional singers must take extra care to keep their vocal cords, throat, and lungs healthy. The most important rule they follow is no smoking. Smoking irritates the vocal cords, causing the tissues to swell up with water. The increased weight of the water makes the vocal cords heavier and lowers the voice's pitch.

FIGURE 15.7

How Breathing Works

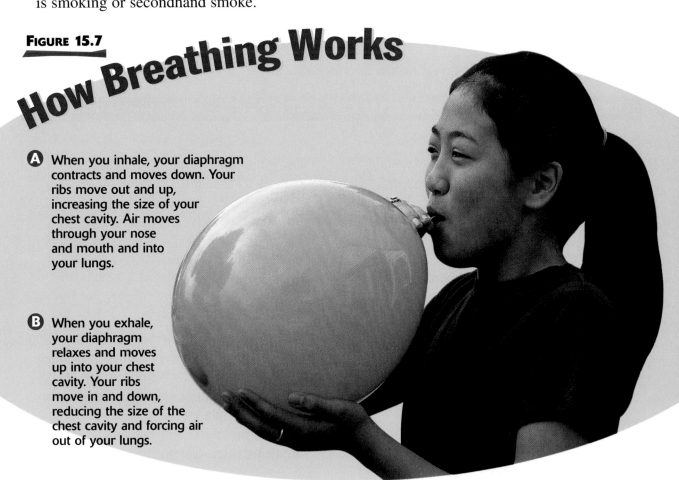

A When you inhale, your diaphragm contracts and moves down. Your ribs move out and up, increasing the size of your chest cavity. Air moves through your nose and mouth and into your lungs.

B When you exhale, your diaphragm relaxes and moves up into your chest cavity. Your ribs move in and down, reducing the size of the chest cavity and forcing air out of your lungs.

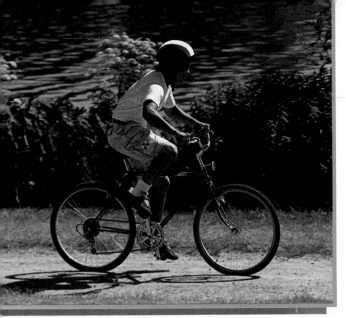

Care of the Respiratory System

You can keep your respiratory system working at its peak by following some commonsense practices.

- **Stay active.** Regular physical activity strengthens your lungs and helps keep other parts of your respiratory system clear. It also strengthens your diaphragm, making it easier for you to breathe.
- **Avoid smoking and secondhand smoke.** Smoking cigarettes, cigars, pipes, or marijuana puts you at increased risk for lung cancer, emphysema, and other respiratory diseases.

You can reduce your exposure to polluted air by avoiding areas with heavy traffic. *Where in your community is the air healthy for outdoor activity?*

- **Avoid polluted air.** When you breathe air that is polluted, you get less oxygen with each breath than you otherwise would. If you ride your bike, for example, choose a road with lighter traffic so you breathe cleaner air.
- **Reduce your risk of respiratory infection.** The respiratory system is highly susceptible to infection by bacteria and viruses—many of which are carried on your hands. To reduce the risk of infection, wash your hands regularly with soap and water and avoid touching your nose and mouth.

Lesson 4 Review

Using complete sentences, answer the following questions on a sheet of paper.

Reviewing Terms and Facts

1. **List** What are the two important jobs of the respiratory system?
2. **Vocabulary** Define the words *epiglottis* and *trachea*.
3. **List** Name three parts of the respiratory system. Name the parts that exchange oxygen for carbon dioxide.
4. **Recall** How does physical activity promote the health of the respiratory system?

Thinking Critically

5. **Synthesize** What happens when you inhale? What happens when you exhale?

Draw a simple diagram showing the path of air through your respiratory system and explain what is happening.

6. **Summarize** List and give a brief explanation of the diseases of the respiratory system that are caused by tobacco smoke.

Applying Health Skills

7. **Refusal Skills** While walking home from school, Nick was offered some inhalants by an older student. Write a script in which Nick applies refusal strategies for avoiding inhalants and points out the damage that these substances can cause to the respiratory system.

Your Nervous System

The Nerve Center

What do riding a bicycle, reading this book, and recognizing the face of a friend have in common? They all result from the activity of your body's control center—your nervous system. The *specialized cells that make up the nervous system* are called nerve cells or **neurons** (NOO·rahnz). Neurons carry information. In **Figure 15.8**, you can see that neurons send messages from the body to the brain, and from the brain to the body. These messages are in the form of electrical signals.

FIGURE 15.8

HOW THE NERVOUS SYSTEM WORKS

Neurons are specialized cells that send quick messages through the brain and body.

Quick Write

Write down at least five different kinds of information you are taking in with your senses right now.

LEARN ABOUT...

- how the nervous system works.
- the different parts of the nervous system.
- protecting your nervous system from injury.

VOCABULARY

- neurons
- central nervous system (CNS)
- peripheral nervous system (PNS)
- somatic system
- autonomic system

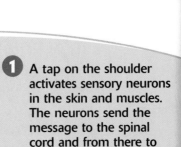

1 A tap on the shoulder activates sensory neurons in the skin and muscles. The neurons send the message to the spinal cord and from there to the brain.

2 One part of the brain interprets the message received as a touch.

3 Another part of the brain sends a message to motor neurons in muscles in the body. Muscles in the head and neck are activated, and the head turns.

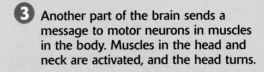

Parts of the Nervous System

Your nervous system has two main parts, as shown in **Figure 15.9**. The **central nervous system (CNS)** includes *the brain and spinal cord.* It is the body's main control center. The **peripheral nervous system (PNS)** includes *the nerves that connect the CNS to all parts of the body.* A nerve is a bundle of long extensions of many neurons. A nerve acts like an electrical cord, moving electrical signals through the nervous system.

FIGURE 15.9

THE NERVOUS SYSTEM

The nervous system controls all of your body's actions. The central nervous system (yellow) and the peripheral nervous system (blue) work together. Shown here are 31 pairs of spinal nerves that branch off from the spinal cord. Each pair serves a particular part of the body.

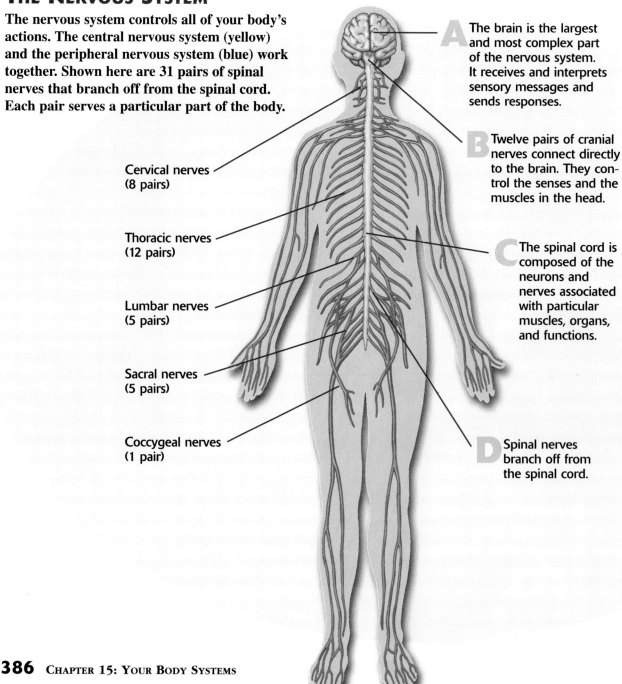

Cervical nerves
(8 pairs)

Thoracic nerves
(12 pairs)

Lumbar nerves
(5 pairs)

Sacral nerves
(5 pairs)

Coccygeal nerves
(1 pair)

A The brain is the largest and most complex part of the nervous system. It receives and interprets sensory messages and sends responses.

B Twelve pairs of cranial nerves connect directly to the brain. They control the senses and the muscles in the head.

C The spinal cord is composed of the neurons and nerves associated with particular muscles, organs, and functions.

D Spinal nerves branch off from the spinal cord.

Central Nervous System

The central nervous system (CNS) controls two kinds of actions. Involuntary actions are those that you do not control by thinking about them, such as your heartbeat and certain digestive processes. Voluntary actions are those, such as walking and talking, that you can control.

The CNS has two main parts. The brain, shown in **Figure 15.10**, is composed of about 10 billion neurons that control all actions, thoughts, and memory. It weighs about 3 pounds and is encased in the bones of your skull.

The spinal cord is a long bundle of many nerves and associated neurons that extends from the base of the brain to the bottom of the backbone. The spinal cord relays messages from the brain to the body and from the body to the brain. Your spinal cord, which is less than 2 feet long and about the same diameter as your index finger, is protected by your backbone.

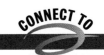

CONNECT TO

Science

BREATH CONTROL
Some automatic functions such as breathing and heartbeat occur in a regular rhythm. Breathing, unlike heartbeat, can be controlled consciously. Breathe naturally and count your breaths for a 60-second period. Then for a second 60-second period, breathe more slowly and count your breaths. *How much control does it take to override your body's natural breathing rhythm?*

FIGURE 15.10

PARTS OF THE BRAIN

Like a computer, the brain is composed of many distinct parts, each with a different function.

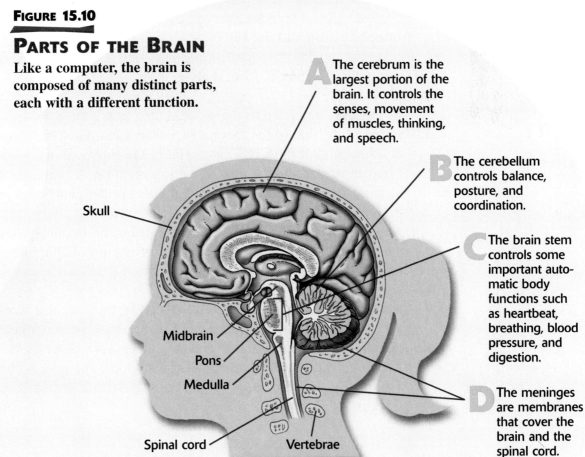

A The cerebrum is the largest portion of the brain. It controls the senses, movement of muscles, thinking, and speech.

B The cerebellum controls balance, posture, and coordination.

C The brain stem controls some important automatic body functions such as heartbeat, breathing, blood pressure, and digestion.

D The meninges are membranes that cover the brain and the spinal cord.

Skull

Midbrain
Pons
Medulla
Spinal cord   Vertebrae

Reading Check

Write *Central Nervous System* in a rectangle. Add *Problems* and *Care* in two ovals branching from the rectangle. List examples of each branching from these ovals.

Peripheral Nervous System

The peripheral nervous system is composed of neurons throughout the body and the nerves that connect them to the central nervous system. The PNS has two main parts. The **somatic** (soh·MA·tik) **system** is *a system dealing with actions that you control.* The nerves that lead to and from muscles in your arms and legs are part of the somatic system. The second part, the **autonomic** (aw·tuh·NAH·mik) **system**, is *a system dealing with actions you do not usually control,* such as digestion and breathing.

Problems of the Nervous System

Several diseases and disorders—most resulting from injury—can affect the nervous system.

- **Head injury** is usually caused by a blow to the head. It can also follow violent jarring of the head, causing the brain to hit the interior of the skull. This injury is called a concussion. Head injuries kill brain neurons, which cannot be replaced. A physician should immediately evaluate a person who sustains a head injury.
- **Spinal cord injury** can result from damage to the head, neck, or body. If the spinal cord is damaged or severed, paralysis of all or part of the body may result.
- **Nerve inflammation** can follow a minor injury. This condition, often called a "pinched nerve," causes pain in a single part of the body, such as the elbow or shoulder. A physician may suggest resting the affected area and may prescribe medicine to reduce pain and inflammation.

Diseases unrelated to injuries can also attack the nervous system. Infection of the meninges, called meningitis, or infection of other parts of the CNS, can result in life-threatening situations. Many infections can be treated with medication. A brain tumor is an abnormal growth of tissue that kills normal neurons around it. Some brain tumors are surgically removed or treated in other ways. In the disease epilepsy, a small area of brain damage causes the person to have seizures—episodes of uncontrollable muscle activity. Epilepsy is usually controlled with medication.

Some diseases are degenerative—that is, they become worse over time. In multiple sclerosis (MS), the protective outer coating of nerves is damaged, and nerves no longer work properly. Alzheimer's disease, which affects mostly older people, is characterized by inflamed areas in the brain and death of neurons.

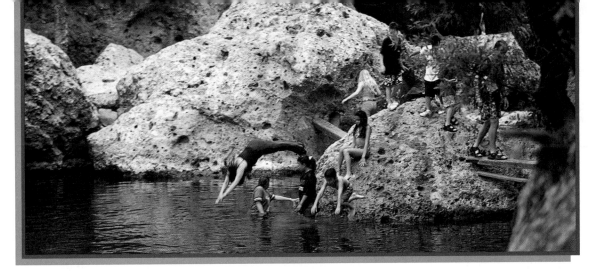

Care of the Nervous System

Following the strategies listed below can help protect the nervous system and prevent many head and spinal cord injuries.

- **Get enough sleep.** Your nervous system needs rest and sleep to function correctly.
- **Avoid alcohol and other drugs.** Alcohol and many other drugs may destroy brain cells, disturb automatic body functions such as breathing, and interfere with thoughts and emotions.
- **Play safely.** Wear appropriate safety helmets and equipment for sports.
- **Wear a safety belt.** Whenever you are in a moving vehicle, fasten your safety belt.
- **Obey all traffic safety rules.** Whether you are on a bike, scooter, or skateboard, or out walking, obey all traffic signs and rules.

Diving into shallow water can cause serious head or spinal cord injury. Never dive into water unless you know its depth. *What are two other behaviors that can maintain the health of your nervous system?*

Lesson 5 Review

Using complete sentences, answer the following questions on a sheet of paper.

Reviewing Terms and Facts

1. **Vocabulary** What are *neurons?* What do they do?
2. **Compare** What is the difference between the somatic system and the autonomic system?
3. **Describe** What is a concussion? What causes it?
4. **Summarize** What are five ways to avoid injury to your nervous system?

Thinking Critically

5. **Apply** Explain what happens in your nervous system when you catch a ball.
6. **Analyze** How can strategies such as getting enough sleep and avoiding alcohol and other drugs help protect the nervous system from accidental injury?

Applying Health Skills

7. **Advocacy** Write and perform a skit to demonstrate to younger children how to protect their nervous systems.

Your Digestive and Excretory Systems

The Digestive System

Food is the fuel you eat to give your body energy. **Digestion** (dy·JES·chuhn) is *the changing of food you eat into substances the body can use.* Your **digestive system** is *an organ system that converts food to a form useful to the body.* As food is digested, chemical energy in the food is unlocked. Moreover, the body uses some substances in foods to repair and make new cells.

The Mouth and Teeth

Digestion begins in the mouth. Your teeth cut and grind food into smaller pieces. At the same time, saliva moistens and softens food. **Saliva** (suh·LY·vuh) is *fluid produced by the salivary glands.* Saliva is about 99 percent water, but it also contains enzymes that begin chemical digestion. **Figure 15.11** shows what happens when you swallow.

FIGURE 15.11

THE PROCESS OF SWALLOWING

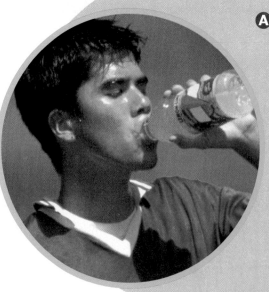

A Before Swallowing
Air passages from the nose and throat to the trachea, or windpipe, are open, allowing air into the lungs.

B During Swallowing
Air passages are closed by two flaps of skin at the back of your throat. The uvula (YOO·vyuh·luh) closes the airway to the nose. The epiglottis closes the opening to the trachea, or windpipe.

The Stomach and the Small Intestine

See **Figure 15.12** and trace the path food takes in the digestive system. When you swallow, food enters your esophagus, a muscular tube that pushes food down into the stomach. The stomach is a muscular sac that collects food and churns it, much like a food processor does. Glands in the walls of the stomach secrete gastric juices—an acidic enzyme mixture. These enzymes begin to chemically break down proteins.

From the stomach, the partially digested food moves into the **small intestine**, *a coiled, tubelike organ that is about 20 feet long.* The small intestine absorbs the digested nutrients, which are used by the body for growth, energy, and repair. Most digestion takes place in the duodenum (doo·uh·DEE·nuhm), the first section of the small intestine.

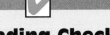

Reading Check

Create a sequence chart. Use the text and the diagrams to write captions explaining the order of the digestive process.

FIGURE 15.12

THE DIGESTIVE SYSTEM

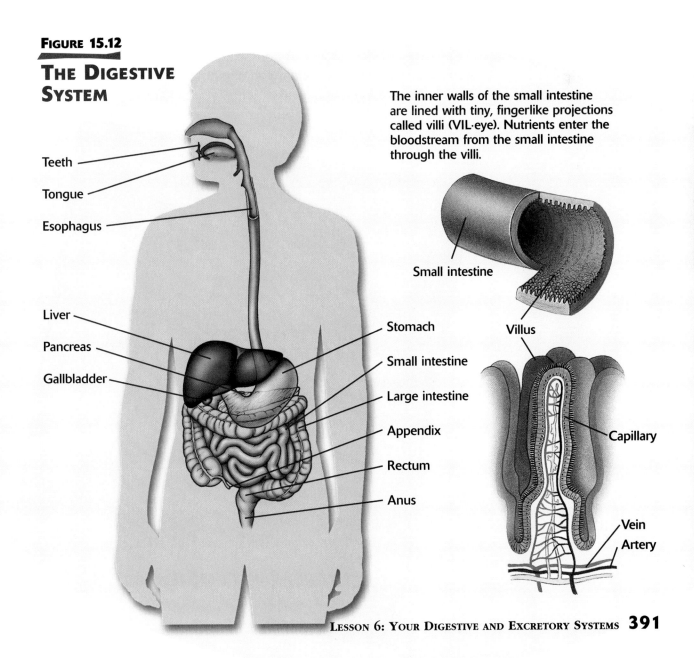

Teeth

Tongue

Esophagus

Liver

Pancreas

Gallbladder

Stomach

Small intestine

Large intestine

Appendix

Rectum

Anus

The inner walls of the small intestine are lined with tiny, fingerlike projections called villi (VIL·eye). Nutrients enter the bloodstream from the small intestine through the villi.

Small intestine

Villus

Capillary

Vein

Artery

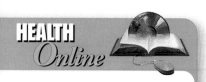
The Liver, Gallbladder, and Pancreas

The digestive system includes three important organs through which food does not pass. These are:

- **Liver.** *A large gland that has many digestive functions* is the **liver**. It produces bile, a substance that aids in the digestion of fats.
- **Gallbladder.** *A small, saclike organ that stores bile* is the **gallbladder**. It releases bile as needed into the small intestine.
- **Pancreas.** *An organ that produces enzymes that assist in digestion* is the **pancreas**. Enzymes are released directly into the small intestine.

The Excretory System

Your **excretory system** is *a system that removes wastes from the body.* Your body produces wastes in the form of solids, liquids, and gas. Solid waste is composed of the parts of foods that could not be digested. For example, humans do not digest cellulose, found in fruits and vegetables. Liquid and gaseous wastes are by-products of the activity of body cells. The skin excretes some wastes through its pores when you perspire. Your lungs expel carbon dioxide, a gaseous waste, when you exhale.

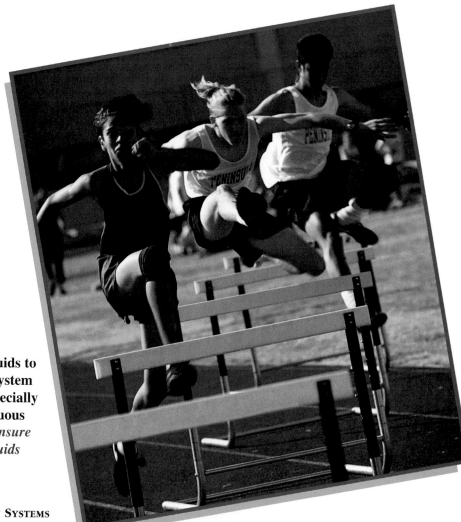

You need plenty of fluids to keep your excretory system working properly, especially if you engage in strenuous activity. *How do you ensure that you get enough fluids when exercising?*

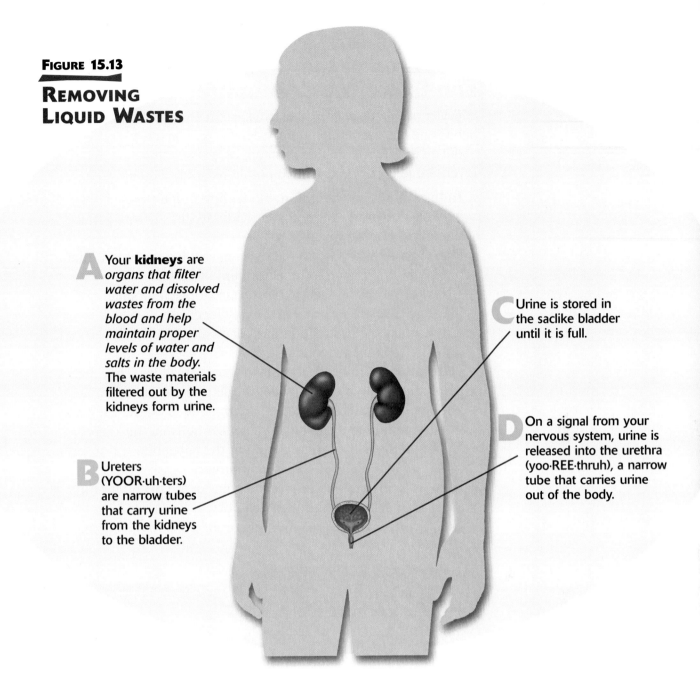

FIGURE 15.13

REMOVING LIQUID WASTES

A Your **kidneys** are *organs that filter water and dissolved wastes from the blood and help maintain proper levels of water and salts in the body.* The waste materials filtered out by the kidneys form urine.

B Ureters (YOOR·uh·ters) are narrow tubes that carry urine from the kidneys to the bladder.

C Urine is stored in the saclike bladder until it is full.

D On a signal from your nervous system, urine is released into the urethra (yoo·REE·thruh), a narrow tube that carries urine out of the body.

The Colon, Kidneys, and Bladder

Excretion (ek·SKREE·shuhn) is *the process of removing wastes from the body.* Remains of food that your body cannot digest pass into the **colon** (KOH·luhn), that is, *the large intestine.* The lining of the colon absorbs most of the liquid from undigested material. The solids that are left are called *feces* (FEE·seez). When the large intestine is full, nerves signal muscles in the walls of the colon to contract. This action pushes feces through the *anus* (AY·nuhs) and out of the body.

Many wastes produced in your body are dissolved in water. The organs involved in removing liquid wastes are shown in **Figure 15.13**.

Problems of the Digestive and Excretory Systems

Most problems of the digestive system are related to eating habits and are usually temporary. However, consult a physician about a persistent digestive problem or one accompanied by a fever. Some common digestive problems are listed below.

- **Indigestion** is an uncomfortable feeling in the stomach that may result from eating spicy or acidic foods, or from eating too quickly or too much.
- **Diarrhea**—watery feces—may be caused by bacteria in food or may be a symptom of another kind of disease.
- **Ulcers** are sores on the interior of the stomach or small intestine. They are painful and may bleed.
- **Cirrhosis** is the destruction of liver tissue, usually caused by drinking too much alcohol.
- **Gallstones** are mineral crystals in the gallbladder. They are painful and may block passage of bile to the small intestine.
- **Kidney stones**, like gallstones, are mineral crystals. They may be very painful and can block exit of urine from the kidney.
- **Appendicitis** is the inflammation of the appendix. It is a serious condition that requires emergency surgery.
- **Hemorrhoids** are swelling of the veins at the opening of the anus. They may be painful and can bleed.
- **Colon cancer** is the growth of abnormal cells in the colon.

HEALTH SKILLS ACTIVITY

ADVOCACY

Encouraging Healthy Eating

Problems of the digestive system often result from eating the wrong foods, from eating on the run, or from other unhealthful eating behaviors. Encourage healthful eating by getting reliable information and by spreading the word to those who could benefit from it.

- **LEARN MORE ABOUT NUTRITION.** Invite a speaker, such as a registered dietician, to talk to your class about common digestive problems and about the role of nutrition in preventing them. In advance, prepare questions about nutrition for teens and teen athletes.

- **GATHER RELIABLE HEALTH INFORMATION.** Use reliable Web sites to gather information about promoting healthy digestion.

WITH A GROUP
Make a poster about nutrition for teens that shows choices that will promote healthy digestion. Ask for permission to display your poster in the school cafeteria.

Care of the Digestive and Excretory Systems

Follow the simple guidelines below for maintaining the health of your digestive and excretory systems.

- **Eat a variety of foods.** Choose low-fat and high-fiber foods from all food groups. Fiber helps keep materials moving through the digestive tract. Include many fruits and vegetables.
- **Eat complete meals.** Eating breakfast is especially important.
- **Do not rush your meals.** Take the time to relax and enjoy your food.
- **Chew food thoroughly.** Do not try to wash large pieces of food down with a beverage.
- **Drink plenty of water.** Your digestive system needs water to work properly. Drink six to eight 8-ounce glasses each day.
- **Get regular dental checkups.** Strong, healthy teeth are essential to the first step in digestion—breaking food into small pieces.

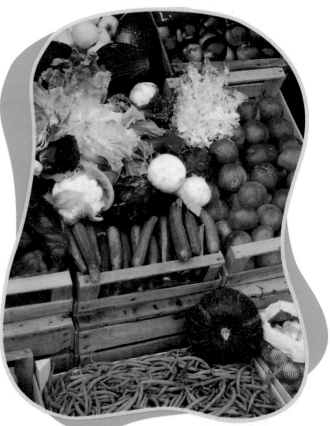

One of the best ways to prevent digestive problems is to eat foods that are high in fiber, such as fruits, vegetables, and dried beans. *What are some of your favorite high-fiber foods?*

 Lesson 6 Review

Using complete sentences, answer the following questions on a sheet of paper.

Reviewing Terms and Facts

1. **Vocabulary** What is *digestion?* Where does it begin?
2. **Identify** How does the liver aid digestion?
3. **Explain** What does the excretory system do?
4. **Summarize** List five mealtime guidelines that help promote healthy digestion.

Thinking Critically

5. **Synthesize** Describe the path of a meal through the digestive system.
6. **Explain** How can healthy teeth contribute to healthy digestion?

Applying Health Skills

7. **Accessing Information** Find a recent article in a magazine, health newsletter, or newspaper about the causes of ulcers. What is the current thinking about the main causes of ulcers? How are ulcers treated? Share your findings with the class. Tell what source you used and how you know it is reliable.

Your Endocrine System

Quick Write

Think about an event that caused you stress. Describe your physical reactions to the stress.

LEARN ABOUT...

- the functions of the endocrine system.
- how your endocrine system prepares your body for stress.
- disorders of the endocrine system.

VOCABULARY

- endocrine system
- gland
- pituitary gland

Regulating Body Functions

Your nervous system has been described as your body's control center. Working closely with your nervous system is the **endocrine** (EN·duh·krin) **system**, *a chemical communication system that regulates many body functions.* During adolescence, the endocrine system plays an important role in growth and development. It is composed of a network of glands located throughout your body.

A **gland** is *a group of cells, or an organ, that secretes a chemical substance.* The endocrine glands secrete chemicals called hormones directly into the bloodstream. The blood carries the hormones directly to the tissue they are targeted to affect. Some hormones are produced continuously, while others are produced only at certain times.

Glands of the Endocrine System

Each type of hormone produced by the endocrine system has a specific job. **Figure 15.14** shows the locations of the endocrine glands and tells what each one does.

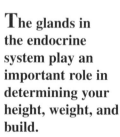

The glands in the endocrine system play an important role in determining your height, weight, and build.

The endocrine glands work by taking signals from the brain or from other glands. The brain receives electrical and chemical messages from the body about the presence of substances in the blood. The **pituitary** (pi·TOO·I·tehr·ee) **gland** at the base of the brain is *a gland that signals other endocrine glands to produce hormones when needed.*

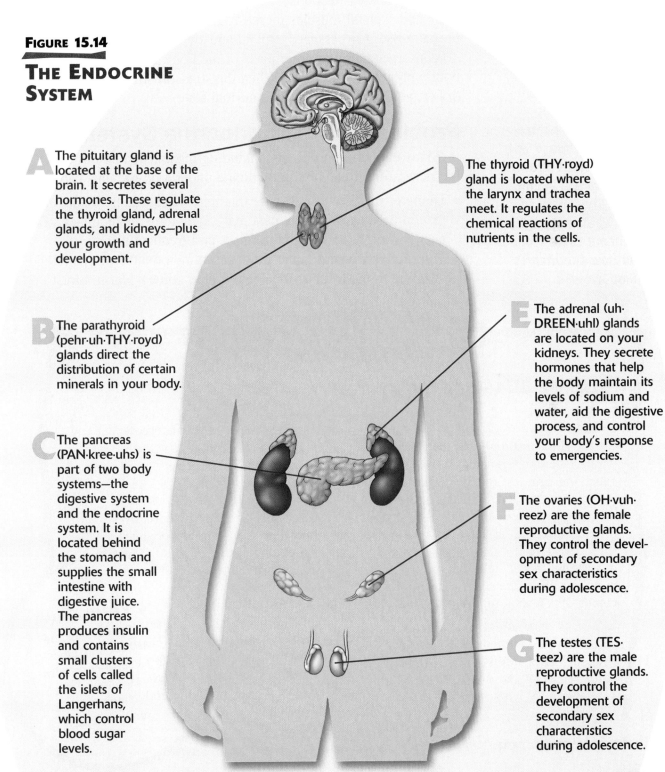

FIGURE 15.14

THE ENDOCRINE SYSTEM

A The pituitary gland is located at the base of the brain. It secretes several hormones. These regulate the thyroid gland, adrenal glands, and kidneys—plus your growth and development.

B The parathyroid (pehr·uh·THY·royd) glands direct the distribution of certain minerals in your body.

C The pancreas (PAN·kree·uhs) is part of two body systems—the digestive system and the endocrine system. It is located behind the stomach and supplies the small intestine with digestive juice. The pancreas produces insulin and contains small clusters of cells called the islets of Langerhans, which control blood sugar levels.

D The thyroid (THY·royd) gland is located where the larynx and trachea meet. It regulates the chemical reactions of nutrients in the cells.

E The adrenal (uh·DREEN·uhl) glands are located on your kidneys. They secrete hormones that help the body maintain its levels of sodium and water, aid the digestive process, and control your body's response to emergencies.

F The ovaries (OH·vuh·reez) are the female reproductive glands. They control the development of secondary sex characteristics during adolescence.

G The testes (TES·teez) are the male reproductive glands. They control the development of secondary sex characteristics during adolescence.

The Body's Response to Stress

Remember the last time you were excited or anxious? You may have had sweaty palms or a pounding heart. When your brain recognizes a stressful situation, your adrenal glands respond by releasing the hormone adrenaline. This hormone prepares your body to respond to stress.

During a stress response, heart rate and the blood flow to the brain and skeletal muscles increase. Blood sugar levels and blood pressure rise. Air passages expand and sweat production increases. To conserve energy in other parts of the body, digestion and other bodily processes may slow. When the stressful stimulus withdraws, your body returns to its normal state.

Problems of the Endocrine System

Many endocrine problems, including those listed below, can be successfully treated with medicine under a physician's care.

- **Diabetes mellitus** is a disease that may be caused by inadequate insulin production by the pancreas. Symptoms include lack of energy, weight loss, extreme thirst, and frequent urination.
- **Overactive thyroid** gland produces symptoms that may include swelling in the front of the neck (called goiter), warm, moist

HEALTH SKILLS ACTIVITY

STRESS MANAGEMENT

Protecting Your Body

The stress response enables you to cope with a hazardous situation. It is sometimes called the fight-or-flight response because it prepares your body to take on danger or to get away from it quickly. The stress response becomes harmful if it goes on for too long, or if it occurs too often and in response to situations that are not hazardous. Here are some strategies for coping with a stressful event or situation.

- **TAKE A DEEP BREATH AND THINK IT THROUGH.** Is this situation serious enough to be upset over? Will it have long-term effects on your life or your relationships with others?

- **REDIRECT THE STRESS RESPONSE.** Go for a bike ride or a run. Shoot baskets in the driveway. Physical activity is a great way to defuse stressful feelings.
- **PUT THINGS INTO PERSPECTIVE.** If you find yourself repeatedly upset over small things, make a habit of stopping and putting each situation in perspective.
- **GIVE YOURSELF BREAKS.** Allow yourself some quiet time. Listen to your body and pay attention to signs of stress.

ON YOUR OWN
Poll students on the healthful strategies they use to cope with stress. Choose one and demonstrate it for the class.

skin, trembling hands, nervousness, increased sweating, disturbed sleep, and weight loss.

- **Underactive thyroid** gland can cause a dull facial expression, hoarse voice, facial puffiness, coarse, dry skin and hair, and weight gain.
- **Growth extremes** are caused by abnormal amounts of growth hormones. Too little growth hormone results in a very short person; too much growth hormone results in a very tall person.

Care of the Endocrine System

The best thing you can do for your endocrine system is to keep your body functioning at peak performance. The tips listed below remind you how to do that.

- **Eat balanced meals.** This ensures that you get the nutrients you need.
- **Get enough sleep.** Fatigue is often related to stress.
- **Engage in regular physical activity.** This keeps your body strong and helps manage stress.
- **Keep things in perspective.** Do not get overly upset about things that are not very important.
- **Have regular medical checkups.** Some hormonal disorders have subtle or unusual symptoms. Your doctor can do medical tests to establish that your hormone function is normal.

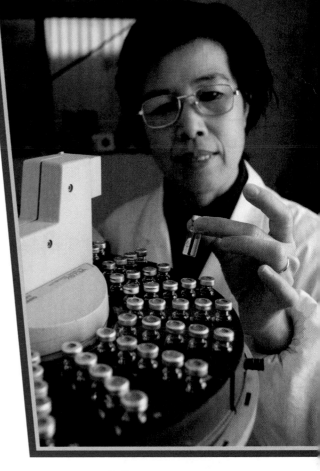

Modern technology makes it easier to identify and treat problems of the endocrine system. However, preventive care is the best way to make sure your endocrine system stays healthy.

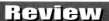

Lesson 7 Review

Using complete sentences, answer the following questions on a sheet of paper.

Reviewing Terms and Facts

1. **Vocabulary** What is a *gland?* Explain the role of glands in the endocrine system.
2. **Review** What is the main function of the pituitary gland?
3. **Identify** Which gland is part of the endocrine system and the digestive system?
4. **Recall** What gland regulates the chemical reactions of nutrients in the cells? Where is it located?

Thinking Critically

5. **Hypothesize** Do you think the fight-or-flight response is less necessary today than in the past? Why or why not?

Applying Health Skills

6. **Accessing Information** Use reliable sources to research how the endocrine system influences growth and development during adolescence. Describe your findings in a brief report.

Your Reproductive System

Quick Write

Why is it important to understand the functioning of both the male and the female reproductive systems?

LEARN ABOUT...

- how sperm are produced.
- the stages of the menstrual cycle.
- ovulation and fertilization.
- keeping your reproductive system healthy.

VOCABULARY

- reproductive system
- sperm
- ovulation
- menstruation
- menstrual cycle
- menopause

The Reproductive System

Reproduction is the process by which life is continued from one generation to the next. A new human life results from the union of two specialized cells, one from a male and the other from a female. These cells, shown in **Figure 15.15**, are produced by the **reproductive** (ree·pruh·DUHK·tiv) **system**, *the organs that make possible the production of offspring*.

Unlike other body systems, the reproductive systems of males and females are not the same. As a result, the potential problems for each system are different. In addition, each system requires different care.

FIGURE 15.15

CELLS OF THE REPRODUCTIVE SYSTEM

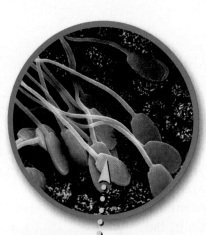

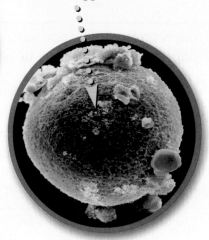

The egg cell in this photograph is magnified. At birth, a female has hundreds of thousands of immature eggs in her ovaries.

The sperm in this photograph are magnified. Approximately 400 million sperm are present in the semen released during a single ejaculation.

The Male Reproductive System

The male reproductive system produces the *male reproductive cells,* called **sperm**. Males begin to produce sperm when they reach puberty, usually between the ages of 12 and 15. The male reproductive system, shown in **Figure 15.16**, includes organs involved in the production and storage of sperm and the release of sperm outside of the body.

Sperm are produced in the testes and mature in the epididymis. From there, they travel through the vas deferens, where they are mixed with seminal (SE·mi·nuhl) fluid, which is produced by the seminal vesicles, the prostate gland, and Cowper's glands. This mixture of sperm and seminal fluid is called semen (SEE·muhn). Muscular contractions force semen through the urethra and out of the body, a process called ejaculation (I·ja·kyuh·LAY·shuhn).

FIGURE 15.16

MALE REPRODUCTIVE SYSTEM

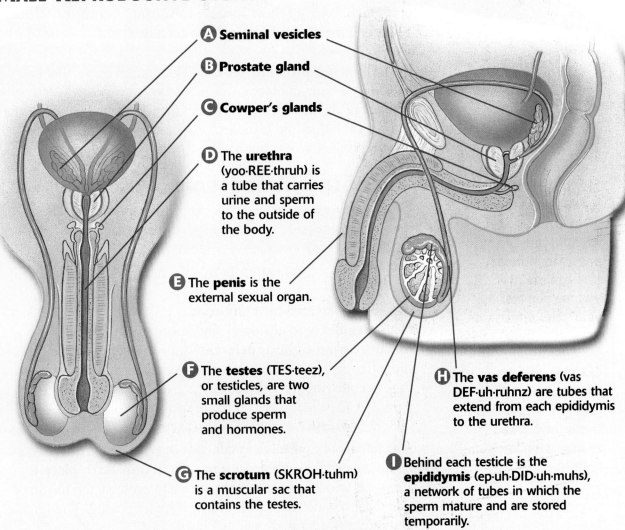

A **Seminal vesicles**

B **Prostate gland**

C **Cowper's glands**

D The **urethra** (yoo·REE·thruh) is a tube that carries urine and sperm to the outside of the body.

E The **penis** is the external sexual organ.

F The **testes** (TES·teez), or testicles, are two small glands that produce sperm and hormones.

G The **scrotum** (SKROH·tuhm) is a muscular sac that contains the testes.

H The **vas deferens** (vas DEF·uh·ruhnz) are tubes that extend from each epididymis to the urethra.

I Behind each testicle is the **epididymis** (ep·uh·DID·uh·muhs), a network of tubes in which the sperm mature and are stored temporarily.

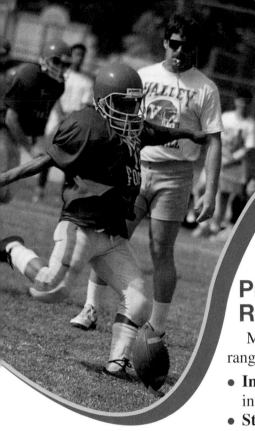

Male teens who engage in any contact sports are advised to use protective equipment to protect their external sexual organs. *For which sports would such equipment be needed?*

Problems of the Male Reproductive System

Males can experience problems with their reproductive systems ranging from merely uncomfortable to very serious.

- **Inguinal hernia** is a tissue separation that allows part of the intestine to push into the scrotum. It may follow heavy lifting.
- **Sterility** is the inability to produce enough healthy sperm to reproduce. It may follow illness or exposure to drugs.
- **Enlarged prostate gland** is a common problem associated with aging.
- **Sexually transmitted diseases (STDs)** are diseases that are spread by sexual contact.
- **Cancer** is uncontrolled cell growth that destroys healthy tissue. Cancer can affect the testicles, prostate, or less often, other male reproductive organs.

Care of the Male Reproductive System

Males should have regular checkups by a physician. The following list provides specific suggestions to help males take good care of their reproductive system.

- **Practice self-examination** of the scrotum and testicles once a month, checking for unusual lumps or swelling. Any change should be evaluated by a physician.
- **Bathe regularly** to ensure cleanliness.
- **Avoid wearing tight underwear**, and wear a protective cup or supporter during athletic activities to prevent accidental injuries.
- **Practice abstinence** from sexual activity before marriage.

The Female Reproductive System

The female reproductive system has many functions. It produces female sex hormones; it stores egg cells; it provides a place for fertilization to occur. It then nourishes and protects the fertilized egg as it grows and matures into a new human being. The female reproductive system is shown in **Figure 15.17**.

Developing Good Character

Responsibility

Take responsibility for your health and learn how to perform a testicular self-examination if you are male, a breast self-examination if you are female. Ask your school nurse or personal physician for information on self-examination. Mark your calendar so that you remember to perform a self-examination each month.

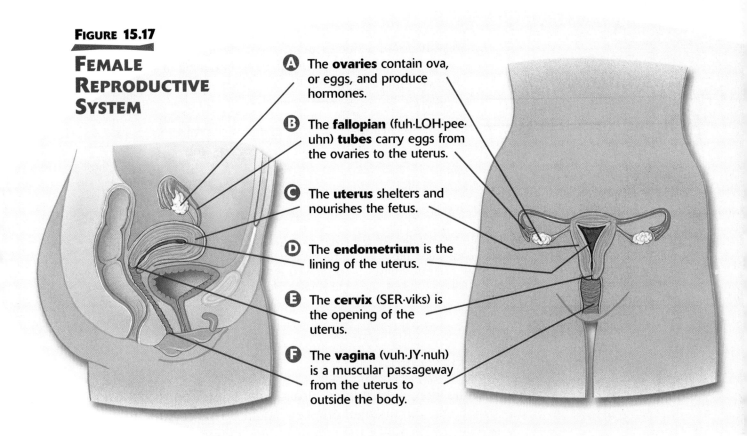

FIGURE 15.17

FEMALE REPRODUCTIVE SYSTEM

A The **ovaries** contain ova, or eggs, and produce hormones.

B The **fallopian** (fuh·LOH·pee·uhn) **tubes** carry eggs from the ovaries to the uterus.

C The **uterus** shelters and nourishes the fetus.

D The **endometrium** is the lining of the uterus.

E The **cervix** (SER·viks) is the opening of the uterus.

F The **vagina** (vuh·JY·nuh) is a muscular passageway from the uterus to outside the body.

The Menstrual Cycle

As a female reaches puberty, hormones cause egg cells to mature in her ovaries. **Ovulation**, *the release of one mature egg cell each month,* begins. The uterus thickens in preparation to receive and begin to nourish a fertilized egg. If fertilization does not occur, the thickened lining breaks down and is expelled. *The flow of the uterine lining out of the body* is called **menstruation**.

The **menstrual cycle** is *the sequence of events in the reproductive system that occurs from one menstruation to another.* Menstruation itself usually lasts from five to seven days. **Figure 15.18** on the next page shows the events of an average menstrual cycle. A cycle usually lasts about 28 days, but it varies from one female to another. Stress or illness may affect the length of the menstrual cycle. Female teens often have irregular cycles.

Most females begin menstruation between the ages of 9 and 16. For the first months or few years, the times of ovulation and menstruation may vary widely. This is not a cause for concern. The degree of cramps and fatigue associated with the menstrual cycle also may vary from one female to another. Menstruation occurs from puberty until menopause. **Menopause**, which usually occurs between age 40 and 60, is *a period marking the end of a female's reproductive years.*

FIGURE 15.18

AN AVERAGE MENSTRUAL CYCLE

The stages of a 28-day menstrual cycle are shown here. Actual cycles vary in length from female to female, especially during the teen years.

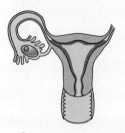 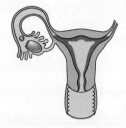 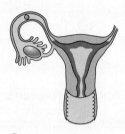 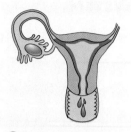

A On days 1 through 13 of the cycle, a new egg cell is maturing inside the ovary.

B On day 14 of the cycle, ovulation occurs and the mature egg is released into one of the fallopian tubes.

C From day 15 through day 20, the egg travels through the fallopian tube.

D On day 21, the egg enters the uterus. After 7 days, if the egg has not been fertilized, menstruation begins.

Fertilization

Fertilization is the joining of male and female reproductive cells to make the first cell of a new human. This cell, the fertilized egg, then moves down the fallopian tube and into the uterus. The fertilized egg attaches to the wall of the uterus and begins to grow. In the early stages, it is called an embryo. After eight weeks of development, it becomes a fetus. The uterus has layers of tissue and a rich blood supply to nourish the developing fetus. The mother's body supplies the fetus with food and oxygen.

After about 40 weeks, the fetus is mature and ready to be born. The walls of the uterus begin to contract. The contractions open the cervix and push the baby out of the uterus and through the cervix. The baby passes through the vagina and out of the female's body.

Problems of the Female Reproductive System

Females can experience problems with their reproductive systems ranging from merely uncomfortable to very serious.

- **Premenstrual syndrome (PMS)** is a collection of physical and emotional changes before and during menstruation.
- **Toxic shock syndrome** is a rare but serious bacterial infection associated with incorrect tampon use. It may produce a fever and a sunburn-like rash, and requires immediate medical care.
- **Infertility** is the inability to reproduce. It may be due to blocked fallopian tubes or failure to produce eggs.
- **Ovarian cysts** are growths on the ovary. Any pain, swelling, abdominal bloating, or feeling of heaviness in the abdomen

should be evaluated by a physician.

- **Sexually transmitted diseases (STDs)** are diseases that are spread during sexual contact.
- **Cancer** is uncontrolled cell growth that destroys healthy tissue. Cancer can affect the breasts, ovaries, uterus, or cervix.

Care of the Female Reproductive System

The following tips will help females take good care of their reproductive systems.

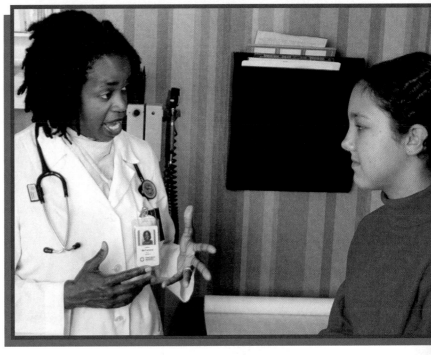

- **Examine your breasts.** Check once a month for unusual lumps or thickening. Any breast changes should be evaluated by a physician.
- **Bathe regularly.** During menstruation, change tampons and sanitary pads frequently.
- **Record your menstrual periods.** Your doctor will want to know when they occur and how long they last.
- **Practice abstinence.** Abstain from sexual activity before marriage.

A gynecologist is a physician who specializes in the care of the female reproductive system. Female teens are advised to have their first visit with a gynecologist once they turn 18, or sooner if they have any concerns.

Lesson 8 Review

Using complete sentences, answer the following questions on a sheet of paper.

Reviewing Terms and Facts

1. **Explain** In which part of the male reproductive system are sperm produced? In which part do they mature?
2. **List** What are four ways for males to care for their reproductive systems?
2. **Vocabulary** Define *ovulation* and *menstruation.*
4. **Review** Describe the path of an egg after it is fertilized.

Thinking Critically

5. **Compare and Contrast** What happens in the uterus if an egg is fertilized? What happens if it is not fertilized?
6. **Analyze** Identify several reasons why it is important to practice sexual abstinence.

Applying Health Skills

7. **Advocacy** With a partner, write a skit in which you present a discussion you might have with a younger sibling who is nearing puberty. Include questions and answers about the body changes to expect, along with information on behaviors that promote good health.

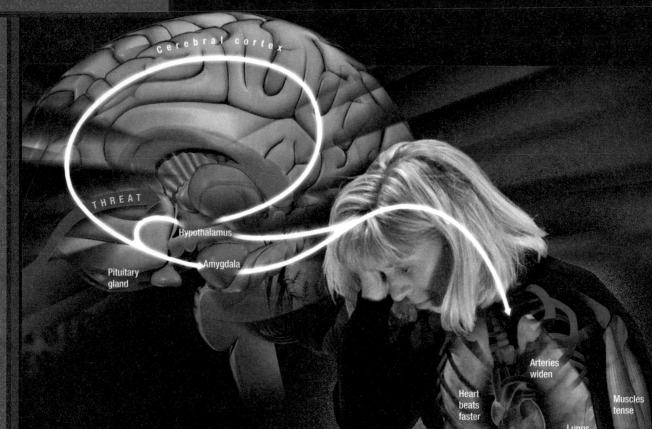

Cerebral cortex

THREAT

Hypothalamus

Amygdala

Pituitary gland

Arteries widen

Heart beats faster

Muscles tense

Lungs ventilate faster

Adrenal glands release hormones

Stomach, digestion shuts down

How Stress Takes Its Toll

Ordinary stress can be harmful to the body as well as the mind.

1. A stress response starts in the brain...

When the brain detects a threat, a number of areas, including the hypothalamus, amygdala, and pituitary gland, go on alert and exchange information with each other. They send signaling hormones and nerve impulses through the nervous system to the rest of the body to prepare for fight or flight.

Stress comes in two forms, each with its own chemistry:

ACUTE A response to immediate danger, acute stress turbocharges the system with powerful hormones that can damage the cardiovascular system.

CHRONIC Caused by constant emotional pressure that the victim can't control, chronic stress produces hormones that can weaken the immune system and damage bones.

2. ...and the body unleashes a flood of hormones...

Adrenal glands react to the alert by releasing the hormone adrenaline (also called epinephrine). This makes the heart pump faster and the lungs work harder to flood the body with oxygen.

The adrenal glands also release extra cortisol and other glucocorticoids, hormones that help the body convert sugars into energy.

Nerve cells release the hormone norepinephrine, which tenses the muscles and sharpens the senses to prepare for action. Digestion shuts down.

3. ...that can cause significant damage

When the threat passes, epinephrine and norepinephrine levels drop, but if danger returns frequently, increased levels of these hormones can damage the arteries. Chronic low-level stress keeps the glucocorticoids in circulation, leading to a weakened immune system, loss of bone mass, suppression of the reproductive system, and memory problems.

FIGHT OR FLIGHT

Our physical reaction to stress, known as the "fight-or-flight" response, probably evolved to help our primitive ancestors deal with a dangerous world. When faced with peril, the body had to be instantly ready to defend itself or run like the wind.

To cope, the terrified brain would signal the adrenal glands, located on top of the kidneys, to release hormones, including adrenaline (also called epinephrine) and glucocorticoids (see the diagram for more on these). The brain would also signal nerve cells to release norepinephrine. These powerful chemicals made the senses sharper, the muscles tighter, the heart pound faster, and the bloodstream fill with sugars for ready energy. Then, when the danger passed, the response would turn off.

Unfortunately, in the modern world, there are some situations that we cannot fight or flee from, such as tensions at home or at school. So our bodies' response mechanisms stay turned on for longer periods of time. Elevated levels of stress and glucocorticoids can lead to serious problems down the road.

TIME TO THINK...

About the Stress Response

The "Fight or Flight" sidebar cites tensions at home or at school as two types of situations that you cannot usually "fight" or "flee" from. Brainstorm specific situations (such as worrying about a big test that's a month away) that you can't "fight" or "flee" from, and put them in one column. In another column, list possible ways of coping with each of these situations. Share your list with the rest of the class.

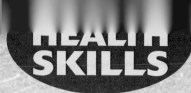
FINDING FACTS ABOUT YOUR BODY

Model

Paul had always been interested in how things work. When he fell and broke his arm, he was curious to know what was going on beneath the cast that the doctor applied. He also wanted to make sure that he did all that he could to heal as quickly as possible.

To get the information he needed, he checked the family medical guide, and then followed up by visiting a medical site on the Internet. From these sources, he discovered that the X rays had enabled the doctor to find the location of the break. The cast was intended to immobilize the arm while it healed. The bone in his arm would produce new cells and blood vessels that would rebuild the broken part. Good nutrition and rest were recommended to aid healing. Reassured, Paul resigned himself to six weeks in a cast.

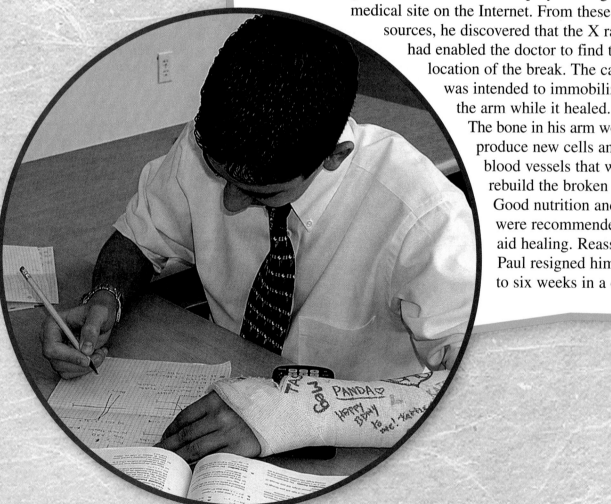

Practice

Read about Mandy's situation. Then answer the questions that follow.

When Mandy learned that her grandmother had suffered a stroke, she had no idea what had happened. Her parents told her that her grandmother would need special care when she came home from the hospital. Mandy thought that the best thing she could do was gain a better understanding of what a stroke was. That way she would be able to help her grandmother recover.

1. If you were in Mandy's position, where would you look for information?
2. How many sources would you use?
3. How would you make sure the information was reliable?

Apply/Assess

Choose a body system or part of a body system that you want to know more about. For example, if you know someone who has diabetes, you might want to learn more about the pancreas. If you have a friend with asthma, you might be interested in how the lungs work. Use reliable print and Internet sources to research the system or body part that you choose. Write down at least three facts that you did not know before you began your research. Prepare a "Facts about . . ." card like the one shown here, presenting the facts and the sources you used. Post your card on a classroom bulletin board.

Facts about . . . the Appendix

1. It is about 3½ inches long and seems to have no function in humans. (AMA Family Medical Guide)
2. In appendicitis, the appendix becomes swollen, inflamed, and painful. (AMA Family Medical Guide)
3. Appendicitis affects about 1 in 500 Americans every year. (Mayo Clinic Web site)
4. The standard treatment for appendicitis is surgical removal. (Mayo Clinic Web site)

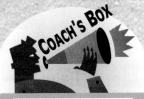

COACH'S BOX

Accessing Information

Using the skill of accessing information involves
● seeking information from reliable sources.
● checking the accuracy of the sources that you use.

Self-√Check

● Did my "Facts About . . ." card contain at least three facts not included in this book?
● Did I show where I found the facts?
● Did I find reliable sources?

After You Read

Use your completed Foldable to review the information on the parts, problems, and care of the skeletal system.

FOLDABLES
Study Organizer

Reviewing Vocabulary and Concepts

On a sheet of paper, write the numbers 1–14. After each number, write the term from the list that best completes each sentence.

- arteries
- capillaries
- circulatory
- contracts
- extend
- calcium
- cartilage
- muscular
- pulmonary
- marrow
- smooth
- systemic
- skeletal system
- veins

Lesson 1

1. The _____ is an internal system made up of bones, joints, and connective tissue.
2. Red and white blood cells are made by _____, a tissue in the center of some bones.
3. _____ is tissue that cushions the joints.
4. Foods high in _____ are essential for building and maintaining strong bones.

Lesson 2

5. The _____ system enables body parts to move.
6. When a muscle shortens, it _____.

7. When a muscle lengthens, it is said to _____.
8. The muscles that line the stomach and intestines are called _____ muscles.

Lesson 3

9. The body's internal transport system is called the _____ system.
10. _____ circulation is the flow of blood from the heart to the lungs and back to the heart.
11. _____ circulation is the flow of blood to all of the body tissues except the lungs.
12. Blood vessels that carry blood away from the heart to other parts of the body are called _____.
13. Blood vessels that carry blood from the body back to the heart are called _____.
14. The tiny tubes that carry blood from your arteries to your body's cells, and then back to your veins, are called _____.

On a sheet of paper, write the numbers 15–26. Write *True* or *False* for each statement below. If the statement is false, change the underlined word or phrase to make it true.

Lesson 4

15. A person can live only a <u>few minutes</u> without air.
16. Air enters lungs through the <u>trachea</u>.
17. When you <u>inhale</u>, your diaphragm relaxes and moves up into your chest cavity.
18. Influenza and colds are caused by <u>bacteria</u>.
19. Smoking cigarettes increases a person's risk of developing <u>lung cancer</u>.

Lesson 5

20. The <u>central nervous system</u> includes the brain and spinal cord.

21. The <u>somatic</u> system deals with actions that you do not usually control.

22. If the spinal cord is damaged or severed, <u>paralysis</u> may result.

Lesson 6

23. Most digestion takes place in the <u>stomach</u>.

24. The liver produces <u>a gastric juice</u>, which helps digest fats.

25. <u>Excretion</u> is the process of removing wastes from the body.

26. Eating spicy or acidic foods may result in <u>gallstones</u>.

On a sheet of paper, write the numbers 27–35. After each number, write the letter of the answer that best completes each sentence.

Lesson 7

27. The gland that is located at the base of the brain is the
   a. adrenal gland.
   b. parathyroid gland.
   c. pituitary gland.
   d. pancreas.

28. Development of secondary sex characteristics in females is controlled by the
   a. thyroid gland.
   b. ovaries.
   c. goiter.
   d. testes.

29. During a stress response,
   a. blood flow increases.
   b. air passages expand.
   c. digestion may slow down.
   d. all of the above.

30. Diabetes is characterized by inadequate production of
   a. amino acids.
   b. adrenaline.
   c. sugar.
   d. insulin.

Lesson 8

31. Sperm are produced in the
   a. seminal vesicle.
   b. Cowper's glands.
   c. sperm glands.
   d. testes.

32. From the epididymis, sperm travel through the
   a. prostate gland.
   b. testes.
   c. urethra.
   d. vas deferens.

33. The female reproductive system functions to
   a. store eggs.
   b. provide a site for fertilization.
   c. nourish and protect a fertilized egg.
   d. all of the above.

34. The opening of the uterus is the
   a. fetus.
   b. cervix.
   c. endometrium.
   d. ovary.

35. A blocked fallopian tube can result in
   a. infertility.
   b. PMS.
   c. STDs.
   d. toxic shock syndrome.

Thinking Critically

Using complete sentences, answer the following questions on a sheet of paper.

36. **Explain** What do calcium and phosphorous do for your bones?

37. **Predict** How would a person's ability to move change if the backbone were a single bone instead of 24 separate bones?

38. **Analyze** In what ways are smooth muscles and skeletal muscles different?

39. **Compare** What is the difference between pulmonary and systemic circulation?

40. **Apply** Why do you need to know your blood type?

41. **Explain** Why does regular handwashing reduce your risk of catching a respiratory infection?

42. **Summarize** Which diseases of the respiratory system are particularly associated with smoking?

43. **Analyze** How are voluntary actions, such as wiggling your toes, and involuntary actions, such as breathing, related to your brain?

44. **Explain** Why is it important to wear a helmet when riding a bike or playing a contact sport?

45. **Apply** How does fiber contribute to the health of your digestive and excretory systems?

46. **Synthesize** What is the relationship between the brain and the endocrine system?

47. **Deduce** Why is the stress response sometimes harmful instead of helpful?

48. **Explain** Why does the menstrual cycle stop when a female is pregnant?

49. **Contrast** Compare and contrast changes in the male and female reproductive systems.

50. **Apply** Identify and list five appropriate sources of health services for the variety of illnesses and disorders covered in this chapter.

Career Corner

Physical Therapist Would you like to help people prevent or overcome physical impairments? Then you might be interested in a career as a physical therapist. These professionals help patients use physical activity and movement to recover from injuries or illnesses that affect their bodies' ability to move. They also teach patients to use crutches, wheelchairs, or artificial limbs. This profession requires a four-year degree in a related field, such as genetics or biology, and a master's degree from a physical therapy program. Learn more about this and other health careers by clicking on Career Corner at health.glencoe.com.

Reading & Writing

Read the paragraphs below and then answer the questions.

When you close your eyes to the world outside, you open them to the world of dreams.

Throughout history, people have felt both fear and fascination when it comes to the mystery of dreams. Some cultures developed ways to not only protect sleeping people from the evil spirits in their dreams, but also to attract pleasant dreams. The North American indigenous people hung "dream-catchers" above sleeping infants to keep out bad dreams and to allow in good ones. Parents in China gave their children double-headed tiger pillows to scare off any evil spirit who might approach through a dream. The Japanese created a mythological creature called a Baku who ate bad dreams. In Europe, a stone hung on a red ribbon and tied to a bedpost was said to protect the sleeper from bad dreams.

Good or bad, our dreams are a part of our lives—interesting mysteries.

1. What is the second paragraph of the passage mainly about?
   - **A** how dreams predict the future
   - **B** how to interpret dreams
   - **C** the meaning of dreams in history
   - **D** dreams in different cultures

2. Which of these statements best reflects the author's attitude toward dreams?
   - **A** Dreams can predict the future.
   - **B** Dreams are always pleasant.
   - **C** Dreams are myths.
   - **D** Dreams are an interesting part of life.

3. Write a paragraph describing a dream, and then explain if you think it means something. Explain why or why not.

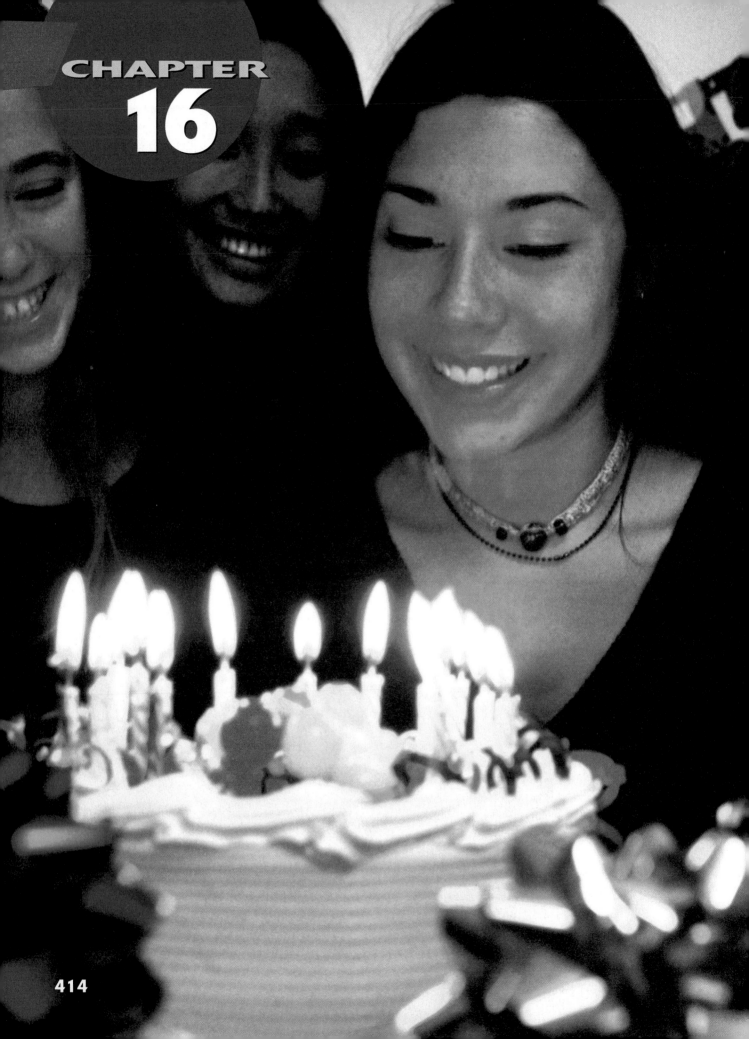

Growth and Development

HEALTH *Online*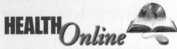

Do your choices and attitudes show that you are preparing for the role of an adult? Find out by taking the Chapter 16 Health Inventory at health.glencoe.com.

FOLDABLES™ Study Organizer

Before You Read

Make this Foldable to help you organize what you learn about the building blocks of life in Lesson 1. Begin with a plain sheet of 8½" × 11" paper.

Step 1

Fold the sheet of paper along the long axis, leaving a ½" tab along the side.

Step 2

Turn the paper. Fold in half, then fold in half again.

Step 3

Unfold and cut the top layer along the three fold lines. This makes four tabs.

Step 4

Turn the paper vertically and label the tabs as shown.

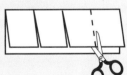

Cells

Tissues

Organ

Body System

As You Read

Under the appropriate tab, write down major concepts related to cells, tissues, organs, and body systems.

The Beginning of Life

Quick Write

Write down what you know about how a baby gets food and oxygen as it grows inside its mother.

LEARN ABOUT...

- how life begins.
- the development of a fetus.
- the birth of a healthy baby.

VOCABULARY

- fertilization
- egg cell
- sperm cell
- tissues
- organs
- uterus
- embryo
- fetus
- placenta
- umbilical cord
- cervix

Building Blocks of Life

You began your life as a single microscopic cell. That cell divided over and over again until it formed the trillions of cells that now make up your body. These cells are organized into tissues, which are organized into organs, which in turn are organized into systems, as shown in **Figure 16.1**.

Fertilization

A unique human body begins as a single cell that is the result of fertilization. **Fertilization** is *the joining together of two special cells, one from each parent.* It takes place inside the mother's reproductive system. *The cell from the mother that plays a part in fertilization* is called an **egg cell**. *The cell from the father that enters the egg cell during fertilization* is called a **sperm cell**.

Sometimes a newly fertilized egg cell separates into two fertilized egg cells. Each of these egg cells then grows into a new body. This results in identical twins of the same gender. When two different egg cells are fertilized at the same time by two different sperm cells, twins are also produced. These fraternal twins do not look exactly alike. They may be two girls, two boys, or one girl and one boy. They are no more similar than other siblings.

Identical twins come from one fertilized egg that separated in two before it began to grow. *What is the difference between identical and fraternal twins?*

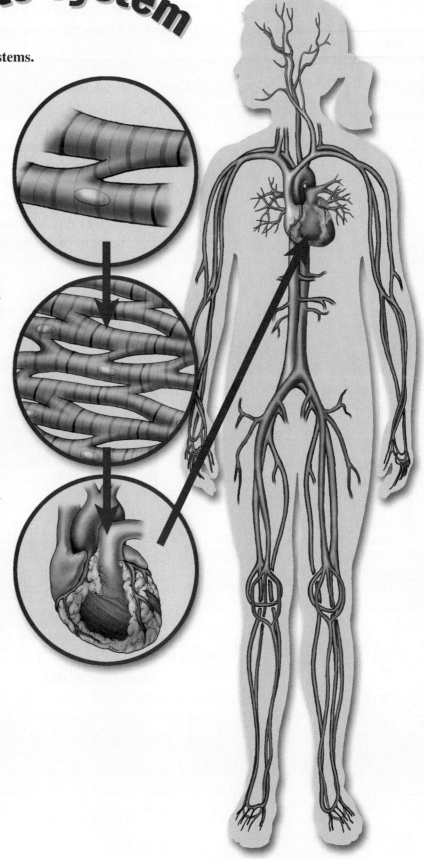

FIGURE 16.1

From Cell to System

Cells form tissues, organs, and systems.

A **Cell**
The basic units, or building blocks, of life are called cells. There are many different kinds of cells in the human body. Each kind of cell does a specific job. This cell is a heart muscle cell. Some other kinds of cells in the body are blood, nerve, and skin cells.

B **Tissue**
Cells that do similar jobs make up **tissues**. Several kinds of tissues are found in the body. The heart muscle tissue, shown here, contains heart muscle cells. Brain tissue contains nerve cells.

C **Organ**
Different kinds of tissues are combined in larger structures called organs. **Organs** are *body parts that perform particular functions*. Heart muscle tissue is the main kind of tissue in the heart, the organ shown here. The brain, liver, and kidneys are other organs in the body.

D **System**
Groups of organs that work together form systems. There are a number of systems in the body, such as the circulatory system, shown here. The heart is the main organ of the circulatory system. Grouping organs into systems makes it easier to understand their functions. However, systems do not function all by themselves. All your body systems work together to keep you alive and active.

Reading Check

Understand sentence structure. Compare the sentences in Figure 16.2 with those in the text. How do they differ?

Growth During Pregnancy

Soon after fertilization, the cell begins to divide. It forms a cluster of cells that attaches itself to the inside wall of the uterus. The **uterus** (YOO·tuh·ruhs) is *a pear-shaped organ inside a female's body where a fetus is nourished.* The cluster of cells is now called an **embryo**, the *name for the developing organism from fertilization to about the eighth week of development.* These cells continue to divide and form cells that do specific jobs.

Over time, cells that do similar jobs combine into tissues, tissues with similar jobs combine into organs, and organs with similar jobs combine into systems. A **fetus** is *the name for the developing organism from the end of the eighth week until birth.* The baby is born about nine months after fertilization. **Figure 16.2** shows the development of the embryo and fetus during these nine months.

FIGURE 16.2

Nine Months of Development

In a remarkable process, a single cell develops into a full-grown baby.

A **End of First Month**
About ⅓ inch long. Heart, brain, and lungs are forming.

B **End of Second Month**
About 1 inch long. All other organs are developing. Arms, fingers, legs, and toes are forming. Heart is beating.

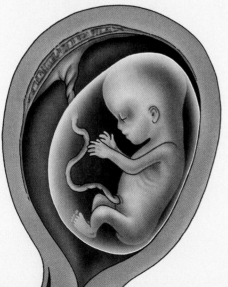

Staying active and eating healthy foods are just as important during pregnancy as they are at all other times.

C **End of Third Month**
Weighs about 1 ounce and is about 3 inches long. Fetus begins to move around.

D **End of Fourth Month**
Weighs about 6 ounces and is about 5 inches long. Facial features are well formed. Mother can feel the fetus move.

E **End of Fifth Month**
Weighs about 1 pound and is just under 10 inches long. Eyelashes and nails appear. Heartbeat can be heard.

Growth Inside the Uterus

A fetus needs food and oxygen in order to grow and develop. The **placenta** (pluh·SEN·tuh) is *a thick, rich lining of tissue that builds up along the walls of the uterus and connects the mother to the fetus*. Food and oxygen in the mother's blood are carried to the fetus through a blood vessel in the **umbilical** (uhm·BIL·i·kuhl) **cord**, *a tube that connects the fetus and the mother's placenta*. Harmful substances, such as alcohol, nicotine, and other drugs, can cross the placenta and harm the fetus.

The umbilical cord also carries the fetus's wastes away. The waste products enter the mother's body, which then gets rid of them. After birth, the cord is cut. The place where the cord was attached to the fetus becomes the baby's navel.

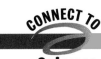

CONNECT TO

Science

CHANGES DURING PREGNANCY
A pregnant female experiences many physiological and emotional changes. *Use reliable resources to find out more about these changes. In a brief paragraph, describe some physiological and emotional changes that occur during pregnancy.*

F End of Sixth Month
Weighs about 1.5 pounds and is about 12.5 inches long. Can open and close mouth and swallow. Develops ability to kick. Fetus can hear sounds.

G End of Seventh Month
Weighs 2 to 2.5 pounds and is about 14.5 inches long. Arms and legs can move freely. Eyes open.

H End of Eighth Month
Weighs about 4 pounds and is almost 18 inches long. Hair gets longer. Skin becomes smoother.

I End of Ninth Month
Weighs 7 to 9 pounds and is 18 to 20 inches long. Body organs have developed to function on their own.

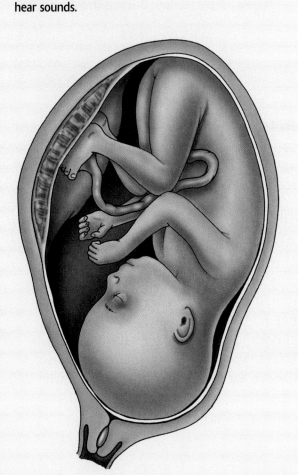

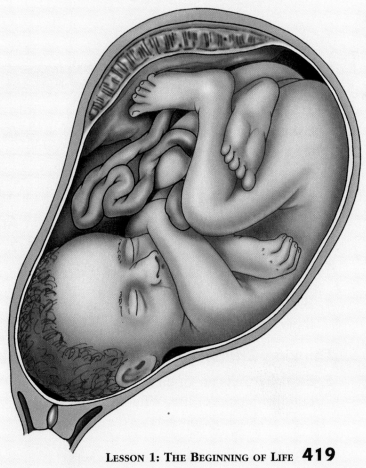

Stages of Birth

About nine months after fertilization, a fetus is fully developed and ready to be born. The birth process occurs in three stages:

- **Stage one.** Mild contractions, which are tightenings in the muscles of the uterus, signal the beginning of the first stage. At this point, *the entrance of the uterus,* called the **cervix**, begins to open.

- **Stage two.** By the time this stage of birth begins, the cervix is open to a width of about 4 inches. The contractions are very strong and are occurring more frequently. At the end of stage two, the contractions push the baby through the cervix and out of the mother's body.

- **Stage three.** Contractions continue after the baby is born until the placenta is pushed out of the uterus. The placenta is no longer needed. In fact, it could cause serious infection if it were not completely removed from the uterus.

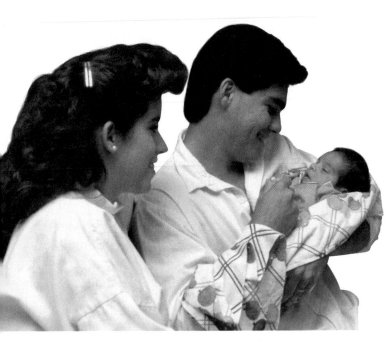

After nine months of pregnancy, a female goes through three stages of birth to deliver a baby. *Which stage results in the baby's birth?*

Lesson 1 Review

Using complete sentences, answer the following questions on a sheet of paper.

Reviewing Terms and Facts

1. **Vocabulary** Define the term *fertilization.*
2. **Describe** What is a fetus like at the end of three months? At the end of six months?
3. **Recall** Describe how a growing fetus gets food and oxygen.
4. **Summarize** What happens during the three stages of birth?

Thinking Critically

5. **Explain** Cells are often referred to as the building blocks of life. Why is this an appropriate description?

6. **Relate** Why are pregnant females advised to avoid alcohol, nicotine, and other drugs and to talk to their doctor before using any medicine?

Applying Health Skills

7. **Accessing Information** Find out about classes that prepare expectant parents for childbirth and parenthood. During what month of pregnancy do classes normally begin? What topics are covered in the classes? Does your community offer different types of classes, such as exercise classes for pregnant females, childbirth education, and baby care classes? How do they differ?

Heredity and Environment

The One and Only You

Every individual is unique. Each has his or her own particular looks, abilities, and personality. A number of factors influence the way a person develops. These factors can be grouped into two major categories: heredity and environment.

Heredity

Heredity is *the passing of traits from parents to their children.* Some examples of inherited traits are eye color, face shape, and even freckles. Tiny structures that are present inside human cells carry the information that enables traits to be inherited.

Quick Write

What advice would you give a pregnant female to protect the health of her developing baby?

LEARN ABOUT...

- how characteristics are inherited.
- environmental factors that can affect the developing fetus.
- different types of birth defects.
- ways a pregnant woman can protect the health of her fetus.

VOCABULARY

- heredity
- chromosomes
- genes
- genetic disorder
- environment
- prenatal care
- obstetrician
- birth defects

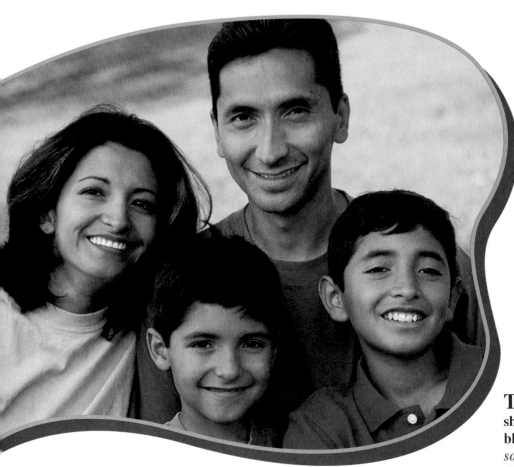

The members of some families share a strong physical resemblance to one another. *What are some of the characteristics that these family members share?*

Traits are passed on through the following structures:

- **Chromosomes.** *The threadlike structures found within the nucleus of a cell that carry the codes for inherited traits* are **chromosomes** (KROH·muh·sohmz). Most cells in the human body have 46 chromosomes, which occur as 23 pairs. One chromosome of every pair comes from each parent. A sperm cell from the father has 23 chromosomes, and an egg cell from the mother has 23 chromosomes. The fertilized egg cell that results from the joining of these two cells has 46 chromosomes.
- **Genes.** *The basic units of heredity* are called **genes.** Genes are sections of chromosomes. They carry codes for specific traits, such as hair color and eye color. Children of the same parents inherit different combinations of chromosomes and genes.

Scientists are working hard to understand and solve genetic problems. *Why is genetic research important?*

Genetic Disorders

Sometimes genes carried by one or both parents can be flawed. When this happens, a baby may be born with a **genetic** (juh·NE·tik) **disorder.** This is *a disorder that is caused partly or completely by a defect in genes.*

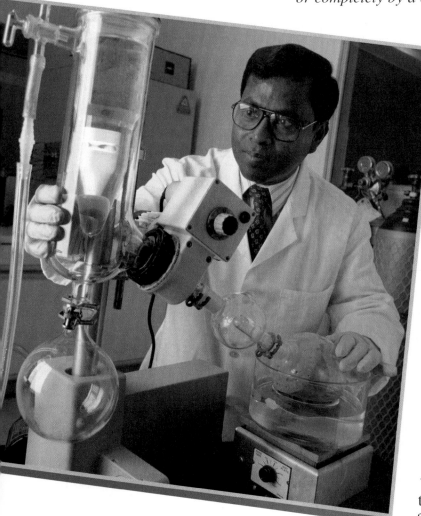

Some genetic disorders occur when a fertilized egg cell has more than 46 chromosomes. For example, people with Down syndrome have an extra chromosome and tend to have characteristic facial features and learning disabilities. Other genetic disorders are caused by abnormal genes. Albinism is a genetic disorder that results in a person's skin, hair, and eyes having no color.

Phenylketonuria (FEE·nuhl·kee·toh·NOOR·ee·uh), or PKU, is a genetic disorder that can prevent the brain from developing normally. Scientists eventually discovered that keeping certain proteins out of the child's diet prevents the brain damage associated with PKU. Today, all children in the United States are tested at birth for PKU.

Environment

The second factor that can affect the health of a developing fetus and of a newborn child is environment. **Environment** is *the sum total of a person's surroundings.* The environment of a developing fetus is its mother's uterus. The health of the baby is affected directly by the activities and overall health of its mother.

Prenatal Care

A healthy mother improves her chances of having a healthy baby. This is why it is extremely important for a female to begin a program of prenatal care as soon as she finds out she is pregnant. **Prenatal** (pree· NAY·tuhl) **care** includes *steps taken to provide for the health of a pregnant female and her baby.*

Important to prenatal health care are regular visits to a health clinic, family doctor, or **obstetrician** (ahb·stuh·TRI·shuhn). This is *a doctor who specializes in the care of a pregnant female and her developing fetus, and who is present at the birth of the baby.* Other steps related to good prenatal health care include:

- Eating nutritious foods.
- Getting enough rest.
- Participating in moderate exercise.
- Avoiding the use of tobacco, alcohol, and other drugs, as well as all medicines except those advised by the health care provider.

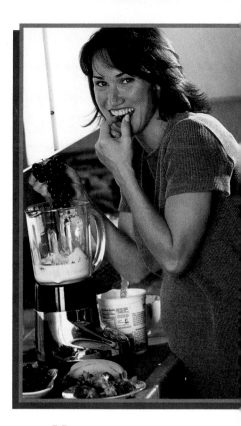

Nutritious foods are particularly important during pregnancy. *How can a pregnant female make sure she is getting the nutrients she and her baby need?*

Hands-On Health

PRENATAL CARE BROCHURE

In this activity, you will create a brochure that will encourage a pregnant female to take steps to ensure that she has a healthy baby.

WHAT YOU WILL NEED
- heavy writing paper
- printed reference materials or access to the Internet
- scissors
- pens, colored markers, glue

WHAT YOU WILL DO
Gather reliable information on prenatal care topics such as nutrition, exercise, and medical checkups. Find pictures to illustrate your brochure. Plan the layout of your brochure. Then write down information, glue on pictures, and use markers to add finishing touches.

IN CONCLUSION
Make your brochure available to a pregnant female in your family or community.

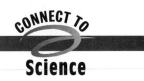
Ultrasound equipment, which uses sound waves to make pictures, allows doctors to see images of a fetus in the uterus. Such images enable them to check the size and position of the fetus and the amount of fluid surrounding the fetus. Ultrasounds taken at intervals in a pregnancy help monitor the progress of the fetus.

Birth Defects

Getting medical care, eating properly, getting enough rest and exercise, and avoiding harmful substances contribute to the health of the developing fetus and help prevent birth defects. **Birth defects** are *abnormalities present at birth that cause physical or mental disability or death.* Some birth defects are caused by a genetic disorder or by harmful substances in the fetus's environment. Certain infections during pregnancy can also lead to birth defects.

Problems in the Fetal Environment

Listed below are some of the environmental factors that can contribute to birth defects:

- **Poor nutrition.** A fetus gets all of its nourishment from its mother. If a pregnant female doesn't follow a healthy eating plan, the baby may be born too early, have a low birth weight, or both. These babies have a greater chance of having mental or physical problems.

- **Alcohol.** When a pregnant female drinks alcohol, it enters her blood, passes through the placenta, and into the blood of her baby. This can lead to fetal alcohol syndrome (FAS), a pattern of physical and mental problems in children whose mothers drank alcohol during pregnancy. Females who are pregnant or who are trying to become pregnant should avoid alcohol completely.

- **Medicines and other drugs.** A pregnant female should avoid all medicines and other drugs, unless their use has been approved by her physician. Even over-the-counter medicines can harm a developing fetus. When a pregnant female takes certain illegal drugs and prescription drugs, her baby may be born addicted to the drug.

An important part of prenatal care is regular checkups. *Why are checkups important for both a pregnant female and her unborn baby?*

- **Tobacco.** Tobacco use during pregnancy can seriously harm the fetus's growth. The baby can be born prematurely or with a low birth weight. Females who are pregnant should also avoid breathing secondhand smoke.
- **Infections.** Rubella, or German measles, can cause deafness or other serious health problems in a baby born to a female who has this disease while pregnant. A female can avoid passing rubella to her fetus by being vaccinated against the disease before she becomes pregnant.
- **STDs.** Certain sexually transmitted diseases (STDs) can also be passed from mother to fetus. STDs can cause brain damage, blindness, and even death. A pregnant female who is infected with HIV, the virus that causes AIDS, can pass the virus to her unborn child. A pregnant female should tell her doctor about any possible STDs.

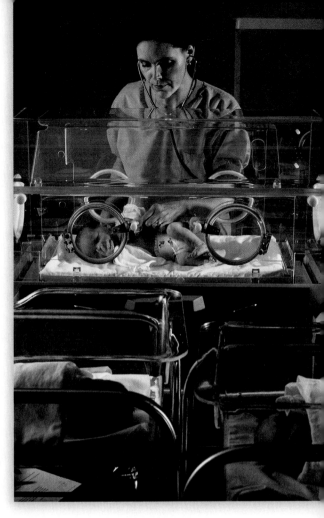

Tobacco use during pregnancy can result in premature birth and a low birth weight. *What are some other factors that can harm the health of a newborn?*

Lesson 2 Review

Using complete sentences, answer the following questions on a sheet of paper.

Reviewing Terms and Facts

1. **Vocabulary** What is a *genetic disorder?*
2. **Give Examples** List four steps a pregnant female can take to protect her own health and the health of her developing fetus.
3. **Summarize** What are five factors in the fetal environment that can contribute to birth defects?

Thinking Critically

4. **Explain** Both heredity and environment influence the way a fetus develops. Over which of these does a pregnant female have the most control? Why?

5. **Relate** Why do you think it is a good idea for a female to develop a nutritious eating plan, to eliminate all use of alcohol and other drugs, and to start an exercise program before she becomes pregnant?

Applying Health Skills

6. **Advocacy** Encourage a pregnant female to practice healthful behaviors by preparing a daily log for her to complete during her pregnancy. Include blanks to write down foods eaten at different meals and snacks. Prepare a summary section at the end where the female can place a check mark next to healthful behaviors she practiced that day.

From Childhood to Adolescence

Stages of Development

The life cycle of human beings can be divided into different stages. A number of different theories exist about how babies develop into adults. Some focus on physical growth. Others look mainly at mental or emotional growth. One widely accepted view is that of scientist Erik Erikson. Erikson divided the human life cycle into eight stages of development. These stages are described and illustrated in **Figure 16.3**.

Many aspects of social growth are defined by **developmental tasks**. These are *events that need to happen in order for you to continue growing toward becoming a healthy, mature adult.* Each stage of growth has its own specific developmental tasks.

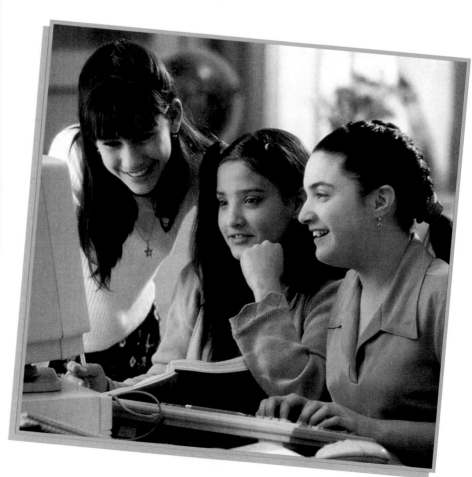

An important develop-mental task of adolescence is to develop a sense of self. Think of some of the interests and talents that define you as a unique individual.

FIGURE 16.3

ERIKSON'S STAGES OF LIFE

Each stage is associated with a developmental task that involves a person's relationship with other people.

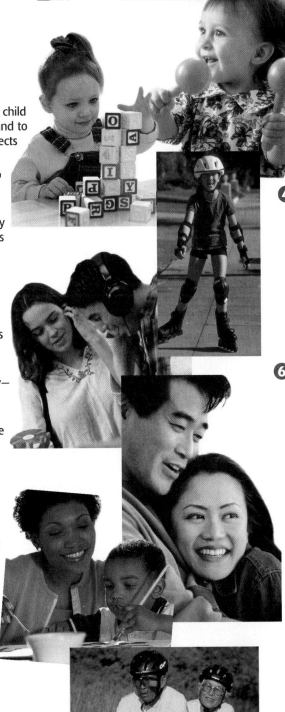

① Infancy
Birth to 1 year

Characteristic of stage: child is completely dependent on others to meet his or her needs

Developmental task: to develop trust

If not mastered: could result in mistrust

② Early Childhood
1 to 3 years

Characteristics of stage: child is learning to separate from parents

Developmental task: to develop ability to do tasks oneself

If not mastered: could result in lack of confidence

③ Middle Childhood
3 to 5 years

Characteristics of stage: child begins to make decisions and to think of and carry out projects

Developmental task: to develop initiative—ability to create one's own play

If not mastered: could result in guilt—feeling guilty about the actions one takes

④ Late Childhood
6 to 11 years

Characteristics of stage: child explores surroundings and masters more and more difficult skills

Developmental task: to develop interest in performing activities

If not mastered: could result in feelings of inferiority

⑤ Adolescence
12 to 18 years

Characteristic of stage: adolescent searches for his or her own identity

Developmental task: to develop one's own identity—a sense of who one is

If not mastered: could result in confusion over the many roles one plays

⑥ Young Adulthood
19 to 30 years

Characteristic of stage: person tries to develop close personal relationships

Developmental task: to develop intimacy—forming a strong relationship with another person

If not mastered: could result in isolation—being alone

⑦ Middle Adulthood
31 to 60 years

Characteristics of stage: person tries to achieve something in work and is concerned with the well-being of others

Developmental task: to develop the sense of having contributed to society

If not mastered: could result in self-absorption

⑧ Maturity and Old Age
61 years to death

Characteristic of stage: person tries to understand meaning of own life

Developmental task: to develop integrity—feeling satisfied with one's life

If not mastered: could result in despair—feeling that one's life has not been satisfying

Stages of Childhood

The theories of early physical and mental/emotional growth can be combined to describe four stages of childhood. These stages are infancy, early childhood, middle childhood, and late childhood. They are illustrated in **Figure 16.4**.

Infancy

The period of fastest physical growth in a human's life occurs during **infancy**, the *first year of life.* A child's weight typically triples and his or her height increases by about 50 percent during this year. When an infant's needs are met in a loving way, he or she learns to trust people and feel safe.

Early Childhood

Children between the ages of one and three who are learning to walk and talk are known as **toddlers**. At this stage they begin to feel proud of their achievements and are eager to do more things by themselves. Failing now and then when trying to do something new is an important part of learning and growing.

FIGURE 16.4

The Growth Years

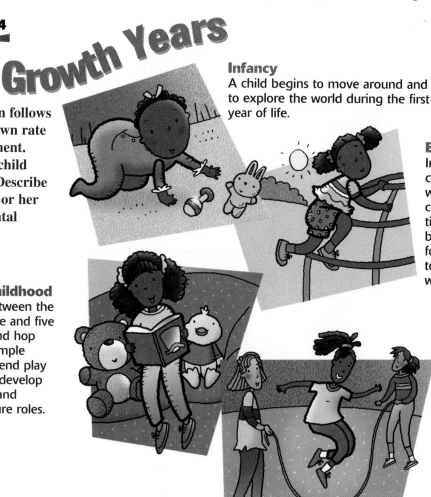

Each person follows his or her own rate of development. Think of a child you know. Describe some of his or her developmental activities.

Infancy
A child begins to move around and to explore the world during the first year of life.

Early Childhood
In early childhood, children learn to walk, run, and climb stairs. At this time, children also begin to do things for themselves and to communicate with others.

Middle Childhood
Children between the ages of three and five can jump and hop and draw simple shapes. Pretend play helps them develop social skills and practice future roles.

Late Childhood
The physical skills of children improve steadily between the ages of 6 and 11. In late childhood, friends are important in building social skills and self-esteem.

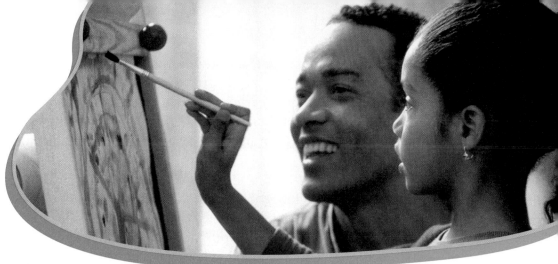

Middle Childhood

Children between the ages of three and five are often referred to as **preschoolers**. This is a period of rapid growth during which the child becomes more coordinated in his or her movements. Playing make-believe and imitating adults are favorite activities. Children of this age often show how fast their minds are growing by asking many questions.

How adults respond to a child's behavior is important. When parents encourage new activities and questions, they promote the child's self-esteem. Parents who are impatient with a child's attempts to do things independently may make the child feel guilty about starting new activities and lower the child's self-esteem.

Late Childhood

Children between the ages of 6 and 11 grow at a more even rate than when they were younger. At this stage, school usually becomes a very important part of a child's life. Physical and mental skills steadily increase.

Children often spend a lot of time making things. If a child's creative efforts are appreciated and rewarded, pride in her or his work increases. A child's success or failure in any of the stages of childhood affects emotional development at that stage. By succeeding at later stages, a child may overcome any setbacks of earlier stages and gain self-esteem.

Adolescence

After infancy, the second fastest period of physical growth is adolescence, the time of life between childhood and adulthood. It usually begins between the ages of 8 and 14. Girls typically enter adolescence earlier than boys do. During this time many physical, mental/emotional, and social changes take place. All of these changes are interrelated, and each individual goes through them at his or her own rate. Try to recognize and accept the differences in levels of maturation.

When parents encourage a child's creativity, the child feels a sense of pride. *Why is it important to encourage a sense of pride at this stage of development?*

Reading Check

Practice paraphrasing. Rewrite the lists in Figure 16.5 in your own words.

Physical Development

Adolescence begins with **puberty**, *the time when you begin to develop certain physical traits of adults of your own gender.* Many of these physical changes are shown in **Figure 16.5**. The exact age of puberty varies from person to person.

Emotional and Social Development

Emotional changes are a normal part of adolescence. Many of them are related to the activity of hormones as they prepare your body for adulthood. Mood swings, during which you feel happy one moment and unhappy the next, are common. You may find yourself wanting to spend time with members of the opposite gender. Such feelings may be confusing and even frightening.

Adolescence is a busy and challenging time. It involves important developmental tasks that you need to accomplish so that you can move successfully into adulthood. Here are some of those tasks:

- Become more independent of parents and other adults
- Learn more about who you are
- Define your values
- Learn how to think, reason, and solve problems in an adult way
- Accept your body and its characteristics
- Gain a masculine or feminine view of yourself
- Form more mature relationships with people of both genders
- Develop an interest in and a concern for your community

HEALTH SKILLS ACTIVITY

STRESS MANAGEMENT

Coping with Mood Swings

Mood swings during adolescence are common and normal. Here are some ways to help deal with mood swings.

- **TALK IT OUT.** Talk to friends and family members you trust.
- **WRITE IT DOWN.** Record your feelings in a diary or journal.
- **DO SOMETHING FUN.** Start working on a project or spend time with a friend.
- **STAY ACTIVE.** Physical activity can improve your mood and clear your thoughts.

- **GET SOME REST.** Things often look better after a quick nap or a good night's sleep.
- **TAKE TIME FOR YOURSELF.** Get away from noise and confusion for a while.
- **TALK TO A PROFESSIONAL.** See a school counselor or doctor if you feel depressed.

ON YOUR OWN

Make a list of ways to cope with mood swings. Choose one strategy and demonstrate it for the class in the form of a role-play.

FIGURE 16.5

PHYSICAL CHANGES DURING PUBERTY

Compare and contrast changes in males and females.

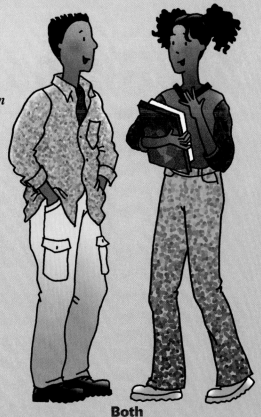

Male
Male hormone production increases.

Facial hair appears.

Larynx enlarges and the voice deepens.

Shoulders broaden.

Muscles develop.

Sperm production begins.

Temporary breast tenderness and enlargement can occur.

Female
Female hormone production increases.

Breasts develop.

Hips widen.

Uterus and ovaries enlarge.

Ovulation occurs.

Menstruation begins.

Body fat increases.

Both
Growth spurt occurs.

Acne may appear.

Most permanent teeth have come in.

Underarm hair appears.

Perspiration increases.

Pubic hair appears.

External genitals enlarge.

Lesson 3 Review

Using complete sentences, answer the following questions on a sheet of paper.

Reviewing Terms and Facts

1. **Vocabulary** Define *developmental tasks*.
2. **Recall** List Erikson's eight stages of the life cycle.
3. **Identify** Which are the two periods of fastest physical growth in humans?
4. **Identify** During which stage of growth do people define their values and learn to solve problems in an adult way?

Thinking Critically

5. **Hypothesize** Why is it important to recognize and accept differences in maturation levels?

6. **Analyze** How are the physical, mental/emotional, and social changes of adolescence interrelated?

Applying Health Skills

7. **Analyzing Influences** Select a teen magazine and find the ways that the articles, pictures, and advertisements try to influence teens. In what ways are teens encouraged to buy things? Why are products advertised so widely to teens?

Adulthood and Aging

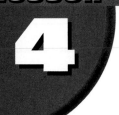

Quick Write

Describe an older person whom you admire. What qualities do you like in that person? What does that person teach you about aging?

LEARN ABOUT...

the three stages of adulthood.
three different ways to measure age.
aging as a positive experience.

VOCABULARY

chronological age
biological age
social age

Stages of Adulthood

The adult years are made up of three main stages: early, middle, and late adulthood. Each stage is marked by certain milestones, such as starting a career, marrying, raising children, and so on. While most people follow these stages in a predictable sequence, many do not. Some adults choose not to marry, or they marry later in life. Some choose to have no children. Many adults change careers several times. Some retire early, while others choose to continue working as long as they are able.

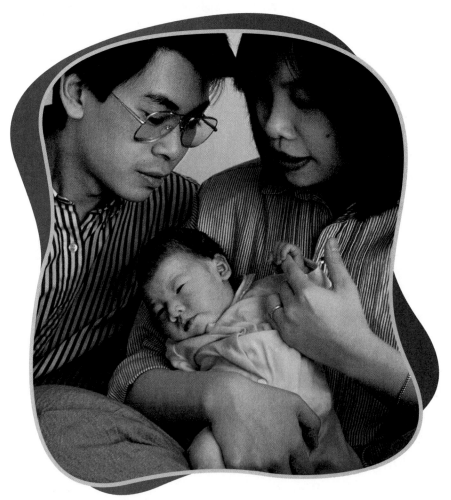

For many people, early adulthood is the time to marry and start a family. *What do you expect to do when you reach early adulthood?*

Early Adulthood

In early adulthood, most people begin working for a living. This is also the time when many people want to begin sharing their lives with another person. That desire is often met by marrying and beginning a family. However, some couples choose to have children in their thirties.

Middle Adulthood

For some people, advancing in their jobs is a major goal in their thirties, forties, and fifties. Many are also raising their children. People in middle adulthood often have a great desire to help young people, and they gain a lot of satisfaction from doing so. The middle adult years can present many demands, however. Some people find themselves stretched by building a career, caring for home and children, and caring for aging parents.

Late Adulthood

People in their mid-sixties and beyond often look forward to retirement so they can pursue interests they didn't have time for when they were busy with their careers and children. Others continue to work, and some change careers. Many choose to stay active by doing volunteer work in their community. Today, Americans are living longer than ever before. As a result, most people can look forward to many years of late adulthood. Those who take good care of their health throughout their adult life are more likely to enjoy the benefits of good health as they age.

The life cycle of humans includes aging, dying, and death. It is important to be comfortable talking about dying and death, as they are a natural part of the life cycle.

Developing Good Character ★

Respect

Although some older adults are slowed by age, most enjoy active and vital lives. It is a mistake to underestimate their abilities or treat them as frail. Describe strategies to show respect for older adults.

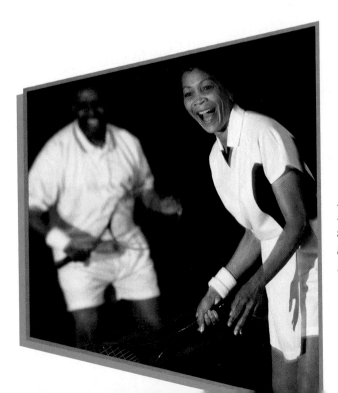

Physical activity and good nutrition are important at any age. *How are these adults contributing to their lifelong health?*

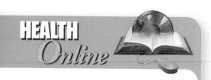

Measuring Age

Have you heard the expression "You're only as old as you feel"? It recognizes that some people feel younger than their years indicate. As **Figure 16.6** shows, age can be measured in three different ways:

- **Chronological** (krah·nuh·LAH·ji·kuhl) **age.** *Age measured in years* is **chronological age**. This is the number of your most recent birthday. We have no control over this measure of age.
- **Biological age.** *Age determined by how well various body parts are working* is **biological age**. It is affected by heredity and by health habits. People who make healthful choices throughout life show fewer signs of physical aging as they grow older.
- **Social age.** *Age measured by your lifestyle and the connections you have with others* is **social age**. Social age has to do with the activities that society expects you to perform at particular points in life. As a teen, you are expected to be in school, learning and preparing for adulthood. Later, you are expected to work, possibly have a family, and contribute to your community.

FIGURE 16.6

CHRONOLOGICAL, BIOLOGICAL, AND SOCIAL AGE

A person's chronological, biological, and social age may not all advance at the same rate. *How can your actions as a teen affect your lifelong health?*

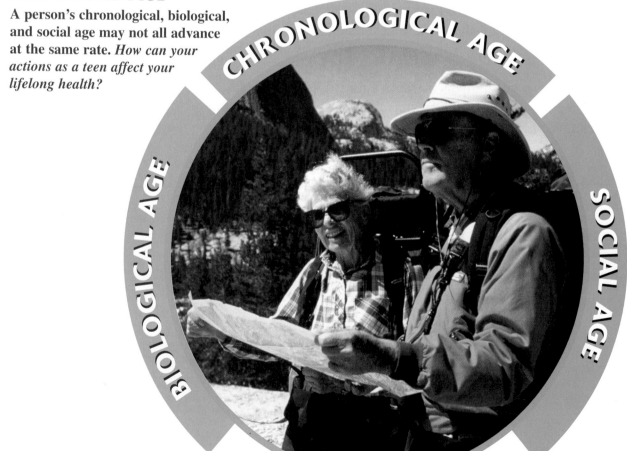

Aging: A Positive Experience

The health triangle is just as useful for older people as it is for you. Paying attention to all three sides of the triangle can help make the later years a rewarding and productive stage of life.

- **Physical health.** Older people who stay physically active, get enough rest, and follow a sensible eating plan are less likely to experience illnesses and disabilities that prevent them from enjoying themselves. Their biological age is lower than their chronological age.
- **Mental and emotional health.** Older people who keep mentally active by reading, working, and challenging themselves mentally will continue to learn. Those who have learned to be resilient are more likely to handle any changes that accompany their later years.
- **Social health.** Older people who maintain contact with family and friends have less difficulty adjusting to the later years and to the loss of loved ones. Many older people benefit from becoming involved in community programs that can use their talents and life experiences.

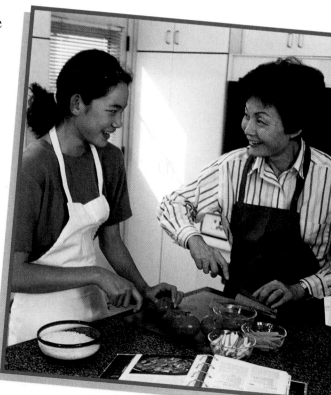

When you form friendships with older adults, both of you benefit. *What are some ways that your life might be made richer by having a close relationship with an older adult?*

Lesson 4 Review

Using complete sentences, answer the following questions on a sheet of paper.

Reviewing Terms and Facts

1. **Identify** What are the three stages of adulthood?
2. **Explain** What might make middle adulthood particularly demanding?
3. **Vocabulary** Define the terms *chronological age, biological age,* and *social age.*
4. **Restate** Using the information in this chapter, describe the life cycle of human beings, including birth, dying, and death.

Thinking Critically

5. **Analyze** Why might a person's chronological, biological, and social ages be different?
6. **Hypothesize** Why do you think that some older people get much more enjoyment out of their later years than others?

Applying Health Skills

7. **Practicing Healthful Behaviors** Talk to some older adults in your community. Find out what behaviors they have followed to maintain a high level of wellness. Then ask what advice they would give to teens who want to live a long and healthy life.

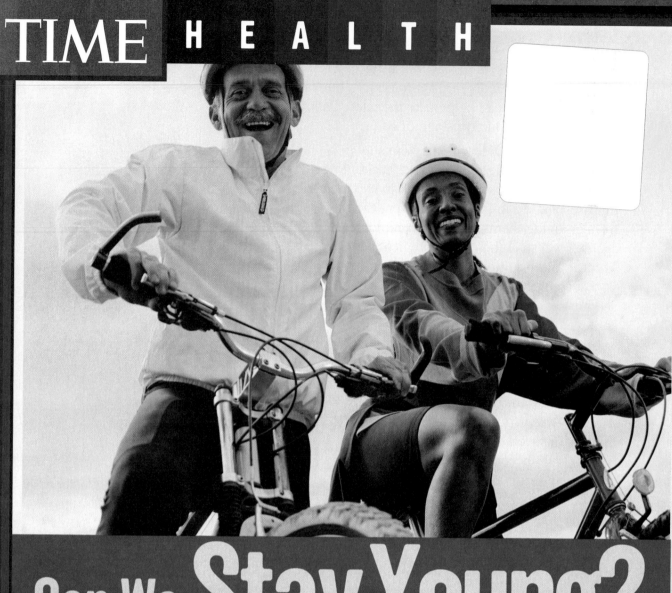

Can We Stay Young?

Scientists are just beginning to unlock the mysteries of aging.

Today, some researchers believe that many people will live beyond age 100. How much further than 100 is it possible to go? Is 150 reasonable? What about 200? If not, why not? To answer these questions, researchers are investigating different factors in the mysterious process of aging.

Free Radicals

Like all organisms, our bodies' cells give off waste as they produce energy. One such waste product is an oxygen molecule known as a free radical—an ordinary molecule with an extra electron. The addition of the electron creates an imbalance that the molecule tries to fix by moving around, attempting to bond with other molecules or structures, including deoxyribonucleic (dee-ahk-see-REYE-boh-noo-KLAY-ik) acid (DNA), the chemical unit that makes up chromosomes. A lifetime of this movement can damage cells, which may lead to a range of disorders, including cancer and the more general signs of aging such as wrinkles and arthritis.

FREE RADICALS

Inside cells' energy-generating structures, metabolism produces unstable oxygen molecules known as free radicals. These molecules bounce around the cells, damaging DNA and other structures.

Cell
Free radicals
DNA
Energy-generating structure

CARAMELIZATION

Excess sugars can bind with proteins, forming a sticky, weblike coating. Over time, the buildup of this substance can stiffen joints, block arteries, and cloud clear tissue.

Sugar
Protein

In recent years, some nutritionists have called for diets rich in fruits and vegetables that contain carotenoids (kar-AH-ten-oids), such as carrots, broccoli, and cantaloupe. These substances act as antioxidants—that is, they grab free radicals and carry them out of the body. Reducing the number of free radicals in the body may slow down the aging process.

Caramelization

When foods such as turkey, bread, and caramel are heated, proteins bind with sugars, causing the surface to darken and, in some cases, turn soft and sticky. In the 1970s, researchers wondered if the same reaction might occur in the bodies of people with diabetes, as excess glucose combined with proteins during the process of metabolism. When sugars and proteins bond, they attract other proteins. This forms a sticky, weblike network, which could stiffen joints, block arteries, and cloud clear tissues like the lens of the eye, leading to cataracts. Researchers call this process caramelization.

What does this have to do with aging? As we get older, we all experience the effects of caramelization, such as joint pain, circulatory disease, and poor vision. Researchers hope that if they can reduce caramelization, they will extend the human life span.

Telomeres

Researchers have been studying genes to find the key that will unlock the secrets of aging. Some have focused on an area at the tip of chromosomes called a telomere. Telomeres keep strands of chromosomes from unraveling, functioning much like the plastic cuff at the end of a shoelace.

As cells divide, telomeres almost always appear to grow shorter. So each time the cell splits, the daughter cells have a little less telomere to play with. When the cell reaches 100 or so replications, the telomere is reduced to a mere nub. At this point, the cell stops replicating.

Some researchers think that the genes covered by the telomere become exposed and active. This might produce proteins that trigger the tissue deterioration that is part of aging.

With a little more progress in studying telomeres, caramelization, free radicals, and other aspects of aging, researchers believe today's adults can hope to live to 120. ■

TIME TO THINK...

About Aging

Using reliable sources on the Internet or in your school's media center, research inventions, discoveries, and trends over the last century that have helped to lengthen (and shorten) the average life span. Have a class discussion about which items are important. Use the entries that the class agreed upon to create a large time line on poster paper about life expectancy in the United States during the last 100 years.

RESOLVING CONFLICTS WITH PARENTS

Model

As you develop your personal identity during your teen years, you will begin to be more independent. You will do more things on your own, without help from your parents. Conflicts with parents can arise when teens believe they are ready to do things that their parents do not want them to do yet. Read about how a teen named Denise uses the T.A.L.K. strategies to resolve a conflict with her parents.

Denise's parents have told her that she is not allowed to go out on dates until she is 16 years old. Denise is upset because she wants to go to a movie with her friend Todd on Friday night. She takes some time out and goes to her room to think. Then she comes back and asks her parents to talk about the situation. She explains that she thinks 14 is old enough to start dating and that some of her classmates are allowed to date. Her parents point out that Denise's friends usually date in groups, not as couples. Denise asks if it would be okay for her to go to the movies with Todd if they invited some other friends along too. Her parents agree to this compromise.

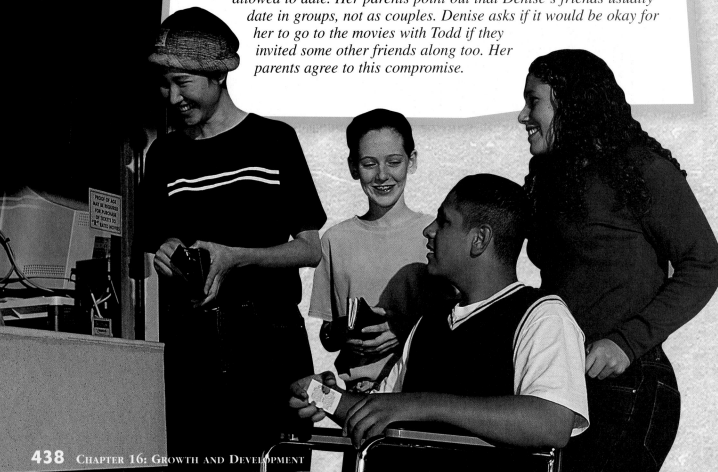

Practice

Read the following scenario and answer the questions that follow.

Fourteen-year-old Logan has a curfew—his parents expect him to be home by 9 o'clock every night. Logan thinks this is too early. He understands why a 9 p.m. curfew might be reasonable on school nights, but most of his friends like to hang out until 11 p.m. or midnight on weekends, and he hates having to leave early.

1. What does Logan want?
2. What do his parents want?
3. How could Logan use the T.A.L.K. strategies to reach a compromise with his parents?

Apply/Assess

Think of a situation that could cause conflict between teens and parents. You can use a personal situation, one that you have invented, or one of the situations described below. Write your scenario on an index card. Then team up with two other students. Choose one of your three scenarios and use it to create a role-play. One of you will play a teen, while the other two will play the teen's parents. In your role play, show how the teen and his or her parents use conflict resolution skills (T.A.L.K.) to find a solution that satisfies everyone. Present your role-play to the class.

Parents think teen plays music too loud.

Parents object to one of teen's friends.

Teen objects to having to keep room tidy.

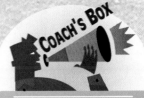

COACH'S BOX

Conflict Resolution

These steps can help you resolve conflicts:

T **Take a time out.**
A **Allow each person to talk.**
L **Let each person ask questions.**
K **Keep brainstorming to find a solution.**

Self-✓Check

- Did we portray a realistic conflict?
- Did we show the steps for conflict resolution?
- Did the characters find a solution that was acceptable to all parties?

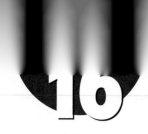

After You Read

Use your completed Foldable to review the information on cells, tissues, organs, and body systems.

FOLDABLES™
Study Organizer

Reviewing Vocabulary and Concepts

On a sheet of paper, write the numbers 1–12. After each number, write the term from the list that best completes each sentence.

- cervix
- genes
- embryo
- fetus
- genetic disorder
- organs
- placenta
- prenatal care
- tissues
- umbilical
- uterus
- heredity

Lesson 1

1. Cells that do similar jobs form _____.
2. Different kinds of tissues are combined in larger structures called _____.
3. The pear-shaped organ in which a fetus is nourished is called the _____.
4. The name of the developing organism from fertilization to about the eighth week of development is the _____.
5. The name for the developing organism from the end of the eighth week until birth is the _____.
6. The thick, rich lining of tissue that builds up along the walls of the uterus and connects the mother to the fetus is called the _____.
7. A cord that connects the fetus to its mother is called the _____ cord.
8. The opening of the uterus is called the _____.

Lesson 2

9. _____ is the passing of traits from parents to their children.
10. The basic units of heredity are called _____.
11. Down syndrome is an example of a(n) _____.
12. _____ refers to steps taken to provide for the health of a pregnant female and her fetus.

Lesson 3

On a sheet of paper, write the numbers 13–15. After each number, write the letter of the answer that best completes each statement.

13. Erikson believed that people pass through _____ developmental stages of life.
    a. two
    b. four
    c. eight
    d. ten
14. The time when you begin to develop traits of adults of your own gender is called
    a. middle adulthood.
    b. early adulthood.
    c. puberty.
    d. late childhood.
15. The emotional changes of adolescence are related to the body's production of
    a. hormones.
    b. toxins.
    c. calcium.
    d. muscle.

Lesson 4

On a sheet of paper, write the numbers 16–18. Write *True* or *False* for each statement below. If the statement is false, change the underlined word or phrase to make it true.

16. The physical signs of aging occur at <u>the same time</u> in different adults.
17. A person's <u>biological age</u> is his or her age measured in years.

18. Social age is measured by a person's lifestyle.

Thinking Critically

Using complete sentences, answer the following questions on a sheet of paper.

19. Analyze Write a set of questions you think a pregnant female might ask her doctor about what she could do to have a healthy baby.

20. Hypothesize How do you think an older adult's biological age might be affected by not being involved in a variety of social groups?

Career Corner

Geneticist Geneticists are scientists who study the ways that parents' genes affect their children. Their research can reveal the causes of genetic disorders. Couples who have a genetic disease in their family may ask a geneticist to determine any risks to their unborn children. Geneticists need at least a master's degree in genetics. Some positions require a doctoral degree. If you have an interest in the study of inherited diseases, go to Career Corner at health.glencoe.com to find out more about this and other health careers.

Standardized Test Practice

Reading & Writing

Read the paragraphs below and then answer the questions.

You may have heard of the terms "left brained" and "right brained." These terms refer to the fact that your brain has two sides, or hemispheres. While each hemisphere has different functions, they work together to help you think, feel, and perform the activities of daily life.

Scientists have learned that the brain's two hemispheres are specialized, with each side being better at different tasks. The left hemisphere, for example, is good with sequencing and language skills. The right hemisphere is more visual and is good at seeing relationships and patterns.

People don't use just one side of the brain, and one side does not control or dominate the other. Both sides are needed for most activities.

1. What phrase from the passage helps readers understand the meaning of the word *hemisphere*?

A work together

B two sides

C different functions

D good with sequencing

2. How does the author organize the ideas in the second paragraph?

A comparing the functions of both sides of the brain

B listing events in the order that they occur

C explaining events in order of their importance

D using cause and effect to explain the two sides of the brain

3. Write a paragraph describing your personality or the personality of a friend or family member.

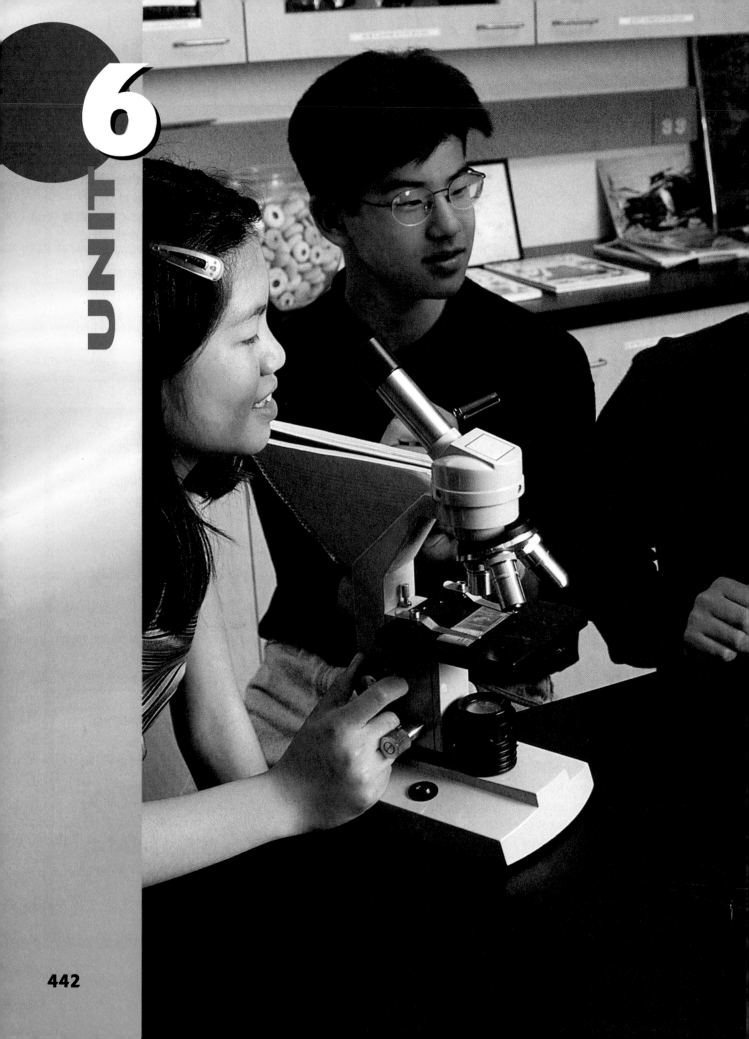

Diseases and Disorders

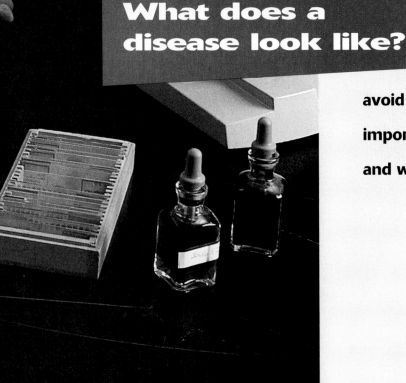

HEALTH in Action

You can't see it in a microscope. Instead, you recognize a disease by its signs, or symptoms, like a fever or a runny nose. Even more important than learning to identify diseases, however, is learning to identify ways to avoid or to manage them. That's an important part of maintaining health and wellness!

What does a disease look like?

Our
Battle
Against
AIDS

The Fight That Keeps
Many Like Magic Johnson
Living and Being Positive

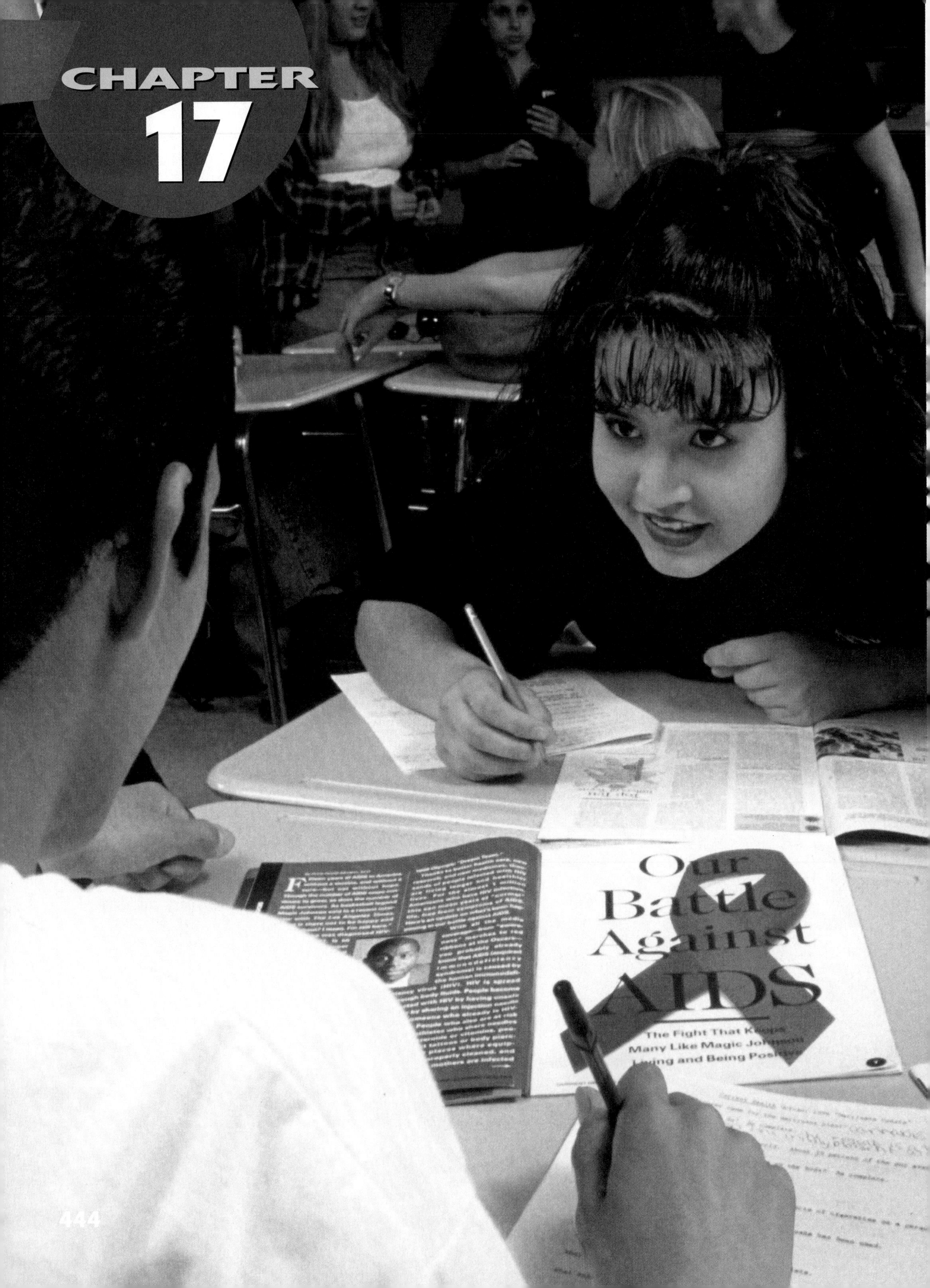

Communicable Diseases

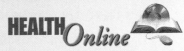

HEALTH Online

Do you make healthful choices when it comes to avoiding and preventing the spread of diseases? Find out by taking the Chapter 17 Health Inventory at health.glencoe.com.

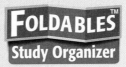

FOLDABLES™ Study Organizer

Before You Read

Make this Foldable to help you record what you learn in Lesson 1 about pathogens and preventing the spread of disease. Begin with a plain sheet of 11" × 17" paper.

Step 1

Fold the short sides inward so that they meet in the middle.

Step 2

Fold the top to the bottom.

Step 3

Open and cut along the inside fold lines to form four tabs.

Step 4

Label the tabs as shown.

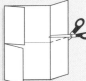

Pathogens and Disease | Types of Pathogens

How Pathogens Are Spread | Preventing the Spread of Disease

As You Read

Under the appropriate tab, summarize the main ideas about pathogens and preventing the spread of communicable diseases.

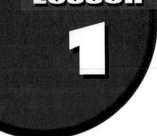

Preventing the Spread of Disease

Quick Write

What do you think is the single most important action you can take to help prevent the spread of disease in your home and school?

LEARN ABOUT...

- causes of communicable diseases.
- the organisms that cause diseases.
- how diseases are spread.

VOCABULARY

- communicable disease
- pathogens
- infection
- bacteria
- virus
- fungi
- protozoa
- rickettsias
- vector
- contagious period

What Is Disease?

When you are healthy, you feel good both physically and mentally. Sometimes, however, a disease might prevent you from feeling your best. A disease is an illness that affects the proper functioning of the body or mind. *A disease that can be passed to a person from another person, animal, or object* is called a **communicable** (kuh·MYOO·ni·kuh·buhl) **disease**.

Diseases that cannot be caught from people, animals, or objects are called noncommunicable diseases. Noncommunicable diseases may be caused by lifestyle factors, conditions that people are born with, or environmental hazards. **Figure 17.1** shows how a communicable disease and a noncommunicable disease can have similar symptoms. Noncommunicable diseases are discussed in Chapter 18.

Causes of Communicable Diseases

The *tiny organisms that cause communicable diseases* are called **pathogens**. You will also hear them called germs. When pathogens enter the body, an infection may result. An **infection** is *a condition that occurs when pathogens enter the body, multiply, and damage cells.* There are many different types of pathogens.

Bacteria

Many communicable diseases are caused by bacteria. **Bacteria** are *tiny one-celled organisms that live nearly everywhere.* Most types of bacteria are harmless, and many types live on and inside the human body. In fact, your body needs certain bacteria to work properly. Common diseases caused by bacteria include strep throat, tooth decay, boils, bacterial pneumonia, and impetigo.

Viruses

A **virus** is *the smallest disease-causing organism.* Colds, flu, and hepatitis are caused by viruses. Viruses also cause diseases of childhood and adolescence, such as measles, mumps, and chicken pox. It is important to know whether a disease is caused by a virus or by another pathogen so that the right treatment can be given.

FIGURE 17.1

COMMUNICABLE OR NONCOMMUNICABLE?

Communicable diseases and noncommunicable diseases require different treatments.

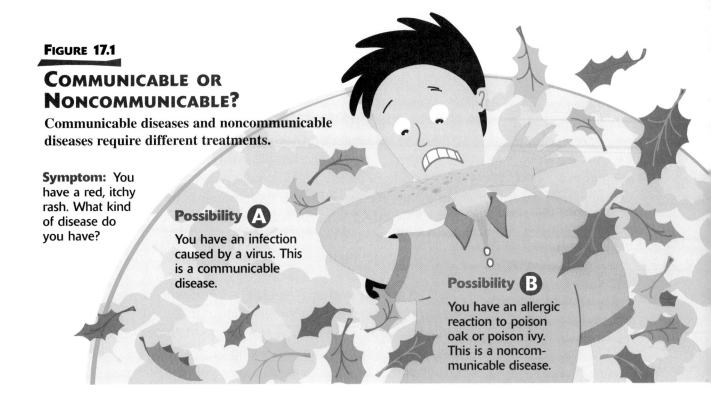

Symptom: You have a red, itchy rash. What kind of disease do you have?

Possibility A

You have an infection caused by a virus. This is a communicable disease.

Possibility B

You have an allergic reaction to poison oak or poison ivy. This is a noncommunicable disease.

In general, bacterial infections can be treated with antibiotics but viral infections cannot. Some viral infections are now treated with prescribed medications.

Other Types of Pathogens

Listed below are three other types of pathogens that cause communicable diseases.

- **Fungi** (FUHN·jy) are *primitive life-forms that feed on organic materials.* Certain fungi live in the hair, nails, and skin. Fungi cause ringworm, an infection of the scalp and skin, and athlete's foot, an infection of the skin between the toes.
- **Protozoa** (proh·tuh·ZOH·uh) are *single-celled organisms that are usually harmless but that can cause certain diseases.* Malaria is a disease caused by protozoa that live in certain kinds of mosquitoes. If an affected mosquito bites a human, the person will be infected. Water contaminated with protozoa can also cause infections.
- **Rickettsias** (rik·ET·see·uhz) are *disease-causing organisms that resemble bacteria but multiply like viruses.* They enter humans from the bites of insects such as fleas or lice. They can cause diseases such as typhus and Rocky Mountain spotted fever.

Athlete's foot is an irritating but usually harmless condition caused by fungi. *What can you do to avoid getting athlete's foot?*

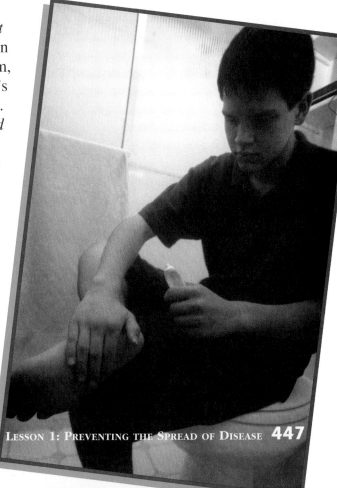

Reading Check

Separate these words into groups: *good hygiene, vaccinations, sharing glasses, ticks, insect repellent, direct contact, undercooked meat, handwashing.* Label each group and add other words.

How Pathogens Are Spread

Illness can occur when a pathogen enters your body. Here are some risk factors associated with communicable diseases:

- **Direct contact with an infected person.** You can pick up pathogens on your skin by coming into direct contact with an infected person. For example, you can pick up the strep throat bacteria by kissing someone who has strep throat. Some pathogens, such as HIV, are spread mainly by sexual contact.

- **Indirect contact with an infected person.** Some pathogens are spread through the air. Pathogens can also enter your body if you share eating utensils or drinking glasses with an infected person.

- **Contact with a vector.** A **vector** is *an organism, such as an insect, that transmits a pathogen.* Mosquitoes, for example, spread malaria. Ticks spread two serious diseases—Lyme disease and Rocky Mountain spotted fever.

- **Other contacts.** Pathogens can enter your body if you drink water or eat food that contains them. Improperly stored food and undercooked meat are dangerous for this reason. Another way to become infected is to receive blood that carries pathogens.

Hands-On Health

HABITS FOR HEALTH

How healthy are your habits? This activity will help you find out.

WHAT YOU WILL NEED
- pencil and paper

WHAT YOU WILL DO
Write yes or no for each statement.
1. I wash my hands after using the bathroom and before preparing or serving food.
2. I cover my nose and mouth when I cough or sneeze.
3. I avoid sharing eating utensils or drinking glasses with others.
4. I avoid drinking water from streams and lakes.
5. I make sure food is properly stored.
6. I avoid sharing combs, brushes, and towels with others.
7. When I'm sick, I avoid others during the contagious period.
8. When I'm sick, I get medical care.
9. I avoid contact with people who have diseases that I could catch.
10. I have received all the recommended vaccinations.

IN CONCLUSION
Give yourself 1 point for each yes. A score of 8–10 is very good. A score of 6–8 is good. A score of 4–6 is fair. If you score below 4, you need to work on improving your health behaviors.

Preventing the Spread of Disease

Preventing the spread of disease involves good personal hygiene, and that starts with hand washing. Wash your hands frequently and always before handling food. Use clean utensils when preparing food, and keep preparation surfaces clean. Do not share utensils or drinking glasses with others.

When outdoors, wear suitable clothing and use insect repellent to avoid bites from ticks and mosquitoes. Examine your body for ticks after you have been in an area where they might be found. Avoid contact with a contagious person until he or she is better. Finally, make sure you have had the vaccinations recommended for your age.

Protecting others involves taking actions to prevent the spread of pathogens. Again, wash your hands frequently. Cover your mouth and nose when you cough or sneeze. If you are sick, determine the **contagious period**, that is, *the length of time that a particular disease can spread from person to person.* Stay home from school and away from other people during this period.

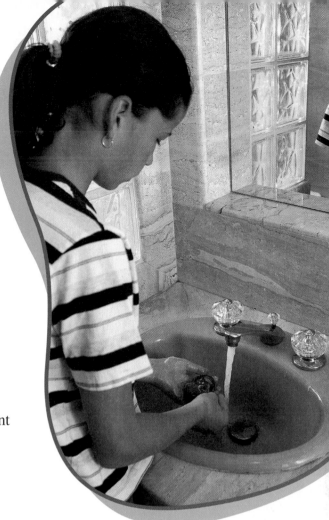

One of the easiest and most effective ways to avoid getting sick is to wash your hands frequently.

Lesson 1 Review

Using complete sentences, answer the following questions on a sheet of paper.

Reviewing Terms and Facts

1. **Vocabulary** Define the terms *pathogens* and *infection.*
2. **Recall** Besides bacteria and viruses, what are three other types of pathogens?
3. **Distinguish** What are four risk factors associated with communicable diseases?
4. **Recall** What is a *vector?* Give two examples of vectors.

Thinking Critically

5. **Summarize** What actions can you take to protect yourself and others from disease?
6. **Explain** Why is it important to know the contagious period for a disease?

Applying Health Skills

7. **Practicing Healthful Behaviors** Help prevent the spread of disease in your school. In small groups, prepare lists of guidelines that can be posted in classrooms, in bathrooms, and in the school cafeteria.

Lesson 2

The Body's Defenses Against Infection

Quick Write

Describe the symptoms you have when you get a cold or the flu. What causes those symptoms?

LEARN ABOUT...

- the body's defenses against pathogens.
- the nonspecific, or general, immune response.
- specific immune responses.
- the difference between natural and acquired immunity.

VOCABULARY

- immune system
- immunity
- lymphatic system
- antigens
- antibodies

The Body's Defenses

Although bacteria, viruses, and other pathogens live all around you, most of them never get a chance to make you sick. That's because your body has many different ways to defend itself. Your first line of defense—your skin and body fluids—forms a barrier between you and pathogens, as shown in **Figure 17.2**.

FIGURE 17.2

THE FIRST LINE OF DEFENSE: STOP AT ENTRY

Your body's first line of defense works to prevent pathogens from entering your body.

Eyes
Tears wash pathogens from your eyes. Tears also contain chemical compounds that kill pathogens.

Skin
The tough, outer layer of skin protects you from pathogens. However, they can enter the body if you have a cut, burn, or scrape.

Stomach
Gastric juices produced by the lining of your stomach help kill pathogens that enter the body through food or drink.

Mucous Membranes and Saliva
Mucous membranes line your nose, mouth, and throat and secrete a fluid called mucus that traps pathogens. In the mouth, saliva washes germs from your teeth. Saliva also contains chemicals that kill many pathogens.

The Main Line of Defense

Sometimes pathogens get past the first line of defense and enter your body. Then your body's main line of defense is activated, and the pathogens are confronted by your immune system. The **immune system** is *a combination of body defenses made up of cells, tissues, and organs that fight off pathogens and disease.* The immune system has two major kinds of defense strategies—a nonspecific, or general, response and a specific response. Together, they offer **immunity**—*your body's ability to resist the germs that cause a particular disease.*

Nonspecific Response

Whenever pathogens invade the body, the immune system launches a nonspecific, all-purpose response. It begins with inflammation, or increased blood flow, to the affected area. Inflammation signals chemical messengers to summon special white blood cells to speed to the affected area and destroy invading pathogens.

If pathogens spread, the inflammation may result in a fever. The higher body temperature causes the body to produce still more white blood cells. The fever also slows the growth of pathogens that cannot survive at high temperatures.

Specific Response

If invading pathogens survive the nonspecific response, a specific response is set in motion. The response targets the pathogen in a more specialized manner. It also gives the body the ability to recognize the same pathogen if it invades again. The body responds in this way to vaccinations as well as to developed diseases.

CONNECT TO

Science

A HEALTHY RESPONSE
When you cut or burn yourself, the area around the wound rapidly becomes red, swollen, and painful to the touch. This inflammation helps wounds heal. Blood vessels enlarge, bringing more germ-fighting white blood cells to the site.

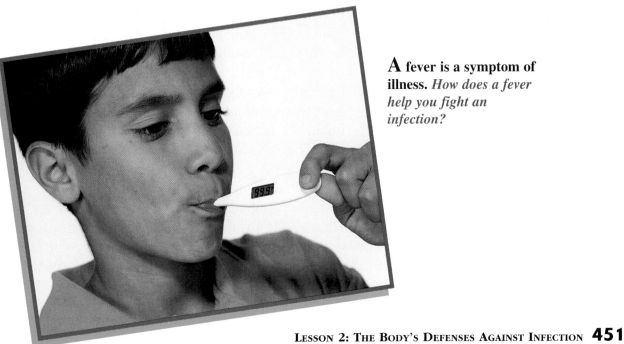

A fever is a symptom of illness. *How does a fever help you fight an infection?*

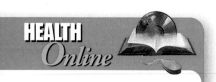
The Lymphatic System and the Immune Response

The **lymphatic** (lim·FA·tik) **system** is *a secondary circulatory system that helps the body fight pathogens and maintain its fluid balance.* The lymphatic system carries a fluid known as lymph and produces white blood cells known as lymphocytes. Two kinds of lymphocytes—B cells and T cells—are involved in the specific immune response. B cells are formed in bone marrow, and T cells are produced in the thymus gland.

Lymphocytes react to **antigens**, *substances released by invading pathogens.* To fight antigens, B cells release **antibodies**, *proteins that attach to antigens, keeping them from harming the body.* B cells produce a specific antibody for each specific antigen. The antibodies remain in your blood and become active if the same pathogen invades your body at a later time.

T cells, produced in the thymus gland, are lymphocytes that attack pathogens directly and that stimulate the production of B cells. There are two main types of T cells. Killer cells attach to invading pathogens and destroy them. Helper cells activate the production of antibodies by B cells. B cells and T cells play critical roles in the immune system.

Immunity

Your natural immunity is present at birth. It includes general immune reactions such as those of skin and mucous membranes and of white blood cells that engulf pathogens.

In contrast, acquired immunity develops over a person's lifetime. It begins when antibodies pass from a pregnant female's body to her developing fetus. Breastfeeding transfers other antibodies to an infant. These events are examples of passive immunity—receiving antibodies to fight pathogens. Another type of acquired immunity is active immunity. In active immunity, your body makes specific antibodies in response to invasion by a pathogen.

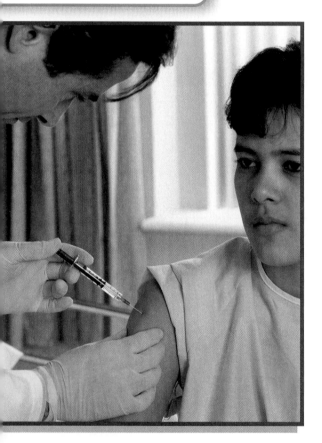

A tetanus vaccine is a preparation of a toxin produced by the bacteria that cause tetanus. *What kind of immunity does this provide?*

The body also makes antibodies when a vaccine is used. As you learned in Chapter 11, a vaccine is a preparation of dead or weakened pathogens (germs) that causes the immune system to produce antibodies. These germs will not cause illness, but will trigger the body to make antibodies for them.

Vaccinations

Vaccinations are also known as immunizations. Some vaccinations, such as those for hepatitis B, must be given as a series over a period of months. Others, such as the vaccination for tetanus, can protect you for several years but must be repeated on a regular basis throughout your lifetime. Keeping vaccinations current protects both the person who is vaccinated and those around him or her. **Figure 17.3** shows recommended vaccinations for children and teens.

FIGURE 17.3

VACCINATION SCHEDULE

Vaccine	Recommended Ages for Vaccination
Hepatitis B	Birth–2 months, 1–4 months, 6–18 months, or 11–12 years if previous doses were missed or given too early
Diphtheria, tetanus, pertussis (DTP)	2 months, 4 months, 6 months, 15–18 months, 4–6 years, with a tetanus booster at 11–16 years
HIB (*H. influenzae* type b)	2 months, 4 months, 6 months, 12–15 months
Polio	2 months, 4 months, 6–18 months, 4–6 years
Measles, mumps, rubella	12–15 months, 4–6 years, or 11–12 years if previous doses were missed or given too early
Varicella (chicken pox)	12–18 months, or 11–12 years if previous dose was missed or given too early
Hepatitis A	24 months–18 years (in selected areas)

Source: American Academy of Pediatrics, 2000

Lesson 2 Review

Using complete sentences, answer the following questions on a sheet of paper.

Reviewing Terms and Facts

1. **Identify** Name the parts involved in the body's first line of defense.
2. **Vocabulary** Define *immune system*. What are its two major kinds of defensive actions?
3. **Explain** How does fever fight disease?
4. **Contrast** What is the difference between antigens and antibodies?

Thinking Critically

5. **Distinguish** How does the nonspecific immune response differ from specific immune system responses?

Applying Health Skills

6. **Accessing Information** Plan an imaginary vacation to a country on another continent. Do research on the Web or in your library to find out what immunizations are required to travel to that destination.

Communicable Diseases

Quick Write

If you have a cold or the flu, what actions do you take to prevent others from catching your disease?

LEARN ABOUT...

- what causes colds, and how they can be treated.
- symptoms of some common communicable diseases.
- good health habits that protect you from disease.

VOCABULARY

- hepatitis
- mononucleosis

The Common Cold

The common cold is the most familiar communicable disease. A cold is caused by one of several hundred different viruses. The symptoms of a cold include mild fever, runny nose, itchy eyes, sneezing, coughing, mild sore throat, and headache.

You can help prevent a cold by limiting your exposure to cold viruses and by keeping yourself healthy enough to resist pathogens. If you do get a cold, take an active role in the management of the disease by getting plenty of rest and drinking lots of fluids. Some OTC medicines may help relieve symptoms. Even if the medicines make you feel better, you should stay home for at least 24 hours after cold symptoms appear. That is when your cold is most contagious, and when you are most likely to pass the virus on to other people.

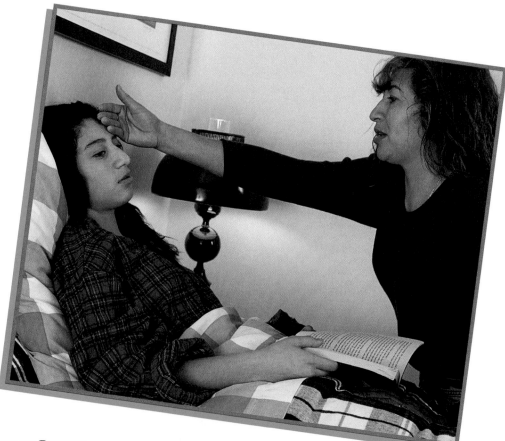

The best way to deal with a cold is to stay home, rest, and drink plenty of fluids. *How do these actions show that you are accepting responsibility for the treatment of disease?*

Other Common Diseases

Some of the most common communicable diseases are described in the list below. Several other diseases are listed in **Figure 17.4**.

- **Influenza, or "the flu."** This disease is caused by one of three broad types of influenza viruses, each with several different strains. Flu symptoms include fever, exhaustion, chills, headache, and body ache. Yearly vaccination against the flu is recommended for older people and for people who have chronic diseases. Because the virus changes frequently, a vaccine that kills an old strain may not harm a new one.

- **Strep throat.** This infection is caused by streptococci bacteria that produce a very sore throat, fever, muscle pain, and enlarged lymph nodes in the neck. Left untreated, strep throat can lead to serious complications, including heart damage. That is why your doctor may order a strep test if your tonsils and throat are inflamed. Strep throat can be cured with antibiotics.

Reading Check

Compare and contrast. Choose two diseases from this page. List their similarities and their differences.

FIGURE 17.4

SOME COMMUNICABLE DISEASES

This figure shows the symptoms and contagious periods of several communicable diseases. *In a paragraph, determine when treatment of these illnesses at home is appropriate and when and how to seek further help when needed.*

Disease	Symptoms	Contagious Period	Vaccine
Chicken pox	Itchy rash, fever	One to five days before symptoms appear to when spots crust over	Yes
Pneumonia	High fever, chest pain, cough	Varies	For some types
Rubella	Swollen lymph nodes, rash, fever	Seven days before rash starts to five days after	Yes
Measles	Fever, runny nose, cough, rash	Three to four days before rash starts to four days after	Yes
Mumps	Fever, headache, swollen areas in neck and under jaw	Seven days before symptoms to nine days after	Yes
Whooping cough	Fever, runny nose, dry cough (with a whooping sound)	From inflammation of mucous membranes to four weeks after	Yes
Tuberculosis	Fever, fatigue, weight loss, coughing blood	Varies	Yes

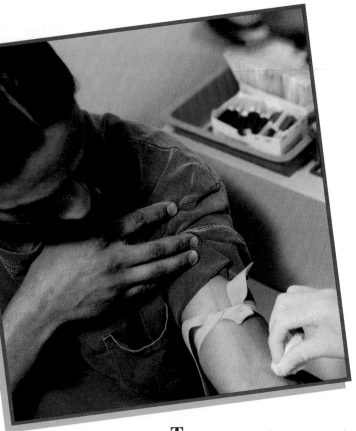

The symptoms for mononucleosis are similar to those for flu. A blood test determines if a patient has mono.

- **Hepatitis** (hep·uh·TYT·uhs). *A viral disease of the liver characterized by yellowing of the skin and the whites of the eyes* is known as **hepatitis**. There are different types of hepatitis, each caused by a different virus. They are hepatitis A, B, and C.
- **Mononucleosis** (mahn·oh·noo·klee·OH·sis). *A viral disease whose symptoms include swollen, tender areas in the neck and a sore throat* is **mononucleosis**. Mononucleosis, often called "mono," is most common in teens and young adults and is spread by direct contact. People who have mono generally feel weak and have little energy. Treatment includes complete bed rest. Recovery can take three or more weeks, and the disease can recur during the year after the first attack.

HEALTH SKILLS ACTIVITY

ACCESSING INFORMATION

Can I Catch What's in the News?

Local newspapers or news programs often report on new diseases or outbreaks of an existing disease. To find out if you are at risk, ask these questions and get the answers from reliable sources.

- **IS THE DISEASE COMMUNICABLE?** If it is, are you likely to come in direct or indirect contact with an infected person?
- **DOES THE DISEASE HAVE AN ENVIRONMENTAL CAUSE?** Some diseases arise from exposure to environmental hazards or from eating certain foods. Have you been exposed to these?

- **WHO IS AFFECTED BY THE DISEASE?** Some diseases affect certain groups of people, such as those of a specific age or gender. Are you in a vulnerable category?
- **IS THE DISEASE CONFINED TO A CERTAIN GEOGRAPHICAL AREA?** Some diseases are focused on a particular place. Do you live in that place, or have you recently traveled there?

ON YOUR OWN

Find a news report about a disease. Using these guidelines, analyze your risk for contracting the disease based on these factors: age, behavior, culture, environment, genetics, and pathogen exposure.

Good Health Habits

Good health habits reduce your chances of illness. When your body is strong and healthy, it is better able to fight off pathogens.

- Follow a sensible eating plan to maintain your overall health. A strong, healthy immune system can fight pathogens better than a weak one.
- Get plenty of rest. Fatigue reduces the effectiveness of your immune system.
- Get regular physical activity, especially when you feel stressed.
- Avoid tobacco, alcohol, and other drugs.
- Drink water only from approved water supplies. Do not drink from streams, lakes, and rivers.
- Avoid sharing personal items such as towels, toothbrushes, hairbrushes, and makeup.

Protecting your health with good nutrition and regular physical activity will help you fight diseases. *What other measures improve your overall health?*

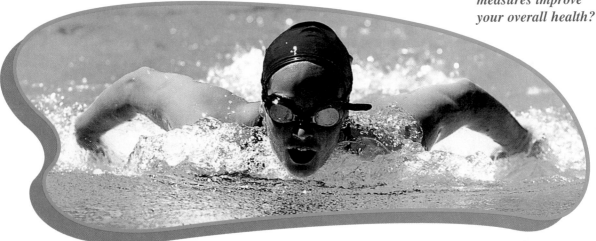

Lesson 3 Review

Using complete sentences, answer the following questions on a sheet of paper.

Reviewing Terms and Facts

1. **Explain** Why should you stay home when cold symptoms first appear?
2. **Explain** What are the symptoms of strep throat? Why do they need to be treated?
3. **Recall** Which communicable disease is identified by swelling in the neck and under the jaw?
4. **List** What are the symptoms of hepatitis and mononucleosis?

Thinking Critically

5. **Summarize** Your friend Chloe has mono. What advice would you give her?
6. **Explain** How does practicing good health habits protect you from disease?

Applying Health Skills

7. **Accessing Information** Select one of the diseases mentioned in this lesson. Use reliable sources of information in the library or on the Internet to learn more about the disease. Prepare a pamphlet that gives detailed information about the causes, symptoms, and treatment of the disease.

Sexually Transmitted Diseases

Quick Write

Write down three questions that you have about sexually transmitted diseases.

LEARN ABOUT...

- sexually transmitted diseases (STDs).
- why abstinence is the best way to avoid getting an STD.
- some common STDs and the problems they cause.
- how some STDs can be treated.

VOCABULARY

- sexually transmitted diseases (STDs)

What Are STDs?

Sexually transmitted diseases, or **STDs**, are *infections spread from person to person through sexual contact*. STDs are sometimes referred to as sexually transmitted infections, or STIs. In the United States, STDs are a major health problem for teens. Each year, one-quarter of all new cases of STDs occur among 15- to 19-year-olds. STDs take a toll on young people because many lack knowledge about STDs and how they are transmitted. **Figure 17.5** summarizes important facts about STDs.

FIGURE 17.5

WHAT YOU SHOULD KNOW ABOUT STDS

Learning the facts about STDs will help you avoid them.

- Most STDs are spread only through sexual contact.
- You cannot tell if someone has an STD by his or her appearance.
- A person with an STD may have no symptoms.
- Many STDs can be treated, but early diagnosis is vital.
- Because treatments for STDs vary, they must be accurately identified.
- STDs can recur because the body does not build up immunity to them.
- STDs are serious diseases that can cause sterility, blindness, deafness, insanity, and death.

Practicing Abstinence

When you practice abstinence, you avoid the serious consequences of contracting an STD. This prevention is critical because STDs differ from other communicable diseases in two important ways. First, there are no vaccines for any STDs except hepatitis B. Second, your body cannot build immunity to STDs.

The only sure way to avoid getting an STD is to practice abstinence from sexual activity. Deciding to say no to sexual activity will be one of the most important health choices you ever make. Make a commitment to abstain from sexual activity. Demonstrate your commitment to abstinence through your words and behavior.

Responsible Behavior

Your actions and body language will tell others that you practice abstinence.

- Choose your friends carefully. They should share your values and support your decision about practicing sexual abstinence.
- Avoid being alone with a date. Group activities remove pressure for sexual activity.
- Know your limits and communicate them with your date before you go out.
- Say no through your words *and* your actions.
- Seek advice from a trusted adult on handling difficult situations.

Effective Communication

Below is a list of statements that someone might make to pressure you into sexual activity. Beside each statement is a sample response that shows your commitment to abstinence.

- If your date says, "If you really care for me, you would have sex with me," you can say, "If you really care for me, you would respect my decision."
- If your date says, "Sex can be safe," you can say, "Abstinence from sex is the only sure way to be safe."
- If your date says, "Everyone else is doing it," you can say, "The only thing that matters to me is what *I* choose to do. Besides, most teens *aren't* having sex."

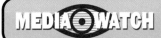

MEDIA WATCH

STDs IN THE MEDIA

Sexual situations and images are very common on television, but how often are STDs mentioned? In a small group, brainstorm some ways in which the media could take a more responsible role in delivering factual information about STDs.

Group activities are a good way to have fun while avoiding pressure to engage in sexual activity. *What group activities do you and your friends enjoy?*

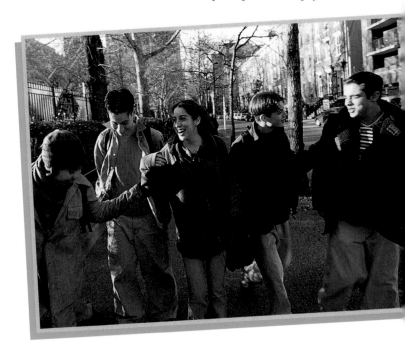

COMMUNICATION SKILLS

Helping a Friend Choose Abstinence

Rick and Jerome play on the school soccer team. In the locker room after practice, Rick listened to some of the other guys on the soccer team. They were boasting about their sexual experiences. Then they teased Rick about his inexperience.

On their way home from practice, Jerome wanted to talk about the incident. He thinks that most of the boys were lying about their experiences. He believes that abstinence is the best decision. What should he say to Rick?

What Would You Do?

Apply the skills for good communication to this situation. With a classmate, role-play a conversation between Jerome and Rick. The teen playing Jerome should state why he believes that abstinence is the best choice of behavior for all teens.

SPEAKING SKILLS

- Use "I" messages.
- Make clear, simple statements.
- Be honest with thoughts and feelings.
- Use appropriate body language.

LISTENING SKILLS

- Use appropriate body language.
- Use conversation encouragers.
- Mirror thoughts and feelings.
- Ask questions.

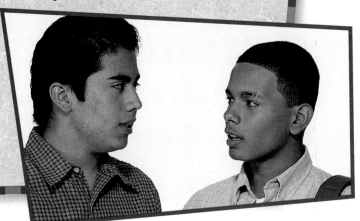

Feel Good About Your Decision

Dating should be fun, and abstinence helps teens enjoy healthy relationships. Also, teens who practice abstinence do not have to worry about STDs or pregnancy.

Common STDs

Each year, about 4 million teens contract an STD. However, many fail to get medical attention because they do not recognize the symptoms or are too embarrassed to ask for help. In all cases, diagnosis and treatment are necessary. **Figure 17.6** on page 462 lists several common STDs, along with their symptoms and treatments. HIV/AIDS, another serious STD, is discussed in Lesson 5.

Here is some general information about the most common STDs.

- **Chlamydia** (klah·MID·ee·ah) is a very common STD. It is a "silent" STD—many infected people have no symptoms. If left untreated, it can seriously damage the reproductive organs in both males and females.

- **Genital herpes** is caused by the virus herpes simplex type 2 (HSV-2). Herpes cannot be cured, and it results in periodic bouts of painful blisters on the genitals. Herpes can be passed to another person even when the blisters are not apparent.
- **Genital warts** are caused by the human papillomavirus (HPV). HPV has been linked with cervical cancer and skin cancer. It is thought that the virus may disable the skin's defenses against ultraviolet radiation from the sun.
- **Gonorrhea** is caused by bacteria. Infection can affect the entire body, causing joint pain. Some people, especially females, may not have symptoms until the disease is advanced.
- **Nongonococcal urethritis (NGU)** is an inflammation of the urethra—the tube that transports urine from the bladder. It is caused by bacteria different from those that cause gonorrhea. NGU is more common in men than in women.
- **Pelvic inflammatory disease (PID)** is a general infection of the female reproductive organs. Most women with PID became infected as a result of another STD, such as chlamydia or gonorrhea. If left untreated, PID may worsen over time and cause sterility.
- **Syphilis** is a very serious STD. If left untreated, the bacteria that cause syphilis invade the entire body, damaging the internal organs. Advanced syphilis may cause blindness, paralysis, insanity, and death.

✓ Reading Check

Understand abbreviations. Which disease names are abbreviated with capital letters? Determine how each abbreviation is formed.

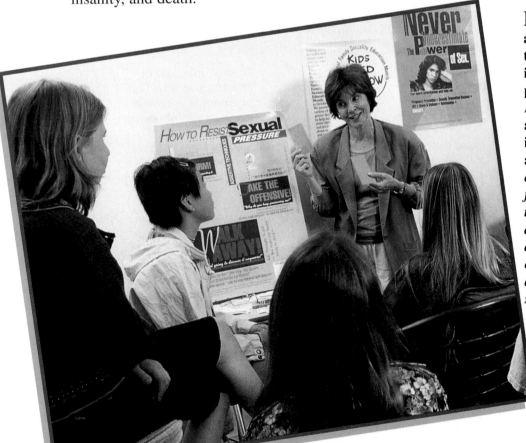

Learning the facts about STDs will help teens make the important decision to practice abstinence. Abstaining from sexual activity before marriage is the only sure way to avoid STDs. *Write an essay summarizing the facts related to STDs. In the essay, analyze why abstinence from sexual activity is the preferred choice of behavior for all unmarried persons of school age.*

FIGURE 17.6

FACTS ABOUT COMMON STDS

Disease (Cause)	Symptoms	Treatment	What Could Happen
Chlamydia (bacteria)	Burning during urination; irritation of genitals; discharge; females may have mild or no symptoms	Antibiotics	Sterility from scarring of reproductive organs; infection of developing fetus in pregnant females
Genital herpes (HSV-2) (virus)	Painful, itchy blisters in genital area; fever; burning when urinating during outbreak	No cure; medication can relieve symptoms	Increased risk of HIV infection; brain damage or death of newborns of infected mother
Genital warts (virus)	Painless warts in genital area three weeks to six months after exposure to infected person	Topical medication; freezing or surgery to remove warts	Cancer of reproductive system; urinary blockage in males; cervical cancer in females; infection of newborn during birth
Gonorrhea (bacteria)	Discharge; swollen lymph nodes in groin; burning during urination; females may have mild or no symptoms	Antibiotics, but some strains of bacteria are drug resistant	Sterility; permanent damage to joints and body organs; infection of developing fetus in pregnant females
Hepatitis B (HBV) (virus)	Fatigue; loss of appetite; nausea; yellowing of the skin; joint pain	Prevented by vaccination; no treatment otherwise	Liver damage; liver cancer; infection of developing fetus in pregnant females
Nongonococcal urethritis (NGU) (bacteria)	Urethral discharge and discomfort in males; irritation of vagina or no symptoms in females	Antibiotics	Sterility; infection of reproductive organs; pneumonia in females; eye infection of newborn
Pelvic inflammatory disease (PID) (females only) (bacteria)	Foul-smelling discharge; tenderness in abdomen; backache; fever; vomiting; heavy menstrual periods	Antibiotics	Sterility from scarring of reproductive organs; constant pelvic pain
Pubic lice (crabs) (small insects)	Itching; presence of lice and eggs in pubic hair	Medicated soaps; washing of all bed linens and clothes	No lasting effects
Syphilis (bacteria)	Red sores in genital area; body rash; flulike symptoms; symptoms may disappear though disease is still active	Antibiotics	Increased risk of HIV infection; damage to cardiovascular system, liver, kidneys, and nervous system; blindness; insanity; death; birth defects in developing fetus of pregnant females
Trichomoniasis (protozoa)	Foul-smelling, yellowish discharge and itching in females; males may have no symptoms	Antibiotics	Infections of the bladder and urethra

Other Infections to Watch For

Other types of infections may have symptoms similar to those of STDs. Urinary tract infections (UTIs) are caused by several different pathogens. In both males and females, a UTI can cause pain and burning during urination. If a urinary tract infection follows sexual activity, it might be an STD.

In females, vaginal yeast infections are fairly common. Yeasts are fungi. If they grow uncontrolled in the vagina, they produce a white discharge accompanied by itching and burning. While a vaginal yeast infection *may* result from sexual activity, not all do. Anyone who has the symptoms of a urinary or vaginal infection should see a physician for diagnosis and treatment.

If You Need Help

If you are concerned that you might have an STD, you must seek treatment right away. Most STDs respond to treatment if diagnosed early. Left untreated, they can lead to severe health problems, or even death. Talk to a responsible and caring adult about your concerns.

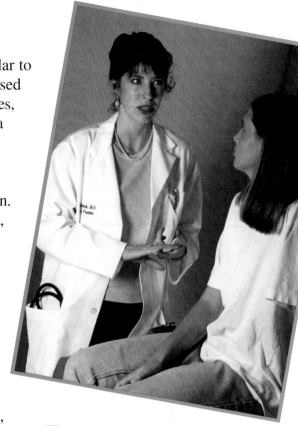

Early detection is the best way to treat an STD. If you suspect that you have one, you can talk confidentially with a health professional.

Lesson 4 Review

Using complete sentences, answer the following questions on a sheet of paper.

Reviewing Terms and Facts

1. **Vocabulary** Using your own words, define *sexually transmitted disease.*
2. **Recall** List four facts about STDs that teens need to know.
3. **Explain** What is the only sure way to avoid getting an STD?
4. **Summarize** Name six STDs and list a fact related to each one.

Thinking Critically

5. **Synthesize** Why should people seek medical help if they think they have been exposed to an STD, even though they have no symptoms?
6. **Discuss** Why is abstinence from sexual activity the only method that is 100 percent effective in preventing STDs?

Applying Health Skills

7. **Refusal Skills** On index cards, write as many lines as you can think of that might be used to pressure someone to be sexually active. With your teacher's approval, put all the cards from the class into a box. Take turns pulling out cards and reading them. Along with your peers, suggest appropriate refusal lines.

HIV/AIDS

LEARN ABOUT...

- AIDS and what causes it.
- how HIV is spread and how it is not spread.
- how to avoid getting HIV.

VOCABULARY

- acquired immunodeficiency syndrome (AIDS)
- human immunodeficiency virus (HIV)
- carrier
- opportunistic infection

What Is AIDS?

AIDS, or **acquired immunodeficiency syndrome**, is *a deadly disease that interferes with the body's natural ability to fight infection. The virus that causes AIDS is called* **HIV**, or **human immunodeficiency virus**. The only way a person can tell if he or she has been infected with HIV is through a blood test. There is currently no vaccine to prevent infection with HIV, and there is no cure for AIDS. It is usually fatal.

A person can be a carrier of HIV without having AIDS. A **carrier** is *a person who appears healthy but is infected with HIV and can pass it to others.* A person infected with HIV may be a carrier for ten or more years before starting to show symptoms of AIDS. **Figure 17.7** shows that people in various age groups might carry HIV without knowing they are infected. AIDS can affect men and women, children, and senior citizens. The primary way HIV is spread is through sexual activity with an infected person. Thus, AIDS can be prevented by practicing sexual abstinence.

FIGURE 17.7

U.S. AIDS CASES AT AGE OF DIAGNOSIS, 1999

AIDS develops months or years after infection with HIV. *How might this long time period make the spread of disease harder to control?*

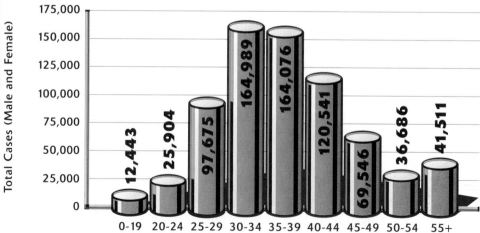

Centers for Disease Control and Prevention-Divisions of HIV/AIDS Prevention: Basic Statistics—Cumulative Cases, 1999

What HIV Does to the Body

HIV attacks the immune system. As you learned earlier, T cells play an important role in the body's immunity function. They start the process of antibody production by activating B cells. HIV seeks out and destroys T cells. The damaged immune system can no longer fight the pathogens that a healthy immune system would destroy.

Shortly after being infected with HIV, some people have flulike symptoms. These symptoms may disappear for months or years, to be followed by the onset of AIDS itself. A person with AIDS may have swollen lymph nodes, fatigue, diarrhea, weight loss, and fever. To diagnose AIDS, doctors determine whether the person's T cell count is below normal.

Another signal that AIDS has developed is the presence of opportunistic infections. An **opportunistic infection** is *an infection that rarely occurs in a healthy person.* With a weakened immune system, a person with AIDS is susceptible to opportunistic infections. For example, many AIDS patients develop a type of pneumonia that can eventually cause death.

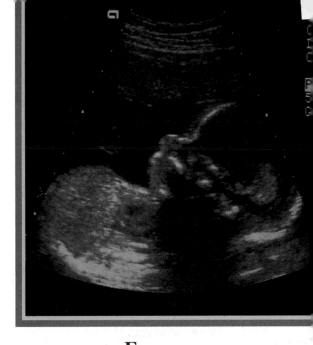

Females infected with HIV can pass the disease on to their babies. *Why should pregnant females be tested for HIV?*

How HIV Is Spread

HIV cannot survive in the air. It is passed from one person to another only in body fluids—including blood, semen, and vaginal secretions. HIV infection can occur in the following ways:

- **Unprotected sexual contact with an infected person.** Infection with HIV can follow *one* incident of sexual activity, even if it is the first one. People who have multiple sex partners are at greatest risk.
- **Piercing the skin with a needle that was previously used by an infected person.** Many injecting drug users who share needles have contracted HIV. Drug use is not the only risky behavior, however. Any skin puncture by a contaminated needle or blade can cause HIV infection. Tattoos and body piercings performed with nonsterile materials greatly increase the risk of HIV infection.
- **Passage of HIV during pregnancy.** HIV transmission from mother to child may occur before or during birth, as well as through breast-feeding. New drug therapies have reduced the rate of HIV infection of the fetus during pregnancy.
- **Transfusions.** All donated blood is tested for HIV. The blood of a newly infected person, however, may not yet contain the antibodies that signal the presence of HIV.

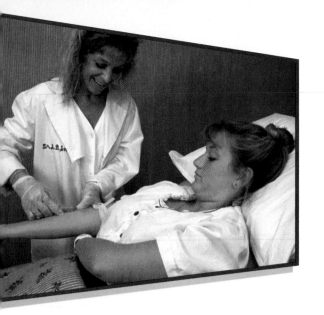

How HIV Is Not Spread

Unfortunately, false ideas about how HIV is spread have led to the social isolation of people with AIDS. Myths have also made some people reluctant to donate blood. Here are the facts:

- **HIV is not spread through the air.** HIV must remain in body fluids to survive. Breathing the same air as an infected person—even being coughed or sneezed on by an infected person—poses no risk of HIV infection.
- **HIV is not spread through kissing.** Kissing with the mouth closed is considered safe. In theory, open-mouthed kissing could transmit HIV if both persons have a cut or sore in the mouth.
- **HIV is not spread through casual contact with an infected person.** Shaking hands or having other casual contact with an infected person poses no risk of HIV infection.
- **HIV is not spread by mosquitoes that have bitten an infected person.** Although some bloodborne pathogens can be spread by mosquito bites, HIV is not one of them.
- **HIV is not spread by sharing eating utensils with an infected person.** You might catch another infection this way, but not HIV.
- **HIV is not spread by donating blood.** In the United States, the needles used to collect blood are sterile and used only once, then discarded. Blood donation in this country presents no risk of HIV infection.

When donating blood in the United States, needles are used only once and then thrown away. *What are some other ways in which HIV is not spread?*

HEALTH SKILLS ACTIVITY

ADVOCACY

Get the Message Out

Education is one of the most effective means of preventing the spread of HIV and AIDS. Here's what you can do.

- **LEARN MORE.** Invite a speaker to your school to discuss HIV/AIDS. You might ask the school nurse, a local physician, or an official of your state or local health department to share his or her knowledge.
- **SPREAD THE WORD.** Help others learn more about HIV/AIDS education and prevention. You might create a poster or write an article for the school newspaper. Create a public service announcement and submit it to a local radio station.
- **VOLUNTEER TO HELP.** Many communities have volunteer organizations that support people with AIDS. Some organizations deliver meals to patients. Others raise money for AIDS research.

AS A GROUP
Brainstorm additional ways to become an active member in the battle to conquer AIDS. Share your ideas with the class.

Testing and Treatment

People who believe that they might be infected need to be tested for HIV. Blood tests detect the presence of antibodies to HIV. Be aware, however, that it may take up to six months after infection for a blood test to detect antibodies.

AZT is an antiviral medicine that slows the progress of HIV in the body. Newer treatment involves combining medicines called protease (PROH·tee·ayz) inhibitors and reverse transcriptase (tran·SKRIP·tayz) inhibitors. These medicines have allowed many AIDS patients to live with their disease and keep it under control. Despite antiviral medication, the HIV-infected individual can still infect others.

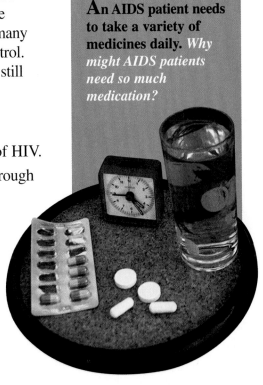

An AIDS patient needs to take a variety of medicines daily. *Why might AIDS patients need so much medication?*

Preventing the Spread of HIV

Following two basic guidelines will prevent the spread of HIV.

- **Avoid sexual contact.** Many HIV infections are spread through sexual contact. Protect yourself by practicing abstinence.
- **Avoid drug use.** Drugs, including alcohol, impair your judgment and make you more likely to take risks. Drug users who share contaminated needles account for a large proportion of HIV infections.

Although great progress has been made in treating AIDS patients, HIV infection is still incurable and AIDS is fatal. This is why it is extremely important to refrain from behaviors that place you at risk for HIV infection.

Lesson 5 Review

Using complete sentences, answer the following questions on a sheet of paper.

Reviewing Terms and Facts

1. **Vocabulary** What term describes a person who has HIV but has not developed AIDS?
2. **Vocabulary** What is an *opportunistic infection?*
3. **Identify** List four ways that HIV infection *can* occur.
4. **Identify** List four ways that HIV infection *cannot* occur.

Thinking Critically

5. **Differentiate** Explain the difference between HIV and AIDS.
6. **Explain** Summarize the facts related to HIV infection and tell why HIV cannot be spread through casual contact with an infected person.

Applying Health Skills

7. **Communication Skills** Write a dialogue to discuss why abstinence from sexual activity is the only method that is 100 percent effective in preventing the sexual transmission of HIV.

Healthy Germs

What's new at the health-food store? Bacteria that fight diarrhea and other illnesses.

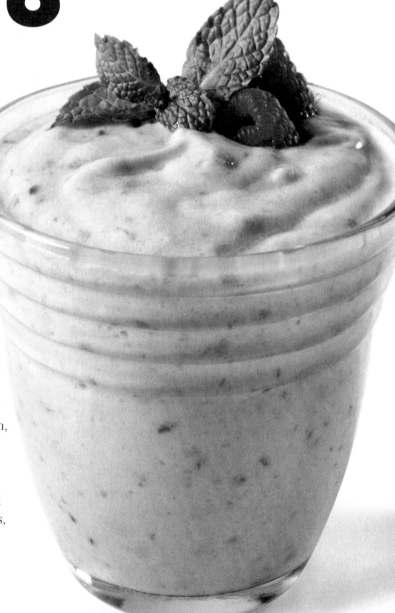

Say the word *bacteria*, and most people think of nasty germs that can make you really sick. Actually, most bacteria aren't bad for you. In fact, eating extra amounts of some bacteria can actually promote good health!

These beneficial bacteria are available without a prescription in drug and health-food stores—and in foods like yogurt. So far, the best results have been seen in the treatment of diarrhea, particularly in children. Researchers are looking into the possibility that beneficial bacteria may cure vaginal infections in women, prevent some food allergies in children, and lessen symptoms of Crohn's disease, a fairly rare but painful intestinal disorder.

Gut Reaction

Where are these good germs lurking? In your intestines! They're commonly found in the colon, which holds at least 400 species of bacteria. Which ones you have depend mostly on your environment and diet. An abundance of good bacteria in the colon usually crowds out any bad bacteria that you have ingested in food. At times, however, this balance can shift. For example, antibiotic treatment for an ear infection can kill normal intestinal germs, allowing the bad bacteria to outnumber the good. The result is often diarrhea.

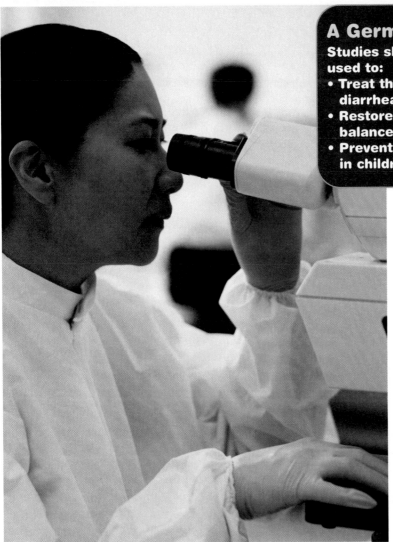

upsets caused by antibiotics. L-GG also seems to work against some viruses, including one of the most common causes of diarrhea in children.

Pediatricians at Johns Hopkins University in Baltimore, Maryland, are studying a different bacterium. It's called Bb-12, and it stimulates the immune system. Infants who are breastfed have large amounts of these bacteria in their intestines. They also have fewer intestinal upsets. Dr. José Saavedra and his fellow researchers have found that Bb-12 prevents several types of diarrhea in hospitalized infants.

Living Bacteria in Food

For generations, people have restored the balance by eating yogurt, buttermilk, or other products made from fermented milk. These foods contain living bacteria that are good for you. Nowadays, you can also swallow a few pills that contain freeze-dried germs. These preparations are called probiotics to distinguish them from antibiotics.

However, you can't always be sure that the bacteria in the products you buy are the same strains as those listed on the label—or even that they're still alive. Heat and moisture can quickly kill the bacteria in probiotics.

Among the most promising probiotics is L-GG, discovered by Dr. Sherwood Gorbach and biochemist Barry Goldin. L-GG has been used to treat traveler's diarrhea and intestinal

TIME TO THINK...

About Beneficial Bacteria

Pretend that you work for an advertising agency. Your big account is a company that produces foods made from fermented milk, which contains bacteria that are beneficial to humans. Create an ad campaign for your key products. The ads can be for magazines, billboards, radio, or TV—but they must both inform consumers about the products' health benefits and be entertaining enough to grab their attention. Present your ad campaign to the class.

PROTECTING YOURSELF AND OTHERS

Model

Tony hates being sick because it means he can't take part in all his favorite activities. Read how Tony tries his best to protect himself from communicable diseases.

Tony avoids sharing eating utensils and drinking cups—especially with people who are sick—and he never shares combs, hats, or towels. When he takes his lunch to school, Tony uses a special lunch box that keeps cold food cold and hot food hot. He washes his hands often, especially after using the bathroom and before handling food. Tony loves to go hiking with his friends, so he knows all about how to protect himself from ticks. He always wears long pants for hiking and tucks them into his socks. After the hike, he examines himself carefully for ticks.

Tony knows that avoiding pathogens is only half the battle, however. He also needs to keep his immune system strong so that it can fight off the germs that get through. To do this, he eats healthful foods, stays active, and gets enough rest. When he does get sick, he stays home and rests until he feels better. Even though he hates missing out on the activities he enjoys, he knows that he will only feel worse if he doesn't take care of himself.

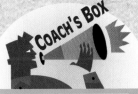
Practice

Annie has just come down with a cold. She is upset because if she stays home, she will miss the tryouts for the school play. On the other hand, she doesn't want to spread pathogens to any of her friends. Read the statements below about Annie's situation. On your own paper, write down the behaviors that can help Annie avoid spreading her pathogens to anyone else. The first one has been completed for you. Then list some other actions Annie could take to protect others from her cold.

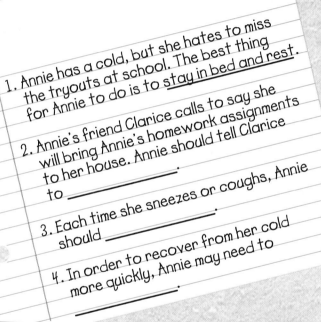

1. Annie has a cold, but she hates to miss the tryouts at school. The best thing for Annie to do is to stay in bed and rest.

2. Annie's friend Clarice calls to say she will bring Annie's homework assignments to her house. Annie should tell Clarice to _____.

3. Each time she sneezes or coughs, Annie should _____.

4. In order to recover from her cold more quickly, Annie may need to _____.

Practicing Healthful Behaviors

To prevent common communicable diseases:
● practice good health habits.
● protect yourself.
● protect others.

Apply/Assess

Here's your chance to be creative. Work with a partner or a small group to create a skit about ways to prevent the spread of communicable diseases. The characters in your skit should demonstrate at least two ways to protect themselves from germs, as well as two ways to avoid spreading their own germs to others. They should also illustrate at least two health habits that can keep the immune system strong enough to fight off pathogens. Be prepared to perform your skit for the class.

Self-√Check

● Does our skit show ways to avoid pathogens?
● Does it show ways to avoid spreading pathogens to others?
● Does it show health habits that help the body fight pathogens?

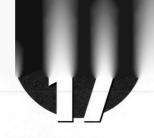

After You Read

Use your completed Foldable to review the information on pathogens and communicable disease.

FOLDABLES
Study Organizer

Reviewing Vocabulary and Concepts

On a sheet of paper, write the numbers 1–9. After each number, write the term from the list that best completes each sentence.

- B cells
- communicable
- viruses
- bacteria
- T cells
- pathogens
- inflammation
- immunity
- fungi

Lesson 1

1. A(n) _____ disease can be passed to a person from another person, animal, or object.
2. _____ are tiny organisms that cause communicable diseases.
3. Tiny one-celled organisms that live nearly everywhere are called _____.
4. Colds, flu, and hepatitis are caused by _____.
5. Ringworm and athlete's foot are examples of diseases caused by _____.

Lesson 2

6. _____ is your body's ability to resist the germs that cause a particular disease.
7. The first nonspecific immune response is _____, or increased blood flow to the affected area.
8. Lymphocytes that produce antibodies are called _____.

9. Lymphocytes that attack pathogens directly and that stimulate the production of B cells are called _____.

On a sheet of paper, write the numbers 10–15. Write *True* or *False* for each statement below. If the statement is false, change the underlined word or phrase to make it true.

Lesson 3

10. Strep throat can be cured with antibiotics.
11. Rubella is a viral disease of the liver characterized by yellowing of the skin.
12. Fatigue has no effect on your immune system.

Lesson 4

13. A person with an STD may have no symptoms.
14. The only sure way to prevent an STD is to practice good hygiene.
15. An STD for which there is no known cure is chlamydia.

Lesson 5

On a sheet of paper, write the numbers 16–18. After each number, write the letter of the answer that best completes each statement.

16. HIV infects and destroys
    a. bacteria.
    b. B cells.
    c. protozoa.
    d. T cells.
17. HIV is passed from one person to another
    a. by mosquitoes.
    b. by shaking hands.
    c. through body fluids.
    d. through the air.
18. HIV is *not* spread by
    a. donating blood.
    b. having sex.
    c. receiving contaminated blood.
    d. sharing needles.

Thinking Critically

Using complete sentences, answer the following questions on a sheet of paper.

19. Apply Relate other drug use to communicable disease: Give three examples of how using drugs can increase the risk of contracting a communicable disease.

20. Synthesize Explain what is wrong with this statement: Once a person gets an STD and receives treatment for it, he or she can never get it again.

21. Analyze How might having a close friend who has HIV influence your attitudes toward people with AIDS?

Career Corner

Nurse Practitioner Would you like to help people stay healthy? Do you like finding answers to health problems? If so, consider a career as a nurse practitioner. These professionals gather medical histories, perform physical examinations, and prescribe medications. To become a nurse practitioner, you need at least a two-year nursing degree and specialized advanced training. Find out more about this and other health careers by clicking on Career Corner at health.glencoe.com.

Standardized Test Practice

Math

Read the paragraph below and then answer the questions.

One communicable disease that is spread by mosquitoes is West Nile virus. Outbreaks occur during times that mosquitoes are active—summer and autumn in temperate climates and all year in warmer climates. Although the symptoms are generally mild, people may become seriously ill or even die from the disease. If you go outside when mosquitoes might be present, use insect repellent to prevent them from biting you.

1. As of September 5, 2003, 174 cases of West Nile virus were reported for 2003 in Texas. Four of these people died. From this information, what is the probability that the disease will be fatal to someone in Texas who becomes ill with West Nile virus?

(A) $2/87$

(B) $1/44$

(C) $87/2$

(D) $44/1$

2. In Ohio, the probability that a person who becomes ill with the West Nile virus will die is $1/15$. Use a proportion to find the number of people who are likely to die if 105 people become ill with the disease.

(A) 5 people

(B) 7 people

(C) 15 people

(D) 105 people

3. As of September 5, 2003, 7 cases of West Nile virus had been reported for 2003 in Georgia, 42 cases in Louisiana, 6 cases in Missouri, 326 cases in Nebraska, and 6 cases in Indiana. What is the mode of these data? Is the mode the best way to interpret these data? What measure might be better to use?

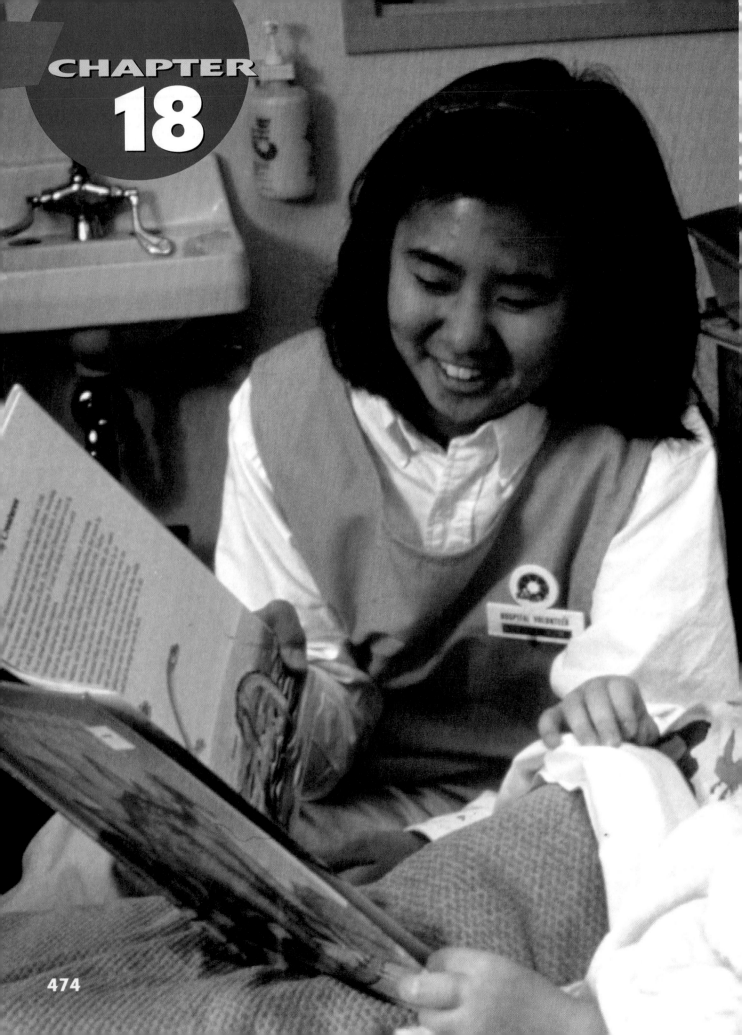

Noncommunicable Diseases

 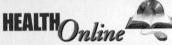
FOLDABLES™
Study Organizer

Before You Read

Make this Foldable to record and collect information on the causes of noncommunicable diseases presented in Lesson 1. Begin with a plain sheet of 11″ × 17″ paper.

Step 1

Fold the sheet of paper into thirds along the short axis.

Step 2

Open and fold the bottom edge up to form a pocket. Glue the edges.

Step 3

Label each pocket as shown.

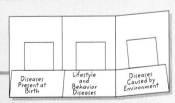

Diseases Present at Birth | Lifestyle and Behavior Diseases | Diseases Caused by Environment

As You Read

Summarize key points on the different types of noncommunicable diseases on index cards or sheets of notebook paper cut into quarter sections. Store these cards in the appropriate pocket of your Foldable.

Noncommunicable Diseases

Quick Write

List three common diseases that you think are *not* passed from person to person. What do you think causes these diseases?

LEARN ABOUT...

- the causes of noncommunicable diseases.
- how lifestyle behaviors can contribute to diseases.
- substances in the environment that can cause diseases.

VOCABULARY

- noncommunicable diseases
- chronic diseases
- degenerative diseases
- risk factors

Causes of Noncommunicable Diseases

As you learned in Chapter 17, communicable diseases are caused by the spread of pathogens. **Noncommunicable diseases**, on the other hand, are *diseases that are not transmitted by pathogens.* Diabetes is one example. You can't catch diabetes from someone who has the disease. **Figure 18.1** provides information about common noncommunicable diseases. In some cases, a noncommunicable disease may be present at birth. In other cases, the disease may develop as a result of a person's lifestyle behaviors. Sometimes the disease develops from the effects of substances in the person's environment. In many cases, the cause is unknown.

Many noncommunicable diseases are **chronic diseases**, *diseases that are present either continuously or off and on over a long time.* Asthma is a chronic disease. Some noncommunicable diseases cause body cells and tissues to break down, or degenerate. *Diseases that cause further breakdown in body cells, tissues, and organs as they progress* are known as **degenerative diseases**. An example is multiple sclerosis.

Diseases Present at Birth

Some babies are born with physical or mental disabilities resulting from birth defects or genetic disorders. The causes of many birth defects are unknown. Some may result from harmful

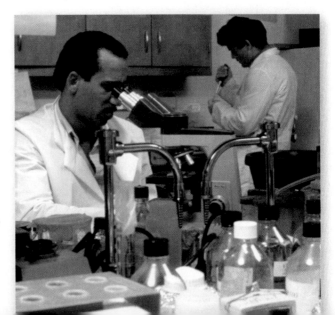

Researchers hope to find new ways of diagnosing, treating, and perhaps even preventing genetic disorders. *Who might benefit from this research?*

476 CHAPTER 18: NONCOMMUNICABLE DISEASES

FIGURE 18.1

COMMON NONCOMMUNICABLE DISEASES

Disease	Description
Allergies	An abnormal reaction by the body to an ordinarily harmless substance. Examples include hay fever, eczema, and food allergies.
Alzheimer's disease	A degenerative brain disorder that causes permanent loss of memory and other brain functions; mainly affects people 60 and older.
Arthritis	A group of diseases that cause body joints to swell, making movement painful and difficult; affects people of all ages.
Asthma	A disorder characterized by attacks of coughing, wheezing, and shortness of breath; results from an overreaction of respiratory airways to specific factors such as pets, foods, and pollen.
Cancer	A group of about 100 diseases that involve uncontrolled growth of abnormal cells; can affect any body tissue.
Cardiovascular disease	A group of diseases that affect the heart and blood vessels. Common forms include high blood pressure and hardening of the arteries, which can cause heart attack and stroke.
Cerebral palsy	A group of conditions that damage the brain around or before the time of birth or during the first year of life.
Cystic fibrosis	An inherited disease characterized by the production of thick, sticky mucus that clogs the respiratory system and digestive tract.
Multiple sclerosis (MS)	A disorder of the brain and spinal cord that causes serious problems with the use of limbs and with vision; can result in paralysis.
Muscular dystrophy	A group of inherited diseases characterized by a weakening of muscle tissue, especially skeletal and cardiac muscles.
Sickle-cell disease	An inherited disease of the blood that causes anemia and extreme pain; mainly affects certain ethnic groups.

substances in the environment. If a pregnant female is exposed to X rays, for example, the developing fetus may be harmed. Other birth defects are caused by lifestyle behaviors of the mother. A pregnant female who drinks alcohol, for example, may give birth to a child with fetal alcohol syndrome (FAS).

Genetic disorders are caused by a defect in genes. Genes carry hereditary information from parents to their children. Examples of genetic disorders include sickle cell disease and Down syndrome. There is no cure for most birth defects and genetic disorders. However, many people with diseases present at birth can be treated with medicine, therapy, or surgery.

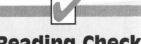

Reading Check

Study charts and graphs. What types of information are provided for the diseases listed in Figure 18.1?

Caring

People with serious noncommunicable diseases often have special health needs. In small groups, identify some of these needs and discuss ways to acknowledge and support them. How can you demonstrate care and concern for someone at school or in the community who has a serious noncommunicable disease? Give two examples.

Lifestyle Behaviors and Disease

In general, it is difficult to predict who will develop a particular disease. For some diseases, however, researchers have identified certain **risk factors**. These are *characteristics that increase a person's chances of developing a disease.* Heredity, age, gender, and ethnic group are risk factors over which people have no control.

Fortunately, people do have control over a major group of risk factors—lifestyle behaviors. Examples include your eating habits, the amount of physical activity you get each day, and the amount of sleep you receive each night. Many diseases are the direct or indirect result of harmful lifestyle behaviors, such as using tobacco or eating too many fatty foods. Healthful lifestyle behaviors, on the other hand, can help prevent, control, or reduce the risk of certain diseases. Lifestyle behaviors may be influenced by cultural factors. For example, cultural traditions may include eating high-fat foods or a variety of fresh fruits and vegetables. Cultural influences can increase or decrease a person's risk for disease.

Although healthful lifestyle behaviors do not guarantee against noncommunicable diseases, they do help. By eating foods low in salt, for example, a person with a family history of high blood pressure can minimize his or her risk.

HEALTH SKILLS ACTIVITY

ADVOCACY

Promoting a Healthful Lifestyle

Be a role model by practicing healthful lifestyle behaviors. Here are some tips.

- **EAT HEALTHFUL FOODS.** Eat plenty of whole grains, fruits, and vegetables. Go easy on foods high in fat, sugar, or salt.
- **STAY PHYSICALLY ACTIVE.** Regular physical activity strengthens all body systems and helps the heart and lungs function better.
- **MAINTAIN A HEALTHY WEIGHT.** Keep your weight within the recommended range for your gender, height, age, and body frame.
- **GET ENOUGH REST.** Teens need at least nine hours of sleep a night.

- **MANAGE STRESS.** Use appropriate time-management and stress-reduction techniques.
- **AVOID TOBACCO AND SECONDHAND SMOKE.** Tobacco causes respiratory and heart diseases and cancer.
- **AVOID ALCOHOL AND OTHER DRUGS.** These substances harm the body and impair judgment.

WITH A GROUP
Working in small groups, select a noncommunicable disease. Prepare an article for the school newspaper emphasizing the role of healthful lifestyle behaviors in preventing that disease.

Diseases Caused by the Environment

The environmental substances listed below can cause serious health problems or make existing health problems worse for some people.

- **Chemical waste** in buried landfills creates fumes that can seep into houses constructed over them. Illness can occur years after initial exposure.
- **Certain construction materials** such as asbestos can cause lung disease after long exposure. Asbestos use is now restricted. Asbestos in existing buildings may be removed or sealed off.
- **Household chemicals,** including paints and solvents, can pollute indoor air and cause health problems.
- **Secondhand smoke** in restaurants, businesses, and homes can be harmful to nonsmokers.
- **Improper waste disposal** by manufacturers of household items such as plastics and paint creates air and water pollution. Improper disposal of household items, such as oil from the car, old paint cans, and old aerosol cans, can pose health risks as well.
- **Radon** is a colorless, odorless gas that is released from soil and rocks that contain tiny amounts of radium. Radon can seep into the air through foundations, basements, and pipes. Exposure to radon over a long span of time increases the risk of lung cancer.
- **Carbon monoxide** is a colorless, odorless gas produced when fuel is burned. It is present in fumes from car exhaust and some furnaces and fireplaces. When fuel-burning appliances do not work properly, they can produce dangerous levels of carbon monoxide. The gas can cause serious illness or even death.

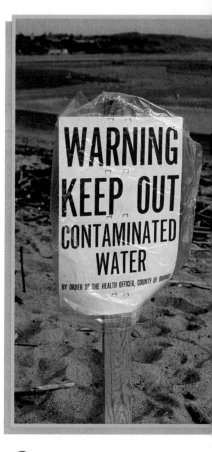

Improper waste disposal can pollute water and pose serious health risks. *How can communities lower the risk of diseases caused by the environment?*

Lesson 1 Review

Using complete sentences, answer the following questions on a sheet of paper.

Reviewing Terms and Facts

1. **Vocabulary** Using your own words, define *chronic disease.*
2. **List** Name five noncommunicable diseases.
3. **Give Examples** Give an example of a lifestyle behavior of pregnant females that could cause their babies to be born with birth defects.
4. **Summarize** What kinds of substances in the environment are harmful to individual and community health?

Thinking Critically

5. **Compare** What are the differences between noncommunicable diseases and communicable diseases?
6. **Evaluate** Distinguish two risk factors associated with noncommunicable diseases. Why is it important to identify these risk factors?

Applying Health Skills

7. **Practicing Healthful Behaviors** Select a noncommunicable disease that may be a risk for you. What steps can you take to reduce your risk?

Allergies and Asthma

LEARN ABOUT...

- what happens during an allergic reaction.
- how allergies are diagnosed and treated.
- what happens during an asthma attack.

VOCABULARY

- allergy
- allergen
- histamines
- hives
- antihistamines
- asthma
- bronchodilator

What Are Allergies?

The immune system reacts to the presence of foreign substances by starting a process to weaken or eliminate the substance. Part of the process is the release of antibodies, which fight foreign substances in the body. Some people develop an **allergy**, or *an abnormal immune reaction to an ordinarily harmless substance. A substance that causes an allergic reaction* is called an **allergen** (AL·er·juhn). When an allergen enters a person's body, the immune system reacts as though it were harmful. Between 40 million and 50 million Americans are affected by allergies.

The most common allergens come from foods, medications, pollens or plants, mold, animals with feathers or fur, insect stings, and synthetic materials. Allergic reactions can affect small areas, such as the part of skin touched by poison oak or poison ivy. In some cases, however, the entire body can be affected. Most allergic reactions occur within seconds or minutes of the time the allergen enters the body. **Figure 18.2** shows the general stages of allergic reaction.

FIGURE 18.2

STAGES OF ALLERGIC REACTION

Some allergens such as poison ivy cause allergic reactions in many people. Almost any substance, however, can set off an allergic reaction in a person who is sensitive to it.

1 Contact is made. Allergens enter the body in three ways: through breathing (dust, smoke); through swallowing (milk, shellfish); and through touching (poison ivy, wool).

2 Attack is launched. When an allergen enters the body, special cells release chemicals (histamines) that cause the symptoms of an allergic reaction.

3 Symptoms appear. Body responses to allergens can involve the eyes, nose, throat, skin, respiratory system, and digestive system.

Reactions to Allergens

The body responds to allergens by releasing histamines. **Histamines** are *chemicals in the body that cause the symptoms of the allergic reaction.* Common symptoms include watery eyes, sneezing, and a skin rash. For some people, an allergic reaction includes **hives**, or *raised bumps on the skin that are very itchy.* **Figure 18.3** shows common body responses to allergens.

Diagnosing and Treating Allergies

How can you tell what causes an allergic reaction? The answer may be as simple as noticing that you break out in a rash whenever you eat peanuts. Perhaps you start sneezing when you are near a cat. Sometimes the cause of an allergic reaction is not easy to identify, however. In these cases, a doctor can perform various tests. In the most common test, the person's skin is scratched and tiny bits of possible allergens are applied. If the person is allergic to one of the substances, the skin in that area will turn red and swell.

Although there is no cure for allergies, there are ways to cope with them. The most basic way is to avoid the allergen. When this is not possible, a person may take **antihistamines**, *medicines that help control the effects triggered by histamines.* For example, antihistamines may relieve itching and redness around the eyes and nose. In severe cases, treatment may involve allergy shots. These provide extremely small quantities of the allergen to help the body build up immunity. This process usually takes about five years.

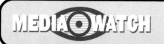

POLLEN COUNT

Every day, the U.S. Environmental Protection Agency measures the amount of pollen in samples of air. This pollen count is reported in local newspapers and on radio and television. Check your local newspaper to find out where the pollen count is listed. *How might people who are allergic to pollen use this information?*

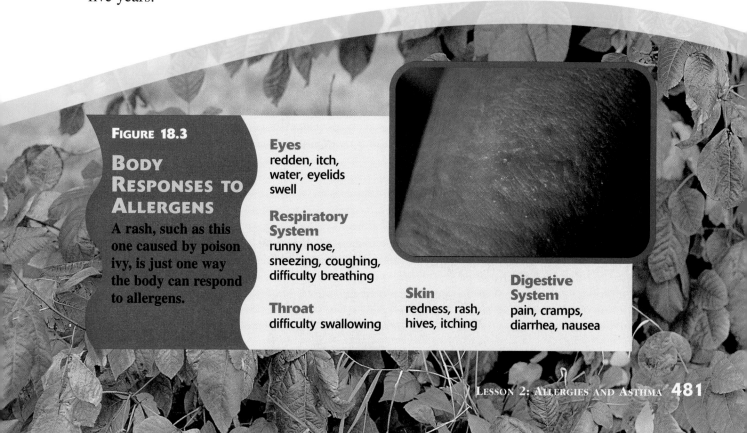

FIGURE 18.3

BODY RESPONSES TO ALLERGENS

A rash, such as this one caused by poison ivy, is just one way the body can respond to allergens.

Eyes
redden, itch, water, eyelids swell

Respiratory System
runny nose, sneezing, coughing, difficulty breathing

Throat
difficulty swallowing

Skin
redness, rash, hives, itching

Digestive System
pain, cramps, diarrhea, nausea

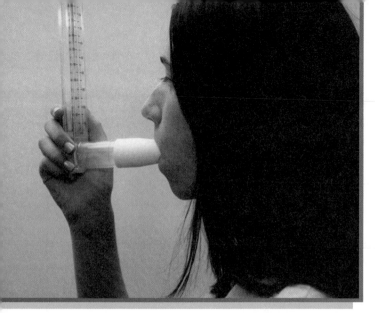

A peak flow meter measures how well a person can blow out air from the lungs. A low reading indicates that an asthma attack may be coming. *Why is it important to remain calm during an asthma attack?*

What Is Asthma?

Asthma (AZ·muh) is *a serious chronic condition that causes air passages in the respiratory system to become narrow or blocked.* More than 17 million people in the United States have asthma. About one-third of these people are under 18 years old. Some people outgrow their asthma at puberty, while others develop it as adults.

The bronchial tubes of people with asthma are unusually sensitive to certain substances. These substances are called asthma triggers. Common triggers include tobacco smoke, air pollution, and certain foods and medicines. When people with asthma come into contact with one of these triggers, they may have an asthma attack. Cold air, strenuous physical activity, strong emotions, and stress can also trigger an asthma attack. A substance that triggers an attack in one person may not affect another person who has asthma. **Figure 18.4** explains what happens during an asthma attack.

Managing Asthma

There is no cure for asthma. However, most people with asthma learn to manage the disease and lead active lives. Even those people whose asthma is triggered by physical activity can usually participate in sports.

FIGURE 18.4

ASTHMA ATTACK

Symptoms of an asthma attack include wheezing, or breathing with a whistling sound; coughing; and tightness in the chest.

A Healthy bronchial tubes are clear and open. Air passes easily through them to fill tiny air sacs in the lungs.

B During an asthma attack, muscles around the bronchial tubes tighten. The tubes narrow and their inner lining swells. Excess mucus clogs airways, making breathing difficult.

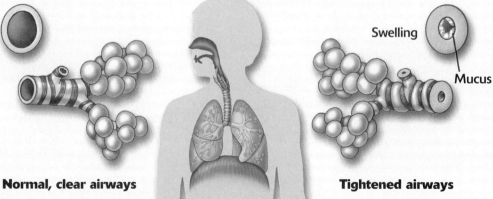

Swelling

Mucus

Normal, clear airways

Tightened airways

Coping with asthma involves avoiding asthma triggers whenever possible. Several types of medicines are also used to treat asthma. Some medicines block swelling in the bronchial tubes and decrease the amount of mucus being produced. Others, called **bronchodilators** (brahn·ko·dy·LAY·terz), are *medicines used to relax the muscles that have tightened around the airways.* When inhaled in a spray, bronchodilators can often bring relief within a few minutes.

HEALTH SKILLS ACTIVITY

DECISION MAKING

Managing Chronic Conditions

Eddie has asthma. This year, he started playing drums in the school marching band. The band has won several awards, and Eddie is proud of the band's accomplishments.

Eddie is especially excited today because his school's band is competing with other bands in the area. However, on his way to school he feels an asthma attack coming on. Eddie wants to play in the competition and does not want to let down his bandmates. He has asthma medicine with him, but is afraid that his performance will be affected anyway.

WHAT WOULD YOU DO?

Apply the skills for decision making to Eddie's situation. What are Eddie's options? What are the possible outcomes? With a classmate, role-play a scene in which Eddie tells his conductor and bandmates about his asthma.

1. STATE THE SITUATION.
2. LIST THE OPTIONS.
3. WEIGH THE POSSIBLE OUTCOMES.
4. CONSIDER VALUES.
5. MAKE A DECISION AND ACT.
6. EVALUATE THE DECISION.

Lesson 2 Review

Using complete sentences, answer the following questions on a sheet of paper.

Reviewing Terms and Facts

1. **Vocabulary** Define the term *allergy.* Use it in an original sentence.
2. **Give Examples** What are three common allergens?
3. **Summarize** List three stages of an allergic reaction.
4. **Recall** For what condition would a bronchodilator be used? What does it do?

Thinking Critically

5. **Hypothesize** Why might it be difficult for someone with allergies to avoid allergens?
6. **Synthesize** What is usually the most helpful step in preventing allergic reactions and asthma attacks?

Applying Health Skills

7. **Communication Skills** Suppose you think you have an allergy. Write a paragraph describing the effective communication skills you could use to discuss this with parents or guardians and health care professionals.

Lesson 3

Cancer

Quick Write

List at least three reasons people get cancer.

LEARN ABOUT...

- causes of cancer.
- cancer's effects on the body.
- treatments for cancer.
- ways to reduce the risk of developing cancer.

VOCABULARY

- cancer
- tumor
- benign tumor
- malignant tumor
- metastasis
- carcinogens
- biopsy
- remission
- recurrence
- mammogram

Skin cancer is the most common form of cancer in the United States. Fortunately, it can be prevented, is easily detected, and can be treated early. *What environmental factor increases the risk for skin cancer?*

What Is Cancer?

Cancer is *a disease characterized by the rapid and uncontrolled growth of abnormal cells.* It can affect people of any age. In the United States, one of every four deaths is from cancer. Thanks to advances in diagnosis and treatment, however, more people are successfully living with cancer than ever before. Everyone can take steps to reduce their risk of developing cancer.

Tumors

The human body has trillions of cells that continually grow and reproduce. Each year, the body forms trillions of new cells. Although the majority of new cells are normal, thousands are abnormal. Most of these abnormal cells are destroyed by the body's immune system. Sometimes, however, an abnormal cell survives. The abnormal cell then starts to reproduce itself, dividing and making more abnormal cells until they form a mass. *A mass of abnormal cells* is called a **tumor**.

There are two kinds of tumors. A **benign** (bi·NYN) **tumor** is *a tumor that is not cancerous.* A **malignant** (muh·LIG·nuhnt) **tumor** is *a tumor that is cancerous.* Cells from a malignant tumor can break away and move through the blood or lymph to other parts of the body. These cells divide and form new tumors. *The spread of cancer from one part of the body to another* is called **metastasis** (muh·TAS·tuh·suhs).

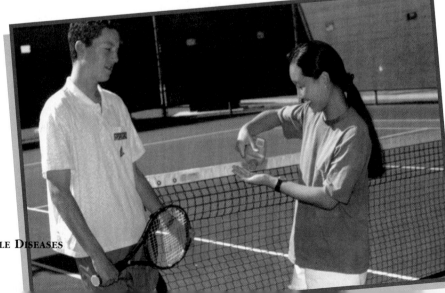

Types of Cancer

Cancer can develop in many parts of the body. Some cancers are more likely to be detected earlier than others because of routine screenings. For example, breast cancer may be detected during a yearly physical exam. Many females detect their own breast cancer while doing a monthly breast self-examination. **Figure 18.5** provides information on common types of cancer.

What Causes Cancer?

Several factors increase a person's risk of developing cancer. One of these factors is heredity. According to the American Cancer Society, between 5 and 10 percent of cancers are hereditary. This means that a person who inherits a particular faulty gene has an increased risk of developing a particular form of cancer.

FIGURE 18.5

COMMON TYPES OF CANCER

Oncology is the medical specialty that studies and treats cancer.

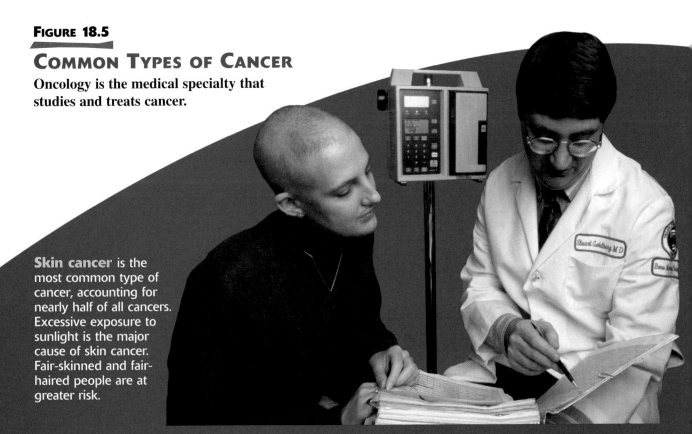

Skin cancer is the most common type of cancer, accounting for nearly half of all cancers. Excessive exposure to sunlight is the major cause of skin cancer. Fair-skinned and fair-haired people are at greater risk.

Breast cancer occurs most often in females over the age of 50. However, younger females can develop breast cancer, and it can also occur in males.

Lung cancer is the leading cause of cancer deaths. Smoking is by far the biggest risk factor for lung cancer for both males and females.

Cancers of the reproductive organs affect both females and males. In females, cancer can occur in the cervix, uterus, and ovaries. In males, it can occur in the prostate and testicles.

Lymphoma is a cancer that starts in the lymphatic system. It weakens the immune system, making the body more susceptible to infection.

Colon and rectum (colorectal) cancer develop in the digestive tract. An eating plan low in fat and high in fiber may decrease the risk of colon and rectum cancer.

Leukemia is a cancer of the white blood cells that starts in the bone marrow. An increase in abnormal white blood cells interferes with the production of healthy cells.

Reading Check

Create your own memory aid. How would you memorize the five types of treatment on page 487?

Other types of cancer are related to lifestyle behaviors. For example, smoking and sunbathing are risk factors for cancer, as are unhealthy eating habits. Many cancers are associated with exposure to **carcinogens** (kar·SIN·un·juhns), which are *substances that cause cancer.* Common sources of carcinogens include

- tobacco, either smoked or smokeless.
- radiation, including X rays in large doses.
- chemicals used in construction and manufacturing, including asbestos and benzene.
- air and water pollution, usually the result of industrial waste.

Warning Signs of Cancer

The earlier cancer is found, the better the chance for successful treatment. Along with having regular physical exams, people can help themselves by watching for any of the warning signs of cancer. For example, females can examine their breasts for lumps. Males can examine their testicles for lumps. Both males and females can watch their skin for changes. **Figure 18.6** shows the general warning signs of cancer.

FIGURE 18.6

WARNING SIGNS OF CANCER

If you notice one of these warning signs, don't wait. Check with your doctor.

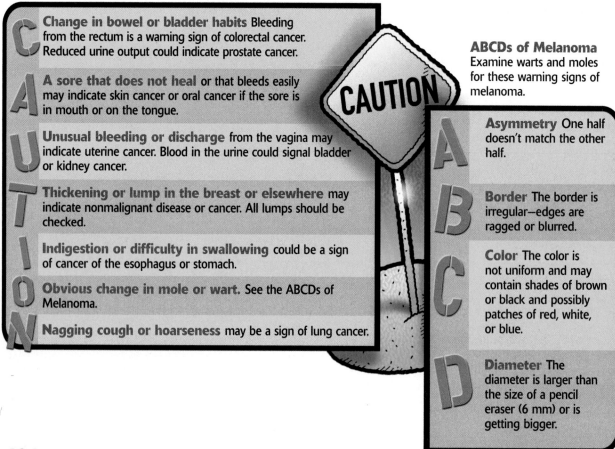

Change in bowel or bladder habits Bleeding from the rectum is a warning sign of colorectal cancer. Reduced urine output could indicate prostate cancer.

A sore that does not heal or that bleeds easily may indicate skin cancer or oral cancer if the sore is in mouth or on the tongue.

Unusual bleeding or discharge from the vagina may indicate uterine cancer. Blood in the urine could signal bladder or kidney cancer.

Thickening or lump in the breast or elsewhere may indicate nonmalignant disease or cancer. All lumps should be checked.

Indigestion or difficulty in swallowing could be a sign of cancer of the esophagus or stomach.

Obvious change in mole or wart. See the ABCDs of Melanoma.

Nagging cough or hoarseness may be a sign of lung cancer.

ABCDs of Melanoma Examine warts and moles for these warning signs of melanoma.

Asymmetry One half doesn't match the other half.

Border The border is irregular—edges are ragged or blurred.

Color The color is not uniform and may contain shades of brown or black and possibly patches of red, white, or blue.

Diameter The diameter is larger than the size of a pencil eraser (6 mm) or is getting bigger.

Diagnosis and Treatment

A person who has one of the warning signs of cancer should see a physician right away for an examination. To diagnose cancer, the doctor will almost always examine samples of tissue under a microscope. *The removal of a tissue sample to see whether cancer cells are present* is called a **biopsy**. The doctor may also order imaging tests, such as ultrasounds, MRIs, or CAT scans. If cancer is diagnosed, the physician will stage the disease. Staging is a process of describing the extent of the cancer and how far it has spread. Staging is used to determine the best treatment.

Types of Treatment

The best way to treat cancer depends on a number of factors. These include the type of cancer, the stage of the disease, and the age and general health of the patient. Doctors follow a detailed plan called a protocol when treating cancer patients. The protocol might involve one or more of the following treatments:

- **Surgery.** During surgery, doctors remove cancer cells from the body.
- **Radiation therapy.** This treatment method involves aiming high-energy rays from radioactive substances at cancerous tissue. These rays destroy or shrink cancer cells. Radiation therapy is often used in combination with surgery.
- **Chemotherapy** (kee·moh·THEHR·uh·pee). With chemotherapy, chemicals are used to destroy cancer cells. Chemotherapy can be used to fight cancers that have spread throughout the body.
- **Immunotherapy.** This treatment method stimulates the body's immune system to fight the cancer. Immunotherapy is most often used in combination with another type of treatment.
- **Hormone therapy.** With this method, cancer is treated with hormones or with medicines that interfere with the production of hormones. Hormone therapy can destroy cancer cells or slow their growth.

When cancer treatment is successful and *when cancer signs and symptoms disappear,* the cancer is in **remission**. Cancer that is in remission is not necessarily cured, however. *The return of cancer after a remission* is called a **recurrence**.

Preventing Cancer

By making healthy lifestyle choices, you can lower your risk of developing certain cancers. Follow these recommendations:

- **Eat nutritious foods.** Choose most of the foods you eat from plant sources. Limit your intake of high-fat foods.

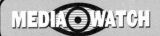

MEDIA WATCH

CELEBRITY CANCER STORIES

The media often feature stories about prominent political, entertainment, and sports figures who have cancer. *Why do you think some public figures choose to publicize their cancer? What are the possible benefits of doing so?*

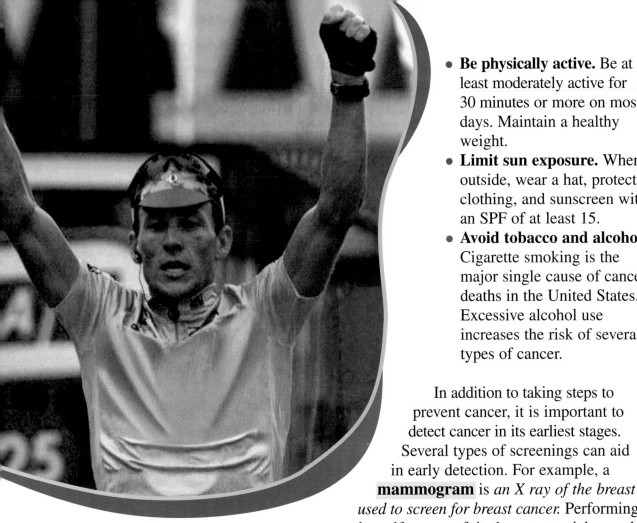

- **Be physically active.** Be at least moderately active for 30 minutes or more on most days. Maintain a healthy weight.
- **Limit sun exposure.** When outside, wear a hat, protective clothing, and sunscreen with an SPF of at least 15.
- **Avoid tobacco and alcohol.** Cigarette smoking is the major single cause of cancer deaths in the United States. Excessive alcohol use increases the risk of several types of cancer.

In addition to taking steps to prevent cancer, it is important to detect cancer in its earliest stages. Several types of screenings can aid in early detection. For example, a **mammogram** is *an X ray of the breast used to screen for breast cancer.* Performing regular self-exams of the breasts, testicles, and skin may also aid in early cancer detection.

Lance Armstrong overcame cancer and went on to win the world's toughest bicycle race—the Tour de France.

Lesson 3 Review

Using complete sentences, answer the following questions on a sheet of paper.

Reviewing Terms and Facts

1. **Vocabulary** What is a *tumor*? Which type of tumor is a more serious health problem: a *benign* or a *malignant* tumor? Explain.
2. **Recall** What is the major cause of skin cancer? Of lung cancer?
3. **Identify** Name three common sources of carcinogens.
4. **Explain** How are the terms *remission* and *recurrence* related?

Thinking Critically

5. **Analyze** Why is it important to discover cancer in its early stages?
6. **Synthesize** What type of foods help lower the risk of colon and rectum cancer?

Applying Health Skills

7. **Goal Setting** Research a health-related profession. Then develop a list of long-term goals and strategies that could help a person have a career in that profession.

Heart and Circulatory Problems

What Is Heart Disease?

Heart disease is any condition that weakens the heart or blood vessels or interferes with the functions they perform. More adults in the United States die from heart disease than from any other cause. Most diseases of the cardiovascular system take many years to develop. Chances of developing heart disease depend partly on age and heredity and partly on lifestyle behaviors. Making wise lifestyle choices during the teen years can help reduce your risk of developing heart disease as an adult.

Arteriosclerosis and Atherosclerosis

Body cells must have a constant supply of fresh oxygen to survive. All tissues and organs depend on the flow of blood through arteries to bring this oxygen. When arteries are healthy, blood flows through them freely. **Figure 18.7** shows how blood flow through arteries can diminish.

FIGURE 18.7

HOW ARTERIES BECOME BLOCKED

As fatty substances build up in the arteries, blood flow is reduced.

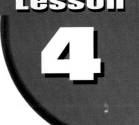

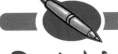

Quick Write

List some behaviors that people can practice to help keep their hearts healthy.

LEARN ABOUT...

- different types of heart disease.
- ways to treat heart and circulatory problems.
- ways to prevent heart disease.

VOCABULARY

- arteriosclerosis
- atherosclerosis
- high blood pressure
- heart attack
- stroke
- pacemaker

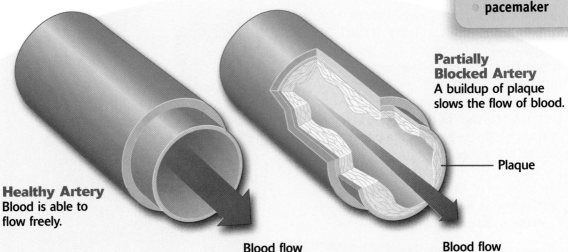

Partially Blocked Artery
A buildup of plaque slows the flow of blood.

Plaque

Healthy Artery
Blood is able to flow freely.

Blood flow

Blood flow

Arteriosclerosis (ar·tir·ee·oh·skluh·ROH·sis) is *a group of disorders in which arteries harden and become more rigid.* Arteriosclerosis reduces the amount of blood that can flow through the arteries. **Atherosclerosis** (a·thuh·roh·skluh·ROH·sis) is *a form of arteriosclerosis in which fatty substances in the blood build up on the walls of the arteries.* The buildup, called plaque, may partially or totally block the flow of blood through the arteries. Buildup in the coronary arteries that lead to the heart carries the risk of heart attack. Buildup in blood vessels leading to the brain increases the risk of stroke.

Hands-On Health

MEASURING BLOOD PRESSURE

This activity will let you hear what a doctor or nurse hears when measuring your blood pressure.

WHAT YOU WILL NEED
- a manual blood pressure measuring device (sphygmomanometer) with a dial
- a stethoscope

WHAT YOU WILL DO
1. Partner A wraps the blood pressure cuff around Partner B's upper arm and tightens the valve. Partner A squeezes the pump to inflate the cuff until the needle on the gauge reaches about 140.
2. Partner A puts the earpieces of the stethoscope in his or her ears. Partner A firmly holds the bell/diaphragm over the large artery in the arm.
3. Partner A opens the valve slightly so that the pressure in the cuff slowly decreases. The needle on the gauge will go down steadily.
4. Partner B watches the gauge and listens. The location of the needle when the first thump is heard is the top blood pressure number. The location of the needle when the last thump is heard is the bottom blood pressure number. Partner B records the reading and removes the cuff.
5. Change roles. Complete the steps again to measure Partner A's blood pressure.

IN CONCLUSION
1. Why might a doctor recommend that a patient monitor his or her own blood pressure at home?
2. Why is it important to learn how to take accurate blood pressure readings?

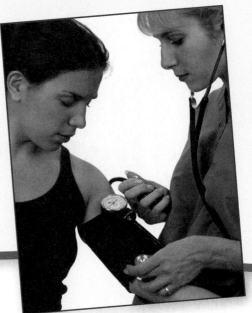

High Blood Pressure

The force of the blood on the inside walls of the arteries is your blood pressure. Blood pressure is expressed as two numbers written like a fraction. The top number is the pressure when the heart beats. The bottom number is the pressure when the heart rests between beats. A blood pressure of less than 120 over 80 is considered normal for adults. Normal blood pressure in teens is lower than in adults, and it varies with age and height.

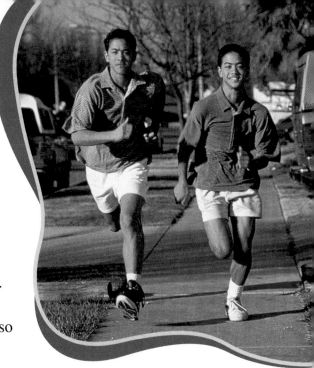

When a person's blood pressure is usually higher than normal for his or her age, the person is said to have **high blood pressure**. High blood pressure, also called hypertension, can lead to heart attack, stroke, and kidney disease.

Heart Attack

A **heart attack** is *a condition in which blood flow to a part of the heart is greatly reduced or blocked.* If the blood is cut off for more than a few minutes, heart muscle cells are damaged and die. The following are possible warning signs of a heart attack:

- Pressure, fullness, squeezing, or pain in the chest
- Pain spreading to the shoulders, neck, or arms
- Chest discomfort with lightheadedness, fainting, sweating, nausea, or shortness of breath

Regular physical activity can help reduce your chance of developing high blood pressure.

Having a heart attack is an emergency situation—every second counts. If someone experiences any of these signs, seek medical assistance immediately.

Sometimes a person experiences chest pain well before a heart attack occurs. Angina pectoris is a painful condition in which blood flow to the heart is adequate to meet normal needs but not increased needs, such as climbing stairs. Angina pectoris is a sign of increased risk of heart attack.

Stroke

A **stroke** is *a condition in which a blood vessel bringing oxygen to the brain bursts or is blocked.* The bursting or blockage prevents blood from reaching part of the brain. Since brain cells cannot live without oxygen, cells in the blocked area can't function and they die. Without these brain cells, the part of the body usually controlled by them no longer functions.

Stroke is a medical emergency. If someone experiences any of the following warning signs, seek medical assistance immediately:

- Sudden numbness or weakness, especially on one side of the body
- Sudden confusion or difficulty with speech or understanding
- Sudden difficulty seeing
- Sudden dizziness, or loss of balance or coordination

Treating Heart and Circulatory Problems

Health care professionals can offer a variety of treatment options for heart and circulatory problems. Some of these include:

- **Medication.** Many problems can be controlled with medicine. For example, people with high blood pressure can take medicine to lower their pressure.
- **Angioplasty.** When there is blockage in a coronary artery, doctors may perform angioplasty (AN·gee·uh·plas·tee). **Figure 18.8** shows the angioplasty procedure.
- **Bypass surgery.** When blockage is life threatening or other treatments do not help, bypass surgery may be necessary. Typically, a healthy vein is taken from the patient's leg or chest and is used to detour around the blockage.
- **Heart valve surgery.** A faulty valve can be replaced with an artificial one made of metal or plastic.
- **Pacemaker.** If a person's heartbeat is irregular, too fast, or too slow, doctors may recommend a **pacemaker**. This is *a small device that sends steady electrical impulses to the heart to make it beat regularly.*

FIGURE 18.8

CLEARING BLOCKED ARTERIES

More than 50 percent of cases of blocked coronary arteries are treated by angioplasty.

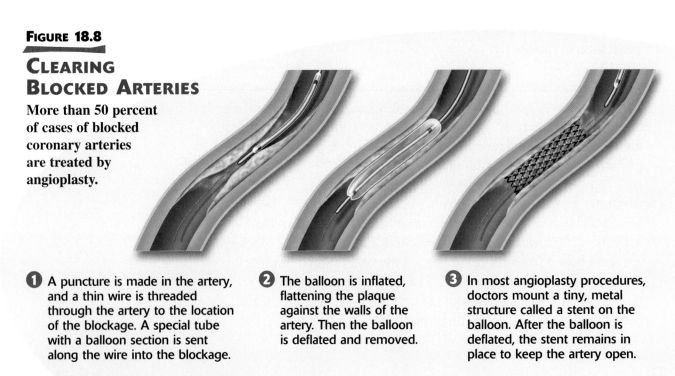

① A puncture is made in the artery, and a thin wire is threaded through the artery to the location of the blockage. A special tube with a balloon section is sent along the wire into the blockage.

② The balloon is inflated, flattening the plaque against the walls of the artery. Then the balloon is deflated and removed.

③ In most angioplasty procedures, doctors mount a tiny, metal structure called a stent on the balloon. After the balloon is deflated, the stent remains in place to keep the artery open.

Preventing Heart Disease

Although symptoms usually don't appear until adulthood, heart disease can begin developing in childhood. The earlier people reduce their risk factors for heart disease, the better their chances for preventing it. Many significant risk factors can be controlled. **Figure 18.9** lists these factors, along with appropriate lifestyle behaviors.

FIGURE 18.9

CONTROLLING RISK FACTORS

Risk Factor	Healthy Lifestyle Behavior
Excess weight	Maintain a healthy weight. Being overweight forces your heart to work harder.
Physical inactivity	Add physical activity to your daily routine. Regular physical activity strengthens your heart and helps you maintain your healthy weight.
Poor eating habits	Follow an eating plan that is high in fiber and low in salt and fat. Too much salt may lead to high blood pressure. Too many fatty foods may contribute to the buildup of deposits in arteries.
Stress	Learn to manage stress in your life. Constant stress can raise your blood pressure.
Tobacco use	Avoid tobacco use and secondhand smoke. Smoking is the most important risk factor for teens.
Alcohol use	Avoid alcohol. Alcohol contributes to arteriosclerosis.

Lesson 4 Review

Using complete sentences, answer the following questions on a sheet of paper.

Reviewing Terms and Facts

1. **Vocabulary** Define *arteriosclerosis* and *atherosclerosis*. How are they related?
2. **Describe** What is the difference between a *heart attack* and a *stroke?*
3. **Identify** List four methods that doctors use to treat heart and circulatory problems.
4. **List** Name six risk factors for heart disease that can be controlled.

Thinking Critically

5. **Analyze** Why is it a good idea to have your blood pressure checked periodically?

6. **Synthesize** How will practicing healthy lifestyle behaviors as a teen help to reduce the risk of heart disease in adulthood?

Applying Health Skills

7. **Practicing Healthful Behaviors** With a family member or friend, try some low-salt, low-fat versions of the foods you normally eat. For example, try low-salt soup, low-fat cookies, or low-fat yogurt. Note which foods you liked and which ones you disliked. Report your findings to your classmates.

Lesson 5

Diabetes and Arthritis

What Is Diabetes?

Diabetes is *a disease that prevents the body from converting food into energy.* In order to get energy from food, the body must break food down into glucose. Glucose—a simple sugar—is the main energy source that cells use to do their jobs. To transport glucose into cells, the body needs **insulin**, *a hormone produced by the pancreas.* Diabetes prevents the body from producing or using insulin. The body's cells cannot get the glucose they need, and glucose builds up in the bloodstream. Diabetes is increasing at an alarming rate. During the 1990s, diabetes rose 70 percent among people in their 30s.

Types of Diabetes

There are two main types of diabetes: type 1 and type 2. **Type 1 diabetes** is *a condition in which the immune system attacks insulin-producing cells in the pancreas.* About 5 to 10 percent of diabetes cases are type 1. **Type 2 diabetes** is *a condition in which the body cannot effectively use the insulin it produces.* The majority of people with diabetes have type 2. Type 2 diabetes is more likely to occur in people who are over the age of 40, obese, and physically inactive. However, type 2 is becoming increasingly common among children and teens.

Diagnosing Diabetes

The only way to diagnose diabetes is with a blood test taken by a health professional. According to the CDC, the following may be symptoms of diabetes:

- Frequent urination
- Excessive thirst
- Unexplained weight loss
- Extreme hunger
- Sudden vision changes
- Tingling or numbness in hands or feet
- Feeling tired much of the time
- Very dry skin
- Sores that are slow to heal
- More infections than usual

Although some people with diabetes may have some or all of these symptoms, others may have no symptoms for years. Untreated diabetes is dangerous because it can lead to serious health problems, including blindness, kidney disease, heart disease, and stroke. If you experience any of the symptoms listed on the previous page, see your doctor as soon as possible.

Preventing and Treating Diabetes

Researchers are making progress in identifying the causes of type 1 diabetes, but there is currently no known prevention. Studies have shown that maintaining a healthy weight and participating in regular physical activity can significantly reduce the risk of developing type 2 diabetes.

There is no cure for diabetes. Treatment for type 1 diabetes involves daily insulin injections. For type 2 diabetes, a daily oral medication may be prescribed or dietary changes may be successful. People with either type of diabetes must monitor their condition carefully and follow their doctor's advice. With medication, a healthful eating plan, and physical activity, most people with diabetes can manage their condition successfully.

What Is Arthritis?

Arthritis is not one disease but many. A person diagnosed with **arthritis** (ar·THRY·tuhs) may have one of *more than 100 conditions marked by pain and swelling in body joints.* Although often thought of as a disease that affects only older people, arthritis can affect people of any age. Two types of arthritis are the most common— rheumatoid arthritis and osteoarthritis.

CONNECT TO

Science

MONITORING GLUCOSE LEVELS
Today's technology provides portable blood glucose monitors that can be used anywhere. Several models give voice instructions— in a choice of languages—to guide the user through the test procedure. The machine then announces the test results. *Who might benefit most from one of these "talking" blood glucose monitors?*

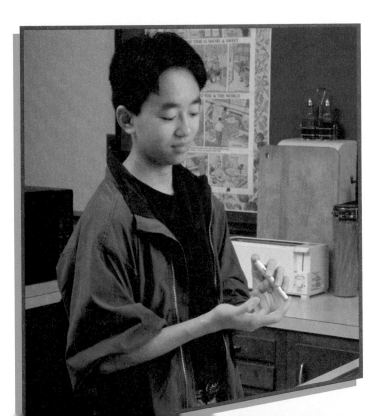

This teen is performing a blood glucose test to check the level of sugar in his blood. *Why do people with diabetes need to monitor their condition carefully?*

Rheumatoid Arthritis

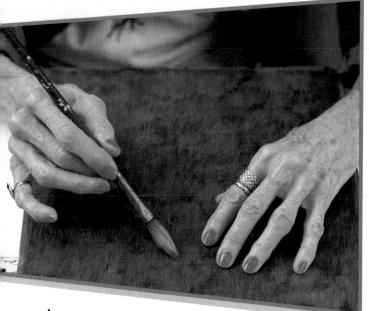

Rheumatoid (ROO·muh·toyd) **arthritis** is *a chronic disease characterized by pain, inflammation, swelling, and stiffness of the joints.* It is the more serious of the two most common forms of arthritis. The joints affected by rheumatoid arthritis often become deformed and no longer function normally. Joints typically affected are those of the hands, feet, elbows, shoulders, neck, knees, hips, and ankles. The effects of rheumatoid arthritis are usually symmetrical—both feet develop the symptoms at the same time and in the same pattern. The cause of rheumatoid arthritis is not known.

Although arthritis can make some activities difficult, medical treatment can help patients live full lives.

Treating Rheumatoid Arthritis

There is no cure for rheumatoid arthritis. Doctors generally treat the disease with medicines to relieve pain, reduce inflammation and swelling, and keep joints functioning as normally as possible. In addition, a combination of exercise, rest, joint protection, and physical therapy is usually recommended.

HEALTH SKILLS ACTIVITY

ACCESSING INFORMATION

Locating Support Groups

Research shows that belonging to a support group can help people with chronic diseases. Many members of support groups not only feel better emotionally but also find that their treatment is more successful. Here are some tips for finding support groups.

- Check with physicians or nurses to see if they know of a local support group.
- Look in the telephone book.
- Call the local hospital and ask for community resources.
- If your town has a Web site, check out any resources listed there.
- Scan the local newspaper for meeting announcements.
- Ask the national organization for the disease, such as the Arthritis Foundation, for help in finding a local support group.

WITH A GROUP
Make a list of local support groups for chronic conditions. Gather information on the activities of the groups, and make it available to other students at your school.

Osteoarthritis

Osteoarthritis (ahs·tee·oh·ahr·THRY·tuhs) is one of the most common types of arthritis. It is a *disease that is characterized by the breakdown of the cartilage in joints.* Cartilage cushions the place where bones meet in a joint. When cartilage breaks down, the bones rub against one another. The result is pain and loss of movement.

The areas most affected by osteoarthritis are the hands and weight-bearing joints such as the knees and hips. Most people affected are over the age of 45.

Treatment of osteoarthritis focuses on relieving pain and improving joint movement. Specific treatment may include medication, heat or cold therapy, and joint protection. Weight reduction may also be recommended to reduce stress on weight-bearing joints.

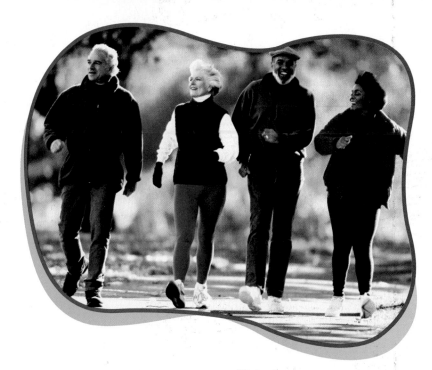

People with rheumatoid arthritis are advised to exercise daily to prevent further stiffness.

Lesson 5 Review

Using complete sentences, answer the following questions on a sheet of paper.

Reviewing Terms and Facts

1. **Recall** Summarize the role of insulin in the body.
2. **Vocabulary** Explain how *type 1 diabetes* differs from *type 2 diabetes.*
3. **Identify** What are five possible symptoms of diabetes?
4. **Vocabulary** Define *arthritis.*

Thinking Critically

5. **Synthesize** What do you think would be most challenging about having diabetes as a teen? Explain your responses in a paragraph.

6. **Compare and Contrast** What are the similarities between rheumatoid arthritis and osteoarthritis? What are the differences?

Applying Health Skills

7. **Analyzing Influences** In small groups, discuss magazine and newspaper ads for products for people with arthritis. What is the major point of each ad? To which age group is the manufacturer appealing? What advertising techniques are used? Do you think people who buy the product will get what they hope for? Why or why not?

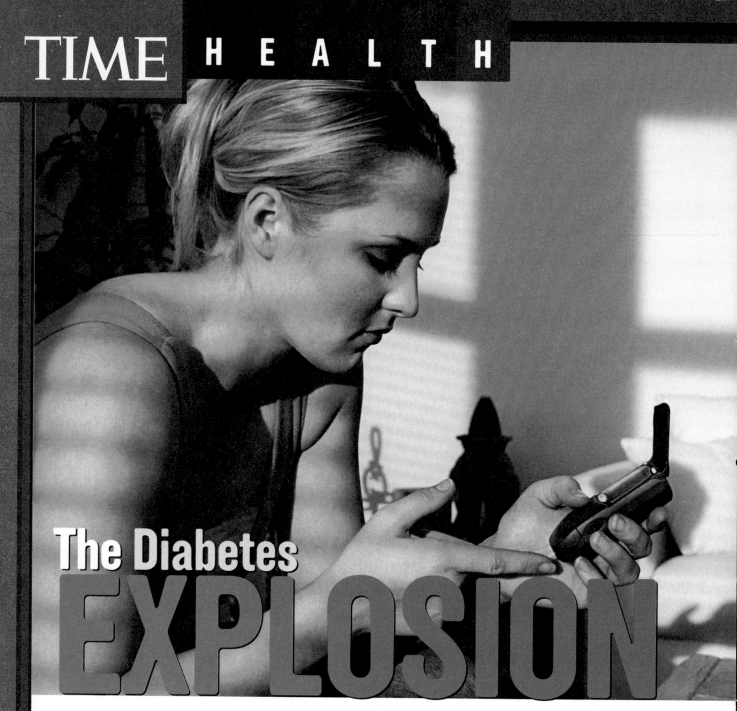

The Diabetes EXPLOSION

As the people in the United States get heavier and heavier, an old disease is showing up in younger and younger victims.

According to a report published in the medical journal *Diabetes Care*, as the population of the United States grows more obese, the number of cases of diabetes is rising, too. The disease is striking more people in younger age groups. Untreated diabetes can result in serious health problems, including blindness, amputations, and heart attacks.

Type 2 diabetes is the most common kind of diabetes. In recent years, the number of Americans with type 2 diabetes has jumped a whopping 33 percent, climbing from 4.9 percent of the population to 6.5 percent.

Younger Victims Than Ever

Though type 2 diabetes has traditionally been seen in people age 45 and older, the greatest increase appears to be among 30- to 39-year-olds. This younger group has seen a stunning 70 percent jump. Among racial and ethnic groups, Hispanics were hit hardest of all, with a 38 percent increase. Caucasians came in next at 29 percent, and African Americans were last at 26 percent.

Dr. Frank Vinicor of the Centers for Disease Control and Prevention finds this rise in the number of diabetes cases ominous: "If that were to happen in a disease like tuberculosis or AIDS, I think there would be a public outcry, and understandably. These trends are very disturbing."

While most public-health threats require a bit of detective work to figure out the cause, this one's a no-brainer. At the same time the diabetes numbers have been climbing, so have the numbers on many people's scales. In 1991 just 12 percent of the U.S. population was considered obese. By 1998 the number had risen to 20 percent. Meanwhile, the number of people considered to be at least "overweight" climbed from 44 percent to 54 percent.

All the added fat appears to make the body less responsive to sugar-processing insulin. As a result, the body produces more and more of that vital hormone. Ultimately, however, the body becomes so unresponsive to certain levels of insulin that injections of more insulin or other medication may become necessary.

Get Off the Couch!

Doctors blame part of the growing problem on America's great pastimes: sitting in front of the TV and surfing the Internet. An increasingly wired country is also becoming an increasingly lazy one, with Web-surfing young people leading the way.

What's the answer? The same as always: Shut down the computer, turn off the TV, and try participating in regular physical activity and eating moderate amounts of nutritious foods. The lecture may be the same as it's always been, but the stakes are becoming higher than ever. ■

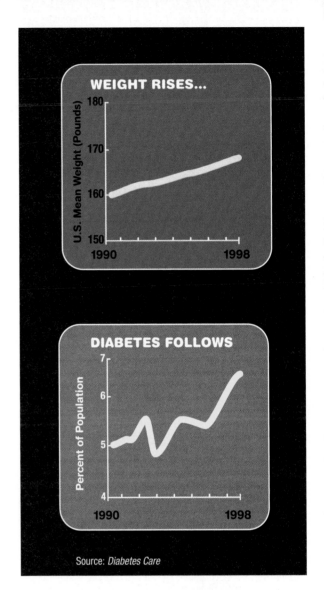

WEIGHT RISES...

DIABETES FOLLOWS

Source: *Diabetes Care*

TIME TO THINK...

About Preventing Type 2 Diabetes

It's important to get the message out to teens about how to reduce their risk of developing type 2 diabetes. In small groups, brainstorm ideas for public service announcements (PSAs) that bring attention to this serious medical condition. The PSAs should encourage teens to get regular physical activity and eat a balanced and nutritious diet. Then transform your ideas into posters that, with your teacher's permission, can be displayed around your school.

MANAGING TEEN STRESS

Model

High stress levels may increase your risk of developing certain noncommunicable diseases. Learning to manage stress reduces your risk of disease and improves your mental and social health, too. Read about Bradley, a teen who had a stressful morning. What sources of stress did he experience? How did he deal with them? Where does Bradley get the support he needs to manage his stress?

Bradley overslept on Monday morning. He didn't have time for breakfast before catching the school bus, so he grabbed a granola bar and a banana to eat on the bus. When he got to school, Bradley discovered that he had left his math homework at home. Instead of hanging out with his friends before school, Bradley went to the library to redo his assignment. He missed seeing his friends, but he figured that having to tell his math teacher he did not have his homework would be even more stressful. He made a point of spending some time with his friends later on between classes. When they teased him about being a "library nerd" that morning, Bradley just joked, "You've discovered my secret." Laughing with his friends helped Bradley relax. His rough morning came to a fairly smooth end.

Practice

Write your name on a sheet of paper. Below that, briefly describe a specific situation you have experienced that caused stress. Exchange papers with another student. Read your classmate's situation and write down a healthy way of dealing with the stress from that situation. Then exchange papers with a different student and repeat the process. Continue trading papers until each paper has suggestions from four different students. Then give each paper back to the person who wrote it.

Read your classmates' suggestions. Circle the ideas you think would work best for you. Share your situation and the responses to it with the class. Do you and your classmates have similar sources of stress? Do you have similar ways of handling stress? Who provides support for you when you are experiencing stress?

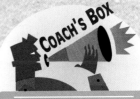

Stress Management

Stress-management strategies include
- identifying sources of stress.
- responding in healthy ways.
- building support systems.

My sister borrows my clothes without asking.

talk to your sister

shoot some hoops or take a long walk to relieve stress

talk to your mom about it

put a sign on your closet door

Self-✓Check

- Did my story identify one or more sources of stress in a teen's life?
- Did my story show healthy ways to manage stress?
- Did my story give examples of people who provide support?

Apply/Assess

Write a short story about a teen who experiences stress. Your story should describe a common source of teen stress, and should show how the character responds to it in healthy ways. Include a description of one or more people who provide emotional support for the teen. Be prepared to present your story to the class.

After You Read

Use your completed Foldable to review the information on causes of noncommunicable disease.

FOLDABLES™
Study Organizer

Reviewing Vocabulary and Concepts

On a sheet of paper, write the numbers 1–8. After each number, write the term from the list that best completes each sentence.

- allergens
- antihistamines
- asthma
- degenerative diseases
- histamines
- hives
- noncommunicable diseases
- risk factor

Lesson 1

1. _____ cause breakdown in body cells, tissues, and organs as they progress.
2. _____, such as diabetes, are not spread through contact with others who have the disease.
3. Heredity is an example of a(n) _____ that may increase a person's chances of developing a certain disease.

Lesson 2

4. Pollen and mold are examples of common _____.
5. _____ are medicines that help control the effects of allergens.
6. _____ are raised bumps on the skin that itch.
7. Chemicals in the body that cause the symptoms of an allergic reaction are called _____.
8. _____ is a chronic condition that causes air passages in the respiratory system to become narrow or blocked.

On a sheet of paper, write the numbers 9–20. Write *True* or *False* for each statement below. If the statement is false, change the underlined word or phrase to make it true.

Lesson 3

9. <u>Metastasis</u> is the term used to describe the spread of cancer in the body.
10. A substance that causes cancer is called a <u>carcinogen</u>.
11. Doctors recommend a <u>biopsy</u>, which is an X ray of the breast, to screen for breast cancer.
12. <u>Cancer</u> is characterized by the rapid and uncontrolled growth of abnormal cells.

Lesson 4

13. <u>Atherosclerosis</u> is a group of diseases in which arteries harden and become more rigid.
14. <u>Arteriosclerosis</u> is a disease characterized by a buildup of plaque in the arteries.
15. An artificial <u>pacemaker</u> can be used to produce the electrical impulses that cause the heart to beat regularly.
16. Hypertension is another term for <u>stroke</u>.

Lesson 5

17. <u>Insulin</u> is a hormone produced by the pancreas.
18. <u>Diabetes</u> affects the body's ability to produce or use insulin.
19. <u>Rheumatoid arthritis</u> is characterized by a breakdown of cartilage in the joints.
20. Pain, inflammation, swelling, and stiffness of the joints are characteristic of <u>osteoarthritis</u>.

Thinking Critically

Using complete sentences, answer the following questions on a sheet of paper.

21. **Apply** How could a teen safely demonstrate care and concern for someone at school or in the community who has a noncommunicable disease?

22. **Suggest** Cole thinks he might be allergic to cats. How can he find out whether his fear is correct?

23. **Recommend** What are some ways to reduce the risk of developing skin cancer?

24. **Analyze** If you had a family history of high blood pressure, what healthy lifestyle choices could help you lower your risk?

25. **Hypothesize** Why might it be difficult for a person who had rheumatoid arthritis to play the guitar?

Career Corner

Occupational Therapist Occupational therapists help people with disabilities regain the skills they need to live independent lives. These professionals may help someone who is physically impaired learn daily living skills such as dressing or cooking. They may also assist patients in using special equipment to perform everyday activities. Occupational therapists need a four-year degree in occupational therapy. Learn more about this and other health careers by clicking on Career Corner at health.glencoe.com.

Standardized Test Practice

Reading & Writing

Read the paragraphs below and then answer the questions.

While we cannot control many of the situations that cause stress, there are actions we can take to prepare for and cope with stress.

Plan: Planning ahead can help you manage your time wisely so that you don't feel overwhelmed. For example, if you know that you have a test on Monday, you might need to study over the weekend and postpone doing something else.

Talk: Talking about your problems with trusted adults and friends can help you discover ways to cope with stress. For example, a teacher might be able to give you tips on how to study.

Relax: Find a healthful activity that you enjoy and take some time to participate in it.

For example, exercising or listening to music are not only fun, they can help reduce stress.

1. Which of the following best describes the organization of the passage?
   A ranking reasons to relieve stress
   B explaining the pros and cons of stress
   C presenting events in the order in which they occur
   D presenting steps and giving examples

2. The reader can tell from the passage that managing stress is
   A easy and fun.
   B challenging but not impossible.
   C not worth doing.
   D complicated and impossible.

3. Write a paragraph describing a stressful situation and explaining how you dealt with it.

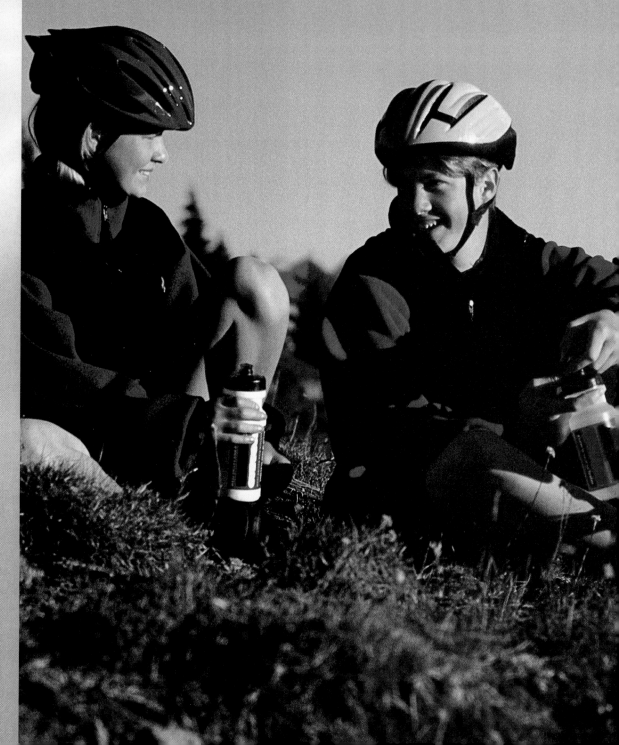

Safety and Environmental Health

HEALTH *in Action*

Our actions don't affect only us; they affect the world around us, too. Staying safe at home and in emergencies are good ways to protect yourself. Other habits you develop, like riding your bike instead of having someone drive you, protect the planet we all share. By behaving carefully and thoughtfully, whether at home, outside, or in traffic, you can prevent many accidents and emergencies—and help keep the skies bright for everyone.

How does riding your bike help keep the sky blue?

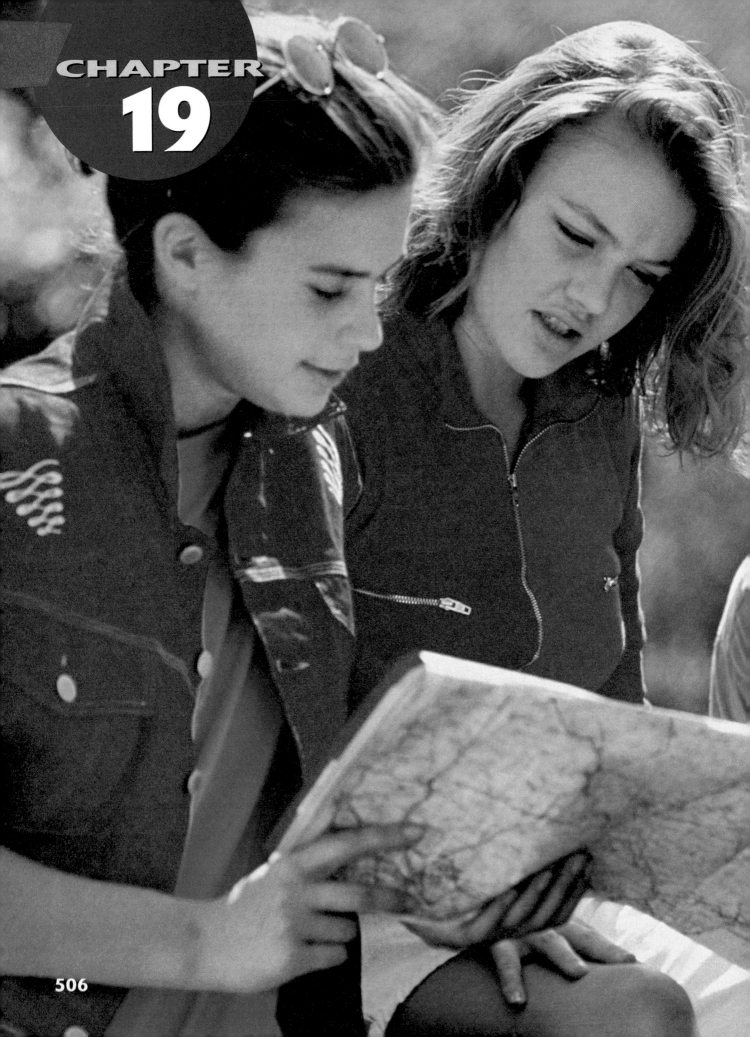

Safety and Emergencies

HEALTH *Online*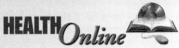

Find out how prepared you are to stay safe and handle emergencies. Take the Chapter 19 Health Inventory at health.glencoe.com.

FOLDABLES™
Study Organizer

Before You Read

Make this Foldable to organize what you learn in Lesson 1 about safety at home and at school. Begin with two sheets of notebook paper.

Step 1

Fold one sheet in half from top to bottom. Cut about 1″ along the fold at both ends, stopping at the margin lines.

Step 2

Fold the second sheet in half from top to bottom. Cut or shave off the fold *between* the margin lines.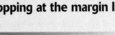

Step 3

Insert the first sheet through the second sheet and align folds.

Step 4

Fold the bound pages in half to make a booklet, and label the cover as shown. Then label each page as instructed by your teacher.

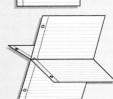

Safety at Home and at School

As You Read

Take notes, define terms, and give examples of home and school safety on the appropriate page of your Foldable.

Safety at Home and at School

Developing Safe Habits

Every hour of every day in the United States, at least one person between the ages of 10 and 19 dies as a result of an injury. About 60 percent of those deaths result from unintentional or **accidental injuries**, which are *injuries resulting from an accident.* An **accident** is *any event that was not intended to happen.* Falling on a slippery floor is an example of an accident. Most accidental injuries could have been prevented.

Injuries often result from a pattern known as an **accident chain**, *a series of events that include a situation, an unsafe habit, and an unsafe action.* Understanding accident chains, such as the one illustrated in **Figure 19.1**, can help you break them. Knowing how accidents happen isn't enough to stay safe, however. You also have to be safety conscious and act safely. Follow these guidelines:

- **Concentrate on what you are doing.** Be extra careful when you are tired, excited, upset, depressed, or in a hurry. Accidents and injuries are most likely to occur during these times.
- **Know your limits.** For example, don't try in-line skating down a steep hill if you are just learning to skate.
- **Think ahead.** Consider possible risks and possible consequences *before* it's too late. Plan ahead so that you won't have to walk home alone after dark.
- **Resist negative peer pressure.** Take responsibility for your own safety. Do what you feel is right, even if it goes against what your friends want you to do.

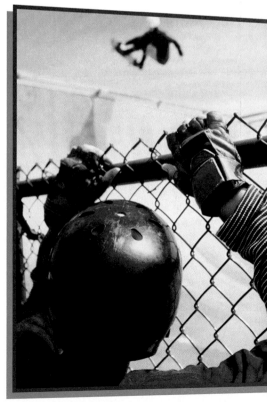

Staying within your limits is not being cowardly—it's being smart.

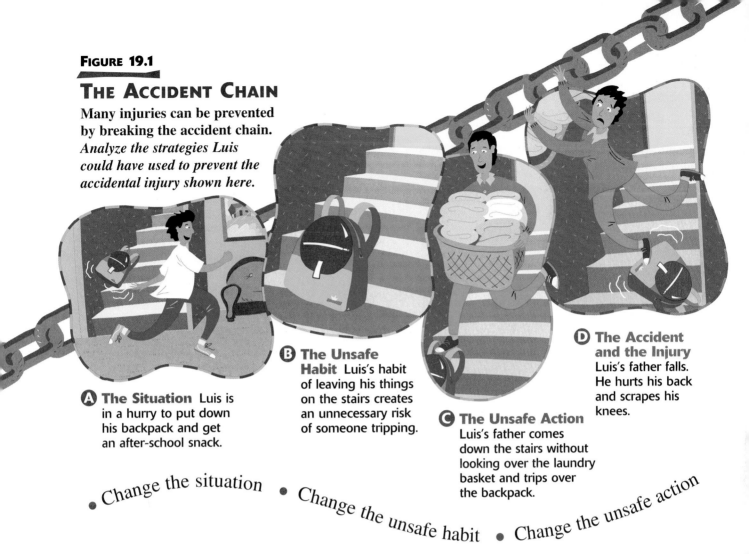

FIGURE 19.1

THE ACCIDENT CHAIN

Many injuries can be prevented by breaking the accident chain. *Analyze the strategies Luis could have used to prevent the accidental injury shown here.*

Ⓐ The Situation Luis is in a hurry to put down his backpack and get an after-school snack.

Ⓑ The Unsafe Habit Luis's habit of leaving his things on the stairs creates an unnecessary risk of someone tripping.

Ⓒ The Unsafe Action Luis's father comes down the stairs without looking over the laundry basket and trips over the backpack.

Ⓓ The Accident and the Injury Luis's father falls. He hurts his back and scrapes his knees.

• Change the situation   • Change the unsafe habit   • Change the unsafe action

Safety in the Home

The most common type of home injury involves falls. Other types of injuries in the home result from poisonings, electrical shocks, and guns. Fires and burns are the third leading cause of unintentional injury and death in the home. The majority of deaths and injuries in the home could have been prevented.

Preventing Falls

Most home falls happen in the kitchen, in the bathroom, and on stairs. To prevent falls in the home, avoid slippery floors by cleaning up spills promptly. Use nonskid rugs, or put a rubber pad under loose rugs to make them safer. Keep stairways well lighted and free from clutter. Many falls result from standing on chairs or furniture to reach high places. Act safely by using a step stool or ladder instead.

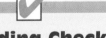

Reading Check

Evaluate your own habits. Think about what you have done this week. Can you change any actions to be more safety conscious?

FIGURE 19.2

PROTECTION FROM POISONOUS PRODUCTS

If there are young children in the home, poisonous substances should be stored out of their reach. *Where are these substances stored in your home?*

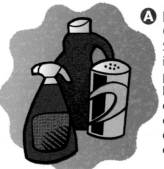

Ⓐ Keep Chemicals Out of Reach
Store cleaning products, insecticides, and other potential poisons in high, locked cabinets that are out of the reach of young children. Use childproof catches on all doors and drawers.

Ⓑ Store Medicines Properly
Keep medicines in their original containers with child-resistant caps. Store them in a locked cabinet out of the reach of young children. Dispose of old medicines that have passed their expiration date by flushing them down the toilet.

Preventing Poisonings

Poisoning can happen by ingestion (swallowing), absorption (through the skin), injection, or inhalation. Young children are particularly susceptible to poisoning by ingestion. Cleaning products and medicines are the most common poisons swallowed by children. **Figure 19.2** shows ways of protecting children from poisoning.

Preventing Electrical Shocks

Electrical items can cause serious injury or death if misused. In the home, replace broken or frayed electrical cords, and never run cords under rugs. Unplug appliances that are not in use or that are not working properly. Keep all electrical appliances and cords away from water. Protect children from electrical shocks by putting safety covers over unused outlets. Follow the procedures shown in **Figure 19.3** for the safe use of electrical outlets.

FIGURE 19.3

PROTECTION FROM ELECTRICAL SHOCK

Prevent electrical shock by connecting appliances safely and using the proper number of cords per outlet. *Why might an overloaded electrical outlet cause a problem?*

Ⓐ Unplug Electrical Devices Safely
Unplug an electrical device by its plug. Never pull a plug out by its cord. Doing so can damage the protective covering on the wire.

Ⓑ Handle Outlets Safely
Do not overload an outlet with too many plugs. Instead, use a multi-outlet power strip that has a reset button to prevent power overload.

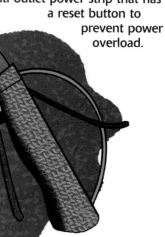

Gun Safety

The best protection against gun accidents in the home is to possess no guns. However, if they are kept in the home, strict safety precautions and strategies should be followed.

- Guns should have trigger locks and should always be stored unloaded in a locked cabinet.
- Ammunition should be stored in a separate locked cabinet.
- Anyone who will handle a gun should be trained in safe gun use.
- Guns should always be handled as if they are loaded.
- Guns should *never* be pointed at anyone.

Fire Safety

The elements needed for a fire—fuel, heat, and air—can be found in any home. For example, rags, wood, gasoline, or newspaper might be fuel. A cigarette, match, or electrical wire can provide heat. Prevent fires in the home by following these safety rules.

- Keep stoves clean to avoid burns and fires. Food particles or grease on a stove or in an oven can catch fire.
- Keep flammable objects at least 3 feet from portable heaters.
- Remind adults who smoke never to smoke in bed or on overstuffed furniture.
- Inspect electrical wires, outlets, and appliances for safety.
- Throw out old newspapers, oily rags, and other materials that burn easily.
- Use and store matches properly. Keep matches and cigarette lighters out of the reach of young children, preferably in high cabinets.
- Install smoke alarms on each level of the home, including the basement. They should be located in hallways outside bedrooms.

Science

GREASE FIRES
If a grease fire starts in a pan on the stove, do not use water to put it out. Oil and grease float on water, causing the flames to spread. The best way to put out a grease fire is to carefully slide a lid over the pan and to turn off the burner. Let the pan cool down completely before you move it or take off the lid. You can also use baking soda to smother the flames.

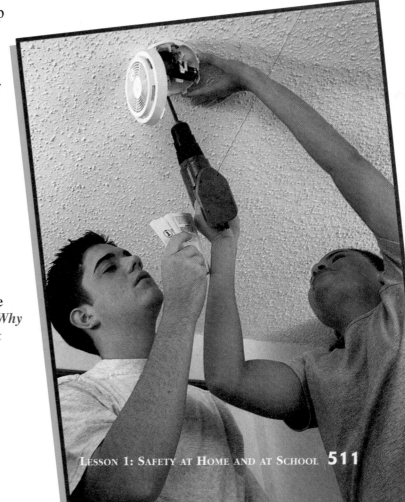

Every home should have working smoke alarms. *Why is it so important to check smoke alarms regularly?*

PRACTICING HEALTHFUL BEHAVIORS

Preparing a Fire Safety Plan

The best protection against injury during a fire is to plan what you will do if one occurs. A good fire safety plan includes the following:

- A floor plan of each level of your home, including doors and windows. Use arrows to indicate escape routes from each room.
- A ladder or coil of rope for escaping through upstairs windows.
- An agreed-on safe location outside the home, where everyone will meet.
- A rule for everyone to leave the house immediately and call the fire department.
- A rule that no one ever goes back into the house for any reason.
- Safety measures to follow, such as testing doors for heat before opening them.

ON YOUR OWN

Develop a fire safety plan with your family, or improve an existing plan. After completing your plan, demonstrate escaping from various rooms and adjust the plan as needed. Encourage your family to practice the plan regularly.

Reducing Risk of Injury in a Fire

Knowing what to do if there is a fire in your home can reduce your risk of injury. Follow these guidelines.

- Leave the house immediately if possible. Call the fire department from a neighbor's house or a cellular phone.
- While you are in the house, stay close to the floor below the smoke, and try to keep your nose and mouth covered.
- Before opening a closed door, feel it. If it is hot, leave the room by another route.
- If your clothing catches fire, stop, drop, and roll, as shown in **Figure 19.4**.
- Never go back into a burning building—for *any* reason.
- Leave firefighting to the experts. Do not try it yourself.

FIGURE 19.4

STOP, DROP, ROLL

If your clothes catch fire, don't run. Stop, drop, and roll. *What might happen if you run?*

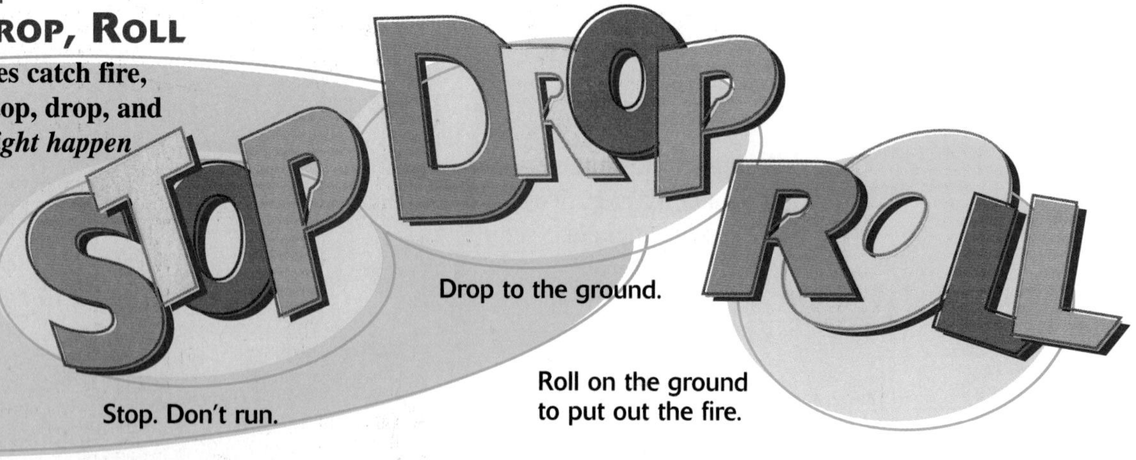

Stop. Don't run.

Drop to the ground.

Roll on the ground to put out the fire.

Safety at School

Because large numbers of people gather at schools, rules are established to protect the health and safety of students and teachers. For example, running isn't permitted in the halls because they are often crowded with people. Here are some strategies for preventing accidental injuries at school:

- **Play by the rules.** Many rules are designed to protect you and others. Follow the rules of the cafeteria, gym, auditorium, halls, and classrooms. It's important to understand and follow rules prohibiting the possession of weapons at school.
- **Report any weapons or unsafe activities.** If you suspect that someone has brought or plans to bring a gun or other weapon to school, report it immediately to a teacher or principal. Do the same if you witness any unsafe behaviors.
- **Wear appropriate safety gear.** Whether in science class or in sports, wear the recommended gear and follow your teacher's directions carefully.

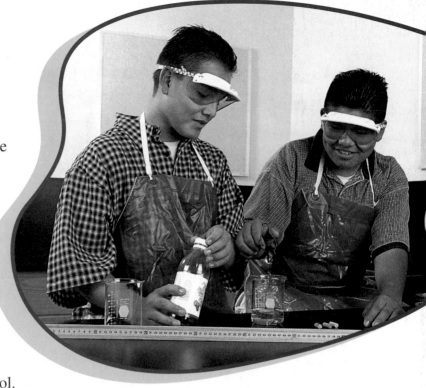

When working with chemicals, be sure to protect your eyes and to follow your teacher's instructions. *Why are these rules important?*

Lesson 1 Review

Using complete sentences, answer the following questions on a sheet of paper.

Reviewing Terms and Facts

1. **Vocabulary** What is an *accidental injury?*
2. **List** Name the sequence of links in an accident chain.
3. **Recall** What strategies can families use to reduce their risk of injuries from guns?
4. **Give Examples** List three strategies for preventing accidental injuries at school. Analyze how each strategy can help people stay safe.

Thinking Critically

5. **Analyze** Review the guidelines for acting safely, on page 508. Briefly describe how each of these factors can reduce the risk of accidents.
6. **Explain** Why is it important to understand and follow the rules prohibiting possession of weapons at school?

Applying Health Skills

7. **Practicing Healthful Behaviors** Work with your family to identify potential hazards that could lead to accidents in your home. Demonstrate corrective action strategies to remove or reduce these hazards and prevent accidental injuries.

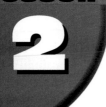

Safety on the Road and Outdoors

Quick Write

List at least five things a bike rider must pay attention to.

LEARN ABOUT...

- safety and traffic rules for bicycles, skates, skateboards, and scooters.
- pedestrian safety.
- avoiding injuries in the water and outdoors.

VOCABULARY

- defensive driving

Traffic Safety

Your behavior as a car passenger can be just as important as a driver's behavior. Motor vehicle collisions cause the largest proportion of all teen injuries. To reduce your risk of injury, use your thinking and decision-making skills as you follow these traffic safety rules.

- **Obey the rules of the road.** When you obey the rules of the road, other people can predict your actions. This helps prevent collisions and injuries.
- **Always buckle up.** Buckling up every time you ride in a car is a simple action that could save your life.
- **Never ride with a driver who has been drinking alcohol or using drugs.** Alcohol is involved in about 35 percent of teen driver deaths. Driving while under the influence of alcohol or drugs is not only high-risk behavior, but also against the law.
- **Never distract a driver.** Driving requires a driver's full attention. If you need to have a discussion or show the driver something, ask the driver to pull over and stop the car.

It takes only a moment to fasten a safety belt. It's a moment that could save a life. *How could a driver encourage passengers to buckle up?*

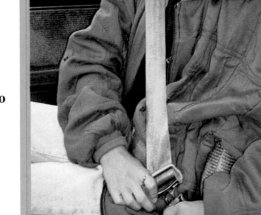

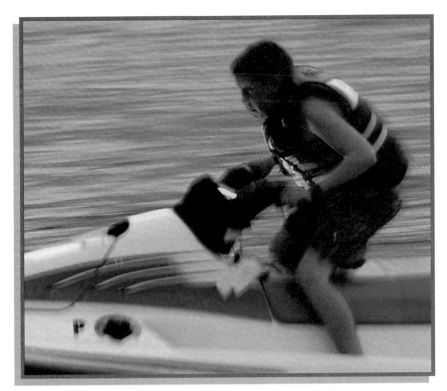

Like bikes and skates, recreational vehicles require a sense of responsibility and a knowledge of safety rules. *How can using thinking and decision-making skills help you avoid high-risk situations when riding motorized recreational vehicles and engaging in other potentially hazardous activities?*

Safety on Wheels and Motorized Vehicles

Many teens enjoy riding bicycles and using skates, skateboards, and scooters. Some even ride all-terrain vehicles, motorized watercrafts, and snowmobiles. These activities are fun, but they come with an increased level of risk. Learning about the risks and taking actions to avoid them can prevent injury.

Bicycle Safety

The first rule of bicycle safety is always to wear a bike helmet. Head injuries are the cause of 70 to 80 percent of the deaths from bicycle accidents. You will reduce your risk of head injury by 85 percent if you wear a helmet every time you ride a bike.

Bicycle riders should follow the rules of the road. These rules include riding with traffic—not against it—and obeying traffic signals and signs. Bicyclists should also practice **defensive driving**, which means not only obeying traffic laws but also *watching out for other people on the road and anticipating unsafe acts.* For good bicycle safety, don't ride at night or in bad weather. If you must do so, be sure to use lights and reflective clothing. You can also reduce your risk of injury by making sure that your bike has the proper safety equipment and keeping your bike in good condition. The tires, for example, should have enough tread to grip the road and should be properly inflated.

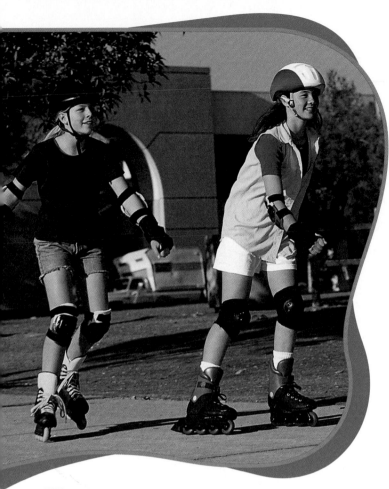

Skates, Skateboards, and Scooters

Skates, skateboards, and scooters can be a lot of fun—if you use them safely. Many skaters and skateboarders who are injured weren't wearing protective gear when they crashed. Follow these guidelines.

- Always wear protective gear: a hard-shell helmet, wrist guards, gloves, elbow pads, and knee pads.
- Keep your speed under control.
- Watch for pedestrians and stay off busy sidewalks.
- Avoid parking lots, streets, and other areas with traffic.
- On a soft surface, practice a safe way to fall—before you head downhill.

Pedestrian Safety

Thousands of pedestrians are injured or killed in traffic accidents every year. Following the do's and don'ts below will help reduce your risk of injury while traveling on foot.

Wearing the right protective gear and maintaining a safe speed are two ways to prevent skating injuries. *What are other ways to prevent skating injuries?*

Do's

- Cross streets at crosswalks and obey traffic signals.
- Look left, right, and left again before crossing the street.
- In daylight, wear bright clothing. At night, wear reflective gear and carry a flashlight.
- If there is no sidewalk, stay to the left side of the road and walk facing oncoming traffic.

Don'ts

- Don't jaywalk, or cross the street in the middle of the block.
- Don't walk into the street from between parked cars.
- Don't enter the street without first looking left, right, and left again.
- Don't assume that a driver will see you just because you see her or him.
- Don't walk in a large group that spills off the sidewalk and onto the street.

Recreational Safety

It's always best to play it safe when you take part in outdoor activities. If you know the risks associated with an activity you enjoy, you can take the necessary preventive actions to stay safe. When outdoors, use your common sense and follow these two general safety rules.

- **Be aware of the weather.** Try to avoid electrical storms and extreme temperatures. If you're caught outdoors in an electrical storm, seek shelter in a building or car, or under a clump of bushes. Avoid isolated trees, and get out of and away from water. If you are outside on a very hot day, drink plenty of water, stay in the shade, and avoid strenuous activity. On a very cold day, dress in layers and protect your fingers, toes, nose, and ears. Also be sure to stay dry and keep active.
- **Use the buddy system.** The buddy system is an agreement between two people to stay together. With a buddy, you can help each other avoid or cope with potentially dangerous situations in healthy ways.

Water Safety

Each year, thousands of people in the United States, including many children, die from drowning. To protect yourself and others, follow these water safety rules.

- Learn how to swim. Take a class to improve your skill.
- Don't swim alone. Always swim with a buddy and only where a trained lifeguard is on duty.
- Always wear a life jacket when boating or waterskiing. If you fall in the water, use the survival techniques shown in **Figure 19.5**.

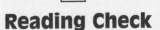

Reading Check

Learn about word parts. Use a dictionary to find the root of the word *pedestrian*.

FIGURE 19.5

SURVIVAL IN COLD WATER

Hypothermia, which is a dangerous drop in body temperature, can be life-threatening to people in cold water. If you fall into the water while boating, assume one of the positions shown here. They will help you stay warm until help arrives. *Why should even strong swimmers always wear a life jacket?*

Ⓐ Lessen heat loss by drawing your knees up to your chest and keeping your upper arms close to the sides of your body. About 50 percent of heat loss is from your head, so try to keep it out of the water.

Ⓑ If you are with one or more other people, huddle close together in a circle to preserve body heat. A child or smaller person who loses heat faster should be placed in the center of the circle.

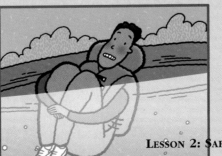

Reading Check

Paraphrase. Rewrite the hiking and camping safety guidelines in your own words.

- If you get caught in a strong current, swim parallel to the shore until the current lessens. Then swim to shore.
- Don't swim when you are tired.
- Dive only into water that you know is deeper than 9 feet and is free of obstacles, such as other swimmers or rocks. Diving into shallow water can result in spinal cord injuries. Never dive into an above-ground pool.
- Avoid drugs and alcohol. About 40 percent of teen drownings involve alcohol.
- Be aware of the weather. If you see lightning or hear thunder, get out of the water right away.

Hiking and Camping Safety

A safe and successful hike or camping trip begins with preparation. Check the weather forecast and take the proper clothing and equipment. Always tell an adult where you will be and when you expect to return. Follow these guidelines:

- **Wear protective clothing.** Wear shoes and socks that protect your feet from the terrain as well as from blisters. Dress in layers and have wet-weather gear on hand. If you will be in grassy areas, wear socks and long pants to help protect against ticks.
- **Bring equipment and supplies.** Make sure that you have a map, compass, first-aid kit, flashlight with extra batteries, and an adequate supply of drinking water.
- **Follow fire safety rules.** Light campfires only where permitted, and never leave the area before the campfire is completely out. Drown it with water or bury it with dirt that is free of debris.
- **Know poisonous plants and animals.** Find out which plants and animals in the area are poisonous. Learn first aid for treating reactions to poisonous plants, insect stings, and snakebites.
- **Have a cell phone.** This will enable you to call someone in an emergency.

Outdoor Sports

Whether you enjoy summer or winter sports, always wear appropriate gear and stay within your ability level. Follow posted signs, and stay in approved locations. In the summer, the sun and heat can cause problems such as sunburn and heatstroke. Protect your skin from sunburn by wearing sunscreen, sunglasses, a hat, and appropriate clothing. During the hottest times of the day (10 A.M. to 4 P.M.), avoid direct sunlight and drink plenty of water. Pay attention to your body's signals. If you feel overheated or tired, take a break and cool down.

When participating in winter sports, keep in mind that ice-skating is safest at supervised ice rinks. Sledding and skiing should take place only on hills that are not too steep and that are free from traffic and obstacles. Winter sports can be dangerous because of the cold weather. Protect yourself by wearing layers of clothing, a hat, mittens or gloves, and appropriate footwear.

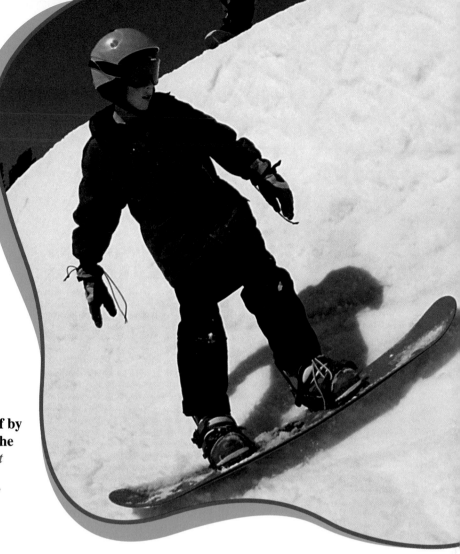

This teen is protecting himself by wearing warm clothing and the appropriate safety gear. *What precautions do you take when participating in winter sports?*

Lesson 2 Review

Using complete sentences, answer the following questions on a sheet of paper.

Reviewing Terms and Facts

1. **List** What are four safety rules that can help reduce your risk of traffic injuries?
2. **Vocabulary** Define the term *defensive driving.* Use it in an original sentence.
3. **Give Examples** List three do's and three don'ts of pedestrian safety.
4. **Identify** Name three items that you should bring when camping or hiking.

Thinking Critically

5. **Explain** How does using the buddy system help keep you safe outdoors?

6. **Analyze** Why do you think it is important to stay within your ability level when playing outdoor sports?

Applying Health Skills

7. **Practicing Healthful Behaviors** Think of a trip that you would like to take, somewhere in the United States. What would you do on your trip? What safety equipment would you need? What safe behaviors would you want to practice? Write a paragraph explaining how you would plan for the trip. List the safety precautions you would follow.

Safety in Weather Emergencies

Quick Write

List the types of weather emergencies that might occur where you live. For each one, write at least two emergency preparations.

LEARN ABOUT...

- staying safe during severe weather.
- protecting yourself during a flood or an earthquake.

VOCABULARY

- tornado
- hurricane
- blizzard
- earthquake

Hazardous Weather and Natural Disasters

Some weather events, such as thunderstorms, can occur anywhere in the United States. Other types of weather and natural disasters, however, are more likely to occur in certain areas and at certain times of the year. For example, tornadoes are found most often in the central states in spring and summer. Hurricanes are a problem along the Atlantic Coast and the Gulf of Mexico. Earthquakes are most common on the West Coast and in southern Alaska.

To protect yourself from dangerous weather risks, stay alert to weather conditions. Listen to local and national weather information. Be especially alert to weather watches and warnings issued by the National Weather Service. A weather *watch* means that severe weather conditions, such as a winter storm or a tornado, are likely to develop. A weather *warning* means that severe weather has been sighted or is about to occur.

Tornadoes

A **tornado** is *a whirling, funnel-shaped windstorm that may drop from the sky to the ground.* The winds of a tornado can reach speeds of more than 300 miles an hour. Tornadoes are extremely dangerous because they can destroy everything in their path. If a tornado warning is issued, the safest action is to go to a basement or cellar that has no windows and stay there until the storm passes. If that is not possible, take the following steps to reduce your risk of injury.

Knowing what to do when a tornado strikes is the key to staying safe. *Why are tornadoes so dangerous?*

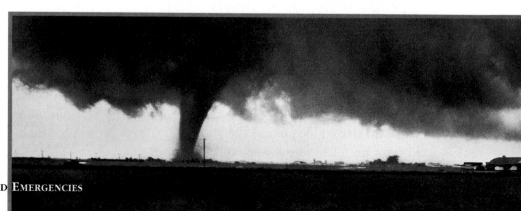

FIGURE 19.6

TRACKING A HURRICANE

Weather experts track the path of a hurricane by recording the coordinates of its location at regular intervals. *How might hurricane tracking help people who live in coastal areas?*

This hurricane curved up through Haiti and Cuba into Florida, Mississippi, and Alabama.

Hurricane Helene occurred in the Atlantic Ocean in September 2000.

- **Avoid windows.** The greatest danger during a tornado is from flying debris. Stay as far away from windows as possible. Go to an inner hallway or a central, windowless room such as a bathroom or closet.
- **Cover yourself.** Get underneath a piece of sturdy furniture such as a heavy table or desk and hold onto it. Another option is to cover yourself with a mattress, blanket, or clothing.
- **Lie down.** If you are outside, lie down in a ditch or other low-lying area.

Hurricanes

A **hurricane** is *a strong windstorm with driving rain that originates at sea.* Hurricanes consist of storm clouds that revolve around the eye, which is a calm area in the center of the storm. Hurricanes can extend over hundreds of miles, and they occur most often in late summer and early fall.

Just as it tracks tornadoes, the National Weather Service also monitors hurricanes. **Figure 19.6** is a map showing the path of a hurricane. To prepare for a hurricane, take the following steps.

- **Secure your home.** Close storm shutters or board up windows to prevent high winds from blowing them in. However, do not stay to board up windows during a storm.
- **Take loose objects indoors.** Bring inside any objects that might be blown away, such as outdoor furniture and toys.
- **Leave the area.** If you live on the coast, go inland. Do not stay to watch the storm.

CONNECT TO

Science

STORM TRACKING
Satellite images are an important tool in forecasting tropical storms and hurricanes. Using computers, forecasters gather information on the direction a storm is going and how it is developing. The newest weather satellites are the GOES series, or Geostationary Operational Environmental Satellite. *Where can people get up-to-date hurricane forecast information?*

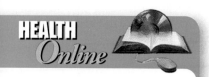
Blizzards

A **blizzard** is *a very heavy snowstorm with winds up to 45 miles per hour.* The wind and heavy snow usually reduce visibility to less than 500 feet, making it easy to get lost. To protect yourself during blizzards or other winter storms, follow these steps.

- **Stay inside.** Indoors is the safest place during a blizzard. If you must go outside, take the following precautions.
- **Wear protective clothing.** Put on several layers of loose-fitting lightweight clothing. Choose outerwear that keeps out wind and moisture, and wrap a scarf around your neck and mouth. Keep your head, nose, ears, fingers, and toes covered.
- **Avoid getting lost.** Use landmarks to find your way, or stay where you are until help arrives.

Floods

If you are in a flood, seek higher ground and stay out of the water. Drowning and electrocution from downed power lines pose serious risks. Never try to swim, walk, ride a bike, or ride in a car through floodwaters.

Most flood deaths are due to flash floods. In a flash flood, water rises very quickly and may move swiftly. Floodwaters can sweep away people, cars, and homes. During a flood, listen to National Weather Service bulletins for updates and advice. If water supplies have been contaminated by overflowing sewage, you may be told to drink only bottled water.

HEALTH SKILLS ACTIVITY

ACCESSING INFORMATION

Local Weather Emergencies

Follow these tips to plan ahead for weather emergencies and natural disasters.

- Identify the weather emergencies likely to affect your community.
- Check with a reliable source for safety measures to take during these types of weather emergencies.
- With family members, develop and maintain a personal and family emergency plan.
- Prepare and maintain an emergency supplies kit. Include a battery-operated radio and a flashlight, both with extra batteries; canned and ready-to-eat food; a can opener; water (1 gallon per person per day); a first-aid kit; and blankets.
- Identify emergency evacuation routes in the local area.

WITH A GROUP
In small groups, choose one weather emergency that occurs in your area. Prepare information sheets on dealing with this type of emergency. Ask parents to post these sheets at home.

Earthquakes

An **earthquake** is *a violent shaking movement of the earth's surface.* In the United States, earthquakes can occur in any of the 50 states. However, they occur most often west of the Rocky Mountains. Although weak earthquakes may cause little or no damage, a severe earthquake can topple buildings and bridges. Most injuries result from collapsing walls and falling debris. If an earthquake strikes, take the following steps to help protect yourself from injury.

- **Stay inside.** If the earthquake begins while you are indoors, stay there. Crouch under a sturdy table or desk, against an interior wall, or in a strongly supported doorway. Stay away from objects that might fall, shatter, or cave in. Cover your head with your arms or a pillow.
- **If you are outdoors, stay in the open.** Keep away from buildings, trees, telephone and electrical lines, streetlights, and overpasses. If you are in a car, the driver should stop and everyone should remain inside the car.
- **Be careful afterward.** After the earthquake is over, stay out of damaged buildings. Be aware that utilities such as electrical or gas lines may have been damaged and could be hazardous. Be prepared for aftershocks—smaller quakes that occur after the main earthquake.

Teens and parents can work together to prepare for natural disasters. For example, securing the water heater to a wall with metal strappings will help keep it from falling over in an earthquake.

Lesson 3 Review

Using complete sentences, answer the following questions on a sheet of paper.

Reviewing Terms and Facts

1. **Compare** Which condition is more serious—a weather *watch* or a weather *warning*? Why?
2. **Vocabulary** Differentiate between a *tornado* and a *hurricane.*
3. **List** Name three steps to take to prepare for a hurricane.
4. **Recall** Why should you stay out of the water during a flood?

Thinking Critically

5. **Analyze** Why is it important to stay indoors during a blizzard?
6. **Synthesize** Why should you stay out of damaged buildings after an earthquake?

Applying Health Skills

7. **Practicing Healthful Behaviors** Choose a weather emergency or natural disaster from this lesson. With a partner, write and perform a skit to demonstrate strategies for staying safe and preventing accidental injuries during your chosen event.

Basic First Aid

Quick Write

Suppose that you witnessed a car accident. List the actions you would take to provide help and the order in which you would take them.

LEARN ABOUT...

○ how to be prepared for emergencies.
○ how to take universal precautions when giving first aid.
○ the basic steps to follow in emergencies.

VOCABULARY

○ first aid
○ universal precautions

What Is First Aid?

First aid is *the immediate temporary care given to an injured or ill person until he or she can get professional help.* Knowing what to do during certain common emergencies can prevent further damage and may even speed recovery. Equally important, though, is knowing what *not* to do. In serious cases, providing the correct first aid can make the difference between life and death. Any time first aid is needed, it's important to stay calm. Doing so will allow you to better help the victim.

Be Prepared

First aid might be needed anywhere, at any time, and without warning. Learning basic first-aid skills will help you handle most common emergencies. Another way to be prepared is to keep a list of emergency numbers near all phones. All family members should know where family health records are kept. If a family member has certain allergies, for example, that information may be needed during an emergency.

It is also important to keep first-aid supplies at home and in the car and to know how to use them. You can assemble your own first-aid kit or buy a packaged kit. **Figure 19.7** provides suggestions for basic first-aid supplies. If a family member has a medical condition, specific medicines may need to be added to the kit.

It's a good idea to take along a first-aid kit when hiking or biking. *For what other types of activities might you bring a first-aid kit?*

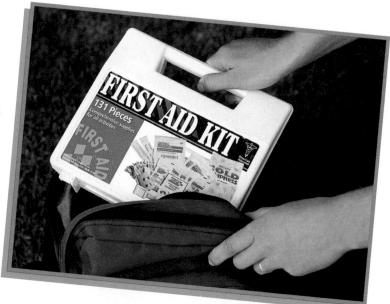

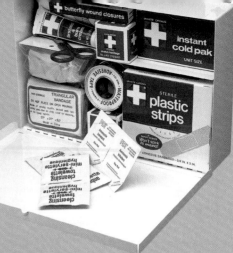

FIGURE 19.7

FIRST-AID SUPPLIES

Keeping a first-aid kit in your home will help your family be prepared for emergencies. *What other supplies might you add to this kit?*

Instruments: tweezers, scissors

Equipment: thermometer, cotton swabs, blanket, cold pack

Medications: antiseptic ointment, sterile eyewash, activated charcoal, syrup of ipecac

Dressings: gauze pads, adhesive tape, adhesive bandages, triangular bandage

Miscellaneous: small flashlight, tissues, hand cleaner, disposable gloves, face mask, plastic bags

Universal Precautions

People infected with HIV or hepatitis B carry the virus in their blood. Because these diseases are communicable, touching contaminated blood carries a risk. For this reason, it is important to protect yourself when giving first aid. Follow **universal precautions**, which are *actions taken to prevent the spread of disease by treating all blood as if it were contaminated.*

Universal precautions include wearing protective gloves when treating a victim. Use a face mask or shield when giving first aid for breathing emergencies. Cover any open wounds on your body with sterile dressings. Avoid touching any object that had contact with the victim's blood. Always wash your hands thoroughly after giving first aid.

The First Steps

Every emergency situation is unique. However, there are four steps to take for most emergencies. The sequence of steps is as follows: recognize the signs of an emergency, decide to act, call for help, and provide care until help arrives.

Recognize the Signs of an Emergency

Your senses of hearing, sight, and smell will alert you to most emergencies. Listen if you hear people calling out. Are they in trouble? Be alert to sudden loud or unusual noises such as shattering glass.

Sometimes the first sign of an emergency is an odor such as the smell of smoke. Also be alert for any strong smell that makes your eyes sting, causes you to cough, or makes breathing difficult. These sensations can signal a chemical spill or toxic gas release.

Developing Good Character ★

Citizenship

As a good citizen, you'll want to be prepared to report accidents, fires, serious illnesses, injuries, and crimes. Check your telephone book to find the number or numbers to call for emergencies in your community. Make a list to keep by the telephone.

Decide to Act

In an emergency, evaluate the situation and decide what action is needed. Then consider your strengths and limitations before you act. For example, unless you are trained in lifesaving, don't dive into a lake to rescue someone who is drowning. Instead, you might throw the person a life preserver or some other object that floats. Your first responsibility in any situation is to protect your own safety. Never put your own life in danger to help someone else.

Some people hesitate to help others because they are afraid of doing something wrong. Almost all states have Good Samaritan laws, which protect rescuers who act responsibly from legal action. In an emergency, one action that is always beneficial is to call for help. Getting help is often the best and only action for you to take, and this alone can save a life.

Call for Help

In most of the United States, the number to call for all emergencies is 911. Dialing 0 for the operator is also an option and may be necessary in some small towns. When you call, stay calm. Be ready to tell the emergency operator the nature of the emergency and the street address or location. The operator will notify the police, fire department, or emergency medical services. If you don't know the address, you can describe the location by using landmarks. Stay on the phone until the operator has the necessary information and tells you that you can hang up.

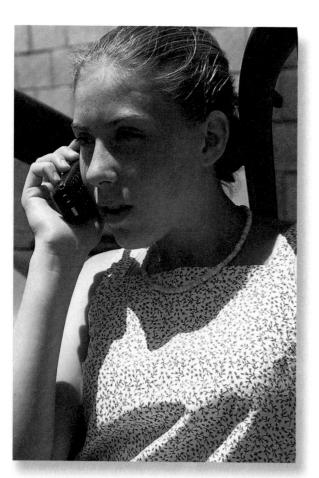

Provide Care Until Help Arrives

Once you have called for help, provide care by staying with the injured person and protecting him or her from further injury. Help the person maintain normal body temperature by providing a coat or blanket for warmth. Carefully loosen any tight clothing, and provide shade from the sun if necessary. Reassure the victim that help is on the way.

In general, you should not try to move a victim. Moving the person could cause pain or further injury. Wait for professional help to arrive. The only situation in which a victim should be moved is if he or she is in danger, such as in the path of oncoming traffic.

If the victim is unconscious and unresponsive, cardiopulmonary resuscitation (CPR) is needed. This technique for dealing with life-threatening emergencies is described in Lesson 6 of this chapter.

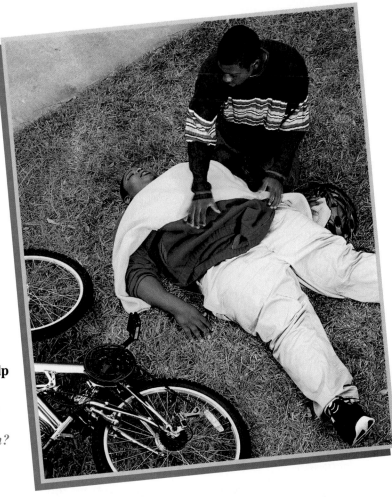

While you wait for medical help to arrive, help the victim stay calm by providing comfort and reassurance. *Why should you avoid moving an injured person?*

Lesson 4 Review

Using complete sentences, answer the following questions on a sheet of paper.

Reviewing Terms and Facts

1. **Vocabulary** Define the term *first aid.*
2. **Recall** What are four universal precautions to take when giving first aid?
3. **Summarize** List the first four steps to take when an emergency occurs.
4. **Identify** Give three examples of ways you can provide help to an injured person until professional help arrives.

Thinking Critically

5. **Analyze** Why is it so important to know basic first-aid strategies for responding to accidental injuries?

6. **Apply** If you come upon an injured person on a jogging path, should you try to drag the person to the side of the path? Why or why not?

Applying Health Skills

7. **Practicing Healthful Behaviors** With family members, discuss your family's preparedness for emergencies. Begin by listing possible emergencies. Then decide what should be done for each situation and how prepared every member is to act. Make a plan of the steps you could take to become more prepared. Demonstrate strategies for responding to accidental injuries by practicing the steps.

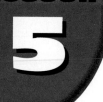
First Aid for Common Emergencies

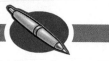

Quick Write

Describe an emergency you experienced or witnessed in which first aid was needed. What help did you or others provide?

LEARN ABOUT...

- how to recognize and evaluate common emergencies.
- first-aid treatments for common emergencies.
- when to call for medical assistance.

VOCABULARY

- sprain
- fracture
- heat cramps
- heat exhaustion
- heatstroke

Common Emergencies

Sprains, bruises, and broken bones are a few of the common emergencies you may experience. Others include insect bites, burns, poisoning, foreign objects in the eye, nosebleed, fainting, heat cramps, and heatstroke. Learn how to properly treat these conditions. Also recognize the difference between a minor condition that you can treat and a more serious condition that needs professional medical assistance.

Sprains

A **sprain** is *a condition in which the ligaments that hold the joints in position are stretched or torn.* Sprains usually result from a sudden force, often a twisting movement. Ankles and knees are the most commonly sprained joints. Swelling and bruising often accompany a sprain. Serious sprains should be treated by a physician. To treat minor sprains, use the R.I.C.E. method:

- **Rest.** Rest the affected joint for 24 to 48 hours.
- **Ice.** Apply ice to reduce swelling and pain. Place a cloth between the skin and the bag of ice in order to reduce discomfort.
- **Compression.** Compress the injured part by wrapping it in an elastic bandage.
- **Elevation.** Elevate, or raise, the injured part above the level of the heart to reduce swelling.

Apply a cold pack to a sprain as soon as possible after the injury to reduce inflammation. *What could you use if you did not have a cold pack available?*

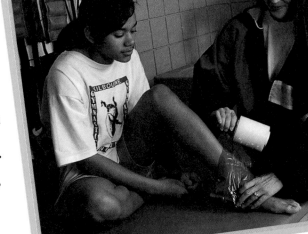

Broken Bones

A **fracture** is *a break in a bone.* An open fracture is a complete break with one or both sides of the bone piercing the skin. A closed fracture does not break the skin and may be difficult to identify. Typical signs of a closed fracture include pain, swelling, and misshapen appearance. Sometimes, however, a broken bone causes no immediate pain. The only way to be sure a bone is broken is to have it X-rayed.

Insect Bites and Stings

Insect bites and stings often cause pain and swelling at the site of the bite or sting. For people who are allergic to bites and stings, however, the situation is much more serious, and possibly life-threatening. If a person develops a rash, has difficulty breathing, shows signs of shock, or is known to be allergic to stings, he or she needs professional medical help immediately.

First aid for insect bites involves washing the affected area and applying a special lotion for bites. For insect stings, you first need to remove the stinger by scraping against it with your fingernail. Once the stinger is out, apply ice or a cold pack to relieve pain and prevent swelling. If a person is bitten by a tick, the tick will burrow into the skin and needs to be removed very carefully. **Figure 19.8** shows the correct procedure for removing ticks.

FIGURE 19.8

HOW TO REMOVE A TICK

If you find a tick on your body, have an adult follow the method shown to remove it.

1 Using a pair of pointed, smooth-tipped tweezers, grasp the tick by the head or mouth parts right where they enter the skin. Do not grasp the tick by the body.

2 Without jerking or twisting, pull firmly and steadily directly outward. Place the tick in alcohol to kill it. Clean the bite wound with disinfectant.

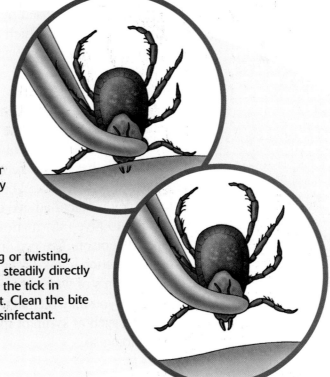

FIGURE 19.9

THREE DEGREES OF BURNS

Treatment for burns depends on the severity of the burn.

Type of Burn	Description	Treatment
First-Degree	Affects only the outer layer of the skin. The skin is usually red, but the outer layer has not been burned through. There may be swelling and pain.	Cool the burn with running water, immerse the burn in cold water, or apply cold compresses for at least 15 minutes. Cover the burn with a sterile bandage.
Second-Degree	Burns through the first layer of skin and burns the second layer of skin. Blisters develop, and the skin looks red and splotchy. Usually there is severe pain and swelling.	A burn no larger than 2 to 3 inches in diameter can be treated as a first-degree burn. If the burn is larger, or is on the hands, feet, face, groin, buttocks, or a major joint, get medical help immediately.
Third-Degree	Involves all layers of skin and may affect fat, muscle, and bone. The burned area may be charred black or appear dry and white. There may be little or no pain felt at this stage.	Call for medical help. While you are waiting, treat the victim for shock as described in Lesson 6. Do not remove burned clothing. Apply cold water to the burn, then cover with a sterile bandage or clean cloth. Keep the victim still and help him or her to sip fluids.

Burns

First aid for burns depends on the amount of skin burned, the location of the burn, and the depth of the burn. Burns to the eye or airway and burns caused by chemicals or electricity require special first-aid procedures, which are not covered here. **Figure 19.9** explains how to recognize and treat three classifications of burns.

Poisoning

A poison is a substance that causes harm when swallowed, breathed in, absorbed by the skin, or injected into the body. About half of all poisonings involve medicines or household products. Anyone who has been poisoned needs immediate treatment. Call the nearest poison control center, a 24-hour hot line that provides emergency medical advice on treating poisoning victims. Be prepared to give information about the victim and about the suspected poison. The person at the poison control center will tell you what action to take. You may be instructed to give the victim large amounts of water or milk to dilute the poison. For some types of poison, you may be told to give the victim something to induce vomiting, such as syrup of ipecac. Read the label on the container before doing so.

If the skin comes into direct contact with a poisonous chemical such as a pesticide or household cleaning agent, remove any clothing that has come into contact with the chemical. Remove as much of the chemical from the surface of the skin as you can by flooding with water for 15 minutes. While the skin is being flooded, call the nearest poison control center.

Foreign Object in the Eye

If you get a foreign object in your eye, don't rub the eye. Rubbing can cause injury. Try to flush the object out of your eye with clean water. Hold the rim of a small, clean glass filled with water against the base of your eye socket. Keeping your eye open, gently pour the water into the eye. If the object isn't washed out, repeat the process. If you cannot clear your eye, get assistance.

To help somebody else who has a foreign object in the eye, first locate the object. Gently pull the lower lid downward while the person looks up. If you do not see the object, hold the upper lid open and examine the eye while the person looks down. If the object is floating on the surface of the eye, lightly touch the object with a moistened cotton swab or the corner of a clean cloth. If you cannot remove the object, seek medical assistance immediately.

Nosebleed

Nosebleeds can be caused by an injury, by being in a very dry place, and even by a cold. If you experience a nosebleed, pinch your nose shut with your thumb and index finger and breathe through your mouth. Keep the nose pinched for 5 to 10 minutes. If bleeding lasts more than 15 minutes or if there is a lot of blood, get medical assistance immediately.

Fainting

Fainting occurs when the blood supply to the brain is cut off for a short amount of time. A person who faints loses consciousness briefly. If you feel faint, lie down or sit down and place your head between your knees. If someone else faints, follow these steps.

- Leave the person lying down. Check the airway. If the person is breathing, raise the legs above the level of the head.

- Loosen any tight clothing.

- If the person does not regain consciousness in one to two minutes, call for help. If the person is not breathing, call for help and start CPR if you are trained (see Lesson 6).

- Losing consciousness after a head injury is not fainting— call for help if this occurs. Immediate CPR is needed if there are no signs of life.

Pinching your nose can help stop your nose from bleeding. *What might cause a nosebleed?*

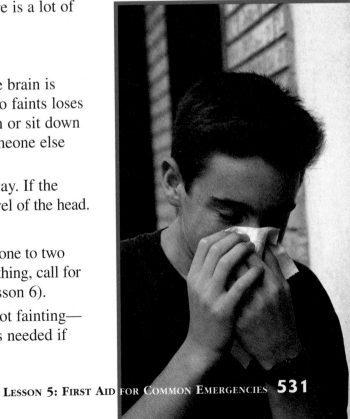

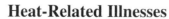

Heat-Related Illnesses

Heat-related illnesses include heat cramps, heat exhaustion, and heatstroke. **Heat cramps** are *painful, involuntary muscle spasms that usually occur during heavy exercise in hot weather.* People who experience heat cramps should rest, cool down, and drink water or a sports drink that contains electrolytes. Gentle stretching exercise and gentle massage may help relieve the cramps.

Heat exhaustion is *a condition characterized by faintness, nausea, rapid heartbeat, and hot, red, dry, or sweaty skin.* Take someone who shows signs of heat exhaustion to a shady or air-conditioned place. Have the person lie down and slightly elevate the feet. Loosen clothing. Have the person drink cold, but not iced, water. Spray the person with cool water and fan him or her. Keep careful watch. Heat exhaustion can quickly become **heatstroke**, which is *the most serious form of heat illness.*

Heatstroke is life-threatening because the body's normal processes for dealing with heat, including sweating, close down. The main sign of heatstroke is a marked increase in body temperature—generally higher than 104°F. Rapid heartbeat and rapid and shallow breathing are other signs. If heatstroke is a possibility, treat the person as for heat exhaustion and call immediately for emergency medical assistance.

It is important to rest, cool down, and drink water when suffering from heat cramps. *What are some common causes of heat cramps?*

Lesson 5 Review

Using complete sentences, answer the following questions on a sheet of paper.

Reviewing Terms and Facts

1. **Vocabulary** Define the terms *sprain* and *fracture.* Use both terms in a sentence that demonstrates their meanings.
2. **Summarize** Explain the process for removing a tick from a person's body.
3. **Recall** What should you do to help someone who has swallowed a poisonous substance?
4. **Describe** What action should you take if you feel faint?

Thinking Critically

5. **Analyze** How would you respond to this accidental injury: a burn about 1½ inches in diameter that had burned through the first layer of skin and burned the second layer of skin? Explain.
6. **Compare and Contrast** How does the treatment for heatstroke differ from that for heat cramps?

Applying Health Skills

7. **Practicing Healthful Behaviors** With a classmate, write a scenario for dealing with a common emergency. Demonstrate strategies for responding to your chosen accidental injury by acting out your scenario for the class.

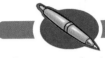
Life-Threatening Emergencies

When Minutes Count

In a life-threatening emergency, a person may have only minutes to live unless the right treatment is provided. If you can provide appropriate first aid in such a situation, you may save a life. For all life-threatening emergencies, try to stay calm, and call for help.

Choking

More than 3,000 people die from choking every year in the United States. Choking occurs when a person's airway becomes blocked by a piece of food or some other object. If the object is not removed, air will not reach the lungs and the person could die. A choking person usually has an expression of fear and may clutch his or her throat—the universal sign for choking. He or she may wheeze or gasp, turn reddish purple, have bulging eyes, and will be unable to speak. If the person can speak or cough, it is not a choking emergency.

A choking person needs immediate help. You may be able to clear the object from an adult's or child's throat by using the maneuver shown in **Figure 19.10** on the next page. This is the **abdominal thrusts** maneuver, which uses *quick, upward pulls into the diaphragm to force out an obstruction blocking the airway.* The first-aid procedure for a choking infant is different from the adult technique. Check with a first-aid manual to learn how to help infants.

This person is demonstrating the universal sign for choking—grabbing the throat with thumb and fingers extended. *How would you respond to someone showing signs of choking?*

Quick Write

In a life-threatening emergency, every second counts. Why is it important to stay calm at such a time?

LEARN ABOUT...

- how to deal with life-threatening emergencies.
- shock, and why it must be considered in any emergency.
- how to provide rescue breathing.
- the ABCs of CPR.

VOCABULARY

- abdominal thrusts
- shock
- CPR

FIGURE 19.10

FIRST AID FOR A CHOKING ADULT OR OLDER CHILD

Before you perform abdominal thrusts, determine if the person is choking. *Why is asking if a person can speak a good way to find out if he or she is choking?*

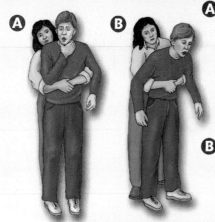

A Stand behind the person who is choking. Wrap your arms around the person's waist and tip the person slightly forward. Make a fist. Place the fist just above the person's navel but below the breastbone. Position the fist so the thumb side is against the victim's abdomen. Grasp your fist with your other hand.

B Quickly, thrust inward and upward. The motion is similar to one you would use if you were trying to lift the person off the ground. Repeat thrusts until the food or object is dislodged. If the person becomes unresponsive, call for medical help and begin CPR.

If you are choking and are alone, give yourself an abdominal thrust. There are two ways to do this. First, make a fist and position it slightly above your navel. Grasp your fist with your other hand and thrust inward and upward into your abdomen until the object pops out. The second technique is to lean over a firm object, such as the back of a chair, and press your abdomen into it.

Shock

Shock is *a life-threatening condition in which the circulatory system fails to deliver enough blood to vital tissues and organs.* The many causes of shock include injury, burns, severe infection, heat, poisoning, blood loss, and heart attack. Because shock can result from a medical emergency, you should look for signs of it when providing first aid.

Signs of shock to watch for include cool, clammy, pale or gray skin; weak and rapid pulse; and slow, shallow breathing. The pupils may be dilated, and the eyes may have a dull look. If conscious, the victim of shock may feel faint, weak, confused, and anxious.

If you think the victim is in shock or in danger of shock, call for medical help and take these precautions.

- Have the person lie down on his or her back. Raise the feet higher than the head. Try to keep the person from moving.
- Loosen tight clothing.
- Keep the person warm. Use a blanket, coat, or whatever is available as a cover.
- Do not give the person anything to drink.
- If the person vomits or bleeds from the mouth, roll the person to his or her side to help prevent choking.

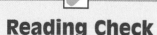

Reading Check

Make connections. The word *artery* comes from a Greek word meaning "way from the chest." One important set of arteries carries blood to the head. Find the name of those arteries on the next page.

FIGURE 19.11

PRESSURE POINT BLEEDING CONTROL

This illustration shows the areas on arms and legs that can be pressed against a bone to stop circulation to the arm or leg.

Arm
Use four fingers to press on the inside of the upper arm at the area circled in the diagram. You will press the artery at this point against the arm bone. To find the artery, feel for a pulse below the round muscle of the biceps.

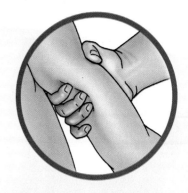

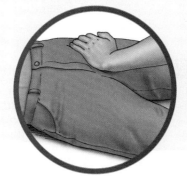

Leg
Keeping your arm straight, use the heel of your hand to press the groin at the area shown in the diagram. You will press the artery at this point against the pelvic bone. You may need to use both hands to apply enough pressure.

Severe Bleeding

To stop severe bleeding, have the person lie down. If possible, raise the site of the bleeding above the level of the heart. When treating bleeding, use protective gloves whenever possible. Bleeding can usually be stopped by applying direct pressure to the wound, using a clean cloth. If that is unsuccessful, apply pressure to the artery that supplies blood to the area of the wound. See **Figure 19.11**.

Hands-On Health

LOCATING PRESSURE POINTS

In addition to the arteries leading to the arms and legs, there are two pressure points on either side of the neck. The carotid arteries, which supply blood to the head and brain, run just below the skin here. Knowing where pressure points are can help you be prepared to quickly check pulse or stop severe blood flow.

WHAT YOU WILL DO
1. Referring to **Figure 19.11**, locate the pressure points for your left and right arm and left and right leg arteries. Feel for the pulse.
2. Referring to the photograph, feel for the pulse at your right carotid. Then find the pulse at your left carotid. The carotid arteries have the strongest pulse.

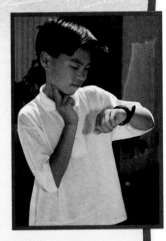

IN CONCLUSION
1. Name the pressure point you would press to stop severe blood flow from the following: left calf, right forearm, right wrist, right ankle.
2. If you needed to check someone's pulse, which pressure point would you use? Why?

FIGURE 19.12

THE ABCs OF CPR

The first steps of CPR involve assessment and rescue breathing. If you have an available breathing mask, follow the directions that came with the mask.

① **Airway.** Look inside the victim's mouth. If you see anything blocking the airway, remove it. Lay the person flat on a firm surface. Gently tilt the head back with one hand and lift the chin with the other. If you suspect head or neck injuries, do not move the victim's head. Open the airway by lifting the jaw instead.

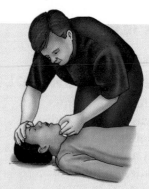

② **Breathing.** Look, listen, and feel to find out if the victim is breathing. *Look* for chest movement. *Listen* at the victim's mouth for breathing sounds. *Feel* for exhaled air on your cheek. If the victim is not breathing, begin rescue breathing. Pinch the person's nostrils shut, take a normal breath and place your mouth over the victim's, forming a seal. Give two slow breaths, each about two seconds long. The victim's chest should rise with each breath.

③ **Circulation.** Check for circulation by watching for some response to your rescue breaths, such as breathing, coughing, or movement. If there are no signs of circulation, a person trained in CPR should begin chest compressions immediately (see **Figure 19.13**). If the victim responds but is not breathing normally, give a rescue breath every five seconds.

CPR

Imagine that you are in an emergency situation in which somebody loses consciousness. You gently shake the victim and shout "Are you OK?" but the victim does not respond. If a victim is unresponsive, he or she needs cardiopulmonary resuscitation (CPR) immediately. **CPR** is *a first-aid procedure that combines rescue breaths with chest compressions to restore breathing and circulation.* Only people who have received the proper training should perform CPR.

The first steps of CPR, as recommended by the American Heart Association, are known as the ABCs—airway, breathing, and circulation. The ABC technique to use for adults and older children is shown in **Figure 19.12**. Check a first-aid manual to learn how to help younger children and infants. **Figure 19.13** illustrates the process for combining rescue breaths with chest compressions.

FIGURE 19.13

CPR FOR ADULTS

CPR involves both chest compressions and rescue breaths. It should be administered only by people who are properly trained and certified.

1 Position your hands. Prepare to start chest compressions by finding a spot on the lower half of the victim's breastbone. Place the heel of one hand on that point, and interlock the fingers with the fingers of the other hand. Do not allow your fingers to rest on the victim's ribs.

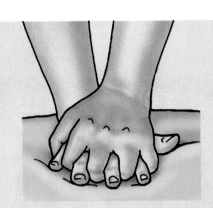

2 Begin chest compressions and rescue breathing. Lean over the victim until your shoulders are over your hands. Lock your elbows, then press down firmly and release, allowing the chest to spring back. Without pausing, give 15 chest compressions at a rate of about 100 per minute. Pause to give 2 rescue breaths (see **Figure 19.12**). Check for signs of circulation after 4 cycles, then every few minutes as you continue. Give CPR until the victim revives or help arrives.

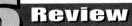

Lesson 6 Review

Using complete sentences, answer the following questions on a sheet of paper.

Reviewing Terms and Facts

1. **Vocabulary** Define *abdominal thrust.*
2. **List** What are the signs of shock?
3. **Summarize** What strategies should you use to respond to an accidental injury that causes severe bleeding?
4. **Explain** What is *CPR?* In what circumstances should it be used?

Thinking Critically

5. **Analyze** A driver walks out after a car crash and says that he is all right. However, his skin is gray, his pupils are dilated, and his breathing is shallow. From what condition might the driver be suffering? What strategies should you use to respond to this condition?

Applying Health Skills

6. **Accessing Information** Research where first-aid procedures, including the choking rescue and CPR, are taught in your community. Find out the location, cost, requirements, and what type of certificates are issued upon completion of the class. Demonstrate basic first-aid procedures by taking the class.

Preventing
Wildfires

Wildfires can be extremely dangerous and destructive. Here are the forces that can drive wildfires and ways to prevent them.

③ Blowing embers allow the fire to jump natural barriers such as rivers and valleys.

① Column of rising hot air creates a void below.

② Fresh air rushes in, bringing more oxygen to fuel the flames.

WIND

WIND

UPHILL BATTLE
Wildfires charge rapidly up mountainsides because the heat from the fire rises and is directed at the fuel uphill, drying it out before the flames arrive.

FUEL
Decades of fighting every forest fire have left many areas dangerously full of fuel—sticks, fallen timber, pine needles, and brush.

TORNADO WINDS
In rare cases, winds within a wildfire create powerful mini-tornados that can shoot spirals of flames into the air and twist apart tree trunks.

SOIL INSULATION
Soil is an excellent insulator that can protect tree roots from a fire's heat, permitting regrowth to begin quickly.

How They Start

Wildfires result when fuel, dryness, and some kind of trigger are all present. Each factor contributes to the severity of the blaze.

- **Fuel** means flammable solids—grass, pine needles, undergrowth, smaller trees—that, with oxygen, feed the fire.
- **Dryness** can be caused by short-term weather patterns with low humidity or by a long drought.
- **Triggers** can be anything from a lightning strike to a campfire to an arsonist.

How They Spread

Weather is the primary force that drives or contains wildfires. However, once they start burning, wildfires create their own weather.

① **Smoke and heat** from fires can rise thousands of feet into the air.

② Then **cooler air** rushes in to fill the void.

③ This movement of air creates **gale-force hot winds** that dry out and preheat fuel ahead of the fire and can propel burning embers as much as half a mile.

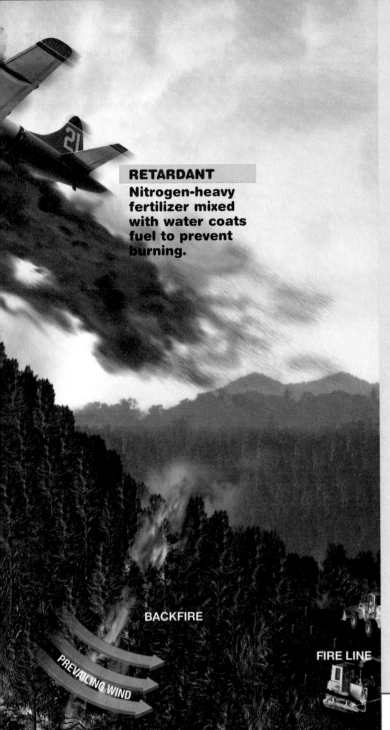

RETARDANT
Nitrogen-heavy fertilizer mixed with water coats fuel to prevent burning.

BACKFIRE

FIRE LINE

PREVAILING WIND

Preventing Wildfires When Camping

- **Build campfires away from overhanging branches, steep slopes, rotten stumps, logs, dry grass, and leaves. Pile any extra wood away from the fires.**

- **Keep plenty of water handy and have a shovel on hand for throwing dirt on the fire if it gets out of control.**

- **Keep the campfire small. Scrape away litter and any flammable material within a 10-foot circle. This will keep a small campfire from spreading.**

- **Be sure your match is out after the fire is lit.**

- **Never leave a campfire unattended. Even a small breeze could quickly cause the fire to spread.**

- **Drown the fire with water. Make sure all embers, coals, and sticks are wet. Move rocks—there may be burning embers underneath. Stir the remains, add more water, and stir again. Be sure all burned material has been extinguished and cooled.**

- **If you do not have water, use dirt. Mix soil or sand with the embers and continue adding and stirring until all material is cooled.**

Source: United States Department of Agriculture-Forest Service and the National Association of State Foresters

How to Fight Them

A fire dies when it is deprived of fuel, heat, or oxygen. The main strategy for fighting wildfires is containment: surround the fire and starve it.

- **Helicopters and tanker airplanes** can drop water or chemical retardants to slow the spread of flames.
- **Firefighters can set up fire lines,** areas cleared of any fuel that allow the fire to spread.
- **Controlled fires** are sometimes set to deny fuel to an approaching blaze. ■

TIME TO THINK...

About Wildfires

With the class, create an ad campaign to warn others about the dangers of wildfires. Include information on how people can prevent wildfires when they're camping. To help campers remember your tips, investigate the word mnemonic (nem-ON-ik) and then create such a device for your campaign.

AVOIDING UNSAFE BEHAVIORS

Model

At times, other teens may urge you to do things that are unsafe. Using refusal skills in these situations can help protect you from injury. Read about a teen named Travis who is out riding his bike with a classmate, Jerry. Note how Travis uses refusal skills to avoid unsafe behavior.

JERRY: Let's go this way. It's a short cut.

TRAVIS: No, we can't go that way. It's private property.

JERRY: So what? No one will see us.

TRAVIS: But it's steep and could be dangerous.

JERRY: I've ridden that way before, and I've never been hurt.

TRAVIS: Better safe than sorry. Why don't we just ride around the long way?

JERRY: Don't be such a baby. I'm going this way.

TRAVIS: I guess I'll meet up with you later, then. I'm going the long way.

JERRY: Oh, all right, have it your way. I'll go with you.

Practice

Read the following scenario and answer the questions at the end.

Several of Gina's teammates have invited her to join them after soccer practice at the local swimming pool. Gina has been swimming there before during the daytime, but she knows that there is no lifeguard there in the evening. When she expresses her concerns, her teammates laugh and say, "Come on, Gina! We've all been swimming there before. We know it's safe."

1. What unsafe behavior are Gina's teammates pressuring her to do?
2. What refusal skills could Gina use to get out of this situation?
3. Give three refusal statements that Gina could make.

Apply/Assess

Working with a partner, create a role-play about a teen who is being pressured to do something unsafe. You can base your role-play on one of the scenarios shown below or make up your own situation. Show how the teen uses refusal skills to avoid the unsafe behavior. Present your role-play to the class.

Lonnie invites Joel to go skateboarding in a nearby parking lot. Joel knows that there are always a lot of cars driving around in the lot, making it unsafe for skating.

Reba and Nadine have made plans to go camping together over the weekend. However, the weather report is now predicting thunderstorms for Saturday night. Nadine does not think it is safe for them to be outside in a thunderstorm.

Jesse has offered to teach Rachel in-line skating. He says that she can borrow his sister's skates and helmet. When Rachel gets to Jesse's house, she finds that Jesse's sister has gone out on her bike and taken her helmet with her.

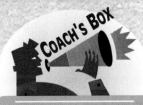

COACH'S BOX

Refusal Skills

You can use just one skill or combine several. You could
S Say no in a firm voice.
T Tell why.
O Offer another idea.
P Promptly leave.

Self-√ Check

- Did our role-play show a teen being pressured to do something unsafe?
- Did our role-play demonstrate how to use refusal skills?
- Did we avoid the unsafe behavior in our role-play?

After You Read

Use your completed Foldable to review the information on home and school safety.

FOLDABLES™
Study Organizer

Reviewing Vocabulary and Concepts

On a sheet of paper, write the numbers 1–5. After each number, write the term from the list that best completes each sentence.

- poisonings
- accident
- helmet
- accident chain
- defensive driving

Lesson 1

1. A(n) _____ is any event that was not intended to happen.

2. A(n) _____ includes a situation, an unsafe habit, and an unsafe action.

3. Cleaning products and medicines are the most common causes of _____ among children.

Lesson 2

4. _____ involves watching out for other people on the road and anticipating unsafe acts.

5. Bikers can reduce their risk of head injury by wearing a(n) _____.

On a sheet of paper, write the numbers 6–14. Write *True* or *False* for each statement below. If the statement is false, change the underlined word or phrase to make it true.

Lesson 3

6. In the event of a <u>hurricane</u>, the safest action is to go to a basement or cellar.

7. The National Weather Service may tell people to drink only bottled water during <u>blizzards</u>.

8. If an <u>earthquake</u> begins while you are indoors, you should crouch under a sturdy table.

Lesson 4

9. <u>Universal</u> precautions are steps taken to prevent disease by treating all blood as if it were contaminated.

10. Your first responsibility in any emergency situation is to <u>act immediately</u>.

11. In general, you should not try to move an accident victim unless the victim <u>asks to be moved</u>.

Lesson 5

12. A break in a bone is a <u>sprain</u>.

13. A <u>fracture</u> is a stretched or torn ligament.

14. The main sign of <u>heat exhaustion</u> is a marked increase in temperature.

Lesson 6

On a sheet of paper, write the numbers 15–17. After each number, write the letter of the answer that best completes each statement.

15. The abdominal thrusts maneuver is used to help a victim of
   a. shock.
   b. heat exhaustion.
   c. severe bleeding.
   d. choking.

16. Signs of shock can include
   a. rapid pulse.
   b. shallow breathing.
   c. faintness.
   d. all of the above.

17. CPR is a procedure that includes
   a. elevating the victim's feet.
   b. rescue breaths and chest compressions.
   c. applying pressure to the wound.
   d. massaging to increase circulation.

Thinking Critically

Using complete sentences, answer the following questions on a sheet of paper.

18. **Explain** How does an understanding of the accident chain help prevent injuries?

19. **Explain** How can you use thinking and decision-making skills to avoid high-risk situations involving motor vehicles? Give three examples.

20. **Analyze** Why is it important to stay tuned to the National Weather Service on the radio during a weather emergency?

21. **Evaluate** How would you evaluate whether a victim needed CPR?

Standardized Test Practice

Reading & Writing

Read the paragraphs below and then answer the questions.

A severe lightning storm hit Norfolk yesterday afternoon, causing a power outage in the western part of town. One bolt struck a tree branch, which fell and injured a Mini Mart employee. The lightning struck during a late afternoon thunderstorm when the Mart was crowded with customers. Power was out for more than two hours after the storm.

When the lightning hit, Mini Mart owner Mike Wojer told customers and employees to stay inside and away from the doors and windows. He turned off the lights and appliances and asked customers not to try to make any phone calls.

"Thankfully, no one in the store was injured by the lightning," said Mr. Wojer.

The injured employee, Tim Yu, was outside the store when the lightning struck. Witnesses said that he was hit by a tree branch that had been struck by the lightning. He is listed in good condition at Norfolk Hospital.

1. What is the news article mainly about?
   - **A** the events of lightning striking near a store
   - **B** the store owner's bravery
   - **C** the damage lightning can cause
   - **D** the injuries caused by lightning

2. From the information in the article, the reader can conclude that
   - **A** lightning is not dangerous.
   - **B** it's safer to be indoors when lightning strikes.
   - **C** lightning only strikes trees.
   - **D** all thunderstorms have lightning.

3. Write a news article about an emergency or a weather-related event.

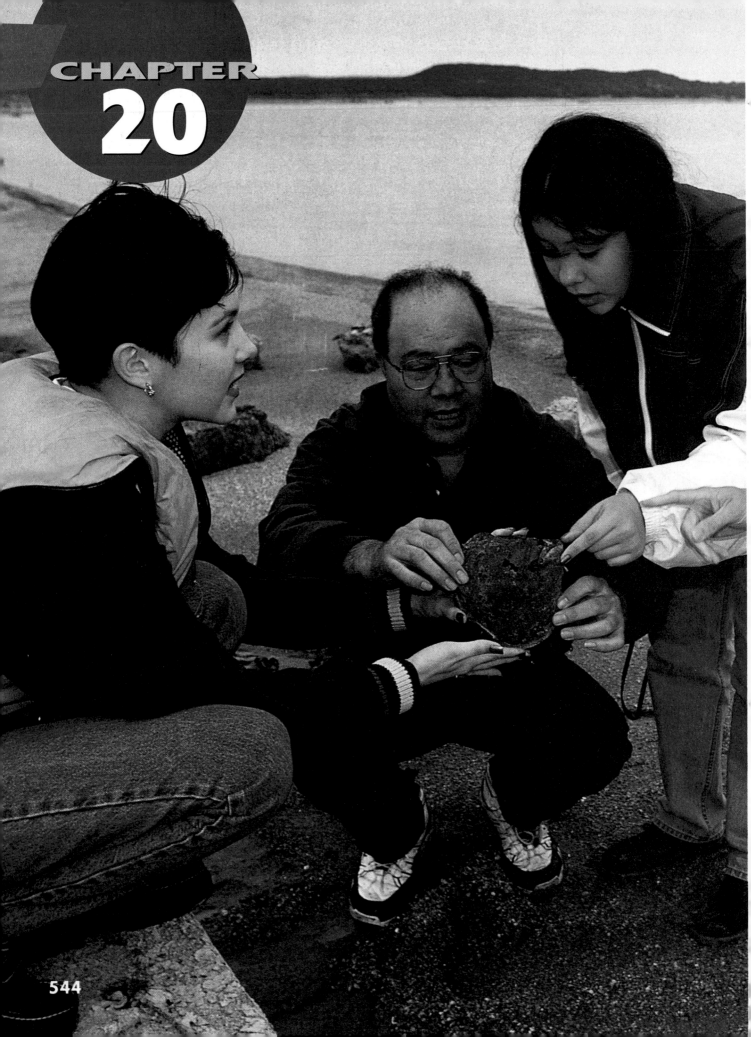

Environmental Health

HEALTH *Online*

How do some of your everyday actions protect the environment? Rate your awareness of environmental concerns by taking the Chapter 20 Health Inventory at health.glencoe.com.

FOLDABLES™ Study Organizer

Before You Read

Make this Foldable to record what you learn about air, water, and land pollution in Lesson 1. Begin with a plain sheet of 8½" × 11" paper.

Step 1

Fold a sheet of paper along the long axis, leaving a 1" tab along the side.

Step 2

Turn the paper and fold it into thirds.

Step 3

Unfold and cut the top layer along both fold lines. This makes three tabs.

Step 4

Label the tabs as shown.

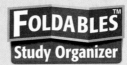

As You Read

Under the appropriate tab, define terms and summarize main ideas on air, water, and land pollution.

1

Pollution and Health

Quick Write

Write down your definition of pollution and give three examples of pollution that you have seen in your community.

LEARN ABOUT...

- what pollution is.
- what contributes to pollution of the air, water, and soil.
- how pollution affects the environment.

VOCABULARY

- pollution
- pesticides
- acid rain
- smog
- ozone layer
- greenhouse effect
- global warming
- landfills
- hazardous wastes

Your Environment

Your environment is everything that surrounds you. On a local level, it includes your home, school, and community. On a broader level, it includes the air you breathe, the water you drink, the trees that grow along the roadside, the climate you live in, and all the living and nonliving elements of the earth.

Without air, water, and land, life on earth would not be possible. Yet people have been polluting the very things that keep us alive. **Pollution** is a broad term that covers *any dirty or harmful substance in the environment.* It affects all living and nonliving things in the environment, and it affects some of the everyday choices you have. For example, when the air is clean, you can go outside and be active knowing your lungs won't be damaged by pollutants. Taking action to protect the environment now will benefit your health and the health of others. Future generations will be able to enjoy the results of your efforts.

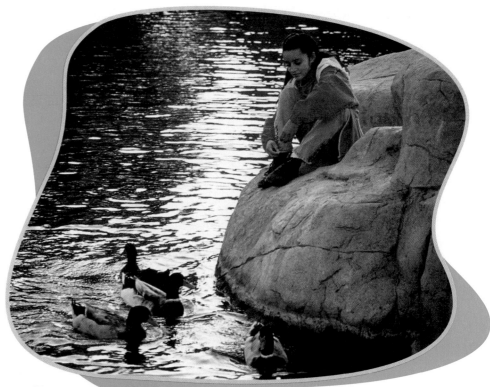

Part of good citizenship is protecting the environment. *What steps can you take to preserve the natural beauty of your surroundings?*

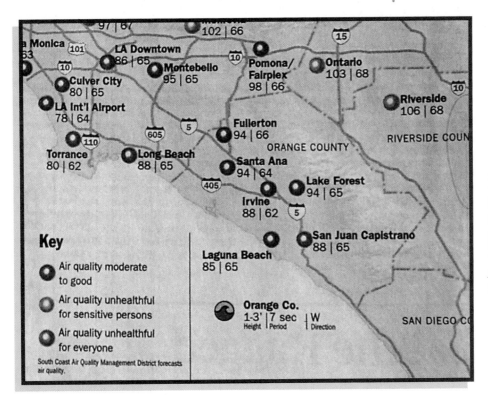

Key

- **Air quality moderate to good**
- **Air quality unhealthful for sensitive persons**
- **Air quality unhealthful for everyone**

South Coast Air Quality Management District forecasts air quality.

Orange Co.
1-3' | 7 sec | W
Height | Period | Direction

Most newspapers publish a daily air quality rating to warn people of air pollution levels. *How would a person with asthma use this information?*

Air Pollution

Natural events, such as an erupting volcano or a dust storm, cause some air pollution. Most air pollution, however, results from human activities that allow gases, dust, soot, and other substances to be released into the air. The major sources of air pollution are described below:

- **Burning fossil fuels.** People depend on energy to run motor vehicles, heat or cool buildings, and carry out countless daily tasks at home and at work. This energy is produced by burning oil, coal, and natural gas. Burning these fossil fuels, however, releases harmful gases such as carbon monoxide, sulfur dioxide, and nitrogen oxides into the atmosphere. Burning oil or coal also produces particulates, tiny particles of soot, ash, and other substances that can remain in the air for a long time.

- **Chemicals.** Many chemicals pollute the air. **Pesticides**, which are *products used on crops to control insects and other pests,* contain harmful chemicals that can get into the air. Chlorofluorocarbons (CFCs), chemicals that have traditionally been used in air conditioners and refrigerators, damage a layer of the atmosphere that protects the earth from dangerous solar radiation. Since 1987, more than 150 countries have signed an international agreement that will eventually phase out the use of CFCs.

- **Other sources.** Natural sources of air pollution include forest and grass fires, dust storms, and volcanic eruptions. Forest fires release carbon monoxide and other gases into the atmosphere that add to air pollution resulting from human activities.

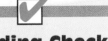

Reading Check

Identify cause and effect. Write your own *If . . ., then . . .* statements about pollution.

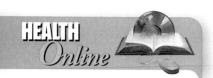
Effects of Air Pollution

Air pollution can have many damaging consequences for the environment. Some of the effects are described below:

- **Acid rain.** *Rain that is far more acidic than normal* is known as **acid rain**. When fossil fuels are burned, they produce sulfur dioxide and nitrogen oxides. These gases mix with water vapor and form weak acids, which then fall to the earth. Over time, the acid in the rain can destroy living things—especially trees, plants, and fish.

- **Smog.** Some gases formed by burning fossil fuels combine to produce ozone, a special form of oxygen. Ozone at ground level is a major component of **smog**, *a yellow-brown haze that forms when sunlight reacts with air pollution.* People with respiratory problems are advised to stay indoors on days when smog levels are high.

- **Destruction of the ozone layer.** Miles above the earth's surface, the **ozone layer** acts as *a shield that protects living things from ultraviolet (UV) radiation.* Certain types of air pollution cause the ozone layer to deteriorate, allowing excessive UV radiation to reach the earth's surface. In humans, this can lead to skin cancer and a weakened immune system.

- **Global warming.** *The trapping of heat by carbon dioxide and other gases in the air* is known as the **greenhouse effect** (see **Figure 20.1**). Without the greenhouse effect, the earth would be too cold to support life. However, air pollution intensifies the greenhouse effect and may be causing an unnatural degree of **global warming**, which is *a rise in the earth's temperatures.* This in turn could affect the water level of oceans and change weather patterns.

FIGURE 20.1

THE GREENHOUSE EFFECT

The heating of earth by gases in our atmosphere trapping heat is similar to how a greenhouse warms.

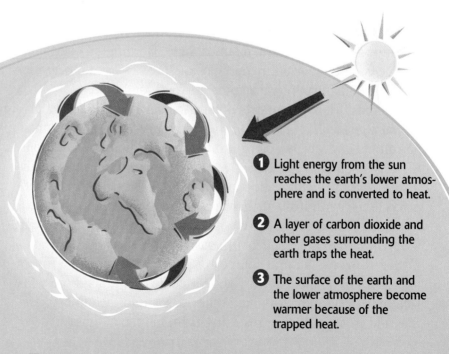

1 Light energy from the sun reaches the earth's lower atmosphere and is converted to heat.

2 A layer of carbon dioxide and other gases surrounding the earth traps the heat.

3 The surface of the earth and the lower atmosphere become warmer because of the trapped heat.

Water Pollution

All forms of life on earth depend on water. The earth's water is polluted by various kinds of wastes, chemicals, and other substances. One form of pollution is sewage—garbage, detergents, and other household wastes washed down drains. Although sewage is treated in the United States, many countries lack the education, money, and facilities needed to treat water properly. Harmful industrial chemicals are another cause of water pollution. Some enter the water from factories. In agricultural regions, pesticides and fertilizers can wash off the land and pollute water.

Oil spills from large tanker ships are a very damaging form of water pollution. Once in the water, oil can destroy plants and animals along with their habitats. Oil can also be spilled on land, resulting in the pollution of nearby lakes, rivers, and wetlands.

CONNECT TO

Science

PESTICIDE PERILS
Prolonged exposure to pesticides has been linked to many serious health problems. *Research the health hazards of exposure to pesticides and ways to avoid this potentially harmful environmental condition.*

Hands-On Health

EFFECTS OF WATER POLLUTANTS

When detergents and garbage get into rivers and lakes, they may cause the amount of algae to change. Algae (AL·jee) are simple organisms that float on the surface of the water and use sunlight to make their food. Some forms of pollution cause algae to multiply rapidly, forming a thick layer that blocks the sunlight. Deprived of light, the algae below the surface die and decay, a process that consumes oxygen. This loss of oxygen can kill fish and other forms of aquatic life. In this activity you will observe the effects of detergents and garbage on the growth of algae.

WHAT YOU WILL NEED
- tap water that has stood uncovered for three days
- water from a pond or aquarium that contains algae
- liquid detergent
- some potato or carrot scraps
- Three clean glass jars (same size, with lids)
- pen or pencil and labels

WHAT YOU WILL DO
1. Label the jars D (detergent), G (garbage), and C (control).
2. Fill each jar halfway with tap water. Add enough pond water to bring the level to three-fourths full.
3. Add a tablespoon of detergent to Jar D and vegetable scraps to Jar G. Do not add anything to Jar C.
4. Place the jars on a windowsill for two weeks.

IN CONCLUSION
1. Observe the jars every other day. Compare and note any changes in the color of the water in each. Which jar had the largest increase of algae? Which jar had the smallest increase?
2. What do your results indicate about the effects of detergent and garbage on algae? How do these results relate to water pollution?

Water polluted with sewage can spread diseases such as typhoid fever and cholera. Although they are rare in the United States, these diseases pose a severe threat in other parts of the world. Eating shellfish from polluted water can cause hepatitis, a disease of the liver. Drinking water that contains lead or mercury can result in serious damage to the brain, liver, and kidneys.

Land Pollution

Land pollution results from littering and the careless disposal of household and industrial garbage. Land pollution impacts the soil, water, and air. This type of pollution includes solid waste and hazardous wastes.

Solid Waste

In the United States, the average person produces about 4.4 pounds of trash, or solid waste, every day! For the nation as a whole, this adds up to millions of tons—enough to fill a professional baseball stadium from top to bottom twice a day. Where does it all go?

Landfills cannot keep up with increasing demand. *What can you do to reduce the amount of waste you personally produce?*

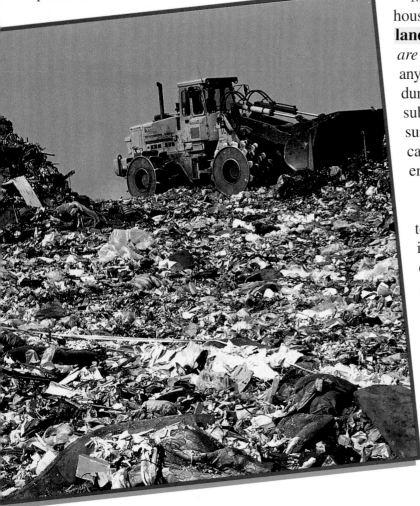

Most solid waste produced by households and businesses goes to **landfills**—*huge pits where wastes are dumped and buried.* At one time, anything and everything could be dumped in a landfill, including harmful substances that could seep into the surrounding land. Today, landfills are carefully regulated to protect the environment.

One alternative to burying trash is to burn it in special furnaces called incinerators. The energy that incinerators produce can be used to make electricity. This cuts down on the burning of fossil fuels. However, incinerators are expensive to operate and can burn only certain materials. Moreover, smoke and ashes from the incinerators contribute to air pollution. For these reasons, many people believe that recycling and reusing materials is a better way to deal with solid wastes.

Hazardous Wastes

In recent decades, advances in science and technology have led to the development of new industries and products. These advances have caused a new problem, however: hazardous wastes. **Hazardous wastes** are *human-made liquid or solid wastes that may endanger human health or the environment.* When hazardous wastes enter and pollute the soil, water, or air, they can cause injury, illness, or even death. All hazardous wastes need special handling.

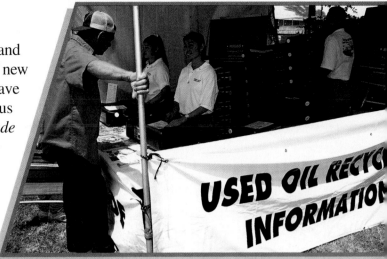

You can play a part in disposing of hazardous materials safely. Find out how your community collects hazardous household items.

Two materials that were once widely used but that are now recognized as hazardous are asbestos and lead. Asbestos is no longer used to insulate buildings because of the discovery that breathing in asbestos particles increases the risk of lung cancer. Exposure to lead affects mental development and performance and kidney function, particularly in young children. Since 1978, lead-based paint has been banned from home use. In addition, most vehicles in the United States now run on unleaded gasoline.

Familiar products that contain hazardous materials include batteries, bleach, insecticides, motor oil, antifreeze, and certain cleaning fluids. If you need to dispose of any hazardous materials, do not throw them out with the regular trash. Instead, contact your local health department or environmental agency to find out how to get these materials safely into hazardous waste storage.

Lesson 1 Review

Using complete sentences, answer the following questions on a sheet of paper.

Reviewing Terms and Facts

1. **Vocabulary** What is *pollution?* Use the word in an original sentence.
2. **List** Name two sources of air pollution and two sources of water pollution.
3. **Explain** How does air pollution affect the ozone layer?
4. **Identify** Name five common products that contain hazardous materials.

Thinking Critically

5. **Synthesize** Explain how fossil fuels are related to the destruction of forests by acid rain.
6. **Explain** Why are hazardous wastes a greater problem now than they were a century ago?

Applying Health Skills

7. **Accessing Information** Use reliable resources to research the dangers of exposure to lead paint and how to avoid this potentially harmful environmental condition. Report your findings to the class.

Preventing and Reducing Pollution

Reduce, Reuse, Recycle

In countries around the world, governments are working to reduce and prevent pollution. The **Environmental Protection Agency (EPA)** is *the agency of the United States government that is committed to protecting the environment.* In addition, many states and countries work to maintain air and water quality by controlling emissions (the gases, including exhaust, that vehicles release into the air) and applying waste management strategies. Waste management involves efforts to dispose of wastes in a way that protects the health of people and the environment.

The best way for individuals to make a difference is to practice the three Rs: reduce, reuse, and recycle. *Reduce* your consumption of energy and other resources. *Reuse* items by repairing them, selling them, or donating them to a charity. *Recycle* materials so that they can be used again in another form.

Today, many people make a conscious effort to reduce the amount of trash that winds up in landfills. Many communities have introduced programs for collecting recyclable materials. The effectiveness of these programs depends on the willingness of individual citizens to cooperate.

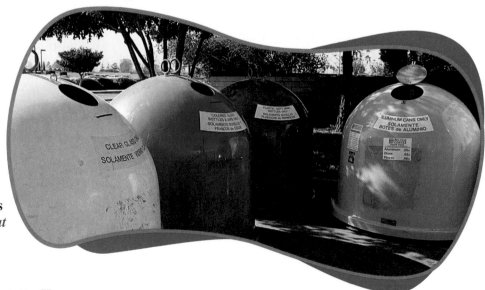

Some communities provide color-coded bins for collecting different kinds of recyclable materials. *What does your community do to encourage recycling?*

Cleaner Air and Water

Anything people do that uses energy produced by burning fossil fuels contributes to air pollution. This includes using electrical appliances, driving a car, and running a power lawn mower. You can help keep the air cleaner by applying these strategies.

- **Walk or bike to nearby places.** When you walk or ride a bike instead of having someone drive you in a car, you help cut down on air pollution, and you get some physical activity too.
- **Use public transportation or carpool.** Buses, trains, and subways transport many people at one time. Carpooling cuts down on the number of cars on the road.
- **Avoid burning trash, leaves, and brush.** Trash should be disposed of by your local waste management facility. Leaves, grass, yard clippings, shredded newspaper, some types of food, and other items can be placed in compost piles, where they will break down naturally.

To keep water clean, use detergents that are **biodegradable**—*broken down easily in the environment.* Discard all waste materials properly. Do not pour hazardous wastes down the drain, on the ground, or into storm sewers, or put them out with the regular trash. Such actions could harm the soil and water supply.

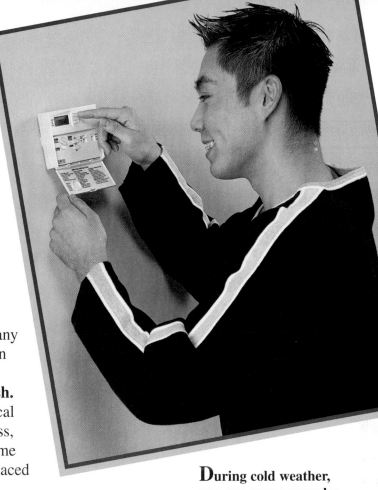

During cold weather, you can save energy by wearing an extra layer of clothing and keeping the thermostat at about 68°F. *How else could you save energy used for heat in your home?*

Conservation

Many natural materials are **nonrenewable resources**—*substances that cannot be replaced once they are used.* Fossil fuels are one example. Once a barrel of oil is burned, it is gone forever. Because nonrenewable resources cannot be replaced, people must use them wisely.

Conservation is *the saving of resources.* The best way to conserve a resource is to use less of it. There are many ways to save energy—and therefore fossil fuels—in the home. In most homes, heating and cooling consume about 70 percent of the energy used; heating water takes another 20 percent; and lighting, cooking, and running small appliances use about 10 percent. **Figure 20.2** on the next page shows some ways to reduce your energy and water use at home.

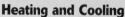

FIGURE 20.2

CONSERVATION IN THE HOME

The best way to conserve a resource is to use less of it. There are many ways to save energy and water at home.

Heating and Cooling

- Seal air leaks around doors, windows, and electric sockets to prevent heat from escaping.
- Keep doors and windows closed during the air-conditioning season, and keep air-conditioning at about 78°F.
- Buy an energy-efficient heating/cooling system that features a thermostat with a timer.

Lighting and Appliances

- Turn off lights when you are not using them.
- Replace traditional lightbulbs with compact fluorescent bulbs. They use less energy and last longer.
- Turn off televisions, computers, fans, and other electric appliances when you are not using them.

Water

- Never let water run unnecessarily.
- Wash clothes in warm or cold water, which uses less energy than hot water.
- Run the washing machine or dishwasher only when you have a full load, and use the short cycle when appropriate.
- If you have an older toilet, place a one-liter bottle filled with water inside your toilet tank. This will reduce the amount of water used for flushing. Another option is to replace an older toilet with a newer model that requires less water per flush.

Cooking

- Don't preheat a conventional oven for longer than necessary.
- Avoid opening the oven while cooking. Instead, use a timer and the oven door window to check if food is done.
- Heat small quantities of food in a microwave, toaster oven, or slow cooker.

Recycling and Precycling

As you learned earlier, recycling involves changing an item in some way so that it can be used again. Recycling conserves energy and natural resources and helps reduce solid waste. The most commonly collected materials for recycling are paper, aluminum, glass, plastics, and yard waste.

How does recycling help conserve energy and natural resources? Think about aluminum soda cans. Energy is needed to mine the ore that is used to make aluminum, to process the ore, and to manufacture the cans. When aluminum cans are recycled, they are changed back into sheets of aluminum. These sheets can then be used to make new cans or other aluminum products. The amount of ore taken from the ground is reduced, and much less energy is needed.

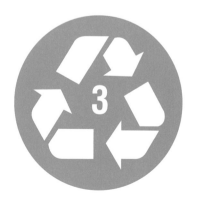

The symbol pictured here showing three curved arrows is a familiar sight on many kinds of products. It shows that an item can be recycled or that it is made of recycled materials. On plastic materials the symbol includes a number in the center. It is a code identifying the type of material. At recycling facilities, plastic objects can be sorted according to their number.

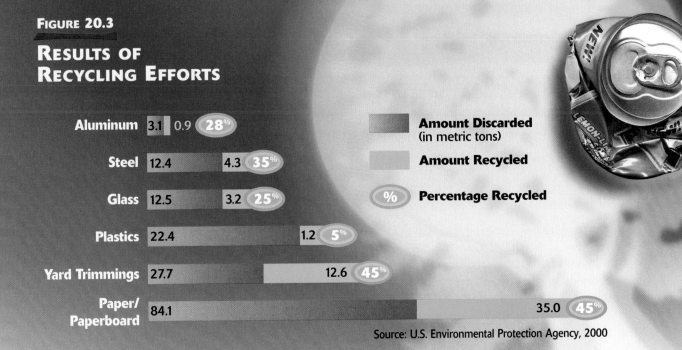

FIGURE 20.3

RESULTS OF RECYCLING EFFORTS

	Amount Discarded (in metric tons)	Amount Recycled	Percentage Recycled
Aluminum	3.1	0.9	28%
Steel	12.4	4.3	35%
Glass	12.5	3.2	25%
Plastics	22.4	1.2	5%
Yard Trimmings	27.7	12.6	45%
Paper/Paperboard	84.1	35.0	45%

Source: U.S. Environmental Protection Agency, 2000

In general, recycling has been an enormous success story in terms of getting people involved. Today, thanks to recycling centers and curbside recycling programs, more than 28 percent of the solid waste produced in the United States is recycled. **Figure 20.3** illustrates the recycling efforts in the year 2000.

As Figure 20.3 also demonstrates, however, plastics recycling has not kept pace with other recycling efforts. Most recycling programs accept plastics, but not necessarily all types of plastics. Some people may be put off recycling plastics by the need to check the code number on the recycling symbol. Others may not bother to recycle because they think that plastic items break down easily in the environment. This is not so. Plastic recycling needs a boost, and almost every household could improve its recycling effort.

In addition to recycling, you can reduce your consumption of resources by **precycling**—*reducing waste before it occurs.* Below are some basic guidelines for precycling.

- Buy products in packages made of materials that can be reused or recycled, such as glass, metal, and paper.
- Look for products in refillable containers.
- Bring a cloth or reusable plastic bag to the store to carry your purchases.

HEALTH SKILLS ACTIVITY

PRACTICING HEALTHFUL BEHAVIORS

Environment-Friendly Shopping

Every time you shop, you have the chance to help the environment. Below are some tips to help you become an environmentally conscious consumer.

- **PLAN.** Make a shopping list. It will help you buy only what you need.
- **BUY IN BULK.** Look for larger packages of foods such as cereal and snacks. Buying in larger quantities cuts down on the amount of packaging you throw away.
- **BE AWARE OF PACKAGING.** Choose products that are packaged in materials that break down easily or can be recycled.

For example, when possible, buy beverages and other food items that come in glass or aluminum containers.

- **READ LABELS CAREFULLY.** Some common household products, such as oven cleaners and paint thinners, contain substances that are harmful to humans. Look for safer commercial products or research alternative substances.

IN A GROUP

Brainstorm other ideas for environment-friendly shopping. List all the ways you can think of that will save energy, packaging, and waste. Combine all the ideas into one list that can be printed and posted on a bulletin board.

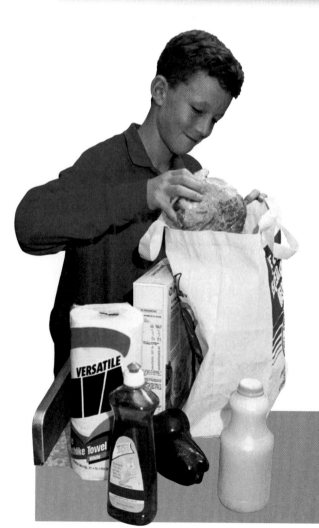

Protecting the Environment

Everyone can play a part in protecting the environment. By your everyday actions you can make a difference. Start locally by taking steps to combat pollution in your school and neighborhood, and then branch out from there. You can help others understand the importance of becoming involved. Here are some suggestions.

- **Take charge of your family's recycling effort.** Find out what recyclables are collected in your community and set up a system that the family can follow.

Some grocery stores offer a cash discount to customers who use their own shopping bags. *Why would stores encourage this practice?*

- **Advocate for greater environmental awareness.** Evaluate advertising, labels, contents, and packaging as it relates to the environment. Give feedback to companies on positive ways they can affect the environment. Write letters to newspapers, and seek opportunities to express your opinions about the environment.
- **Join a conservation organization.** Ask several organizations to provide you with resources about current environmental issues. By becoming part of such a group, you can discover ways to make a difference in your community.

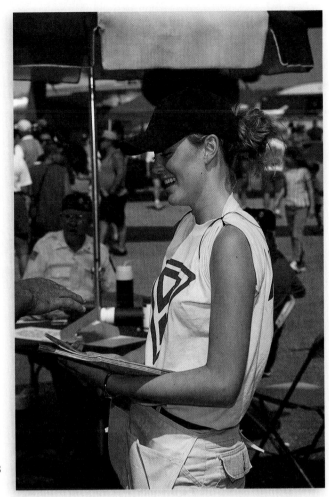

An important step toward a healthier environment is to get involved locally. Find out what environmental programs exist in your community.

Lesson 2 Review

Using complete sentences, answer the following questions on a sheet of paper.

Reviewing Terms and Facts

1. **Identify** What are the 3 Rs? How are they related to your health?
2. **Give Examples** Give three examples of actions you can take to help keep the air clean.
3. **Vocabulary** Define the term *nonrenewable resource*. Give an example of a nonrenewable resource.
4. **List** What are four ways that you can conserve energy and water in your home?
5. **Compare** What is the difference between *recycling* and *precycling?*

Thinking Critically

6. **Apply** Briefly describe how each of the following strategies helps protect the environment: emission control, monitoring water quality, and waste management.

Applying Health Skills

7. **Goal Setting** Set a goal to improve your family's record for reducing, reusing, and recycling. Analyze your family's current approach to the 3 Rs. Then set specific goals and, working with family members, figure out ways to meet those goals.

Mean Clean
Machines

Getting around doesn't have to pollute the atmosphere. Here are some better ways to go.

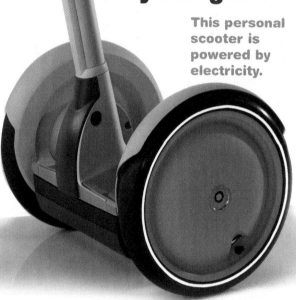

This personal scooter is powered by electricity.

Thanks to new types of fuel and construction materials, driving a car promises to become more environmentally friendly, stylish, and fun. In the near future, we may not be whizzing around in flying cars like the Jetsons, but we will be traveling in ways never before imagined.

The best way to conserve energy and reduce pollution would be to phase out cars in favor of mass transportation. That probably isn't going to happen. Most people want a private, comfortable way to get around, and so our love of the automobile is as strong as ever. Manufacturers sell more than 17 million cars each year in the United States.

Because people won't give up their four-wheelers, the challenge is to reduce the auto emissions that contribute to everything from respiratory distress to global warming. The key is to find a better power source.

The first solution, which was introduced a few years ago, was battery-powered electric cars. However, electric cars have less range than gas-powered cars, and recharging the batteries isn't convenient. The newer gasoline-electric hybrid cars recharge themselves and go much farther on a gallon of gas than do conventional cars—but they aren't pollution free.

The Hydrogen Solution

Many experts believe that hydrogen will one day power electric cars. Special fuel cells can combine hydrogen with oxygen to produce electricity. The electricity, in turn, would drive a motor that can spin the wheels of the car much more quietly than a gas engine can. The only thing spewing from the tail pipe would be water that is pure enough to drink. Because fuel cells and electric motors are more compact than bulky internal-combustion engines, the new technology will allow cars to have revolutionary shapes and designs.

One of the most innovative approaches to fuel-cell cars is the Hy-wire prototype. It eliminates the engine, transmission, and gas tank found in today's internal-combustion cars. In their place is a skateboard-like platform—just 6 inches thick—that houses the fuel cells, the hydrogen tank, and all the electronics needed to power the car. Electric motors placed inside each wheel get the car rolling.

A Serious Scooter

Eliminating cars altogether might be another solution to the pollution problem. After all, "it is still very energy intensive to move a 2,000- or 3,000-pound machine," says Dean Kamen, founder of DEKA Research in Manchester, New Hampshire. His solution: the $8,000 scooter that goes up to 13 miles per hour. The scooter is powered by an electric motor and runs on just a nickel's worth of electricity a day. One of the machine's coolest features is its steering and braking system: Lean forward and it accelerates; lean backward and it stops.

The Wheel Deal

For those on a tighter budget or who want to get some healthful exercise, there is always the

bicycle, which appears to be mounting a come-back. After a slump in the mid-1990s, bicycle production leaped to more than 100 million units in 2000, compared with just 62 million in 1980. What about couch potatoes who refuse to pedal? At least two manufacturers think they have the answer: Have the classic two-wheeler propel itself with the help of a fuel cell! ◼

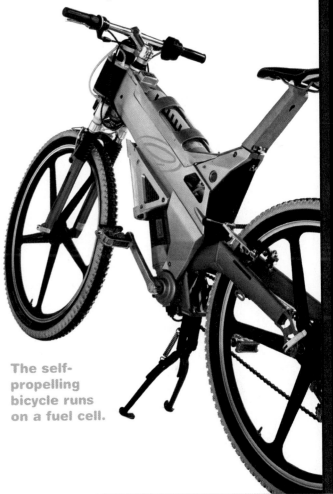

The self-propelling bicycle runs on a fuel cell.

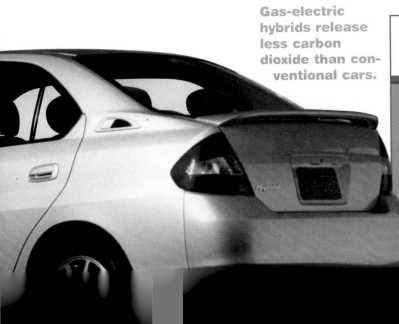

Gas-electric hybrids release less carbon dioxide than conventional cars.

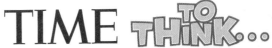

MAKE THE MOST OF IT

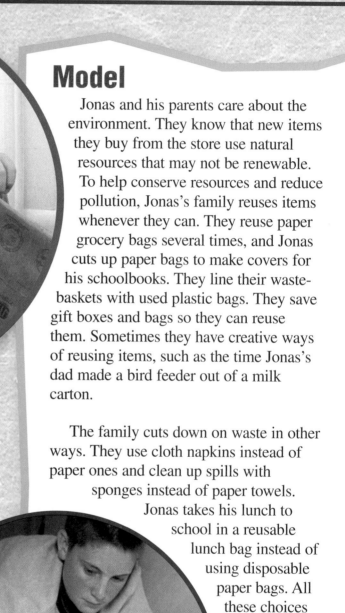

Model

Jonas and his parents care about the environment. They know that new items they buy from the store use natural resources that may not be renewable. To help conserve resources and reduce pollution, Jonas's family reuses items whenever they can. They reuse paper grocery bags several times, and Jonas cuts up paper bags to make covers for his schoolbooks. They line their waste-baskets with used plastic bags. They save gift boxes and bags so they can reuse them. Sometimes they have creative ways of reusing items, such as the time Jonas's dad made a bird feeder out of a milk carton.

The family cuts down on waste in other ways. They use cloth napkins instead of paper ones and clean up spills with sponges instead of paper towels. Jonas takes his lunch to school in a reusable lunch bag instead of using disposable paper bags. All these choices help Jonas's family protect the environment.

Practice

Form small groups. Each group will discuss ways to reuse an item from the following list:

- Paper and plastic bags
- Cardboard boxes
- Bottles and jars
- Metal cans
- Old clothes
- Paper goods
- Old tires
- Plastic milk cartons

Brainstorm all the different ways you can think of to reuse this type of item. Make a list of your group's ideas and share it with the class. Then, as a class, brainstorm ways that you could reuse or repair damaged items and replace disposable items with reusable ones.

Apply/Assess

Put your ideas to work by creating a chart about reducing waste. Divide a large sheet of paper or poster board into three columns. Label the first column "Items we throw away." Keep track of all the items you throw away throughout the day. Use the first column of your chart to list the items you threw away that could be reduced, reused, or repaired. Also list all the disposable items that could have been replaced with reusable items.

Label the second column "Ways to reduce and reuse." Use it to list the changes that you could make so that you would not have to throw away as many items. For example, you could replace the paper napkin you threw away at lunch with a reusable cloth napkin. You might also limit the number of napkins used. Finally, use the third column to list the advantages of reducing, reusing, and recycling items. You could describe savings of money as well as benefits to the environment. Label this column "Why it matters." Share your chart with the class.

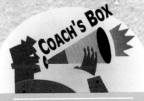

COACH'S BOX

Practicing Healthful Behaviors

You can reduce waste by
- reusing items.
- reducing the number of items used.
- repairing broken items.
- replacing disposable items with reusable ones.

Self-√Check

- Did I identify items that I threw away unnecessarily?
- Did I describe ways to reduce and reuse these items?
- Did I explain the benefits of reducing, reusing, and recycling?

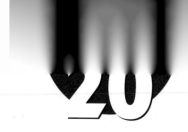

After You Read

Use your completed Foldable to review the information on air, water, and land pollution.

FOLDABLES™
Study Organizer

Reviewing Vocabulary and Concepts

On a sheet of paper, write the numbers 1–10. After each number, write the term from the list that best completes each sentence.

- landfills
- acid rain
- fossil fuels
- water pollution
- greenhouse effect
- asbestos
- smog
- hazardous wastes
- ozone layer
- pesticides

Lesson 1

1. The burning of _____ is a major source of air pollution.
2. Chemicals that are intended to kill or control insects are known as _____.
3. Rain that is far more acidic than normal and that destroys plants and trees is called _____.
4. When sunlight reacts with air pollution, _____, a yellow-brown haze, forms.
5. The _____ is a shield that protects living things from ultraviolet radiation.
6. The _____ is the trapping of heat near the earth's surface.
7. Sewage, industrial chemicals, and oil spills are some of the causes of _____.
8. Most solid waste produced by households and businesses is buried in _____.
9. Advances in science and technology have led to the problem of _____, or waste products that can cause illness, injury, or death.
10. _____ is a hazardous product that was once used as insulation in buildings.

Lesson 3

On a sheet of paper, write the numbers 11–15. After each number, write the letter of the answer that best completes each statement.

11. The United States government works to prevent and reduce pollution through which of the following agencies?
    a. The National Safety Council
    b. The Environmental Protection Agency
    c. Centers for Disease Control and Prevention
    d. Agency for Healthcare Research and Quality
12. You can help to keep the water clean by using detergents that are
    a. biodegradable.
    b. available in tablet form.
    c. available only in liquid form.
    d. nonrenewable.
13. Substances that cannot be replaced once they are used are
    a. precycled.
    b. nonrenewable.
    c. sustainable.
    d. radioactive.
14. Which of the following strategies will help promote clean air?
    a. using public transportation
    b. burning trash in bonfires
    c. leaving lights on when not in use
    d. burning oil instead of coal
15. The practice of reducing waste before it occurs is called
    a. presorting.
    b. precycling.
    c. recycling.
    d. reconstructing.

Thinking Critically

Using complete sentences, answer the following questions on a sheet of paper.

16. **Apply** What lifestyle changes could you make or develop in the future to conserve energy and reduce air pollution?

17. **Explain** Why is the disposal of hazardous wastes more of a problem than the disposal of other solid wastes?

18. **Hypothesize** Does precycling conserve more energy than recycling? Explain.

19. **Explain** Why is it necessary for people to become actively involved in protecting the environment? What might happen if people ignore environmental problems?

Career Corner

Ecologist If you're interested in the environment, you might want to consider becoming an ecologist. These health scientists study the environment. They explore the relationships among human, animal, and plant life. They also study the effects of environmental change. To enter this profession, you'll need a degree in biology or environmental science. Find out more about this and other health careers by clicking on Career Corner at health.glencoe.com.

Standardized Test Practice

Reading & Writing

Read the paragraphs below and then answer the questions.

Air, water, and land pollution can harm the health of both people and the environment. Air pollution can worsen symptoms in people with respiratory problems. Water pollution can contaminate drinking water, making people ill and killing plants and aquatic life. Hazardous substances in common products such as batteries can leak into the surrounding soil when these products are discarded improperly.

These facts make it clear—working to reduce pollution is worthwhile. Some ways to reduce pollution include using mass transit if it's available and disposing of household products properly. For example, don't pour household products such as bleach or motor oil down drains.

1. Which sentence from the passage represents the author's opinion?

   A Air, water, and land pollution can harm the health of both people and the environment.

   B Air pollution can worsen symptoms in people with respiratory problems.

   C These facts make it clear—working to reduce pollution is worthwhile.

   D Water pollution can contaminate drinking water, making people ill and killing plants and aquatic life.

2. The author probably wrote the editorial

   A to explain why pollution occurs.

   B to criticize people who litter.

   C to describe the steps he or she takes to reduce pollution.

   D to persuade readers to take steps to reduce pollution.

3. Write a paragraph describing additional ways to reduce pollution.

Glossary

The Glossary contains all the important terms used throughout the text. It includes the **boldfaced** terms listed in the "Vocabulary" lists at the beginning of each lesson and that appear in text and art.

The Glossary lists the term, the pronunciation (in the case of difficult terms), the definition, and the page on which the term is defined. The pronunciations here and in the text follow the system outlined below. The column headed "Symbol" shows the spelling used in this book to represent the appropriate method.

PRONUNCIATION KEY

Sound	As In	Symbol	Example
ă	hat, map	a	abscess (AB·ses)
ā	age, face	ay	atrium (AY·tree·uhm)
a	care, their	eh	capillaries (KAP·uh·lehr·eez)
ä, ŏ	father, hot	ah	biopsy (BY·ahp·see)
ar	far	ar	cardiac (KAR·dee·ak)
ch	child, much	ch	barbiturate (bar·BI·chuh·ruht)
ĕ	let, best	e	vessel (VE·suhl)
ē	beat, see, city	ee	acne (AK·nee)
er	term, stir, purr	er	nuclear (NOO·klee·er)
g	grow	g	malignant (muh·LIG·nuhnt)
ĭ	it, hymn	i	bacteria (bak·TIR·ee·uh)
ī	ice, five	y	benign (bi·NYN)
		eye	iris (EYE·ris)
j	page, fungi	j	cartilage (KAR·tuhl·ij)
k	coat, look, chorus	k	defect (DEE·fekt)
ō	open, coat, grow	oh	aerobic (e·ROH·bik)
ô	order	or	organ (OR·guhn)
ȯ	flaw, all	aw	palsy (PAWL·zee)
oi	voice	oy	goiter (GOY·ter)
ou	out	ow	fountain (FOWN·tuhn)
s	say, rice	s	dermis (DER·mis)
sh	she, attention	sh	conservation (kahn·ser·VAY·shuhn)
ŭ	cup, flood	uh	bunion (BUHN·yuhn)
u	put, wood, could	u	pulmonary (PUL·muh·nehr·ee)
ü	rule, move, you	oo	attitudes (AT·i·toodz)
w	win	w	warranty (WAWR·uhn·tee)
y	your	yu	urethra (yu·REE·thruh)
z	says	z	hormones (HOR·mohnz)
zh	pleasure	zh	transfusion (trans·FYOO·zhuhn)
ə	about, collide	uh	addiction (uh·DIK·shuhn)

564

Abdominal thrusts Quick, upward pulls into the diaphragm to force out an obstruction blocking the airway. (page 533)

Abstinence Not participating in high-risk behaviors. (page 17)

Abuse The physical, emotional, or mental mistreatment of one person by another. (page 177)

Accident Any event that was not intended to happen. (page 508)

Accident chain A series of events that include a situation, an unsafe habit, and an unsafe action. (page 508)

Accidental injuries Injuries resulting from an accident. (page 508)

Acid rain Rain that is far more acidic than normal. (page 548)

Acquired Immunodeficiency Syndrome (AIDS) A deadly disease that interferes with the body's natural ability to fight infection. (page 464)

Active listening Hearing, thinking about, and responding to another person's message. (page 37)

Addiction A physical or psychological need for a drug. (pages 277, 304)

Addictive Capable of causing a user to develop intense cravings. (page 300)

Adjustment An adaptation or change in behavior. (page 130)

Adolescence The time of life between childhood and adulthood. (page 9)

Adrenaline A hormone that gives the body extra energy. (page 40)

Advertising Sending out messages designed to interest consumers in buying a product or service. (page 59)

Aerobic exercise Rhythmic, nonstop, moderate to vigorous activity that requires large amounts of oxygen and works the heart. (page 222)

Alcohol A drug that is produced by a chemical reaction in fruits, vegetables, and grains. (page 320)

Alcoholism A progressive, chronic disease involving a mental and physical need for alcohol. (page 326)

Allergen (AL·er·juhn) A substance that causes an allergic reaction. (page 480)

Allergy An abnormal immune reaction to an ordinarily harmless substance. (page 480)

Alternatives Other ways of thinking or acting. (page 333)

Alveoli (al·VEE·uh·ly) Microscopic air sacs in the lungs. (page 382)

Amino acids Small units that make up protein. (page 197)

Amphetamine (am·FE·tuh·meen) A drug that stimulates the central nervous system. (page 278)

Anabolic steroids Drugs that cause muscle tissue to develop at an abnormally fast rate. (page 241)

Anaerobic exercise Intense physical activity that requires little oxygen but uses short bursts of energy. (page 222)

Anorexia nervosa An eating disorder characterized by self-starvation leading to extreme weight loss. (page 256)

Antibiotics (an·ti·by·AH·tiks) Medicines that reduce or kill harmful bacteria in the body. (page 272)

Antibodies Proteins that attach to antigens, keeping them from harming the body. (page 452)

Antigens Substances released by invading pathogens. (page 452)

Antihistamines Medicines that help control the effects triggered by histamines. (page 481)

Anxiety An overwhelming feeling of dread, much like fear. (page 92)

Anxiety disorder A disorder in which intense anxiety or fear keeps a person from functioning normally. (page 96)

Appetite The psychological desire for food. (page 193)

Appropriate weight The weight that is best for your body. (page 250)

Arteries Blood vessels that carry blood away from the heart to other parts of the body. (page 378)

Arteriosclerosis (ar·tir·ee·oh·skluh·ROH·sis) A group of disorders in which arteries harden and become more rigid. (page 490)

Arthritis (ar·THRY·tuhs) More than 100 conditions marked by pain and swelling in body joints. (page 495)

Assertive Behaving with confidence and clearly stating your intentions. (page 149)

Asthma (AZ·muh) A serious chronic condition that causes tiny air passages in the respiratory system to become narrow or blocked. (page 482)

Atherosclerosis (a·thuh·roh·skluh·ROH·sis) A form of arteriosclerosis in which fatty substances in the blood build up on the walls of the arteries. (page 490)

Attitude Feelings and beliefs. (page 18)

Autonomic (aw·tuh·NAH·mik) **system** The part of the nervous system that deals with actions you do not usually control. (page 388)

Bacteria Tiny one-celled organisms that live nearly everywhere. (page 446)

Balance A feeling of stability and control. (page 221)

Battery The beating, hitting, or kicking of another person. (page 177)

Benign (bi·NYN) **tumor** A tumor that is not cancerous. (page 484)

Binge drinking The consumption of several alcoholic drinks in a very short period of time. (page 322)

Binge eating disorder Compulsive overeating. (page 258)

Biodegradable Broken down easily in the environment. (page 553)

Biological age Age determined by how well various body parts are working. (page 434)

Biopsy The removal of a tissue sample to see whether cancer cells are present. (page 487)

Birth defect Abnormality present at birth that causes physical or mental disability or death. (page 424)

Blended family A family that consists of a parent, a stepparent, and the children of one or both parents. (page 126)

Blizzard A very heavy snowstorm with winds up to 45 miles per hour. (page 522)

Blood alcohol concentration (BAC) The amount of alcohol in a person's bloodstream. (page 322)

Body composition The ratio of body fat to lean body tissue, such as bone, muscle, and fluid. (page 228)

Body image The way you see yourself. (page 250)

Body language The use of body movements and gestures to communicate a message. (page 35)

Body Mass Index (BMI) A measurement that allows you to assess your body size, taking your height and weight into account. (page 251)

Bronchi (BRAHN·ky) Passages through which air enters the lungs. (page 382)

Bronchodilators (brahn·ko·DY·lay·terz) Medicines used to relax the muscles that have tightened around the airways. (page 483)

Bulimia A condition in which a person eats large amounts of food and then tries to purge. (page 257)

Calories Units of heat that measure the energy used by the body and the energy that foods supply to the body. (page 192)

Cancer A disease characterized by the rapid and uncontrolled growth of abnormal cells. (page 484)

Capillaries Tiny tubes that carry blood from the arteries to the body's cells, and then back to the veins. (page 378)

Carbohydrates The sugars and starches that provide your body with most of its energy. (page 196)

Carbon monoxide A colorless, odorless, poisonous gas that is produced when tobacco burns. (page 300)

Carcinogens (kar·SIN·un·juhns) Substances that cause cancer. (page 486)

Cardiac muscle Muscle found in the walls of your heart. (page 373)

Cardiovascular (KAR·dee·oh·VAS· kyoo·ler) **system** Organs and tissues that transport essential materials to body cells and remove their waste products. (page 376)

Carrier A person who is infected with a virus and who can pass it on to others. (page 464)

Cartilage (KAHR·tuhl·ij) Strong, flexible tissue that provides cushioning at the joints. (page 370)

Central nervous system (CNS) The brain and spinal cord. (page 386)

Cervix The entrance of the uterus. (page 420)

Character The way in which a person thinks, feels, and acts. (page 119)

Character trait A quality that demonstrates how a person thinks, feels, and acts. (page 119)

Chromosomes (KROH·muh·sohmz) The threadlike structures found within the nucleus of a cell that carry the codes for inherited traits. (page 422)

Chronic diseases Diseases that are present either continuously or off and on over a long time. (page 476)

Chronological (krah·nuh·LAH·ji·kuhl) **age** Age measured in years. (page 434)

Cilia Tiny, hairlike structures that protect the lungs. (page 300)

Circulatory (SER·kyuh·luh·tohr·ee) **system** Organs and tissues that transport essential materials to body cells and remove their waste products. (page 376)

Cirrhosis (suh·ROH·sis) Scarring and destruction of the liver. (page 321)

Citizenship The way you conduct yourself as a member of a community. (page 120)

Clinical depression A mood disorder in which people lose interest in life and can no longer find enjoyment in anything. (page 98)

Clique A group of friends who hang out together and act in similar ways. (page 144)

Cold turkey Term used to describe quitting a habit, such as smoking, all at once. (page 311)

Colon (KOH·luhn) The large intestine. (page 393)

Commitment A pledge or a promise. (page 129)

Communicable (kuh·MYOO·ni·kuh·buhl) **disease** A disease that can be passed to a person from another person, animal, or object. (page 446)

Comparison shopping A method of judging the benefits of different products and services by measuring and comparing several factors, such as quality, features, and cost. (page 60)

Compromise To give up something in order to reach a solution that satisfies everyone. (page 168)

Conflict A disagreement between people with opposing viewpoints, ideas, or goals. (page 164)

Conflict resolution Solving a disagreement in a way that satisfies both sides. (page 168)

Consequences Outcomes or effects that may occur as a result of a decision or an action. (page 154)

Conservation The saving of resources. (page 553)

Consumer Anyone who purchases products or services. (page 58)

Contagious period The length of time that a disease can spread from person to person. (page 449)

Cool-down A period of low to moderate exercise to prepare your body to end a workout session. (page 234)

Coordination The smooth and effective working together of your muscles and bones. (page 221)

Cornea A clear protective structure of the eye that lets in light. (page 354)

CPR A first aid procedure that combines rescue breathing with chest compressions to restore breathing and circulation. (page 536)

Cross-training Switching between different forms of physical exercise. (page 225)

Cumulative risks Related risks that increase in effect with each added risk. (page 17)

Cuticle (KYOO·ti·kuhl) A fold of epidermis around the fingernails and toenails. (page 348)

Cycle of abuse Pattern of repeating abuse from one generation to the next. (page 179)

Dandruff A flaking of the outer layer of dead skin cells on the scalp. (page 348)

Decibel A measure of the loudness of sound. (page 358)

Decision making The process of making a choice or finding a solution. (page 29)

Defensive driving Watching out for other people on the road and anticipating unsafe acts. (page 515)

Degenerative diseases Diseases that cause further breakdown in body cells, tissues, and organs as they progress. (page 476)

Dehydration Excessive water loss from the body. (page 238)

Depressants Substances that slow down body functions and reactions. (page 279)

Dermatologist (DER·muh·TAHL·uh·jist) A physician who treats skin disorders. (page 345)

Dermis (DER·mis) The thick inner layer of skin. (page 344)

Detoxification (dee·tahk·si·fi·KAY·shuhn) The physical process of freeing the body of an addictive substance. (pages 288, 327)

Developmental tasks Events that need to happen in order for you to continue growing toward becoming a healthy, mature adult. (page 426)

Diabetes A disease that prevents the body from converting food into energy. (page 494)

Diaphragm (DY·uh·fram) A dome-shaped muscle that separates the lungs from the abdomen. (page 382)

Dietary Guidelines for Americans Advice about food choices for all healthy Americans age 2 and over. (page 202)

Digestion (dy·JES·chuhn) The changing of food you eat into substances your body can use. (page 390)

Digestive system An organ system that converts food to a form useful to the body. (page 390)

Distress Negative stress. (page 39)

Divorce A legal end to a marriage contract. (page 130)

Drugs Substances other than food that change the structure or function of the body or mind. (page 270)

Earthquake A violent, shaking movement of the earth's surface. (page 523)

Eating disorder Extreme and damaging eating behavior that can lead to sickness and even death. (page 256)

Egg cell The reproductive cell from the female that joins with a sperm cell to make a new life. (page 416)

Embryo A developing organism from the time of fertilization to about the eighth week of development. (page 418)

Emotional needs Needs that affect a person's feelings and sense of well-being. (page 94)

Emotions Feelings that arise in response to thoughts, remarks, and events. (page 91)

Empathetic (em·puh·THE·tik) Able to identify and share another person's feelings. (page 143)

Empathy The ability to understand and share another person's feelings. (page 92)

Empty calories Calories that come from foods that offer few, if any, nutrients. (page 209)

Endocrine (EN·duh·krin) **system** The body's chemical communication system that regulates many functions. (page 396)

Environment The sum total of a person's surroundings. (pages 49, 423)

Environmental Protection Agency (EPA) The agency of the United States government that is committed to protecting the environment. (page 552)

Epidermis (e·puh·DER·mis) The visible and outermost layer of the skin. (page 344)

Epiglottis (e·puh·GLAH·tis) A flap of tissue that closes over the trachea when you swallow. (page 382)

Escalate To become more serious. (page 165)

Eustachian (yoo·STAY·shuhn) **tube** The part of the ear that allows air to pass from the nose to the middle ear so the air pressure is equal on both sides of the eardrum. (page 358)

Eustress Positive stress. (page 39)

Evaluate To determine the value of something. (page 30)

Excretion (ek·SKREE·shuhn) The process of removing wastes from the body. (page 393)

Excretory system The body system that removes wastes from the body. (page 392)

Exercise Specifically planned and organized session of physical activity that improves or maintains physical fitness. (page 220)

Extended family A person's immediate family plus other relatives such as grandparents, aunts, uncles, and cousins. (page 124)

Eye contact Direct visual contact with another person's eyes. (page 36)

Family The basic unit of society. (page 124)

Family therapy Counseling that seeks to improve troubled family relationships. (page 103)

Fatigue Exhaustion. (page 40)

Feedback A response by the listener to what the speaker has said. (page 37)

Fertilization The joining together of a male sperm cell and a female egg cell. (page 416)

Fetal alcohol syndrome (FAS) A group of alcohol-related birth defects that include both physical and mental problems. (page 323)

Fetus A developing organism from the end of the eighth week of the mother's pregnancy until birth. (page 418)

Fiber The part of fruits, vegetables, grains, and beans that your body cannot digest. (page 199)

Fight-or-flight response The process by which the body prepares to deal with a stressor. (page 40)

First aid The immediate temporary care given to an injured or ill person until professional help is available. (page 524)

Flexibility The ability of your body's joints to move easily through a full range of motion. (page 228)

Food Guide Pyramid A guide for making healthful daily food choices. (page 204)

Foodborne illness Sickness that results from eating food that is not safe to eat. (page 203)

Fracture A break in a bone. (page 529)

Fraud Deliberate deceit or trickery. (page 68)

Fungi (FUHN·jy) Primitive life-forms that feed on organic materials. (page 447)

Gallbladder A small, saclike organ that stores bile. (page 392)

Gang A group of people who associate with one another to take part in criminal activity. (page 173)

Genes The basic units of heredity. (page 422)

Genetic (juh·NE·tik) **disorder** A disorder that is caused partly or completely by a defect in genes. (page 422)

Gingivitis (jin·juh·VY·tis) A common disorder in which the gums are red and sore and bleed easily. (page 353)

Gland A group of cells, or an organ, that secretes a chemical substance. (page 396)

Global warming A rise in the earth's temperatures. (page 548)

Goal setting The process of working toward something you want to accomplish. (page 31)

Greenhouse effect The trapping of heat by carbon dioxide and other gases in the air. (page 548)

Grief The sorrow caused by loss of a loved one. (page 106)

Grief counselor Counselor who teaches coping strategies to deal with grief. (page 109)

H

Hallucinogens (huh·LOO·suhn·uh·jenz) Drugs that distort moods, thoughts, and senses. (page 282)

Hangnail A split in the cuticle along the edge of a fingernail. (page 348)

Hazardous wastes Human-made liquid or solid wastes that may endanger human health or the environment. (page 551)

Health A combination of physical, mental/emotional, and social well-being. (page 4)

Health advocacy Taking action to influence others to address a health-related concern or to support a health-related belief. (page 61)

Health care system All the medical care available to a nation's people, the way they receive the care, and the way the care is paid for. (page 63)

Health fraud The sale of worthless products or services claimed to prevent diseases or cure other health problems. (page 68)

Health insurance A plan in which private companies or government programs pay for part of a person's medical costs. page 66)

Health Maintenance Organization (HMO) An organization that provides health care for a fixed price. (page 66)

Heart and lung endurance The ability of your heart and lungs to work effectively when you exercise and to return to normal when you stop. (page 224)

Heart attack A condition in which blood flow to a part of the heart is greatly reduced or blocked. (page 491)

Heat cramps Painful, involuntary muscle spasms that may occur during heavy exercise in hot weather. (page 532)

Heat exhaustion A condition characterized by faintness, nausea, rapid heartbeat, and hot, red, dry, or sweaty skin. (page 532)

Heatstroke A serious form of heat illness in which the body's normal processes for dealing with heat close down. (page 532)

Hepatitis (hep·uh·TYT·uhs) A viral disease of the liver characterized by yellowing of the skin and the whites of the eyes. (page 456)

Heredity The passing of traits from parents to their children. (page 421)

High blood pressure A condition in which a person's blood pressure stays at a level that is higher than normal. (page 491)

Histamines Chemicals in the body that cause the symptoms of an allergic reaction. (page 481)

Hives Raised bumps on the skin that are very itchy. (page 481)

Homicide The killing of one human being by another. (page 172)

Hormones Chemical substances, produced in glands, that help to regulate many body functions. (page 9)

Hospice care Care provided to the terminally ill that focuses on comfort, not cure. (page 107)

Human Immunodeficiency Virus (HIV) The virus that causes AIDS. (page 464)

Hunger The physical need for food. (page 194)

Hurricane A strong windstorm with driving rain that originates at sea. (page 521)

 I

Immune system A combination of body defenses made up of cells, tissues, and organs that fight off pathogens and disease. (page 451)

Immunity Your body's ability to resist the pathogens that cause a particular disease. (page 451)

Glossary

Individual sports Physical activities that you can do on your own or with a friend. (page 236)

Infancy The first year of life. (page 428)

Infection A condition that occurs when pathogens get inside the body, multiply, and damage body cells. (page 446)

Ingrown toenail A condition in which the nail pushes into the skin on the side of the toe. (page 348)

Inhalant Any substance whose fumes are sniffed and inhaled to produce mind-altering sensations. (page 283)

Insulin A hormone produced by the pancreas. (page 494)

Interpersonal communication The exchange of thoughts, feelings, and beliefs between two or more people. (page 34)

Intoxicated Physically and mentally impaired by the use of alcohol. (page 322)

Iris The colored part of the eye. (page 354)

Joints The points at which bones meet. (page 369)

Kidneys Organs that filter water and dissolved wastes from the blood and help maintain proper levels of water and salts in the body. (page 393)

Landfills Huge pits where wastes are dumped and buried. (page 550)

Larynx (LA·ringks) The upper part of the respiratory system, which contains the vocal cords. (page 382)

Lens A clear flexible structure of the eye that focuses light on the retina. (page 354)

Lifestyle factors Behaviors and habits that help determine a person's level of health. (page 14)

Ligaments (LI·guh·ments) Strong cords of tissue that connect the bones in each joint. (page 370)

Limits Invisible boundaries that protect you. (page 151)

Liver A large gland that has many digestive functions. (page 392)

Lymphatic (lim·FA·tik) **system** A secondary circulatory system that helps the body fight pathogens and maintain its fluid balance. (page 452)

Mainstream smoke Smoke that a smoker inhales and then exhales. (page 306)

Malignant (muh·LIG·nuhnt) **tumor** A tumor that is cancerous. (page 484)

Malnutrition A condition in which the body doesn't get the nutrients it needs to grow and function properly. (page 257)

Mammogram An X ray of the breast used to screen for breast cancer. (page 488)

Marrow A tissue in the center of some bones. (page 368)

Media Various methods for communicating information. (page 59)

Mediation A process in which a third person, a mediator, helps those in conflict find a solution. (page 169)

Medicines Drugs that are used to treat or prevent diseases and other conditions. (page 270)

Menopause A period marking the end of a female's reproductive years. (page 403)

Menstrual cycle The sequence of events in the female's reproductive system that occurs from one menstruation to the next. (page 403)

Menstruation The flow of the uterine lining out of the body. (page 403)

Mental and emotional health The ability to accept oneself and others, adapt to and cope with emotions, and deal with the problems and challenges one meets in life. (page 86)

Metastasis (muh·TAS·tuh·suhs) The spread of cancer from one part of the body to another. (page 484)

Methamphetamine A stimulant similar to amphetamine. (page 278)

Minerals Elements needed in small quantities for forming healthy bones and teeth, and for regulating certain body processes. (page 199)

Mixed message A situation in which your words say one thing but your body language says another. (page 35)

Mononucleosis (mahn·oh·noo·klee·OH·sis) A viral disease whose symptoms include swollen, tender areas in the neck and a sore throat. (page 456)

Mood disorder A disorder in which a person undergoes changes in mood that seem inappropriate or extreme. (page 97)

Muscle endurance The ability of a muscle to repeatedly exert a force over a prolonged period of time. (page 225)

Muscle strength The most weight you can lift or the most force you can exert at one time. (page 225)

Muscular system The group of structures that make your body parts move. (page 372)

Narcotics Specific drugs that are obtainable only by prescription and are used to relieve pain. (page 277)

Neglect The failure to meet a person's basic physical and emotional needs. (page 178)

Neurons (NOO·rahnz) Specialized cells that make up the nervous system. (page 385)

Nicotine An addictive drug found in tobacco leaves and in all tobacco products. (page 300)

Nicotine gum A type of chewing gum that enables a user to give up tobacco while gradually cutting down on nicotine. (page 311)

Nicotine patch A medicated patch placed on the skin that enables a user to give up tobacco while gradually cutting down on nicotine. (page 311)

Noncommunicable diseases Diseases that are not transmitted by pathogens. (page 476)

Nonrenewable resources Substances that cannot be replaced once they are used. (page 553)

Nutrient deficiency A shortage of a nutrient. (page 195)

Nutrient density The amount of nutrients relative to the number of calories they provide. (page 210)

Nutrients Substances in food that your body needs. (page 192)

Nutrition The process of using food and its substances to help your body have energy, grow, develop, and work properly. (page 192)

O

Obstetrician (ahb·stuh·TRI·shuhn) Doctor who specializes in the care of a pregnant female and her developing fetus, and who is present at the birth of the baby. (page 423)

Online shopping Using the Internet to buy products and services. (page 62)

Ophthalmologist (ahf·thuhl·MAHL·uh·jist) A medical doctor who specializes in medical and surgical treatment of the eyes, and who prescribes corrective lenses. (page 356)

Opportunistic infection A disease that attacks a person with a weakened immune system and rarely occurs in a healthy person. (page 465)

Optometrist (ahp·TAHM·uh·trist) A professional who checks vision and prescribes corrective lenses. (page 356)

Organs Body parts that perform particular functions. (page 417)

Orthodontist (or·thuh·DAHN·tist) A dentist who prevents or corrects problems with the alignment or spacing of teeth. (page 353)

Osteoarthritis (ahs·tee·oh·ahr·THRY·tuhs) A disease that is characterized by the breakdown of the cartilage in joints. (page 497)

Over-the-counter (OTC) medicines Medicines that are safe enough to be taken without a written order from a physician. (page 271)

Overweight More than the appropriate weight for gender, height, age, body frame, and growth pattern. (page 251)

Ovulation The release of one mature egg cell each month. (page 403)

Ozone layer A shield above the earth's surface that protects living things from ultraviolet (UV) radiation. (page 548)

P

Pacemaker A small device that sends steady electrical impulses to the heart to make it beat regularly. (page 492)

Pancreas An organ that produces enzymes that assist in digestion. (page 392)

Panic A feeling of sudden, intense fear. (page 93)

Parenting The process of meeting a child's physical, mental/emotional, and social needs. (page 131)

Pathogens Tiny organisms that cause communicable diseases. (page 446)

Peer pressure The influence to go along with the beliefs and actions of other people of your age. (page 147)

Percent Daily Value The percent of the recommended daily amount of a nutrient provided in a serving of food. (page 206)

Periodontal (per·ee·oh·DAHNT·uhl) **disease** Advanced gum disease, in which the periodontium is infected with bacteria. (page 353)

Periodontium (per·ee·oh·DAHN·shee·um) A structure made up of the jawbone, the gums, and connectors called ligaments. (page 350)

Peripheral nervous system (PNS) The nerves that connect the central nervous system to all parts of the body. (page 386)

Personality The unique combination of feelings, thoughts, and behavior that makes one person different from everyone else. (page 87)

Personality disorder A variety of psychological conditions that affect a person's ability to get along with others. (page 97)

Pesticide Product used on crops to kill insects and other pests. (page 547)

Phobia Intense and exaggerated fear of a specific situation or object. (page 97)

Physical activity Any kind of movement that uses up energy. (page 220)

Physical dependence A type of addiction in which the body feels a direct need for a drug. (pages 283, 304)

Physical fitness The ability to handle the physical demands of everyday life without becoming overly tired. (page 220)

Pituitary gland A gland that signals other endocrine glands to produce hormones when needed. (page 397)

Placenta (pluh·SEN·tuh) A thick, rich tissue that lines the walls of the uterus during pregnancy and that nourishes the fetus. (page 419)

Plaque (PLAK) A soft, colorless, sticky film containing bacteria that forms on teeth. (page 351)

Point of Service (POS) plan A health plan that allows members to choose providers inside or outside the plan. (page 66)

Pollution Any dirty or harmful substance in the environment. (page 546)

Precaution A planned action taken before an event to increase the chances of a safe outcome. (page 17)

Precycling Reducing waste before it occurs. (page 555)

Preferred Provider Organization (PPO) A type of health insurance in which medical providers agree to charge less for members of the plan. (page 66)

Prejudice A negative and unjustly formed opinion, usually against people of a different racial, religious, or cultural group. (page 167)

Prenatal (pree·NAY·tuhl) **care** Steps taken to provide for the health of a pregnant woman and her baby. (page 423)

Preschooler A child between the ages of three and five. (page 429)

Prescription medicines Medicines that can be sold only with a written order from a physician. (page 271)

Preventive care Steps taken to keep disease or injury from happening or getting worse. (page 63)

Primary care physician A medical doctor who provides physical checkups and general care. (page 64)

Proteins Nutrients your body uses to build, repair, and maintain cells and tissues. (page 197)

Protozoa (proh·tuh·ZOH·uh) Single-celled organisms that are usually harmless but that can cause certain diseases. (page 447)

Psychiatrist (sy·KY·uh·trist) A medical doctor who treats mental health problems. (page 105)

Psychological dependence An addiction in which the mind sends the body a message that it needs more of a drug. (pages 282, 304)

Psychologist (sy·KAH·luh·jist) A mental health professional who is trained and licensed by the state to counsel. (page 105)

Puberty The time when you begin to develop certain physical traits of adults of your own gender. (page 430)

Public health The protection and promotion of health at the community level. (page 72)

Pulmonary circulation The flow of blood from the heart to the lungs and back to the heart. (page 377)

Pupil The dark opening in the center of the iris. (page 354)

Rape Any kind of sexual intercourse against a person's will. (page 176)

Recovery The process of learning to live an alcohol-free life. (page 327)

Recurrence The return of cancer after a remission. (page 487)

Refusal skills Communication strategies that help you say no effectively. (pages 37, 148)

Relationships The connections you have with other people and groups in your life. (page 118)

Remission A period during which cancer signs and symptoms disappear. (page 487)

Reproductive (ree·pruh·DUHK·tiv) **system** The organs that make possible the production of offspring. (page 400)

Resilience The ability to adapt to and recover from disappointment, difficulty, or crisis. (page 94)

Respiratory system The organs that provide the body with a continuous supply of oxygen and rid the body of carbon dioxide. (page 381)

Retina (RE·tin·uh) A thin layer of nerve cells in the eye that absorb light. (page 354)

Rheumatoid (ROO·muh·toyd) **arthritis** A chronic disease characterized by pain, inflammation, swelling, and stiffness of the joints. (page 496)

Rickettsias (rik·ET·see·uhz) Disease-causing organisms that resemble bacteria but multiply like viruses. (page 447)

Risk behavior An action or behavior that might cause injury or harm to you or others. (page 15)

Risk factors Characteristics that increase a person's chances of developing a disease. (page 478)

Saliva (suh·LY·vuh) Fluid produced by the salivary glands in the mouth. (page 390)

Saturated fats Fats that are solid at room temperature. (page 197)

Schizophrenia (skit·zoh·FREE·nee·uh) A severe mental disorder in which a person loses contact with reality. (page 97)

Secondhand smoke Air that has been contaminated by tobacco smoke. (page 306)

Sedentary lifestyle A way of life that involves little physical activity. (page 16)

Self-concept The view you have of yourself. (page 87)

Self-control Control of your own emotions and desires. (page 18)

Self-esteem The way you feel about yourself, and how you value yourself. (page 87)

Self-respect The positive feeling you have about yourself when you live up to your beliefs and values. (page 154)

Sexual harassment Uninvited and unwelcome sexual conduct directed at another person. (page 178)

Sexually transmitted diseases (STDs) Infections spread from person to person through sexual contact. (page 458)

Shock A life-threatening condition in which the circulatory system fails to deliver enough blood to vital tissues and organs. (page 534)

Side effect Any effect of a medicine other than the one intended. (page 274)

Sidestream smoke Smoke given off by the burning end of a cigarette, cigar, or pipe. (page 306)

Skeletal muscle Muscle attached to bones that enables you to move your body. (page 373)

Skeletal system An internal body system made up of bones, joints, and connective tissue. (page 368)

Small intestine A coiled, tubelike digestive organ that is about 20 feet long. (page 391)

Smog A yellow-brown haze that forms when sunlight reacts with air pollution. (page 548)

Smooth muscle Type of muscle found in organs and in blood vessels and glands. (page 373)

Sobriety Living without alcohol. (page 327)

Social age Age measured by your lifestyle and the connections you have with others. (page 434)

Social health Your ability to get along with the people around you. (page 118)

Somatic (soh·MA·tik) **system** The part of the nervous system that deals with actions that you control. (page 388)

Specialist Doctor trained to handle particular kinds of patients or medical conditions. (page 64)

Sperm Male reproductive cells. (page 401)

Sperm cell The cell from the father that enters the egg cell during fertilization. (page 416)

Sports conditioning Regular physical activity or exercise to strengthen and condition muscles for a particular sport. (page 238)

Sprain A condition in which the ligaments that hold the joints in position are stretched or torn. (page 528)

Stepparent Someone who marries a child's mother or father. (page 126)

Stimulants (STIM·yuh·luhnts) Substances that speed up the body's functions. (page 277)

Stress Your body's response to change. (page 39)

Stress management skills Ways to deal with and overcome problems. (page 41)

Stressor Anything that causes stress. (page 40)

Stroke A condition in which a blood vessel bringing oxygen to the brain bursts or is blocked. (page 491)

Subcutaneous (suhb·kyoo·TAY·nee·uhs) **layer** A layer of fat under the skin. (page 344)

Suicide Intentionally killing oneself. (page 98)

Support system A network of people available to help when needed. (page 47)

Systemic circulation Flow of blood to all the body tissues except the lungs. (page 377)

Tar A dark, thick, sticky liquid that forms when tobacco burns. (page 300)

Tartar A hard coating on the teeth that is difficult to remove. (page 351)

Team sports Organized physical activities with specific rules in which groups of people play together against other groups. (page 237)

Tendons Tough bands of tissue that attach muscles to bones. (page 370)

Therapy Treatment. (page 102)

Time management Strategies for using time efficiently. (page 43)

Tissues Groups of similar cells that perform a specific function. (page 417)

Toddler A child between the ages of one and three who is learning to walk and talk. (page 428)

Tolerance A condition in which a person's body becomes used to the effect of a medicine and needs greater amounts of it in order for it to be effective. (page 274)

Tornado A whirling, funnel-shaped windstorm that may drop from the sky to the ground. (page 520)

Trachea (TRAY·kee·uh) Windpipe that directs air to the lungs. (page 382)

Tumor A mass of abnormal cells. (page 484)

Type 1 diabetes A condition in which the immune system attacks insulin-producing cells in the pancreas. (page 494)

Type 2 diabetes A condition in which the body cannot effectively use the insulin it produces. (page 494)

Umbilical (uhm·BIL·i·kuhl) **cord** A tube that connects the fetus and the mother's placenta. (page 419)

Unconditional love Love without limitation or qualification. (page 132)

Underweight Less than the appropriate weight for gender, height, age, body frame, and growth pattern. (page 251)

Universal precautions Actions taken to prevent the spread of disease by treating all blood as if it were contaminated. (page 525)

Unsaturated fats Fats that remain liquid at room temperature. (page 197)

Uterus (YOO·tuh·ruhs) A pear-shaped organ inside a female's body where a fetus is nourished. (page 418)

Vaccine A preparation of dead or weakened germs that causes the immune system to produce antibodies. (page 272)

Values The beliefs and ideals that guide the way a person lives. (pages 30, 119)

Vector An organism, such as an insect, that transmits a pathogen. (page 448)

Veins Blood vessels that carry blood from the body back to the heart. (page 378)

Violence Any act that causes physical or psychological harm to a person or damage to property. (page 172)

Virus The smallest disease-causing organism. (page 446)

Vitamins Substances needed in small quantities to help regulate body functions. (page 198)

Warm-up A period of low to moderate exercise to prepare your body for more vigorous activity. (page 233)

Warranty A written promise to handle repairs if a product fails to work properly. (page 61)

Wellness An overall state of well-being, or total health. (page 6)

Win-win solution An agreement that gives each party something they want. (page 169)

Withdrawal The physical and psychological symptoms that occur when someone stops using an addictive substance. (pages 287, 305)

Z

Zero tolerance policy A policy that makes no exceptions for anybody for any reason. (page 174)

Glosario

A

Abdominal thrusts/presiones abdominales Presiones rápidas y hacia arriba que se hacen sobre el diafragma para forzar la salida de algo que esté bloqueando la vía respiratoria.

Abstinence/abstinencia No participar en conducta de alto riesgo.

Abuse/abuso El maltrato físico, emocional o mental de una persona a otra.

Accident/accidente Un suceso que ocurre de manera no intencional.

Accident chain/accidente en cadena Una serie de sucesos que incluye una situación, un hábito peligroso y un acto peligroso.

Accidental injuries/Lesiones accidentales Lesiones que resultan de un accidente.

Acid rain/lluvia ácida Lluvia que es mucho más ácida de lo normal.

Acquired immunodeficiency syndrome (AIDS)/síndrome de inmunodeficiencia adquirida (SIDA) Una enfermedad mortal que interfiere con la habilidad natural del cuerpo de combatir infecciones.

Active listening/audición activa Oír el mensaje de otra persona, pensar en el mensaje y responder.

Addiction/adicción La necesidad física o psicológica de una droga.

Addictive/adictivo Capaz de ocasionar que el consumidor desarrolle una necesidad repentina intensa.

Adjustment/ajuste Una adaptación o cambio en la conducta.

Adolescence/adolescencia El periodo de vida entre la niñez y la adultez.

Adrenaline/adrenalina Una hormona que proporciona energía adicional al cuerpo.

Advertising/publicidad El envío de mensajes diseñados para hacer que los consumidores compren un producto o servicio.

Aerobic exercise/ejercicio aeróbico Actividad rítmica ininterrumpida de intensidad moderada a vigorosa que requiere grandes cantidades de oxígeno y hace que el corazón trabaje.

Alcohol/alcohol Una droga producida por una reacción química en frutas, verduras y granos.

Alcoholism/alcoholismo Una enfermedad progresiva y crónica caracterizada por una necesidad mental y física de consumir el alcohol.

Allergen/alergeno Una sustancia que causa una reacción alérgica.

Allergy/alergia Una reacción anormal del sistema inmunológico hacia una sustancia comúnmente inofensiva.

Alternatives/alternativas Diferentes maneras de pensar o actuar.

Alveoli/alveolos Cavidades microscópicas en los pulmones.

Amino acids/aminoácidos Unidades pequeñas que forman las proteínas.

Amphetamine/anfetamina Una droga que estimula el sistema nervioso central.

Anabolic steroids/esteroides anabólicos Drogas que causan que el tejido muscular se desarrolle con rapidez anormal.

Anaerobic exercise/ejercicio anaeróbico Actividad física intensa que requiere poco oxígeno pero exige breves brotes de energía.

Anorexia nervosa/anorexia nerviosa Un trastorno en la alimentación que se caracteriza por autoinanición conducente a una pérdida de peso extrema.

Antibiotics/antibióticos Medicinas que disminuyen o matan bacterias dañinas en el cuerpo.

Antibodies/anticuerpos Proteínas que se adhieren a los antígenos para prevenir que dañen al cuerpo.

Antigens/antígenos Sustancias que liberan los agentes patógenos.

Antihistamines/antihistamínicos Medicinas que ayudan a controlar los efectos que provocan las histaminas.

Anxiety/ansiedad Un sentimiento abrumador de terror, muy parecido al miedo.

Anxiety disorder/trastorno de ansiedad Un trastorno en el cual la ansiedad intensa o el miedo impide que una persona funcione de manera normal.

Appetite/apetito El deseo psicológico de alimentarse.

Appropriate weight/peso apropiado El peso más adecuado para tu cuerpo.

Arteries/arterias Vasos sanguíneos que llevan sangre desde el corazón a otras partes del cuerpo.

Arteriosclerosis/arteriosclerosis Un conjunto de trastornos por el cual las arterias se endurecen y se tornan rígidas.

Arthritis/artritis Más de 100 afecciones que se caracterizan por el dolor y la hinchazón de las articulaciones del cuerpo.

Assertive/firme Comportarte con seguridad y declarar claramente tus intenciones.

Asthma/asma Una grave enfermedad crónica que causa el estrechamiento u obstrucción de las diminutas vías del aparato respiratorio.

Atherosclerosis/aterosclerosis Un tipo de arteriosclerosis por el cual sustancias grasas en la sangre se acumulan en las paredes de las arterias.

Attitude/actitud Sentimientos y creencias.

Autonomic system/sistema autónomo La parte del sistema nervioso que se ocupa de las acciones que generalmente tú no controlas.

Bacteria/bacterias Organismos diminutos unicelulares que viven en casi todas partes.

Balance/equilibrio Un sentimiento de estabilidad y control.

Battery/agresión Dar palizas, golpear o dar puntapiés a otra persona

Benign tumor/tumor benigno Un tumor que no es canceroso.

Binge drinking/borrachera El consumo de muchas bebidas alcohólicas en un corto plazo.

Binge eating disorder/trastorno de la alimentación compulsiva Sentirse impulsado a comer demasiado.

Biodegradable/biodegradable Que se descompone fácilmente en el medio ambiente.

Biological age/edad biológica Medida de la edad, determinada según el funcionamiento de varias partes del cuerpo.

Biopsy/biopsia La extirpación de una muestra de tejido para determinar la presencia de células cancerosas.

Birth defect/defecto de nacimiento
Anormalidad presente al momento del nacimiento que causa incapacidad física o mental o la muerte.

Blended family/familia mezclada Una familia que consiste en padre o madre, padrastro o madrastra, y los hijos de uno o ambos padres.

Blizzard/ventisca Una tormenta de nieve fuerte, con vientos que llegan a 45 millas por hora.

Blood alcohol concentration (BAC)/ concentración de alcohol en la sangre La cantidad de alcohol presente en el torrente sanguíneo de una persona.

Body composition/composición del cuerpo La proporción entre la grasa del cuerpo y los tejidos magros, tales como huesos, músculos y líquidos.

Body image/autoimagen La manera en que te ves a ti mismo.

Body language/lenguaje corporal
El uso de movimientos corporales y gestos para comunicar un mensaje.

Body Mass Index (BMI)/Índice de masa corporal Una medida que te permite evaluar el tamaño de tu cuerpo, teniendo en cuenta tu estatura y peso.

Bronchi/bronquios Pasajes a través de los cuales entra el aire en los pulmones.

Bronchodilators/broncodilatadores
Medicinas que se usan para relajar los músculos que se han tensado alrededor de las vías respiratorias.

Bulimia/bulimia Una afección por la cual una persona come grandes cantidades de alimentos y después intenta inducirse el vómito.

Calories/calorías Unidades de calor que miden la energía que el cuerpo usa y la energía que los alimentos aportan al cuerpo.

Cancer/cáncer Una enfermedad que se caracteriza por el desarrollo rápido e incontrolable de células anormales.

Capillaries/capilares Conductos minúsculos que llevan sangre desde las arterias a las células del cuerpo, y de regreso a las venas.

Carbohydrates/hidratos de carbono
Los azúcares y almidones que le proporcionan a tu cuerpo la mayor parte de su energía.

Carbon monoxide/monóxido de carbono Un gas incoloro, inodoro y tóxico que se produce al quemarse el tabaco.

Carcinogens/carcinógenos Sustancias que causan el cáncer.

Cardiac muscle/músculo cardiaco
El músculo en las paredes del corazón.

Cardiovascular system/sistema cardiovascular Órganos y tejidos que transportan materia esencial a las células del cuerpo y eliminan los sus desechos.

Carrier/portador Una persona infectada con un virus que puede contagiar a otras.

Cartilage/cartílago Tejido fuerte y flexible que amortigua las articulaciones.

Central nervous system (CNS)/ sistema nervioso central El cerebro y la médula espinal.

Cervix/cuello del útero La entrada del útero.

Character/carácter La manera en la que una persona piensa, siente y actúa.

Character trait/rasgo del carácter Una cualidad que demuestra la manera en que una persona piensa, siente y actúa.

Chromosomes/cromosomas Las estructuras filiformes dentro del núcleo de las células que contienen los códigos de las características hereditarias.

Chronic diseases/enfermedades crónicas Las enfermedades que están siempre presentes o reaparecen repetidamente durante un largo periodo de tiempo.

Chronological age/edad cronológica La edad medida en años.

Cilia/cilios Estructuras diminutas parecidas al cabello que protegen los pulmones.

Circulatory system/aparato circulatorio Los órganos y los tejidos que transportan materias esenciales a las células del cuerpo y se llevan sus desechos.

Cirrhosis/cirrosis La cicatrización y destrucción del hígado.

Citizenship/ciudadanía La forma en que te comportas como miembro de una comunidad.

Clinical depression/depresión diagnosticada Un trastorno del ánimo por el cual la persona pierde interés en la vida y es incapaz de disfrutar de nada.

Clique/camarilla Un grupo de amigos que salen juntos y que se comportan de manera similar.

Cold turkey/parar en seco Expresión que se usa para describir la acción de abandonar un vicio de una vez, por ejemplo el fumar.

Colon/colon El intestino grueso.

Commitment/compromiso Una promesa o voto.

Communicable disease/enfermedad contagiosa Una enfermedad que se puede propagar a una persona de otra persona, un animal o un objeto.

Comparison shopping/comparación de productos Un método de evaluar los beneficios de diferentes productos y servicios al medir y comparar varios factores, tales como la calidad, las características y el precio.

Compromise/acordar Llegar a un acuerdo en el que se cede algo con el fin de llegar a una solución satisfactoria para todos.

Conflict/conflicto Un desacuerdo entre personas con puntos de vista, ideas o metas opuestos.

Conflict resolution/resolución de un conflicto Resolver un desacuerdo de manera satisfactoria para ambas partes.

Consequences/consecuencias Los resultados o efectos que pueden ocurrir como resultado de una decisión o un acto.

Conservation/conservación El ahorro de recursos.

Consumer/consumidor La persona que compra bienes o servicios.

Contagious period/periodo de contagio El periodo de tiempo en que una enfermedad se puede propagar de una persona a otra.

Cool-down/recuperación Un periodo en el que se realizan ejercicios de intensidad baja a moderada a fin de preparar al cuerpo para terminar una serie de ejercicios vigorosos.

Coordination/coordinación El funcionamiento conjunto de los músculos y los huesos de manera eficiente y sin complicaciones.

Cornea/córnea Una estructura transparente que protege al ojo y deja pasar la luz.

CPR/resucitación cardiopulmonar Un procedimiento de primeros auxilios que combina la respiración de rescate y compresiones sobre el pecho para restaurar la respiración y la circulación.

Cross-training/entrenamiento variado El cambiar de un ejercicio físico a otro.

Cumulative risks/riesgos acumulativos Riesgos relacionados cuyos efectos aumentan con cada uno que se añade.

Cuticle/cutícula Un doblez de epidermis alrededor de las uñas de los pies y las manos.

Cycle of abuse/ciclo de abuso Un patrón de repetición del abuso de una generación a la siguiente.

Dandruff/caspa Las escamas de piel muerta en la superficie del cuero cabelludo.

Decibel/decibel Una medida del volumen del sonido.

Decision making/tomar decisiones El proceso de hacer una selección o de hallar una solución.

Defensive driving/conducir de manera defensiva Estar atento a las otras personas en la carretera y anticipar acciones peligrosas.

Degenerative diseases/ enfermedades degenerativas Enfermedades que causan la destrucción progresiva de las células, tejidos y órganos del cuerpo a medida que avanzan.

Dehydration/deshidratación Pérdida excesiva del agua del cuerpo.

Depressants/depresivos Sustancias que disminuyen las funciones y reacciones del cuerpo.

Dermatologist/dermatólogo Médico que trata trastornos de la piel.

Dermis/dermis La capa gruesa e interna de la piel.

Detoxification/desintoxicación El proceso físico de liberar al cuerpo de una sustancia adictiva.

Developmental tasks/tareas requeridas para el desarrollo Sucesos que deben ocurrir para que continúes desarrollándote hasta llegar a convertirte en un adulto saludable y maduro.

Diabetes/diabetes Una enfermedad que impide que el cuerpo convierta los alimentos en energía.

Diaphragm/diafragma Un músculo en forma de domo que separa los pulmones del abdomen.

Dietary Guidelines for Americans/ Pautas alimenticias para los estadounidenses Consejos sobre los alimentos para todos los estadounidenses saludables de 2 años de edad en adelante.

Digestion/digestión El proceso de convertir los alimentos que comes en sustancias que tu cuerpo pueda usar.

Digestive system/aparato digestivo Un sistema de órganos que convierten los alimentos en una forma útil para el cuerpo.

Distress/angustia El estrés negativo.

Divorce/divorcio Un fin legal a un contrato matrimonial.

Drugs/drogas Sustancias, que no sean alimentos, que cambian la estructura o el funcionamiento del cuerpo o la mente.

Earthquake/terremoto El sacudimiento violento de la superficie de la tierra.

Eating disorder/trastorno en la alimentación Costumbre en la alimentación por la cual una persona come de manera extrema y nociva y que puede causar enfermedades y aun la muerte.

Egg cell/óvulo La célula reproductora femenina que se une con el espermatozoide para crear una nueva vida.

Embryo/embrión Un organismo en desarrollo desde la fecundación hasta aproximadamente la octava semana del desarrollo.

Emotional needs/necesidades emocionales Las necesidades que afectan los sentimientos y el bienestar de una persona.

Emotions/emociones Sentimientos que surgen en respuesta a pensamientos, comentarios y sucesos.

Empathetic/tener empatía Capaz de identificar y compartir los sentimientos de otra persona.

Empathy/empatía La habilidad de entender y compartir los sentimientos de otra persona.

Empty calories/calorías vacías Calorías que provienen de alimentos con poco, o ningún, valor nutritivo.

Endocrine system/sistema endocrino El sistema químico de comunicaciones del cuerpo que regula varias funciones.

Environment/medio ambiente La suma total de lo que rodea a una persona.

Environmental Protection Agency (EPA)/Agencia de Protección Ambiental La agencia del gobierno de Estados Unidos a cargo de la protección del medio ambiente.

Epidermis/epidermis La capa visible y más externa de la piel.

Epiglottis/epiglotis Una tapa de tejido que cubre la tráquea cuando tragas.

Escalate/intensificar Llegar a ser más grave.

Eustachian tube/trompa de Eustaquio La parte del oído que deja pasar aire desde la nariz al oído medio para que la presión del aire sea igual en ambos lados del tímpano.

Eustress/estrés positivo Tensión positiva.

Evaluate/evaluar Determinar el valor de algo.

Excretion/excreción El proceso de eliminar desechos del cuerpo.

Excretory system/sistema excretor El sistema del cuerpo que elimina desechos del cuerpo.

Exercise/ejercicio Actividad física específica, planeada y organizada que mejora o mantiene la condición física.

Extended family/familia extensa La familia nuclear y otros parientes tales como abuelos, tías, tíos y primos.

Eye contact/contacto visual El mirar directamente a los ojos de otra persona.

Family/familia La unidad básica de la sociedad.

Family therapy/terapía familiar Asesoramiento cuyo propósito es mejorar relaciones problemáticas entre familiares.

Fatigue/fatiga Agotamiento.

Feedback/reacción Una respuesta del oyente a lo que el orador ha dicho.

Fertilization/fecundación La unión de un espermatozoide y un óvulo.

Fetal alcohol syndrome (FAS)/ síndrome alcohólico fetal Un conjunto de defectos de nacimiento causados por el alcohol que incluyen problemas físicos y mentales.

Fetus/feto El organismo en desarrollo desde el final de la octava semana del embarazo de la madre hasta el momento del nacimiento.

Fiber/fibra La parte de las frutas, verduras, granos y frijoles que tu cuerpo no puede dirigir.

Fight-or-flight response/respuesta de lucha o huida El proceso mediante el cual el cuerpo se prepara a enfrentarse con un estresante.

First aid/primeros auxilios El cuidado inmediato y temporal que se le proporciona a una persona herida o enferma hasta que reciba ayuda profesional.

Flexibility/flexibilidad La habilidad de mover las articulaciones del cuerpo con facilidad a través del arco completo de movimiento.

Food Guide Pyramid/Pirámide Nutricional Una guía para la selección diaria de alimentos sanos.

Foodborne illness/enfermedad producida por un alimento Enfermedad que proviene de haber comido un alimento no sano.

Fracture/fractura Una rotura de un hueso.

Fraud/fraude Engaño o decepción deliberado.

Fungi/hongos Organismos primitivos que se alimentan de materias orgánicas.

Gallbladder/vesícula biliar Pequeño órgano en forma de bolsa que almacena bilis.

Gang/pandilla Un grupo de personas que se relacionan para tomar parte en actividades criminales.

Genes/genes Las unidades básicas de la herencia.

Genetic disorder/trastorno genético Un trastorno causado parcial o totalmente por defectos en los genes.

Gingivitis/gingivitis Un trastorno común que se caracteriza por el enrojecimiento y dolor de las encías que sangran con facilidad.

Gland/glándula Un grupo de células, o un órgano, que secreta una sustancia química.

Global warming/calentamiento del planeta Un aumento en las temperaturas de la Tierra.

Goal setting/establecer metas El proceso de esforzarte para lograr algo que quieres.

Greenhouse effect/efecto invernadero La retención del calor por la presencia de dióxido de carbono y otros gases en el aire.

Grief/pena El pesar provocado por la muerte de un ser querido.

Grief counselor/consejero especializado en la pena Consejero que enseña estrategias para superar una pena.

Hallucinogens/alucinógenos Drogas que alteran el estado de ánimo, los pensamientos y los sentidos.

Hangnail/padrastro Una grieta en la cutícula al lado del borde de la uña.

Hazardous wastes/desechos peligrosos Desechos líquidos o sólidos generados por los seres humanos, que pueden perjudicar la salud de las personas o el medio ambiente.

Health/salud Una combinación de bienestar físico, mental/emocional y social.

Health advocacy/promoción de la salud Tomar medidas para influir en las personas de manera que dirijan sus esfuerzos a un asunto de la salud o que apoyen una creencia relacionada con la salud.

Health care system/sistema de asistencia sanitaria Toda la asistencia médica al alcance de los ciudadanos de una nación, la manera en que ellos reciben la asistencia, y la manera en que se paga por la asistencia.

Health fraud/fraude contra la salud La venta de productos o servicios inútiles que se afirma que protegen contra enfermedades o curan otros problemas de la salud.

Health insurance/seguro de salud Un plan en el que una compañía privada o programa del gobierno paga parte de los gastos médicos de una persona.

Health maintenance organization (HMO)/organización para el mantenimiento de la salud Una organización que proporciona asistencia médica a un precio fijo.

Heart and lung endurance/ resistencia cardiaca y respiratoria La capacidad de corazón y pulmones de funcionar con eficacia cuando haces ejercicio y de regresar al ritmo normal cuando paras.

Heart attack/ataque cardiaco Una afección en la cual el flujo de sangre a una parte del corazón está considerablemente reducido u obstruido

Heat cramps/calambre debido al calor Dolorosos espasmos involuntarios de los músculos que pueden ocurrir al realizar ejercicio vigoroso cuando hace mucho calor.

Heat exhaustion/agotamiento debido al calor Una afección caracterizada por el desmayo, la náusea, el ritmo cardiaco rápido y la piel caliente, roja, seca o sudorosa.

Heatstroke/insolación Un tipo de enfermedad debido al calor grave en que los procesos normales del cuerpo que controlan los efectos del calor dejan de funcionar.

Hepatitis/hepatitis Una enfermedad vírica del hígado que se caracteriza por el color amarillo de la piel y del blanco de los ojos.

Heredity/herencia La transferencia de características de los padres a sus hijos.

High blood pressure/presión arterial alta Una afección en la que la presión arterial de una persona se mantiene a un nivel más alto de lo normal.

Histamines/histaminas Sustancias químicas en el cuerpo que provocan los síntomas de una reacción alérgica.

Hives/urticaria Granos en la piel que pican mucho.

Homicide/homicidio El acto en que una persona mata a otra.

Hormones/hormonas Sustancias químicas, producidas por glándulas, que ayudan a regular varias funciones del cuerpo.

Hospice care/asistencia para enfermos desahuciados Asistencia para personas con enfermedades incurables que apunta a brindar comodidad, no una cura.

Human immunodeficiency virus (HIV)/virus de inmunodeficiencia humana (VIH) El virus que causa el SIDA.

Hunger/hambre La necesidad física de alimentos.

Hurricane/huracán Una tormenta de vientos y lluvia torrencial que se origina en alta mar.

Immune system/sistema inmunológico Una combinación de las defensas del cuerpo, compuesta de células, tejidos y órganos que combaten patógenos y enfermedades.

Immunity/inmunidad La habilidad del cuerpo de resistir los patógenos que causan una enfermedad en particular.

Individual sports/deportes individuales Actividades físicas que puedes realizar solo o con otra persona.

Infancy/infancia El primer año de vida.

Infection/infección Una afección que se produce cuando agentes patógenos invaden el cuerpo, se multiplican y dañan las células del cuerpo.

Ingrown toenail/uña encarnada Una afección en la cual la uña se introduce en la piel al lado del dedo del pie.

Inhalant/inhalante Toda sustancia cuyos gases se aspiran para producir sensaciones alucinantes.

Insulin/insulina Una hormona producida por el páncreas.

Interpersonal communication/ comunicación entre personas El intercambio de pensamientos, sentimientos y creencias entre dos personas o más.

Intoxicated/embriagado Física y mentalmente afectado por el consumo de alcohol.

Iris/iris La parte coloreada del ojo.

Joints/articulaciones Lugares en donde se unen los huesos.

Kidneys/riñones Los órganos que filtran el agua y los desechos disueltos de la sangre y contribuyen a mantener los niveles adecuados de agua y sales en el cuerpo.

Landfills/terraplenes sanitarios Pozos enormes donde se tiran y se entierran desechos.

Larynx/laringe La parte superior del aparato respiratorio que contiene las cuerdas vocales.

Lens/cristalino La estructura transparente y flexible del ojo que enfoca la luz en la retina.

Lifestyle factors/factores del estilo de vida Conductas y hábitos que ayudan a determinar el nivel de salud de una persona.

Ligaments/ligamentos Cuerdas fuertes de tejido que unen los huesos en las articulaciones.

Limits/límites Barreras invisibles que te protegen.

Liver/hígado Una glándula grande que tiene varias funciones digestivas.

Lymphatic system/sistema linfático Aparato circulatorio secundario que le ayuda al cuerpo a combatir patógenos y a mantener el equilibrio de líquidos.

Mainstream smoke/humo directo El humo que el fumador aspira y exhala.

Malignant tumor/tumor maligno Un tumor canceroso.

Malnutrition/desnutrición Una afección por la cual el cuerpo no recibe los nutrientes que necesita para crecer y funcionar bien.

Mammogram/mamografía Una radiografía del seno que se usa para determinar si hay evidencia del cáncer.

Marrow/médula Un tejido en el centro de algunos huesos.

Media/medios de difusión Los diversos métodos de comunicar información.

Mediation/mediación Un proceso en el cual una tercera persona, un mediador, ayuda a otros a encontrar una solución al conflicto entre ellos.

Medicines/medicinas Drogas que se usan para curar o prevenir enfermedades u otras afecciones.

Menopause/menopausia Una etapa que marca el fin de los años reproductivos de una mujer.

Menstrual cycle/ciclo menstrual La serie de sucesos en el aparato reproductor de la mujer que ocurre entre una menstruación y la siguiente.

Menstruation/menstruación La eliminación de materia celular del revestimiento del útero.

Mental and emotional health/salud mental y emocional La capacidad de aceptarse a sí mismo y a otros, de adaptarse a las emociones y sobrellevarlas, y de superar los problemas y retos de la vida.

Metastasis/metástasis La propagación de cáncer de una parte del cuerpo a otra.

Methamphetamine/metanfetamina Un estimulante parecido a la anfetamina.

Minerals/minerales Elementos que se necesitan en cantidades pequeñas para la formación de dientes y huesos saludables, y para regular determinados procesos corporales.

Mixed message/mensaje contradictorio Una situación en que tus palabras expresan algo pero tu lenguaje corporal lo contradice.

Mononucleosis/mononucleosis Una enfermedad vírica cuyos síntomas incluyen hinchazón y dolor en áreas del cuello y dolor de garganta.

Mood disorder/trastorno del estado de ánimo Un trastorno en que la persona cambia de humor de manera aparentemente inapropiada o extrema.

Muscle endurance/resistencia muscular La capacidad que tiene un músculo de ejercer una fuerza repetidamente durante un largo periodo de tiempo.

Muscle strength/fortaleza muscular El peso máximo que puedes levantar o la fuerza máxima que puedes ejercer a la vez.

Muscular system/sistema muscular El grupo de estructuras que permiten el movimiento de las partes de tu cuerpo.

Narcotics/narcóticos Ciertas drogas específicas que se pueden obtener únicamente con receta médica y que se usan para aliviar el dolor.

Neglect/abandono El no satisfacer las necesidades básicas físicas y emocionales de una persona.

Neurons/neuronas Células especializadas que componen el sistema nervioso.

Nicotine/nicotina Una droga adictiva que se encuentra en las hojas del tabaco y en todos los productos del tabaco.

Nicotine gum/goma de mascar con nicotina Un tipo de goma de mascar cuyo efecto es permitir que el consumidor abandone el tabaco mientras el nivel de nicotina baja gradualmente.

Nicotine patch/parche de nicotina Un parche medicado que se pone en la piel y que permite que el consumidor abandone el tabaco mientras el nivel de nicotina baja gradualmente.

Noncommunicable diseases/enfermedades no contagiosas Las enfermedades que no son causadas por agentes patógenos.

Nonrenewable resources/recursos no renovables Sustancias que no se pueden reemplazar una vez que se han usado.

Nutrient deficiency/deficiencia nutricional Una escasez de un nutriente.

Nutrient density/densidad de los nutrientes La cantidad de nutrientes comparados con las calorías que proporcionan.

Nutrients/nutrientes Sustancias en los alimentos que tu cuerpo necesita.

Nutrition/nutrición El proceso de usar alimentos y sus sustancias para ayudar al cuerpo a tener energía, crecer, desarrollarse y funcionar bien.

Obstetrician/obstetra Médico especialista en el cuidado de la mujer embarazada y el feto en desarrollo y que está presente durante el nacimiento del bebé.

Online shopping/compras en Internet El uso de Internet para comprar productos y servicios.

Ophthalmologist/oftalmólogo Médico especialista en el tratamiento médico y quirúrgico de los ojos y también receta lentes correctivos.

Opportunistic infection/infección oportunista Una enfermedad que ataca a una persona con un sistema inmunológico debilitado que rara vez afecta a una persona saludable.

Optometrist/optómetra Un profesional que examina la vista y que receta lentes correctivos.

Organs/órganos Partes del cuerpo que cumplen funciones determinadas.

Orthodontist/ortodoncista Dentista que previene o corrige problemas en el alineamiento de o el espacio entre los dientes.

Osteoarthritis/osteoartritis Una enfermedad que se caracteriza por el deterioro del cartílago en las articulaciones.

Over-the-counter medicines/medicinas sin receta Medicinas inofensivas que se pueden consumir sin receta médica.

Overweight/sobrepeso Más del peso apropiado de acuerdo al sexo, estatura, edad, estructura corporal y ritmo de crecimiento.

Ovulation/ovulación El desprendimiento de un óvulo maduro cada mes.

Ozone layer/capa de ozono Una capa protectora sobre la superficie de la Tierra que protege a los seres vivos de la radiación ultravioleta.

Pacemaker/marcapasos Pequeño aparato que envía pulsaciones eléctricas constantes al corazón, para que los latidos sean regulares.

Pancreas/páncreas Un órgano que produce enzimas que ayudan en la digestión.

Panic/pánico Un sentimiento repentino de miedo intenso.

Parenting/crianza de hijos El proceso de satisfacer las necesidades físicas, mentales, emocionales y sociales de un niño.

Pathogens/patógenos Organismos diminutos que causan enfermedades contagiosas.

Peer pressure/presión de pares La influencia que personas de tu misma edad tienen sobre ti para que adoptes sus creeencias y forma de actuar.

Percent Daily Value/porcentaje del valor diario El porcentaje de la cantidad diaria recomendada de un nutriente en una porción de alimento.

Periodontal disease/enfermedad periodontal Enfermedad avanzada de las encías en la cual el periostio dental se ve infectado por bacterias.

Periodontium/periostio dental Una estructura que consiste en la mandíbula, las encías y los conectadores llamados ligamentos.

Peripheral nervous system (PNS)/sistema nervioso periférico Los nervios que conectan al sistema nervioso central con todas partes del cuerpo.

Personality/personalidad La combinación singular de sentimientos, pensamientos y conducta que hacen a una persona diferente de todas las demás.

Personality disorder/trastorno de la personalidad Una variedad de trastornos psicológicos que afectan la habilidad de una persona para llevarse bien con otras.

Pesticide/pesticida Producto que se usa en las cosechas para matar insectos y otras plagas.

Phobia/fobia Un miedo intenso y exagerado de una situación u objeto específico.

Physical activity/actividad física Todo movimiento que usa energía.

Physical dependence/dependencia física Una adicción en que el cuerpo siente una necesidad directa de una droga.

Physical fitness/buen estado físico La capacidad de cumplir con las exigencias físicas de la vida diaria sin cansarse demasiado.

Pituitary gland/glándula pituitaria Una glándula que señala a otras glándulas endocrinas la necesidad de producir hormonas.

Placenta/placenta El tejido espeso y rico que cubre las paredes del útero durante el embarazo y que nutre al feto.

Plaque/placa bacteriana Una película blanda, incolora y pegajosa que contiene bacterias y que se acumula en los dientes.

Point of Service (POS) plan/plan de lugar del servicio Un plan de salud que permite que sus miembros escojan proveedores que participen o no en el plan.

Pollution/contaminación Toda sustancia sucia o nociva en el medio ambiente.

Precaution/precaución Una acción planeada que se toma con anticipación de un suceso, a fin de aumentar las probabilidades de un resultado no peligroso.

Precycling/prereciclaje El proceso de reducir los desechos antes de que se produzcan.

Preferred Provider Organization (PPO)/organización de proveedores preferidos Un plan de seguro de salud en el cual los médicos participantes cobran menos a los miembros del plan.

Prejudice/prejuicio Una opinión negativa e injusta, generalmente en contra de personas de otro grupo racial, religioso o cultural.

Prenatal care/cuidado prenatal Medidas que se toman para cuidar de la salud de una mujer embarazada y su feto.

Preschooler/niño preescolar Un niño de entre tres y cinco años de edad.

Prescription medicines/medicinas bajo receta Medicinas que sólo se pueden vender con receta de un médico.

Preventive care/cuidado preventivo Medidas que se toman para evitar que ocurran enfermedades o daños o que empeoren.

Primary care physician/médico principal Un médico que proporciona a sus pacientes exámenes y cuidado general.

Proteins/proteínas Nutrientes que el cuerpo usa para crear, reparar y mantener células y tejidos.

Protozoa/protozoos Organismos unicelulares que en general no son dañinos pero que pueden causar ciertas enfermedades.

Psychiatrist/psiquiatra Un médico que trata trastornos de la salud mental.

Psychological dependence/ dependencia psicológica Una adicción por la cual la mente envía un mensaje al cuerpo indicando que necesita mayor cantidad de una droga

Psychologist/psicólogo Un profesional de la salud mental capacitado y autorizado por el estado para aconsejar y guiar.

Puberty/pubertad La etapa de la vida en la cual comienzas a desarrollar ciertas características físicas propias de los adultos de tu mismo sexo.

Public health/salud pública La protección y el fomento de salud al nivel comunitario.

Pulmonary circulation/circulación pulmonar La circulación que lleva la sangre desde el corazón, a través de los pulmones y de regreso al corazón.

Pupil/pupila Una abertura oscura en el centro del iris.

Rape/violación Todo tipo de relación sexual contra la voluntad de la persona.

Recovery/recuperación El proceso de aprender a vivir una vida libre de alcohol.

Recurrence/reaparición El regreso de cáncer después de una remisión.

Refusal skills/destrezas de negación Estrategias de la comunicación para ayudarte a decir no de manera eficaz.

Relationships/relaciones Las conexiones que tienes con otras personas o grupos en tu vida.

Remission/remisión Un periodo durante el cual se desaparecen las señales y síntomas del cáncer.

Reproductive system/aparato reproductor Los órganos que posibilitan la producción de hijos.

Resilience/capacidad de recuperación La habilidad para adaptarse y recuperarse después de una decepción, dificultad o crisis.

Respiratory system/aparato respiratorio Los órganos que proporcionan oxígeno continuamente al cuerpo y que eliminan el bióxido de carbono.

Retina/retina Una capa delgada de neuronas en el ojo que absorben luz.

Rheumatoid arthritis/artritis reumatoide Una enfermedad crónica que se caracteriza por dolor, inflamación, hinchazón y anquilosamiento de las articulaciones.

Rickettsias/rickettsia Organismos que causan enfermedades, que se parecen a bacterias pero que se multiplican como los virus.

Risk behavior/conducta arriesgada Un acto o conducta que puede causarte daño o perjudicarte a ti o a otros.

Risk factors/factores de riesgo Características que aumentan la probabilidad de una persona de contraer una enfermedad.

Saliva/saliva Líquido producido por las glándulas salivales de la boca.

Saturated fats/grasas saturadas Grasas que son sólidas a temperatura ambiente.

Schizophrenia/esquizofrenia Un trastorno mental grave por el cual una persona pierde contacto con la realidad.

Secondhand smoke/humo secundario Aire que ha sido contaminado por el humo del tabaco.

Sedentary lifestyle/estilo de vida sedentaria Un modo de vivir caracterizado por la escasez de actividad física.

Self-concept/autoconcepto La manera en que te ves a ti mismo.

Self-control/dominio de sí mismo Control de tus propias emociones y deseos.

Self-esteem/autoestima La opinión que tienes de ti mismo y cuánto te valoras.

Self-respect/dignidad propia El sentimiento positivo que tienes de ti mismo cuando cumples con tus creencias y valores.

Sexual harassment/acoso sexual Conducta sexual no solicitada y fuera de lugar dirigida a otra persona.

Sexually transmitted diseases (STDs)/enfermedades de transmisión sexual (ETS) Enfermedades que se propagan de una persona a otra a través de contacto sexual.

Shock/choque Una afección que puede causar la muerte en la cual el aparato circulatorio no lleva la suficiente cantidad de sangre a tejidos y órganos vitales.

Side effect/efecto colateral Todo efecto reacción inesperada de una medicina.

Sidestream smoke/humo indirecto El humo producido por la colilla encendida de un cigarrillo, cigarro o pipa.

Skeletal muscle/músculo del sistema osteoarticular Músculo ligado a huesos que te permiten mover el cuerpo.

Skeletal system/sistema osteoarticular Sistema corporal interno compuesto de huesos, articulaciones y tejidos conjuntivos.

Small intestine/intestino delgado Un órgano digestivo enrollado y semejante a un tubo que mide unos 20 pies de largo.

Smog/smog Una neblina de color amarillo-café que se forma cuando la luz solar reacciona con la contaminación del aire.

Smooth muscle/músculo liso Tipo de músculo que se encuentra en los órganos, los vasos sanguíneos y las glándulas.

Sobriety/sobriedad Vivir sin consumir alcohol.

Social age/edad social La edad calculada de acuerdo a tu estilo de vida y las conexiones que tienes con otras.

Social health/salud social Tu habilidad para llevarte bien con las personas que te rodean.

Somatic system/sistema somático
La parte del sistema nervioso relacionada con las acciones que tú controlas.

Specialist/especialista Médico que está capacitado para tratar determinada clase de pacientes o problemas de salud.

Sperm/espermatozoide Células reproductoras masculinas.

Sperm cell/espermatozoide La célula del padre que entra en el óvulo durante la fertilización.

Sports conditioning/entrenamiento deportivo Actividad física normal o ejercicios para fortalecer y entrenar los músculos para un deporte determinado.

Sprain/torcedura Una afección en que los ligamentos que mantienen las articulaciones en su lugar están distendidos o quebrados.

Stepparent/padrastro o madrastra La persona que se casa con la madre o el padre de un niño.

Stimulants/estimulantes Sustancias que aceleran las funciones del cuerpo.

Stress/estrés La reacción de tu cuerpo a cambios.

Stress management skills/habilidad de controlar el éstres Maneras de tratar y superar los problemas.

Stressor/factor estresante Todo lo que provoca el estrés.

Stroke/apoplejía Una afección que ocurre cuando un vaso sanguíneo que lleva oxígeno al cerebro estalla o se obstruye.

Subcutaneous layer/capa subcutánea Una capa de grasa debajo de la piel.

Suicide/suicidio Matarse intencionalmente.

Support system/sistema de asistencia Una red de personas dispuestas a ayudar cuando haya necesidad.

Systemic circulation/circulación sistémica El flujo de sangre a todos los tejidos del cuerpo excepto los pulmones.

Tar/alquitrán Un líquido espeso, oscuro y pegajoso que se forma al quemarse el tabaco.

Tartar/sarro Placa endurecida que se forma en la superficie de los dientes y que es difícil de quitar.

Team sports/deportes en equipo Actividades físicas organizadas, con reglas específicas, en las cuales grupos de personas juegan contra otros grupos.

Tendons/tendones Bandas de tejidos fuertes que unen los músculos y los huesos.

Therapy/terapia Tratamiento.

Time management/organización del tiempo Estrategias para usar el tiempo eficazmente.

Tissues/tejidos Masa de células similares que desempeñan una función específica.

Toddler/niño que empieza a andar Un niño de entre uno y tres años de edad que está aprendiendo a caminar y a hablar.

Tolerance/tolerancia Una afección por la cual el cuerpo de una persona se acostumbra a los efectos de una medicina y necesita mayor cantidad para que ésta sea eficaz.

Tornado/tornado Una tormenta de viento en torbellino, con forma de embudo, que gira en grandes círculos y que puede caer del cielo a la tierra.

Trachea/tráquea Vía respiratoria que dirige el aire a los pulmones.

Tumor/tumor Una masa de células anormales.

Type 1 diabetes/diabetes tipo 1 Una afección por la cual el sistema inmunológico ataca las células productoras de insulina en el páncreas.

Type 2 diabetes/diabetes tipo 2 Una afección que se caracteriza por la inhabilidad del cuerpo para usar de manera eficaz la insulina que produce.

Umbilical cord/cordón umbilical El conducto que conecta el feto a la placenta de la madre.

Unconditional love/amor incondicional Amor sin restricciones ni reservas.

Underweight/de peso insuficiente Por debajo del peso apropiado de acuerdo al sexo, estatura, edad, estructura corporal y ritmo de crecimiento.

Universal precautions/precauciones universales Medidas para prevenir la propagación de enfermedades al tratar toda la sangre como si estuviera contaminada.

Unsaturated fats/grasas no saturadas Las grasas que permanecen líquidas a temperatura ambiente.

Uterus/útero Un órgano en forma de pera dentro del cuerpo de la mujer donde se nutre un feto.

Vaccine/vacuna Un preparado de gérmenes muertos o debilitados que causa que el sistema inmunológico produzca anticuerpos.

Values/valores Las creencias y los ideales que guían la manera en que vive una persona.

Vector/vector Un organismo, por ejemplo un insecto, que transmite un agente patógeno.

Veins/venas Vasos sanguíneos que llevan la sangre desde el cuerpo de regreso al corazón.

Violence/violencia Todo acto que causa daño físico o psicológico a una persona o bien.

Virus/virus El organismo causante de enfermedades más pequeño.

Vitamins/vitaminas Sustancias que el cuerpo necesita en pequeñas cantidades para regular sus funciones.

Warm-up/precalentamiento Un periodo de ejercicio suave que se hace para preparar al cuerpo para actividad más vigorosa.

Warranty/garantía La promesa escrita de reparar un producto si no funciona bien.

Wellness/bienestar general Un estado de bienestar, o salud total.

Win-win solution/situación en que todos ganan Un acuerdo en que todos reciben algo que desean.

Withdrawal/síndrome de abstinencia Los síntomas físicos y psicológicos que ocurren cuando una persona deja de usar una sustancia adictiva.

Zero tolerance policy/normativa de tolerancia nula Una normativa en que no hay excepciones para nadie por ninguna razón.

Index

Note: Page numbers in *italics* refer to art and marginal features.

Hiking safety, 518
Hinge joints, 369
Histamines, 481
HIV (human immunodeficiency virus), 155, 277, 425, 464–467. *See also* AIDS
Hives, 481
HMOs (health maintenance organizations), 66
Home
  conservation of energy in, 553, *554*
  demonstrating character at, 122
  protection from violence in, *175*
  safety in, 509–511
Home health aides, 217
Homicide, 172
Honesty, 36, 87
Hormone therapy, 487
Hormones, 396, *398. See also specific hormones*
  and acne, 345
  and alcohol use, 323
  definition of, 9
  female, 403
  and hair health, 347
  and osteoporosis, 370
  production of, 397
  and stress response, 398
Hospices, 67, 107
Hospitals, 65
Hot lines, 180, 181, 530
Household chemicals, diseases and, 479
HPV (human papillomavirus), 461
HRSA (Health Resources and Services Administration), 73
Human papillomavirus (HPV), 461
Humor, 42
Hunger, 194
Hurricanes, 521
Hype, 70
Hypertension, 241, 252, 379, 380, 491
Hypnotics, 279, *280*
Hypothermia, *517*

I

"I" messages, 35, 36, 136
Identical twins, 416
Identity, personal, 87–88
IHS (Indian Health Services), *73*
Illegal drugs, 281–285
Illness. *See also* Diseases
  of family member, 126, 128
  foodborne, 203
  heat-related, 532
Image, personal, 308
Immediate family, 124
Immune system, 272, 451, 452, 465
Immunity, 451–453
Immunizations, *65*, 453
Immunotherapy, 487
Inadequacy, feelings of, 89
Incinerators, 550
Independence, 309
Indian Health Services (IHS), 73
Indigestion, 394
Individual differences, acceptance of, 123, 429
Individual health. *See also* Personal health care
  billboards influencing, *303*
  and biological age, 434
  and character, 121
  media and technology influencing, 49
  negative relationships influencing, 13
  positive relationships influencing, 13, 47

skills related to. *See* Health skills
  taking responsibility for, 14–19
  and violence in media, *173*
Individual sports, 236
Infancy, *427, 428*
Infants
  risks of teen parenthood to, 132
  and secondhand smoke, 307
Infections. *See also* Sexually transmitted diseases
  and birth defects, 425
  and damage to skeletal system, 370
  definition of, 446
  effects on fetus, 425
  eye, 356, 357
  from ingrown toenails, 348
  medicines fighting, 272
  of nervous system, 388
  opportunistic, 465
  of respiratory system, 384
  from tattoos/piercings, 347
  urinary tract, 463
  viral vs. bacterial, 447
  yeast, 463
Infertility, 404
Inflammation, 451
Influences, 59. *See also* Analyzing influences
Influenza, 383, 455
Information
  accessing. *See* Accessing information
  reliability of, 45
  right to, 61
  unbiased, *59*
Ingestion of medicine, *273*
Ingrown toenails, 348
Inguinal hernia, 402
Inhalants, 283
Inhalation of medicine, *273*
Inhaling, process of, 382
Injection of medicine, *273*
Injuries. *See also* Safety
  accidental, 232, 325, 402, 508
  alcohol-related, 325
  deliberate, *172*
  during earthquakes, 523
  from firearms, 173
  and hallucinogen use, 282
  to nervous system, 388
  to skeletal system, 370
  from sports, 239, 240
  unintentional, 508
Inner ear, *357, 358*
Insect bites/stings, 447, 449, 529
Insulin, *397*, 494
Insulting statements, 123
Insurance, 66, 304, 307
Integrity, 87
Interests
  increased awareness of, 11
  and making new friends, *143*
  in marriage, 130
  romantic, 11
  sharing, 123
Internal influences, *23*, 48, 59, 308–309
Internet, 45, 62. *See also* Health Online
Interpersonal communication, 34–38. *See also* Communication skills; Conflict resolution; Refusal skills
Intestines, 391, 393
Intoxication, 322
Involuntary actions, 387, 388
Involuntary muscles, 373
Iris (eye), *354*
Iron, 194, *198*, 199, 238
Islets of Langerhans, *397*

J

Jealousy, 92
Jogging, 225
Joints, 369
  arthritis in, 495–497
  flexibility of, 228–229
  and stretching exercises, 233
Jumping rope, 225

K

Ketamine, 284
Kidney stones, 394
Kidneys, 257, 393, *397*
Killer cells, 452
Kübler-Ross, Elisabeth, 106

L

Labels
  food, 206, 207
  on over-the-counter medicines, 272
  on prescription medicines, 271
Land pollution, 550–551
Landfills, 550
Language arts connections, *104, 398*
Large intestine, 393
Larynx, *382*
Laser eye surgery, 357
Late adulthood, 433
Late childhood, *427, 428,* 429
Laughter, 42
Laws. *See also* Legal issues
  as external influences, 49
  health-related, *74*
Laxative use, 257
LDL (low-density) cholesterol, 200
Lead, 550, 551
Legal issues
  abuse, 179
  alcohol use, 320, 322, 331
  illegal drugs, 281–285
  physical abuse, 177
  rape, 176
  sale of alcohol, *326*
  sexual abuse, 178
  sexual activity of minors, 154
  sexual harassment, 178
Lens (eye), *354, 355*
"Let the buyer beware," 68
Leukemia, 380, *485*
Lice, 348, *462*
Life cycle, 426
  adolescence, *427,* 429–430, *431*
  adulthood, 432–435
  age and aging, 434–435
  death and dying, 106, 108, 433
  early adulthood, 433
  early childhood, *427*
  fetal development, *418–419*
  infancy, *427,* 428
  late adulthood, 433
  late childhood, *427, 428,* 429
  maturity and old age, *427*
  middle adulthood, *427,* 433
  middle childhood, *427, 428,* 429
  stages of, *427*
  young adulthood, *427*
Life skills. *See* Health skills
Lifestyle
  benefits of active, 221, 223
  for counteracting risk factors, 16
  and noncommunicable diseases, 478
  and nutrition, 194
  sedentary, 16
  and social age, 434

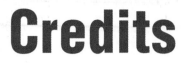
Credits

Photographs

All-Sport Photo: Mike Powell, page 239. Aurora: Jan Sonnenmair, page 134. Comstock: page 424. Corbis: pages 368, 504, 312–313, 361; AFP, page 379; Paul Barton, page 47; Lester Bergman, page 481; Andrew Brooks, page 270; Anna Clopet, page 348; Jim Cummins, pages vi, 31, 165; Michael Kevin Daly, page 28 (bottom right); Jon Feingersh, page 427 (7); Rick Gomez, page 423; Charles Gupton, page 335; John Henley, page 256; Michal Heron, page 234; Reed Kaestner, page 220; Catherine Karnow, pages 334–335; Ronnie Kaufman, pages 12, 279, 421, 427 (6); Chuck Keeler Jr, page 320; Michael Keller, page 427 (3); Raoul Minsart, page 125 (bottom left); Bob Mitchell, pages v (left), 237; Guy Motil, page 479; Mug Shots, page 116; Jose L. Pelaez, pages 204, 248, 331, 426, 427 (2), 429, 452; Gabe Palmer, pages 179, 282; Steve Prezant, page 129; Reuters NewMedia Inc., page 488; RNT Productions, page 255; R.B. Studio, page 125 (right); Bill Ross, page 540; Chuck Savage, pages 151, 427 (5); Norbert Schafer, page 418; M.L. Sinibaldi, page 457; Ariel Skelley, page 32; Leif Skoogfors, page 485; Joseph Sohm, page 218; Dann Tardif, page 466; Tim Wright, page 298; Ed Young, pages 399, 422. Courtesy of Kerisha Harris: page 156. Courtesy Nick Casey: page 156. Custom Medical Stock: pages 447, 482, 533. Ed McDonald Photography: pages 7, 22, 33 (bottom right), 90, 143, 149, 167, 171, 451, 460. Emily Shur: pages 20, 21 (all). Eric Camden Photography: pages v (right), 59 (middle right), 69, 527, 553. FoodPix: Eisenhut & Mayer, page 257; Brian Hagiwara, page 212; John E. Kelly, page 468. Getty Images: page 77, 469; Bruce Ayers, pages 103, 106; Benelux Press, page 96; Christopher Bissell, page 178; Keith Brofsky, page 456; Gary Buss, pages viii, 125 (top left); Ron Chapple, pages 84, 508; Ken Chernus, page 41; Jim Cummins, page 497; Mel Curtis, page 5 (middle); Dale Durfee, page 2; EyeWire, page 433; Rob Gage, pages 119, 296; L. D. Gordon, page 48; David Hanover, page 366; Chip Henderson, page 130; Ziggy Kaluzny, page 177; John E. Kelly, page 193; Howard Kingsnorth, page 262; Klaus Lahnstein, page 506; Lifestock, page 360; Steven Mark Needham, page 197; John Riley, pages 82, 450; Ron Silva Productions, page 190; Don Smetzer, pages 107, 260, 263; Ann Stratton, page 196; SW Productions, pages 5 (middle left), 140; Telegraph Colour Library, pages 35, 86; Arthur Tilley, pages 9, 62; Gandee Vasan, page 340; VCG, pages 5 (middle right), 158; Garry Wade, page 436; David Young-Wolff, pages 254, 414. Image State: page 157. The Image Works: E. Crews, page 101; Bob Daemmrich, pages 8, 122, 272, 285; Sonda Dawes, page 325; M. Eastcott, page 514; J. Greenberg, page 303; Willie L. Hill, page 330; Steve Warmowski, page 276; Mitch Wojnarowicz, page 16. Index Stock: page 76; Steve Dunwell, page 360. Index Stock Imagery: Myrleen Cate, page 1; Thomas Craig, page 467; Lonnie Duka, page 515; Rick Souders, page 208; Bob Winsett, page 519. International Stock: Kirk Anderson, page 28 (top left); Scott Barrow, page 39; James Davis, page 266; Michael Paras, page 459; Patrick Ramsey, pages 71, 112; Peter Langone, page 152. Jim West, page 334. Jim Whitmer Photography: page 395. Judd Pilosoff Photography: page 209. Lon Tweeten, page 406. Masterfile: Zoran Milich, page 94. Matt Meadows Photography: pages vii (top), 34, 52, 126, 153, 172, 181, 184, 287, 374, 375, 396. Painet, Inc.: pages 11, 91, 109, 188, 214. Photo Researchers: A. Glauberman, page 300 (both); Aaron Haupt, page 318; Richard Hutchings, page 132; Ken Lax, page 378; Judy Manna, pages xi (right), 241; Will & Deni McIntyre, page 463; Motta & Familiari/Anatomy Dept./University "La Sapienza", Rome/Science Photo Library, page 400 (right); David M. Phillips, page 400 (left). Photodisc: pages 23, 78 (middle), 554. PhotoEdit: Bill Aron, page 526; Bill Bachmann, page 307; Billy Barnes, page 476; Robert Brenner, pages 93, 108; Myrleen Ferguson Cate, pages 194, 311, 353, 474, 532, 546; David Kelly Crow, page 495; Mary Kate Denny, pages 58, 121, 199, 268, 328, 416, 461; Laura Dwight, pages 362, 432; Tony Freeman, pages 75, 224, 302, 342, 420, 491, 535, 551, 552; Robert Ginn, page 271; Spencer Grant, pages 333, 402; Jeff Greenberg, page 500; Will Hart, page 444; Richard Hutchings, pages 162, 198, 480; Bonnie Kamin, page 560 (all); Richard Lord, pages 142; Felicia Martinez, page 211 (border); Michael Newman, pages 144, 182, 223, 253, 289, 355, 356, 405, 389; Dwayne Newton, page 470; Jonathon Nourok, pages 427 (8), 442; Robin L. Sachs, page 64; Susan Van Etten, page 408; Rudi Von Briel, page 183; David Young-Wolff, pages x, xi (left), 13, 17, 26, 72, 95, 99, 118, 147, 150, 154, 164, 192, 238, 250, 288, 292, 308, 346, 381, 383, 390, 392, 427 (1 & 4), 434, 435, 449, 454, 484, 496, 516, 523, 524, 547, 556. Photographik Company: pages xii, 5 (bottom), 6, 19 (all), 33 (top left), 38 (both), 45, 59 (top), 70, 102, 113, 166 (both), 168, 203, 211 (middle), 221 (all), 235, 252, 274, 305, 329, 334 (both). Phototake, NYC: Yoav Levy, page 490. Photri: Bachmann, page 240; Karen Holsinger, page 277; Michael Yelman, pages ix, 380. PictureQuest: Henryk Kaiser/Index Stock Imagery, page 14; Nicole Katano/Brand X Pictures, pages vii (bottom), 314; Phototake, page 465; SW Production/Index Stock Imagery, page 173. Robin Bowman: 135. SABA: Asnin, pages 50 (all), 51 (all). SEGWAY, page 558. Stock Boston: Mark Burnett, pages 136, 528; Bob Daemmrich, pages 4, 63, 174, 384, 438, 511, 513, 544; Lionel Delevingne, page 176; Judy Gelles, page 371; Leonard Harris, page 323; Jim Harrison, page 236; Lawrence Migdale, page 104; David Simson, page 531. Stan Musilek, page 559. Superstock: pages 37, 67, 124, 128, 349, 358, 425, 520, 525, 550. Susan Parker, page 213. Tim Fuller Photography: page 56. Todd France: page 134. Toyota, page 558–559. U.S. Food and Drug Administration: page 78 (top, bottom). Unicorn Stock: Mike Doyle, page 557. Kyra White: page 61. Workbook Stock: Mark Harmel, page 498.

Illustrations

Art and Science: pages 273, 301, 321, 354, 355, 369, 373, 377, 382, 386, 387, 391 (left), 393, 397, 417, 418, 419, 482, 492, 529, 534, 535, 536, 537. Dan Brawer: pages 243–244. Ed Gabel: pages 538–539. Joe Lertola: page 406, 437. Hilda Muinos: pages 357, 391 (right), 401, 403. Network Graphics: page 404. Parrot Graphics: page 372. Precision Graphics: pages 345, 350, 351, 489. Tim Robinson, pages 110–111. All other illustrations: The Mazer Corporation.